Advance Praise for *Bouncebacks! Critical Care*

What Emergency Physicians are saying about *Bouncebacks! Critical Care*

I have always disagreed with how morbidity and mortality conferences are run; they are retrospective and an unfair dissection of patient cases which resulted in poor outcomes. This book takes a more unique, prospective, and realistic approach in a "talk-aloud" process that helps readers understand what was and what should have been in the mind of the clinician during these critical care encounters.

Michelle Lin, MD
ALiEM Founder and CEO
Professor and Digital Innovation Lab Director
Department of Emergency Medicine
University of California, San Francisco

"Bouncebacks!" has done it again! Mike et al. brings the infamous suspenseful, yet relatable series of cases...this time with a critical care focus. These cases are quick to grab your attention… much like a suspense thriller, the original documentation (with time stamps to boot) literally transport you to the bedside. Like a fly-on-the-wall of the resuscitation room, it is a phenomenal way to see real life cases play out. Regardless of your level of training, "Bouncebacks! Critical Care" teaches and refreshes you on common pitfalls and errors easily made along the way. This book, like the rest of the "Bouncebacks!" Series, gives you the opportunity to learn from subtle clinical presentations and errors that none of us are immune from.

Mizuho Morrison, DO
Editor-in-Chief Hippo Education
Clinical Faculty, LAC+USC Emergency Medicine
Attending Physician, Kaiser Permanente SCPMG

"Bouncebacks! Critical Care" captures the kind of medical education we've always wanted: practical and actionable clinical insight into the necessarily gray-areas of frontline emergency medicine. This book thoughtfully captures and breaks down the meta-cognitive decision-making process of trusted experts and how they think through the critical care decisions we all face.

Paul Jhun, MD
Assistant Clinical Professor, Department of Emergency Medicine
Zuckerberg San Francisco General Hospital, University of California San Francisco
Vice President, Hippo Education
Conference Co-Chair, Essentials of Emergency Medicine

The Bouncebacks books are must reads for emergency medicine learners of all levels and are books I return to again and again, finding new lessons which make me a better clinician and smarter in my documentation. "Bouncebacks! Critical Care" is the clear evolution of the Bouncebacks series. The familiar case-based format we love returns, but is made fresh and exciting by focusing on the bounceback visit in which the patient is SICK! Anchoring medical teaching to specific cases, pausing throughout for discussion and reflection, mirrors the way we learn on shift and allows the reader to learn from these terrifying experiences. This book is exciting, fun to read, and will challenge your thinking today, in a way that will impact your practice tomorrow!

Jenny Beck-Esmay, MD
Assistant Residency Director
Assistant Professor of Emergency Medicine
Mount Sinai St. Luke's - Mount Sinai West

"Bouncebacks" is back, baby!!! This is a must read for any practicing emergency physician, at any point in their career. The cases start from the beginning and walk you through the medical and the legal aspects of high-risk cases that frequently masquerade as benign complaints. The authors provide story pauses at important decision points as possible management strategies are reviewed in a literature-based fashion, all while remaining concise and easily readable.

Salim R. Rezaie, MD
Greater San Antonio Emergency Physicians (GSEP)
Director of Clinical Education Associate
Clinical Professor at University of the Incarnate Word school of Osteopathic Medicine
Senior Editor of Emergency Physicians Monthly Emergency Medicine/Internal Medicine
Creator/Founder of REBEL

Michael Weinstock and his colleagues display an engaging approach to illuminating the key features of serious diagnoses, sprinkled with gems and insight from some of the leading minds in emergency medicine.

Ryan P. Radecki, MD, MS
Clinical Assistant Professor at the University of Texas Medical School at Houston
Physician Lead, Laboratory Appropriateness Committee
NWP Lead, Precision Medicine & Genomics
Chair, Institutional Review Board

This isn't just about the cases, it is a fundamentally different way of looking at how we practice medicine. It doesn't need to be in a fearful litigious-averse way! And it doesn't need to be in the punitive archaic M&M-style way. Dr. Weinstock has leveled-up our thinking and practices to focus on what matters; the patient! THIS is how doctors think and how we learn. You can feel the emotion as the patients get sicker and your brain engages in such a meaningful way. Bouncebacks books are the textbooks of the future, and the latest addition is a huge value-add to the best series in EM!

Jaime Hope, MD
Assistant Professor, Emergency Medicine
Beaumont Health Level 1 Trauma Tertiary Care Center
Harbor Beach Rural Critical Access Hospital

"Bouncebacks! Critical Care" is the perfect complement to the earlier books in the Bouncebacks series. An all-star team of editors and authors take clinicians through the unexpected twists and turns that routinely occur in Emergency Departments and Urgent Care Centers. This book represents an opportunity for practitioners to learn from other's mistakes... without ever making the same mistake yourself.

Alfred Sacchetti, MD, FACEP
Chief Emergency Medicine
Virtua-Our Lady of Lourdes Hospital
Assistant Professor Emergency Medicine
Thomas Jefferson University

It's back, it's Bouncebacks! One of the mostly widely read and highly regarded education series in all of Emergency Medicine. Clinicians fear the medical malpractice landscape, but Mike Weinstock and the team give you all the tools you need to protect yourselves. Documentation people, documentation. Now with a critical care version. Read this book, sleep better at night, as simple as that! Love, love this series!

Mel Herbert, MD, MBBS, BMedSci, FACEP, FAAEM
Professor of Emergency Medicine at the Keck School of Medicine LAC+USC Medical Center
Owner and editor of EM: RAP

I have been reading and recommending the Bouncebacks! series to colleagues and residents since the release of the first edition. The cases contain invaluable "back-to-the-basics" lessons on how to perform an exemplary H&P, how to think critically about our diagnostic and management plans, and how to document responsibly and thoughtfully. The innovative format of this edition forces the reader to consider challenging clinical questions as they work through the case with accompanying expert commentaries which transport the reader into a virtual high quality Educational Grand Rounds environment. Highly recommended reading for emergency physicians regardless of level of training.

Ramin Tabatabai, MD, MACM
Clinical Associate Professor of Emergency Medicine
Program Director, LAC+USC Emergency Medicine Residency

Whether you're a PA or NP just starting to work in the ED or an experienced, EM Board-certified veteran, *Bouncebacks Critical Care* is just packed with page after page of essential information to help keep patients and clinicians safe. It's an easy "read" and should be a key part of every emergency clinician's library.

Rick Bukata, MD
Medical Director, The Center for Medical Education, Inc., Creamery, Pennsylvania
Adjunct Clinical Professor
Los Angeles County / University of Southern California Medical Center

Dr. Weinstock has once again brought together a dream-team of clinical and legal experts to teach clinical reasoning, this time by tackling critical care cases. This is the only book I know of that takes the innovative approach of highlighting the bounceback visit of a recently discharged patient by intertwining patient stories with clinical questions and teaching pearls. The case-based approach makes it read like a novel, with salient interjected comments from editors, as if you're standing at the bedside with three critical care experts dropping pearls in your ear. The stories are memorable, the clinical questions are practical, and the answers are evidence-based. Bouncebacks! Critical Care pushes us not just to meet a legal standard of care, but to push for excellence in the care of critically ill patients. I enjoyed reading it and recommend it to all who take care of sick patients.

Jeff Riddell, MD
Assistant Professor of Clinical Emergency Medicine
Keck School of Medicine of the University of Southern California

Bouncebacks! Critical Care is an absolute must read for EM docs at any stage of their career! This book does a great job of highlighting the errors in the initial visit while at the same time offering literature-based feedback on the treatment provided at the critical care visit. Additionally, this book provides expert commentary relating to the medical and legal aspects of the case. I love this book!

Adam Kessler, DO, FACEP
Assistant Professor of Medicine
Director, Emergency Critical Care Service Line
Department of Emergency Medicine
Department of Anesthesiology Division of Critical Care Medicine
University of Alabama Birmingham

Bouncebacks! Makes it REAL! The refreshing format puts EMDOCS in the moment and at the bedside resuscitating a crashing patient. Bouncebacks! pauses at the time when we are thirsty for the most recent evidence-based answers, and coaches us through by fully exploring every critical decision point! As the case unfolds, it feels like practicing with Legendary BAFERDS guiding decisions with evidence. Oddly, I found myself NOT wanting to put Bouncebacks! down! Thanks guys - you've done it again!

K. Kay Moody, DO, MPH
Adjunct clinical faculty
Pacific Northwest University College of Osteopathic Medicine
Founder EMDOCS

Let's face it – learning from textbooks is out. Thankfully, the Critical Care edition of Bouncebacks (like its predecessors) is the anti-textbook in every way! Engaging cases with compelling clinical lessons and expert commentary from the greatest minds in resuscitation. The teaching points from this book are relevant for every Emergency Physician and are presented in a way that respects how we actually learn – from stories and errors. As the saying goes, "...it's better to learn from the mistakes of others" and Bouncebacks delivers a map to the landmines that lurk in the care of the critically ill.

Joshua Russell, MD, MSc, FACEP
Editor-in-Chief, Journal of Urgent Care Medicine
Associate Editor, Urgent Care: RAP Podcast (HIPPO UC RAP)

Drs. Weinstock and Klauer have assembled an all-star cast for this latest Bouncebacks! installment. These pages contain decades of carefully mined, evidence-based critical care gold. The case-based format, with pauses for expert reflection, implore the reader to simulate their own response, providing the ultimate substrate for growth. I'm reminded of the proverb, "Without consultation, plans are frustrated, but with many counselors they succeed." I recommend it to all our residents-in-training, but even the most seasoned veteran will be sharper for reading it.

Benjamin Cooper, MD, FACEP
Assistant Professor, Associate Program Director, Department of Emergency Medicine
McGovern Medical School, The University of Texas Health Science Center at Houston

BOUNCEBACKS! CRITICAL CARE

AVOID SERIOUS MISTAKES IN THE ED

Michael B. Weinstock, MD
Kevin M. Klauer, DO

Consulting editor:
Scott D. Weingart, MD

Legal commentary:
Gregory L. Henry, MD

Designed and illustrated by:
Hannah Schumick

Anadem Publishing

Anadem, Inc.

INTELLECTUAL PROPERTY RIGHTS

USING THIS BOOK

Bouncebacks! Critical Care does not provide medical advice for specific patients:

The text, information, graphics, images, and other material ("Content") contained in *Bouncebacks! Critical Care* is for informational purposes only. The Content is not intended to replace or be a substitute for professional medical advice, diagnosis, or treatment. Readers of *Bouncebacks! Critical Care* are cautioned to use their own judgment in making clinical decisions and, when appropriate, consult and compare information from other sources.

All information and recommendations are meant to aid in general patient care and are not meant to apply to specific patients or patient care scenarios. Anadem, Inc., its employees, contractors enlisted to assist Anadem, Inc. in preparing this book for publication, or authors, contributors, editors or reviewers do not accept responsibility for the application of the Content in direct or indirect patient care. It is the responsibility of the healthcare provider to ensure that treatment recommendations are appropriate for an individual patient-care situation.

Bouncebacks! Critical Care Content consists of medical cases and contains the opinions and recommendations of authors, commentators, contributors and editors who are medical providers. Their opinions and recommendations expressed in this book are beyond the scope of knowledge or understanding of Anadem, Inc., its employees or contractors. The opinions and recommendations of the authors, contributors, editors and reviewers are their own and do not necessarily reflect any position, policy or recommendation of Anadem, Inc., its employees or contractors.

If you are a consumer, you access *Bouncebacks! Critical Care* at your own risk. Do not rely on *Bouncebacks! Critical Care* as a substitute for professional medical advice or a relationship with a physician or other qualified healthcare professional.

Anadem, Inc.
www.anadem.com
anadem@anadem.com
614-262-2539
BOUNCEBACKS CRITICAL CARE ISBN: 978-1-890018-83-2

ABOUT THE AUTHORS

MICHAEL B. WEINSTOCK, MD

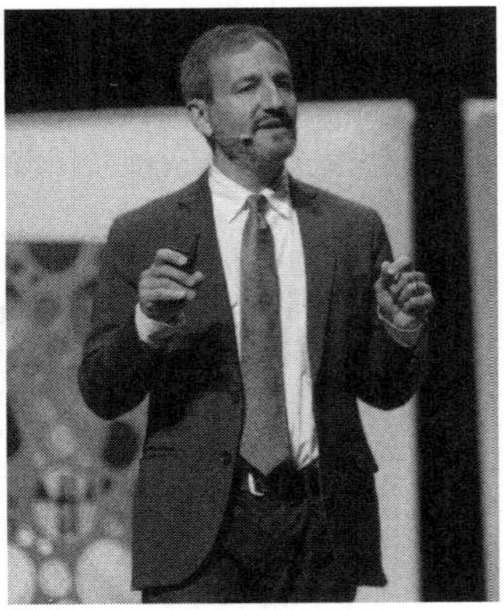

Mike is the Associate Program Director at the Adena Emergency Medicine Residency and Professor of Emergency Medicine, Adjunct at the Wexner Medical Center at The Ohio State University. He has lectured nationally and internationally on medical topics and patient safety issues and is the executive editor for HIPPO's UC RAP, the risk management section editor for EM RAP, and has contributed to ERCast, Risk Management Monthly, and is a chapter author for CorePendium. He has published original research and editorials in multiple journals including Annals of Emergency Medicine, JAMA-IM, The Journal of the American Heart Association, and The Journal of Emergency Medicine. Michael has practiced medicine nationally and internationally including volunteer work in Papua New Guinea, Nepal, and the West Indies.

Research interests include ED evaluation and management of chest pain, patient safety, and EM medical education. He is married to family physician Beth Weinstock, with children Olivia, Eli, Theo and Annie. He is the leader of The Big Rockin' Blues Band.

KEVIN M. KLAUER, DO

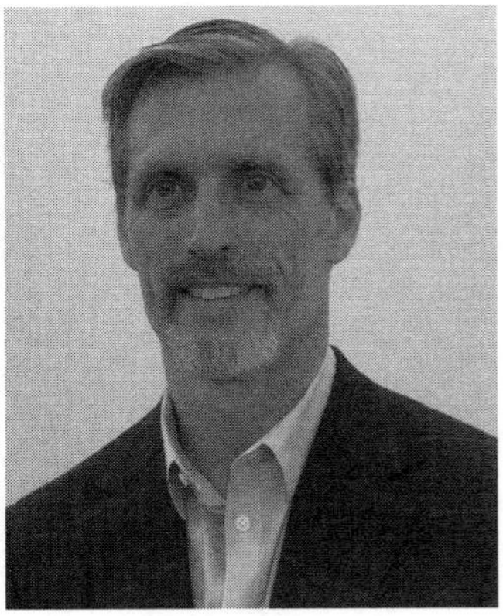

Dr. Klauer is the current CEO of the American Osteopathic Association. He served as Chief Medical Officer, Hospital Based Services, Chief Risk Officer, Executive Director of the Patient Safety Organization, and the Medical Director for the Medical Call Center for TeamHealth. He is a Clinical Assistant Professor at Michigan State University College of Osteopathic Medicine and The University of Tennessee. Dr. Klauer served as the Medical Editor-in-Chief for ACEP Now, ACEP's monthly publication, and as former Editor-in-Chief for Emergency Physicians Monthly publication. He is the Co-Author of three risk management books: Bouncebacks: Pediatrics, Emergency Medicine Bouncebacks: Medical and Legal and Risk Management and the Emergency Department: Executive Leadership for Protecting Patients and Hospitals.

Dr. Klauer also served as the American College of Emergency Physicians Council Speaker and served on their Board of Directors from 2016 through 2019. In 2014, he was the recipient of the American College of Emergency Physicians Honorable Mention Outstanding Speaker of the Year Award and was recognized by the Ohio Chapter of ACEP with the Bill Hall Award for service. In 2016 he was honored with the ACEP Outstanding Speaker of the Year Award, as well as EMRA's highest honor, the Joseph F. Waeckerle award. In 2018, Dr. Klauer was awarded the Janice A. Wachtler Educator of the Year Award by the American College of Osteopathic Emergency Physicians. Dr. Klauer earned his Executive JD, with honors, from Concord Law School in 2011.

SCOTT D. WEINGART, MD

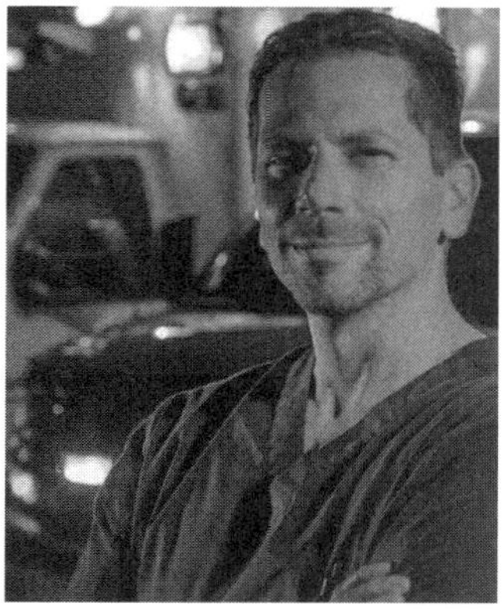

Scott is an ED Intensivist from New York. He did fellowships in Trauma, Surgical Critical Care, and ECMO. He is best known for talking to himself about Resuscitation and Critical Care on a podcast called EMCrit, which has been downloaded > 30 million times.

GREGORY L. HENRY, MD

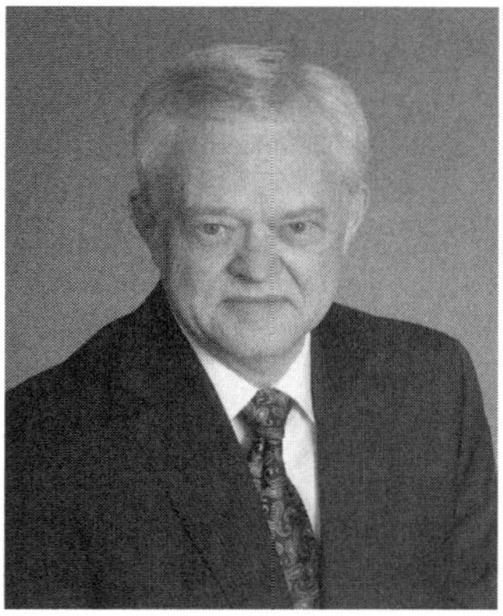

Gregory L. Henry is a former Clinical Professor in the Department of Emergency Medicine at University of Michigan Medical Center. He was the President of the American College of Emergency Physicians (ACEP) from 1995–1996 and is also former President and CEO of Medical Practice Risk Assessment, Inc. and President of Savannah Assurance Limited, LTD. He is on the editorial boards of Emergency Medicine Practice, Emergency Department Management, and Foresight and the Emergency Department Legal Letter. He is the recipient of numerous awards including the "Over the top" lecturer award and the "Outstanding speaker of the Year" award from ACEP. He is the author of Neurologic Emergencies: A Symptom-Oriented Approach, 2nd ed. He is a medical legal expert and has been an expert in many hundreds of cases.

FOREWORD

Rob Orman, MD
Emergency medicine physician
Executive editor: ERcast podcast

"Hey, do you remember that patient you saw last night…"

These are words that fill us with dread. Sometimes, an adverse outcome could not be anticipated, but other times we may have culpability; from anchoring, failing to see the bigger picture, or being rushed. But it is in the pages of the *Bouncebacks!* books that we can pause and reflect on how we might approach a challenging situation without being an actual participant since there are often subtle clues which serve as cautionary tale.

In this, the 4th in the *Bouncebacks!* series, we get to dissect decision points, pitfalls, and errors during the critical care bounceback course with expert guidance along the way. For example, we get to meet a 42-year-old man who presents to an urgent care with upper back pain. When we meet the patient in his next medical encounter, *spoiler alert*, he is in cardiac arrest. What could have avoided this outcome? What is "best care" during a cardiac arrest?

Unique to this book, we see the clues which may have helped to make the correct diagnosis as well as the sequalae. Consider an elderly non-English-speaking woman who presents with fever, headache, neck pain and vomiting and is discharged with a diagnosis of "Bronchitis." As we discover in the chapter by Kalantari and Werley, an accumulation of small cognitive errors can lead to a big miss, with drastic consequences, as evidenced by the bounceback visit 4 days later with tachycardia and hypotension.

One of the best ways to build resilience against cognitive errors is by recognizing they exist in the first place; that is the real lesson to take from this edition of *Bouncebacks!* Sure, you'll get smarter, you'll learn critical care, your brain may even swell with knowledge to degrees of extraordinary magnitude, but what you are really developing is resilience. These cases are real, and as the authors ask you to step into the footsteps of the provider, this has the secondary effect of providing a path to protection against cognitive errors as well as helping build emotional strength during a shift.

And now you will know, even if you've never encountered this situation during an actual shift, you've "been there" and "done that."

PREFACE

In the "*The Times They are a Changin,*" Bob Dylan sang, "You better start swimmin' or you'll sink like a stone…" We took that to heart; in this fourth book in the *Bouncebacks!* series we employ a *fresh* approach. Whereas, the first three *Bouncebacks!* books focus on the initial visit, this edition examines the *bounceback* visit, putting the reader in the footsteps of the clinician as the patient deteriorates. The story pauses at important decision points as possible management strategies are reviewed in a literature-based fashion, followed by a revelation of the path chosen by the actual provider. As the patient's course progresses, we reach additional decision points and address further clinical questions.

In addition to our chapter authors, many with expertise in critical care emergency medicine, we have an all-star lineup of *expert-whisperers*: first an EM/critical care section editor (below) and second, EMCRIT.org's double-boarded critical care guru, Scott Weingart. Their comments are inserted in grey boxes and are intended to give tips and tricks borne of experience and to provide context to the literature, "as if" they are standing over our shoulder and advising during a resuscitation.

SECTION EDITORS (EM/CRITICAL CARE):

Section A – Airway/arrest:
Lillian Emlet – University of Pittsburgh

Section B – Breathing/pulmonary
Don Yealy – University of Pittsburgh

Section C – Cardiac/vascular
John Greenwood – University of Pennsylvania

Section D – Drugs & Delirium
Mike Winters – University of Maryland

Section E – Neuro & sepsis
Tiffany Osborn – Washington University
Evie Marcolini – Geisel School of Medicine at Dartmouth

Section F – Trauma, diabetes, heme, GI, HTN
Joe Shiber – University of Florida

Additionally, there are three chapters where we address the medical-legal aspects of care. Enter Greg Henry MD, past president of The American College of Emergency Physicians (ACEP) and one of the most experienced physician medical-legal experts in the country. He opines on the approach that both the defense and plaintiff would likely pursue and, by extension, how we can make patients safer through our evaluation and documentation before there is an adverse outcome.

Whereas, these chapters contain the actual documentation from the ED chart, a very few chapters have slight modifications to the final aspects of the return visit at decision point 3, to allow for exploration of different critical care scenarios. There is still plenty of commentary on the documentation, missed red-flags, and what could have been done to improve care at the initial visit. Our goal is to make each chapter challenging, dynamic, and realistic… to move us from "standard of care" to "excellence in care."

There are some subjects which we intentionally cover in multiple chapters; for example, the discussion of cutting-edge techniques to manage refractory ventricular fibrillation or indications for emergent cardiac catheterization post-arrest. This redundancy serves to reinforce important concepts through space repetition and to allow authors leeway for their own interpretation of the literature since there are often multiple acceptable approaches to the same clinical problem. There will be times when Weingart, the section editors, and the chapter authors disagree. After all, you are now at the bedside during a difficult resuscitation while being precepted by the best and brightest in the field; it is not surprising that there are different ways to approach the same problem!

Finally, some of these cases have been previously presented in podcasts and lectures. For example, the 47-year-old woman with anaphylaxis in chapter 4 was highlighted in a mock trial performed at Emergency Medicine Grand Rounds at The Ohio State University with OSU and Adena EM residencies, the 53-year-old man with elevated blood pressure was discussed on the podcasts Urgent Care Reviews and Perspectives (UC RAP) and Risk Management Monthly (RMM), and the 41-year-old woman with "multiple complaints" was the subject of a 6-part series on the podcast Emergency Medicine Reviews and Perspectives (EM RAP). A complete listing is on the next page.

Thanks to Anadem, Inc., Will Kuhlmann, Mike Cheadle, Dave Schumick, and Hannah Schumick, for your expertise and advice—we have now been working together for several decades and it has been a fantastic ride!

And thanks to the readers; we hope that you get as much out this book as much as we did by writing it. It is only appropriate to restate what Greg Henry sagely wrote in the first Bouncebacks! book in 2006:

"The smart doctor is not the one who learns from his/her own mistakes. The smart doctor is the one who learns from the mistakes of others. Here's hoping that this book is read by a lot of smart doctors."

Happy reading!!

Michael B. Weinstock
Kevin M. Klauer

CASES ON MEDIA AND PRESENTED AT NATIONAL CONFERENCES:

1. **Chapter 1:** ***A 42-year-old man with a history of IVDU and upper back pain***
    - Mt. Carmel St. Ann's joint M&M conference, Columbus Ohio 2016
2. **Chapter 2:** ***A 53-year-old man with a tracheostomy and shortness of breath***
    - All-LA conference 2014
3. **Chapter 3:** ***A 41-year-old woman with chest pain***
    - Essentials of Emergency Medicine (EEM) 2013
    - EM RAP podcast with a 6-segment series 2014-2015
    - The Journal of Urgent Care medicine September 2020
4. **Chapter 4:** ***A 47-year-old woman with anaphylaxis***
    - The Ohio State University Emergency Medicine OSU mock trial 2018
    - Podcast: http://emcrit.org/emcrit/refractory-anaphylaxis-mock-trial/
5. **Chapter 8:** ***A 78-year-old man with end stage renal disease (ESRD) and shortness of breath***
    - Ohio ACEP resident's assembly 2018
    - UC RAP 2021
    - ERcast 2021
6. **Chapter 13:** ***A 33-year old man with abdominal pain who leaves AMA***
    - ACOEP national mtg 2017
7. **Chapter 17:** ***A 48-year-old suicidal man with beta-blocker overdose***
    - EM RAP podcast 2017
8. **Chapter 21:** ***A 50-year-old woman with flank pain***
    - Essentials of Emergency Medicine (EEM) 2017
    - Dutch North Sea Emergency Medicine Conference, Amsterdam 2018
    - Joint Grand Rounds at Brooke Army Medical Center, San Antonio, TX 2018
    - Adena GME grand rounds, 2020
9. **Chapter 25:** ***A 51-year-old diabetic woman with vertigo***
    - The Ohio State University Emergency Medicine grand rounds 2010
    - EM RAP podcast 2010
10. **Chapter 27:** ***A 53-year-old man with elevated blood pressure***
    - Risk management monthly (RMM) podcast
    - UC RAP podcast 2018
11. **Chapter 28:** ***A 75-year-old woman with head and neck pain and vomiting***
    - Digital Essentials, Los Angeles, CA 2016
    - Adena GME grand rounds, 2020

TABLE OF CONTENTS

SECTION C – CARDIAC / VASCULAR

Section editor: John Greenwood – University of Pennsylvania

SECTION D – DRUGS & DELIRIUM

Section editor: Mike Winters – University of Maryland

BOUNCEBACKS! CRITICAL CARE

The Medical Legal Considerations

Kevin M. Klauer, DO, EJD, FACEP, FACOEP
Chief Executive Officer, American Osteopathic Association
Assistant Clinical Professor, University of Tennessee Health Sciences Center
Assistant Clinical Professor, Michigan State University, College of Osteopathic Medicine

The medical-legal risk associated with critically ill patients centers around three themes:
1. Misdiagnosis
2. Delayed diagnosis
3. Inadequate or inappropriate management

The risk is substantially amplified by an adverse outcome.

Though it seems that the sickest of patients carry the greatest risk, the opposite may be true. When a critically ill patient presents with an obvious diagnosis such as stroke, STEMI, or multi-system trauma, the first theme (above) "misdiagnosis" is mitigated; now the legal risk is limited to the second and third themes, delayed diagnosis and poor management. Additionally, with an obvious critical illness, many patients and their families accept the likelihood of a bad outcome.

Ensuring appropriate expectations, reflected in the documentation, may help to avoid initiation of a legal action. If there is an adverse outcome, constructing a sound defense begins with real-time documentation, but is weakened by trying to fill in gaps with recollection years later.

THE THREE THEMES:

1. Misdiagnosis

Misdiagnosis is a medical-legal house of cards. There are many times when a definitive diagnosis isn't obtainable at the time of the ED visit. However, a well-considered differential diagnosis, inclusive of serious life-threatening entities, should help to justify clinical decisions. For example, discharge of a chest pain patient who is "low-risk" for acute coronary syndrome and without risk factors for venothromboembolic disease may be appropriate, despite the fact that the patient may ultimately experience a major acute coronary event or a pulmonary embolism (PE). Be cautious about documenting a broad differential for the purpose of enhancing medical decision-making complexity purely from a coding and billing perspective; if you haven't truly considered the differential, then don't include those items. The legal system does not give "partial credit."

A common misconception about differential diagnoses is that if a clinical entity is included in the differential, then definitive diagnostics must be used to rule in or rule out those entities; this is simply not true. Many etiologies are often considered but ruled out following the history and physical examination. For instance, a 45-year-old male patient with non-red flag back pain, following lifting a heavy object, does not require imaging, but documenting the consideration of cauda equina syndrome from lumbar disc herniation or spinal epidural abscess, without the aid of diagnostics, is a good idea. However, listing high-risk items in your differential without a definitive diagnostic evaluation requires some explanation. For example:

Ineffective documentation:
Ddx: Cauda equina, malignancy, infected ureteral stone, pyelonephritis
MDM: "The patient has a low back muscular strain as there is pain with palpation on the left low back and the pain is worse with range of motion. He will be treated w/NSAIDS."

Effective documentation:
MDM: "The patient's presentation is most consistent with a low back muscular strain as it started immediately upon lifting, is worse with range of motion and with palpation. Cauda equina syndrome seems very unlikely as there is no fever, history of IVDU or urinary retention, and malignancy would be very unusual with no history of weight loss or history of cancer. The clinical presentation is most consistent with muscular etiology."

The most common reason for a lawsuit is misdiagnosis (Brown 2010, Kachalia 2007). Though no one intends to discharge a patient with a critical illness, in a full career, it does happen. For example, many patients with minor head injury do not need to receive imaging, but if there is a 0.1% chance of hemorrhage, even with a low risk history and exam, it will occasionally happen. It is easier to put a short statement in the chart reflecting that the presentation was not consistent with intracranial injury and which clinical decision instrument was utilized for risk stratification, than to get a CT, check the results, return to discuss with the patient and then discharge. Additionally, this approach is safer for the patient.

2. Delayed diagnosis:
Delayed diagnosis may occur when the initial treating clinician does not make a timely diagnosis or when the correct diagnosis is made by a subsequently treating clinician. Inherent in theme #1, misdiagnosis, is a delay in diagnosis and definitive management. All visits are not created equal; a delay does not automatically equate to poor care or harm, as the initial diagnosis may not have been clear, and the delay might not have resulted in an adverse outcome. The diagnosis may become apparent through subsequent visits and the elapse of time.

- Avoid the use of the term "diagnosis" when the etiology of a patient's presentation is unclear. "Diagnosis" carries with it a legal meaning implying that you are certain the patient has "x." However, terms such as preliminary diagnosis, initial impression and clinical impression reflect that a definitive diagnosis has not been made and more importantly, that the clinician isn't committing to one specific diagnosis.
- A clinician's medical decision-making should reflect reasonableness of action of diagnostic and therapeutic choices throughout the course of the encounter. This is particularly important when a definitive "diagnosis" has not been made.

Many patients experience an appropriate delay in diagnosis due to the time it takes to make the diagnosis; this may occur with thoracic aortic dissection (TAD) or complex stroke presentations.

Retrospectively, the likely diagnosis is suspected, but imaging, consultation, reassessment and transfer may take hours or more to accomplish. The question at hand is whether the steps taken, and the time spent to make the diagnosis, were reasonable.

For example, a decision to evaluate for TAD may be very reasonable, despite the fact that the patient is ultimately diagnosed with acute coronary syndrome (ACS), resulting in a delay of cardiology evaluation. Effective documentation is essential in this regard. For example:

Ineffective documentation:
MDM: "Chest x-ray and CTA of the chest were negative. After reviewing the patient's CT result, the troponin came back positive. Cardiology was consulted."

Effective documentation:
MDM: [date and time] "The initial differential diagnosis included acute coronary syndrome and thoracic aortic dissection. As the troponin was pending and the initial ECG was non-diagnostic, a CTA was performed to rule out dissection. Upon ruling out dissection, the troponin was noted to be positive. Cardiology was promptly consulted as the presentation now is most consistent with acute coronary syndrome."

3. Inadequate or inappropriate treatment/management
When managing patients without a definitive diagnosis, what is the standard of care for the tort of negligence? The answer will be your actions; was your management reasonable for a similarly trained clinician in similar circumstances? For instance, most would agree that sending a hypotensive, 85-year-old patient with severe flank and abdominal pain to radiology for a CT of the abdomen and pelvis is not reasonable due to the potential for decompensation from suspected ruptured abdominal aortic aneurysm. However, sending a 32-year-old with a minor head injury and a GCS of 14 to radiology for a CT of the brain would be reasonable. Even though the latter patient may very rarely decompensate in the CT scanner, the decision to send them there was reasonable and consistent with the standard of care. When the diagnosis is unclear, the documentation should reflect your thought process at critical junctures in the patient's care.

TIPS FOR MINIMIZING LEGAL RISK WITH CRITICALLY ILL PATIENTS:

I. Consultation:

The gateway to much definitive surgical or medical management is consultation. Though we strive to be self-sufficient, seeking expert advice should not be viewed as a sign of weakness or an admission of clinical incompetence. With critically ill patients, earlier consultation may be valuable to obtain timely input and preparation from those clinicians who will ultimately assume care. Due to the high risk of adverse outcomes with this population, gaining and documenting the input of consultants is beneficial and risk-protective. It is very difficult to overcome the perception that delayed consultation does not contribute to bad outcomes with a jury of laypersons. All consultations do not have to occur at the bedside; phone consults should include:

- Name of consultant and time contacted
- The clinical information provided
- Questions asked of the consultant
- Advice provided

Case Example 1
A 26-year-old woman presented to an emergency department (ED) with an unusual and persistent headache. A CT scan of the brain was ordered, which revealed a pituitary adenoma. The CT result also noted "paraclinoid compression of the internal carotid arteries bilaterally, without stenosis." The neurosurgeon was contacted, advised of the normal neurological examination and of the CT findings. The emergency physician (EP) documented that the report was read to the neurosurgeon and asked specifically about obtaining an emergent MRI, admission and/or discharge. The neurosurgeon advised the EP that emergent MRI was not necessary, and the patient should follow up in his office in one week. The patient returned to the ED in 4 days with a massive stroke and the patient was left with severe neurological sequelae.

Discussion: Although a lawsuit was filed, the documentation of the questions asked, the data provided, and the advice given by the neurosurgeon resulted in a defense verdict for the emergency physician. The non-ED co-defendants in the case were not so fortunate.

Case Example 2
A 44-year-old woman presented to the ED, with an unusual headache which started with a near syncopal event with the onset, which was abrupt. A CT was performed and was negative. A lumbar puncture was then performed, noting approximately 1,700 red cells in tube 1 and 1500 in tube 4. The neurosurgeon was contacted who dismissed the findings as a "traumatic tap." The EP's documentation reflected his acceptance of this consultant's opinion and recommendation to discharge the patient without further evaluation. The patient returned 48 hours later with a massive subarachnoid hemorrhage, resulting in death.

Discussion: Due to insurmountable challenges with this case, including the limited documentation of the phone consultation and acceptance of the inappropriate interpretation of the results and the recommendations of the neurosurgeon, the case was settled for well-above policy limits. Interestingly, the neurosurgeon was dismissed from the case following his deposition testimony. He reported, "Had I been more thoroughly informed about the condition of the patient and the concern of the emergency physician about subarachnoid hemorrhage, I would have recommended emergent follow up-studies and I would have come to hospital immediately." Without documentation reflecting the concerns of the EP and the specific questions asked of the neurosurgeon, there was no effective way to refute the neurosurgeon's recollection other than the recollection of the EP, which in this case, appeared conveniently self-serving to the jury.

II. Physical examination:
At the bedside, the presentation of critically ill patients is often clear. For instance, it is not difficult to diagnose a dense left MCA distribution stroke by observation alone. Unfortunately, such obvious clinical presentations are frequently accompanied by a lack of documented physical examination findings. This suggests inattention to detail, despite the fact that the care may have been reasonable, and a thorough examination was actually performed. It's worthwhile to document the detailed and often extensive physical findings that occur in these patients. The documentation should paint a picture of what was seen upon entering the room and during the ED course. The presentation is sometimes not so obvious when the documentation is later reviewed.

III. Boarding:

Boarding of critically ill patients creates considerable professional liability exposure. It is common for the initial treating clinician to step back once the patient is admitted. However, if there has not been a commensurate acceptance of responsibility from the admitting clinician, this may create gaps in care and increased professional liability, as no one is assuming responsibility for the patient. The time of the admission decision is when the transition of care should be determined and documented. In the absence of documentation in the medical record reflecting the transition of care, the location of the patient will be dispositive to the question of ultimate responsibility.

Case Example 3

A 32-year-old man presents to the ED with hypotension, tachycardia, generalized weakness and numerous episodes of vomiting. He had a known history of alcoholism and had been drinking heavily the night before. Although there were some laboratory abnormalities, he did not have a fever and diagnostics did not identify a source of infection. He was treated appropriately and aggressively with intravenous fluids and antiemetics. The care was appropriate, based on the presentation and the diagnostic results available at that time. The hospitalist was contacted for admission to the ICU and agreed to admit the patient. Over six hours transpired prior to the patient's transfer to the ICU. The hospitalist had not seen the patient, and no reassessment note from the emergency physician was documented. Over the following 24 hours, the patient became much more ill and was ultimately diagnosed with sepsis, resulting in a four-limb amputation. In retrospect, there were indications of worsening of condition during that prior six-hour period. It was unclear if and to whom such changes should have been reported by nursing; neither physician was aware.

Discussion: The change in clinical conditions became the focus of this case, resulting in a large seven-figure settlement. The lesson here is that a clear transition of care should be documented, including with whom and at what point in time the responsibility for care transitioned. Prior to that agreed-upon point in time, the current physician is still primarily responsible. Merely accepting a patient for admission is not sufficient evidence of a transition of care or responsibility; document a transition note for your admitted patients, particularly those who will be boarding, and be clear who is primarily responsible and when that responsibility will transition.

IV. Heroic efforts:

As critically ill patients worsen and treatment options become limited, clinicians may become overly creative with their management decisions. This can be very problematic. If a treatment option wasn't indicated earlier, be cautious about offering it later in the patient's course. The late consideration of a formerly non-indicated modality implies that the option was indicated but was merely delayed in delivery. By way of example, decompensating patients with posterior circulation strokes are often given tPA, long beyond the normal time window(s). The clinicians may have noted that tPA was not offered earlier as it was not indicated for posterior circulation stroke. However, due to the patient's worsening condition, it was offered as a last-ditch effort to save them. Unfortunately, this discordance may be the focus of deposition testimony.

Case Example 4

A 38-year-old woman patient presented to the ED with confusion, depressed mental status, intermittent paresthesias and upper extremity weakness, which was not demonstrated on physical examination. The patient received a thorough evaluation from the EP, including a mental health evaluation due to the bizarre and inconsistent nature of her presentation. Documentation also was included that tPA was considered, but her presentation was not consistent with an ischemic stroke at that time. She was admitted to the ICU, where her symptoms evolved, and it became clear that she was experiencing locked-in syndrome from a basilar artery occlusion. Twenty-four hours into the admission, the decision to administer tPA was made, as she was not improving, and the admitting physician documented, "We need to try something."

Discussion: As there is controversy around whether or not tPA is indicated for posterior circulation strokes, the decision not to administer tPA early in her presentation when the diagnosis was unclear was very defensible. However, the lynch pin in this case was that once tPA was given, this removed the question of indication. The plaintiff's counsel asserted that tPA was indicated, but it was given over 24 hours late, as defined by the 3-hour time window defined by the American Heart and Stroke Associations. If heroic efforts, with marginal indication, are being considered, make certain that the purpose of this approach and the therapeutic limitations are noted. If possible, advise patients and families of these limitations and obtain their assent for doing so. To summarize, they should have realistic expectations when you are being creative in circumstances that call for heroic measures but may have limited benefit, and this should be documented in the record.

Conclusion:

The complexities and time-sensitive challenges associated with caring for the critically ill or injured patients should be our focus, as opposed to the risk management implications associated with the horrific outcomes that commonly occur. Despite the severity of patients' illnesses and injuries, the risk associated with caring for these patients can be mitigated by the previously discussed strategies and, most importantly, providing the highest quality of care possible; this is the focus of our book.

References:

- Brown TW, McCarthy ML, Kelen GD, et al. An epidemiologic study of closed emergency department malpractice claims in a national database of physician malpractice insurers. Acad Emerg Med 2010 May;17(5):553-60.
- Kachalia A, Gandhi TK, Puopolo AL, et al. Missed and delayed diagnoses in the Emergency Department: A study of closed malpractice claims from 4 liability insurers. Annals of Emerg Med 2007;49:196-205.

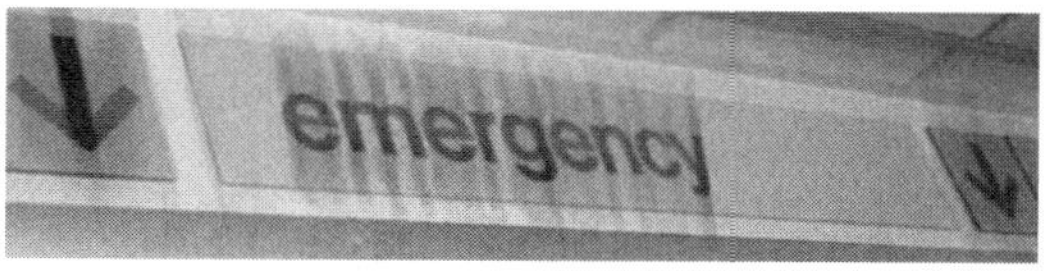

SECTION A – AIRWAY/ARREST

Chapter 1: A 42-year-old man with history of IVDU and upper back pain

Corinne Horan, DO

Attending emergency physician
Our Lady of Lourdes Medical Center
Camden, NJ

Section editor:

Lillian L. Emlet, MD, MS, FACEP, FCCM

Clinical Associate Professor
Depts. of Critical Care Medicine & Emergency Medicine
Associate Program Director
IMCCM Fellowship of the MCCTP
Interim Associate Chief of Staff of Education, VA
University of Pittsburgh School of Medicine
Pittsburgh, PA

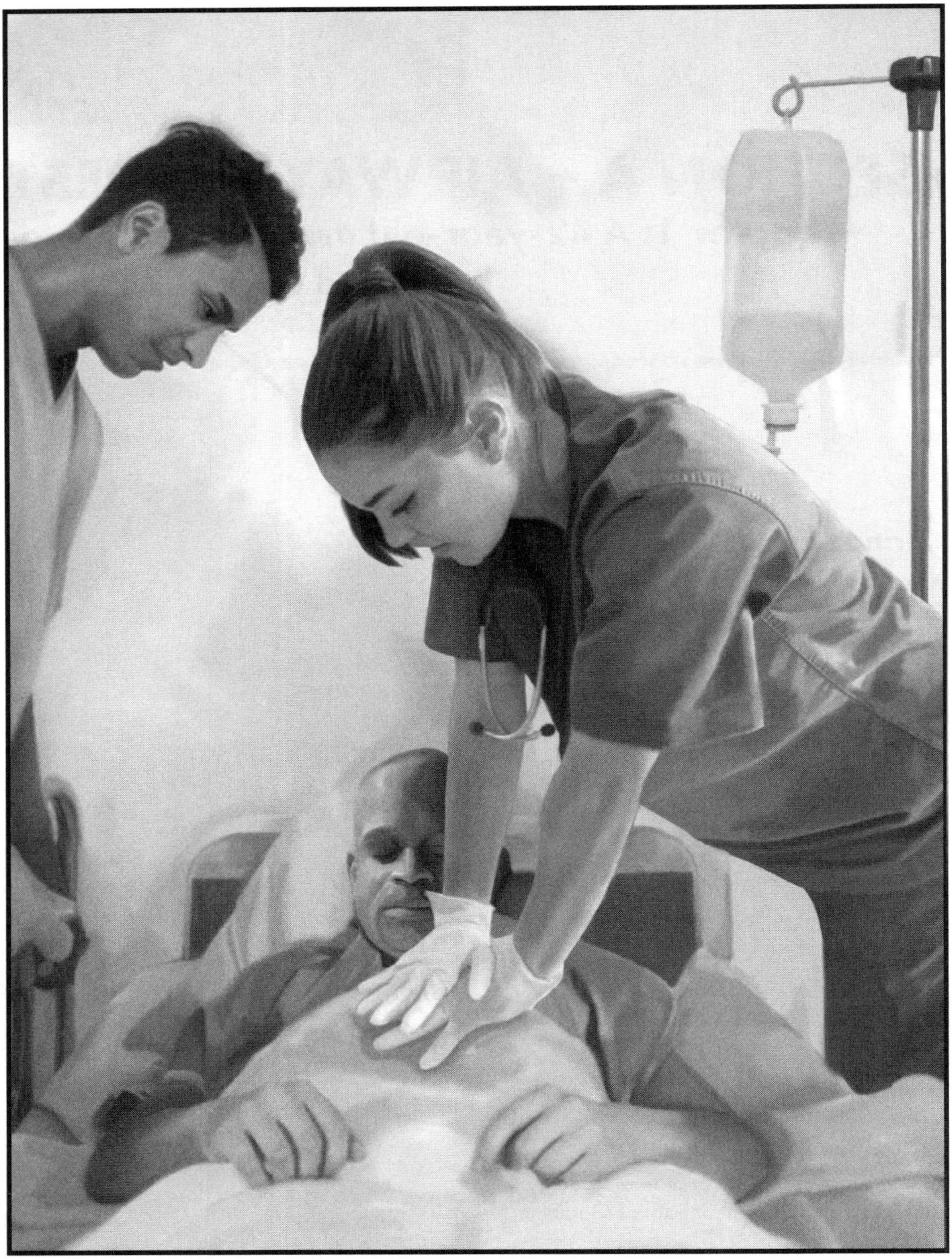

SECTION A /CHAPTER 1

A 42-year-old man with history of IVDU and upper back pain

The patient's story:
After spending 8 months in a refugee camp in a war-torn region of Somalia, Mohammed is approved to emigrate to America; work is scarce, and despite community support, he struggles to get by. He eventually finds a full-time job at a distribution center. He is paid with a yearly salary which includes health benefits, a source of considerable pride. Though he continues to hold down the job, he has assumed some of the habits of previous acquaintances, including drug use.

Spring of 2016 brings much needed warmth and soccer. Mohammed is passionate about the sport, but on a sunny Sunday in April, after a competitive game, he begins to have back pain, which worsens through the day. He decides to seek help from an urgent care center.

URGENT CARE VISIT

CC: Upper back pain

HPI: Pt is a 42-year-old man with c/o heartburn, regurgitation and upper back pain with myalgias. Denies fever, numbness, cp, palpitations, weakness. Rates pain as a 4/10 worse at night and has generalized body aches.
ROS: No fever, malaise, weight change, cp, sob, cough, DOE, syncope, melena, urinary symptoms, leg pain or swelling

NKDA
PMH: Insomnia, GERD, just treated for H. pylori
SH: No tobacco, alcohol, drugs
FH: Neg for CAD, HTN, DM, CA

PE:

Vitals, Afebrile:			
Pulse	Resp	BP	Sat (RA)
98	16	122/78	99%

CONSTITUTIONAL: WNWD, NAD
MENTAL STATUS/PSYCHIATRIC: Affect normal
EYES: PERRLLa
EARS: TMs without and canals normal
NECK: Supple, no sign LAN, thyromegaly

CHEST: CTA
HEART: RRR without m, t, r
ABD: Soft and NT. No HSM or masses
EXT: No cyanosis, clubbing, edema
NEURO: Reflexes nl and 2+ symmetrically knees and Achilles. Gait is WNL

A/P: Myalgias, muscle spasm, GERD
Lansoprazole 30mg PO QD #30/0
Cyclobenzaprine 10mg QHS PRN #10/0
F/U PCP if not improving

Evaluation of back pain: As the vast majority of patients have back pain from a benign cause, it is easy to let down our guard. Pain in the spine and back accounted for 2.9% of emergency department (ED) visits in the U.S. in 2016.[1] Evaluation for serious causes of back pain can be assessed simply through a thorough history and physical exam. Unfortunately, on this patient's initial visit, this was not done.

Serious diagnoses to consider included epidural compression syndrome, aortic dissection, pyelonephritis, ureteral stone, an acute coronary syndrome, and malignancy. Even without consideration of the "worst first" diagnoses, a more thorough history could have at least attempted to support a benign diagnosis (or *any* diagnosis), such as musculoskeletal back pain. Important historical points in our patient included lack of fever, chest pain or shortness of breath, and urinary symptoms, but could have included:

- Acuity of onset
- Exacerbating factors such as pain worsened with range of motion or with exertion
- History of intravenous drug abuse
- Specific history of bowel or bladder incontinence
- Personal history of cancer
- Syncope
- Recent trauma
- Pain that is worst at rest or at night

Documentation: The history of present illness (HPI) only included 3 elements of back pain; location (upper back), severity (4/10), and timing (worse at night). It does not support a likely explanation of the diagnosis ("myalgias, muscle spasm, GERD"), and more importantly, it does not exclude life-threatening etiologies including vertebral fractures with or without spinal cord compression, thoracic aortic dissection (TAD), epidural abscess, osteomyelitis, cauda equina syndrome or acute coronary syndrome.

To make matters worse, the physical exam does not even include a full back exam... OK, that is being kind. It does not include *any* back exam! The examination for back pain should include inspection for zoster/infection/trauma, palpation for muscular pain, and range of motion.

Lack of pain with range of motion or palpation increases suspicion of a visceral or referred cause of pain. A neurologic exam should be part of the back exam, with a focus on deficits attributable to epidural compression.

MDM – putting it all together: While it is difficult to determine if the physician considered some of the possible life-threats, it seems unlikely. The patient was previously treated for *H. pylori* and has a documented history of GERD, but there is no mention if these symptoms were new or chronic. Diagnosing a patient with two separate complaints should also give us pause; it is unlikely that *both* of these diagnoses were coincidentally causing this patient's back pain; a single diagnosis is most often to blame.

Author comments (Weinstock):

The initial evaluation was inadequate. It was a guess at our patient's symptoms without excluding serious, "can't-miss" causes. The practice of "empiric" medicine, i.e. being *usually* right, is not fair to our patients or respectful to our profession; our goal should not be *standard* of care, but *excellence* in care.

ED BOUNCEBACK (2 hours after urgent care visit)

CC per RN (11:49): Cardiac arrest

HPI:42-year-old male presents in cardiac arrest. EMS response to a witness arrest. They came the scene where police were doing CPR they responded and patient did not have a pulse and goes in V. tach and PEA. Patient did receive multiple defibrillations multiple rounds of epinephrine amiodarone and atropine. No other history was taken.

PMH/Social History: per nursing notes

PE:

Vitals:

Time	Temp	Pulse	Resp	Syst	Diast	Sat
11:51	16	0	16 w bagging	0	0	85% (BVM)

CONSTITUTIONAL: Comatose GCS 3T
EYES: Pupil fixed mid dilated, no scleral icterus.
EARS: Normal external ear; normal EAC's and TM's, no hemotympanum
THROAT: Moist oral mucosa; no posterior pharynx erythema
NECK: Supple without mass
RESP: Good bilateral BW w bagging
CARDIO: No heart tones
ABD: Minimally distended, soft, no surgical scars
SKIN: Normal for age and race; warm and dry; mottled

PMH/Social History:
Medical history: No items have been selected or recorded.
Past Medical History: Heroin abuse
Surgical history: No items have been selected or recorded
Family history: No items have been selected or recorded

Author comments (Weinstock):

Through this book, as we consider the "bounceback" critical care encounter, we explore 3–4 multi-question "decision points" followed by a review of the literature and recommendations for management. We next detail what interventions the *actual provider* took, the patient's response, and then move to the next decision point. Intermittently the section editor, consulting editor (Scott Weingart), and/or book author(s) will interject commentary and pearls as "expert whisperers."

For our first case, we are faced with a 42-year-old man with a witnessed arrest who has not responded to the initial rounds of ACLS. You are the team leader at the bedside. We are at:

DECISION POINT A – YOU ARE FACED WITH 7 QUESTIONS:

1. **What is the differential diagnosis of our patient's arrest?**
2. **Is Naloxone indicated for a patient in cardiac arrest?**
3. **What is the best approach to maintaining high-quality CPR?**
4. **If standard defibrillation fails, what options can be pursued?**
5. **Which medications are helpful in cardiac arrest?**
6. **What is the utility of end tidal CO_2 in cardiac arrest patients?**
7. **When should a code be ended?**

What does the literature say?

Q#1: What is the differential diagnosis of our patient's arrest?

As a patient in full arrest rolls into the resuscitation bay, considerations for the code leader including getting report from EMS, confirmation of ET tube placement and adequacy of lines, and consideration of a focused differential diagnosis. The most common cause of cardiac arrest is ischemic heart disease. With our patient and the extremely limited available history, and noting that his initial rhythm was ventricular tachycardia, coronary disease is the likely etiology. Additionally, the classic "Hs and Ts" of cardiac arrest should be considered including hypoxia, hyperkalemia, hypoglycemia, hypothermia, hydrogen ions/acidosis, trauma, toxins, tamponade, tension pneumothorax, and thrombosis. A focused echocardiographic examination can identify reversible causes of the arrest and has been shown to change management when used during CPR or in the peri-resuscitation period in conjunction with ECG analysis.[2] Findings may include:

- Pericardial tamponade
- Presence or absence of cardiac activity
- Cardiac wall motion abnormalities
- Pneumothorax

Caution that point-of-care ultrasound (POCUS) may double the time that chest compressions are paused.[3] Adequate chest compressions and defibrillation remain the primary interventions affecting code outcome; POCUS should not take precedence.

In our patient, there is mention of heroin abuse, but without family available or other confirmation, it is unclear how this information was obtained. In this high acuity patient, it is possible that the arrest was secondary to an overdose of opioids; however, it should not sway consideration of the above differential.

Q#2: Is Naloxone indicated for a patient in cardiac arrest?

If we are to believe that the history of heroin abuse is valid, the next question is "Should we give Naloxone?" With the patient presenting in a ventricular rhythm, the answer is most likely "no." While the use of Naloxone to reverse PEA/asystolic arrest that is clearly caused by opioid overdose has been described, there is no consistent evidence of improved outcome when used as an adjunctive therapy in cardiac arrest. In fact, the catecholamine and resultant sympathetic surge from naloxone administration can theoretically lead to a ventricular dysrhythmia.[4] With our patient already in a ventricular rhythm, particularly one that has been refractory to multiple prehospital defibrillation attempts, using a medication that can increase the myocardial irritability is not advisable. If the cause is thought to be hypoxic arrest, particularly a current O_2 saturation of 85% with BVM, the next step to consider would be an advanced airway placement such as an endotracheal tube or a supraglottic airway. Ideally, a supraglottic airway would have been placed by EMS en route. Advanced airway placement should be performed with minimal interruptions in chest compressions, ideally in less than 10 seconds or during chest compressions by experienced providers.[5]

Section editor comments (Emlet):

Supraglottic device options should have been placed by prehospital providers for continued ACLS on route to ED.

Consulting editor comments (Weingart):

I agree that there is not any real benefit to naloxone; the only reason I would give it to a patient with a suspected opioid overdose once intubated is from the diagnostic perspective, for example "I don't know why this patient is so obtunded, if I give naloxone will they wake up and try to pull out their tube?" But if the idea is "Let's increase their respiratory rate," well, that just seems silly.

Will we harm the patient? I don't think so. Most of the harm from naloxone, the negative pressure pulmonary edema, comes from the fact that the patient is under-ventilated at the time when naloxone is given. We have a patient that's been apneic for a long period of time, their brain keeps secreting enormous amounts of catecholamines and other stress hormones in an attempt to initiate breathing, but because the respiratory center is blocked off, they can't breathe, and naloxone is administered and they take this enormous breath against the closed glottis and then they get this negative pressure pulmonary edema. That shouldn't be happening if you've already ventilated a patient. That's why in New York City when they bag patients down prior to giving the naloxone, it markedly decreases the incidence of naloxone complications. You're probably not going to hurt them; I just don't see a benefit. And if you put them in acute withdrawal, it's going to make your life really annoying!

Q#3: What is the best approach to maintaining high-quality CPR?

While an advanced airway should be considered in our patient, the placement of an airway device should not take precedence over maintaining high quality CPR. Continuous and high-quality compressions are one of the few measures that have been shown to improve the chances of a patient surviving to hospital discharge with good neurologic outcome. Quality compressions can be monitored in several ways, but the best is direct observation by the team leader. Aspects that should be observed include:

- the rate of compressions
- the depth of compressions
- allowing for full chest recoil
- the ventilation rate
- the compression fraction[6]

As a team leader, ensuring high quality chest compressions is *our* responsibility. Use of a mechanical compression device can standardize the depth, rate, and lean of compressions that are applied, but the out-of-hospital use has not been shown to improve hospital survival.[7] The patient's response to quality resuscitative measures is most readily obtained by the use of end-tidal CO_2 monitoring. This measurement often begins in the pre-hospital setting and offers a non-invasive option to monitor the patient's cardiac output. A patient having an increase in the $EtCO_2$ during resuscitation can indicate return of spontaneous circulation (ROSC), whereas a persistently low $EtCO_2 < 10$mmHg is indicative of a futile resuscitation.[6]

Section editor comments (Emlet):

CPR should not be interrupted for IV or airway access. If available, use continued assessment of $EtCO_2$ for CPR quality as well as to determine when to terminate resuscitative efforts. If there is no $EtCO_2$ present the entire time, resuscitation efforts will not be fruitful.

Q#4: If standard defibrillation fails, what options can be pursued?

Optimizing the timing and utilization of defibrillation doesn't seem complicated but it can be tricky. External defibrillation should be delivered with as short of a pause in CPR as possible, with some bold resuscitation teams practicing "hands on" CPR without any breaks in compressions for defibrillation. Though this is not currently recommended, we should continue CPR while charging, then shock, then quickly return to compressions. A peri-shock pause lasting more than 40 seconds, constituting the pause in compressions both pre- and post-shock, has been linked to increased mortality; minimizing this break in compressions improves survival to hospital discharge.[6] Clear communication should occur from the team leader to ensure continued CPR during the charging phase of the defibrillator and monitor the resumption of compressions after defibrillation.

Dual sequence defibrillation: Our patient did, in fact, receive several shocks as well as amiodarone prior to arriving to the hospital. At the time of hospital arrival, he had a non-perfusing ventricular rhythm. Do we have any further options, or is it just more of the same? Refractory ventricular fibrillation, sometimes referred to as electrical storm, is most frequently associated with ischemia secondary to coronary artery disease. When standard therapies fail, dual sequential defibrillation can be attempted. This approach allows the practitioner to apply up to 760J of energy and change the vector that this energy is applied through. By recruiting a second monitor and applying a second set of pads, we can coordinate 2 simultaneous or closely successive defibrillations with a simple count to 3. Dual sequential defibrillation can increase the likelihood of obtaining ROSC, but it hasn't been shown to improve mortality.[8]

Consulting editor comments (Weingart):

Dual sequential is kind of in flux right now. We used to recommend it because really, what's the downside? With conventional defibrillation, you are not getting all of the cardiac myocytes actually shocked in one vector. But if you put two vectors, you have a chance of getting more of them; you need at least 95% to have a successful defibrillation, so boom. But now we're finding out that this can actually destroy the defibrillator, but doing it in a really evil way, in that it still appears to function. When the nurses check, the defibrillators will register as all good, but they won't be delivering shock with efficacy anymore. And the manufacturers obviously will not support fixing that under warranty so a lot of us have pulled back until a company actually creates a manufacturer-supported way of doing more than one set of pads. At this point I am not recommending it, nor am I doing it.

Beta-blockade: If this approach fails, consider adding esmolol, at a dose of 500μg/kg. This loading dose can be followed with a continuous infusion from 50–100μg/kg/min.[9] The goal of esmolol is to provide myocardial sympathetic blockade, with the consideration that sympathetic blockade can assist in decreasing the irritability of an ischemic myocardium. For patients with persistent shockable rhythms despite standard care, esmolol could potentially lead to ROSC or even increased hospital discharge.[10] In a case report of a patient with electrical storm esmolol was used between 2 dual sequential defibrillations and restored the patient to a normal rhythm, allowing the patient to be discharged from the hospital.[11] While these small studies and case reports yield promising results, the use of beta-blockade for refractory ventricular fibrillation needs to be more extensively studied. For our patient, with an observed arrest and refractory V-fib, this technique is worth considering.

Consulting editor comments (Weingart):

Esmolol, on the other hand, while we don't have fantastic evidence—no one has done an RCT yet—makes a lot of sense, especially if a lot of epi has been given. The reason esmolol is considered to be efficacious is that the patient may be in refractory V-fib due to the beta effects of epi. We give epi because we want the alpha, but the beta comes along as an unwanted guest, so if at the end of a code you've given a lot of epi, and the patients are not shocking out of V-fib, trying esmolol may help, as excess sympathetic tone seems to predispose the patient to not shocking out of V-fib. It has also been efficacious in patients who are just in ventricular storm without cardiac arrest. I use 500 micrograms/kilogram as a bolus. If effective, most people recommend starting a drip, which I think is unwieldy, so if I had the patient shock out and then they went back into V-fib and I wanted to give a second dose, I would just repeat that 500 microgram/kg dose.

Section editor comments (Emlet):

One other option to consider is eCPR (extracorporeal CPR), determined by the presence of $EtCO_2$. If the patient is deemed appropriate, transfer to a quaternary center is reasonable with application of a mechanical CPR device (i.e. Lucas) or protocols for cannulation for VA ECMO (veno-arterial ECMO) in the ED. If there are any neurologic signs present including eye opening or awakening during CPR, we should have early consideration with a goal of obtaining femoral access points.

Q#5: Which medications are helpful in cardiac arrest?

While adequate compressions and early defibrillation has been shown to improve outcomes and survival to hospital discharge, the same cannot be said of the code drugs. Though amiodarone or lidocaine are recommended by ACLS protocols to terminate the ventricular rhythm and achieve ROSC, a study by Kudenchuk compared lidocaine, amiodarone, and placebo in out-of-hospital cardiac arrest from shock refractory (> 2 shocks) ventricular fibrillation and found that there was no increase in rate of survival to hospital discharge; even more surprising, there was no statistically significant difference between either of these groups when compared with placebo.[12] While there have been some studies suggesting increased rates of ROSC with amiodarone compared to lidocaine or placebo, these short-term benefits were not sustained; a subgroup analysis did find improved outcomes for those with witnessed arrest. Epinephrine is also recommended by ACLS, with a primary goal to increase coronary and cerebral perfusion pressures. Though it increases the likelihood of achieving ROSC, one study suggested adverse neurological outcomes, primarily with early use.[13]

Q#6: What is the utility of end tidal CO_2 in cardiac arrest patients?

The end-tidal CO_2 acts as a marker for cardiac output by assessing pulmonary blood flow. While a CO_2 detecting device can check tube placement, continuous waveform capnography monitors both the adequacy of compressions and achievement of ROSC. The goal for end-tidal CO_2 should be > 20mmHg during compressions. A sudden increase in end-tidal CO_2 indicates that the patient has achieved ROSC; this can help avoid interruptions in compressions for pulse checks.[6]

Q#7: When should a code be ended?

EMS providers have clear cut indications for not starting resuscitation including decapitation, the presence of rigor mortis or lividity. They also have guidelines for considering termination of resuscitation efforts, including prolonged CPR (> 40–60 minutes), multiple rounds of CPR with a continued non-shockable rhythm, or end-tidal CO_2 that is persistently < 10mmHg during CPR. When a patient arrives in the ED, biases may contribute to the decision to terminate a code including individual provider experience and comfort with resuscitation. Some scenarios where resuscitation may be unsuccessful include elderly patients, multiple medical problems, and those presenting with asystole or PEA, unsuccessful attempts by EMS at resuscitation, or those with an unwitnessed or prolonged down time; a prolonged ED resuscitation is unlikely to improve their chances.[14]

What did the actual provider do?

MDM: 44-year-old male presents in cardiac arrest. Pt. is getting CPR and he is intubated easily with a GlideScope with a 7.5 ET tube. Good bilateral BS after intubation and good color change on the CO_2 detector. Pt. given Epi 1mg. Chest compressions were stopped and Pt. found to be in V-fib and was defibrillated with 360J twice and chest compressions were continued. He was given IVF wide open through 2 IVs and chest compressions continued for another 5 minutes and a second dose of Epi 1mg was given then pulse check was done while monitor was checked. Pt. still in V-fib without a pulse and another defib was done at 360. After this the monitor shows a sinus rhythm and pulse is able to be palpated right femoral.

PE:

Vitals:

Time	Temp	Pulse	Resp	Syst	Diast	Sat
12:12		38	16	86	49	92% (vent)

Author comments (Weinstock):

We have successfully resuscitated the patient! But he remains hypotensive and bradycardic. Our job is not finished... we are at:

DECISION POINT B – YOU ARE FACED WITH 4 QUESTIONS:

1. **Should atropine be given for the bradycardia?**
2. **Which patients benefit from post-arrest cardiac catheterization?**
3. **Which interventions are helpful in the post-arrest period?**
4. **What are the best ventilator settings in the post-arrest period?**

What does the data say?

Q#1: Should atropine be given for the bradycardia?

There is no evidence to suggest that atropine will be helpful for our patient's bradycardia. Post-cardiac arrest syndrome is a condition marked by myocardial dysfunction, reperfusion injury, and cerebral injury. Post-arrest care is aimed at minimizing and reversing these effects. Our patient has initial vitals notable for both bradycardia and hypotension. Now that we have ROSC, an ECG can tell us if the bradycardia is sinus or secondary to heart block. Whereas post-cardiac arrest myocardial dysfunction may cause this rhythm, we need to address other etiologies including potassium, hypoxia, and acidosis.[15] An ECG should be done immediately.

Q#2: Which patients benefit from post-arrest cardiac catheterization?

While coronary artery disease is a main cause of cardiac arrest, not every patient needs an emergent cardiac catheterization post-arrest. Certain indications for emergent catheterization are straightforward, such as a STEMI seen on a post-arrest ECG[16] with the best candidates being those with a witnessed arrest, an initial ventricular rhythm, immediate bystander CPR, and ROSC within 30 minutes. Patients with end-stage renal disease (ESRD), advanced age, non-cardiac cause of arrest such as a drug overdose, drowning, or stroke, and microcirculatory failure may be less likely to benefit from cardiac catheterization.

A 2019 *New England Journal of Medicine* (NEJM) multicenter, randomized trial shed light on the utility of emergent catheterization in the arrest patient *without* a STEMI. Lemkes, et al. randomized 552 post-cardiac arrest patients without STEMI to undergo immediate coronary angiography vs. angiography which was delayed until after neurologic recovery. They found that at 90 days, 176 of 273 patients (64.5%) in the immediate angiography group were alive and 178 of 265 patients (67.2%) in the delayed angiography group were alive. There were no significant differences in the groups between secondary endpoints such as cerebral performance, myocardial injury, markers of shock, duration of mechanical ventilation, major bleeding, or neurologic status when discharged from the ICU.[17]

Patients with a known history of cardiac disease or a history provided by a family member that is concerning for acute coronary syndrome (ACS) in the setting of cardiac arrest warrant a discussion with the interventional cardiologist, regardless of ECG findings,[18] but it is likely most important to continue with medical stabilization and hypothermia protocols until a patient has neurologic recovery.

Q#3: Which interventions are helpful in the post-arrest period?

While the charge nurse may already be looking for an ICU bed, a great deal of post-resuscitation care should begin in the ED:

- Close hemodynamic control with a goal of systolic BP above 90mmHg and MAP above 65mmHg should be achieved with the use of IV fluids and vasopressors. This MAP goal helps maintain cerebral perfusion pressure, which in some observational studies leads to improved neurologic outcomes following arrest. Consider placing an arterial line to accurately monitor blood pressures.
- Targeted temperature management (TTM) can be initiated in the ED using external cooling devices or by packing patient's axilla, neck, and groin with ice packs. Whereas past recommendations targeted cooling to 32–36° C for at least 24 hours in patients not following commands after ROSC, Cronberg, et al. compared 950 cardiac arrest patients in a multicenter, international, parallel group, assessor-masked randomized clinical trial to TTM at 33° F vs. 36° F and found patient recovery similar for patients at either end of the temperature range.[19] A meta-analysis by Schenone, et al. came to a similar conclusion; that there was no evidence to recommend one temperature goal over another. Other studies have also failed to demonstrate an improvement in neurologic outcomes with TTM with one temperature compared to another.[20-22] While hyperglycemia has been associated with worsened neurologic outcomes in post-arrest patients, there is limited evidence for optimal glucose concentrations. Most institutions have protocols for maintaining normal glucose concentrations; the goal is to avoid either hypoglycemia or hyperglycemia.[23]

Patients with seizure disorders can be maintained at a cooler temperature while a patient with a bleeding disorder or sepsis may be kept warmer. Continuous core temperature should be monitored with an esophageal, rectal, or bladder thermometer. Avoidance of hyperthermia is equally as important and patients that are febrile post-arrest should be treated with antipyretics. Initial induction of TTM can cause fluid and electrolyte shifts including potassium, calcium, and magnesium, so these electrolytes should be monitored and corrected.

Consulting editor comments (Weingart):

The goal temp we used on all our brain injury patients is 35° F, which is also my goal with the post-arrest and in the post-surgical patient. I choose a temp of 35 knowing it's not going to affect their bleeding but still get the lion's share of any benefits for TTM. There are some platelet effects at 32–34° F, and maybe at this temperature we are even at the very beginning of affecting coagulation cascade, but cooling to 35–36° F, has no effect whatsoever on platelets or the anticoagulation cascade; it's 100% safe. Regarding the goal, if we stop at 36° F I have found that it's too easy for them to slide up into temps I don't want, so I like a little buffer.

The goal of ventilation is aimed at maintaining normocarbia with an end-tidal CO_2 of 30–40mmHg or a $PaCO_2$ of 35–45mmHg. Several observational studies have noted that hypocarbia has been associated with worsened neurologic outcomes.[24] Normocarbia and normoxia are currently accepted as a reasonable post-arrest goal. Similarly, recommendations regarding oxygenation center around initially providing 100% oxygen until an ABG can confirm that the patient is adequately oxygenated. Oxygen should be titrated as low as possible to maintain saturation > 94%, as severe hyperoxia (PaO_2 > 300mmHg) has been associated with increased mortality. Note that a low pulse ox post-arrest may be an inaccurate representation due to peripheral vasoconstriction.

- Ventilator-associated pneumonia is a leading cause of morbidity and mortality in ICU with a mortality rate ranging from 20–50%. Prevention should start in the ED with good respiratory hygiene. The head of the patient's bed should be kept at 30–40 degrees, an orogastric tube should be placed for gastric decompression, ET tube cuff pressure should be maintained to help prevent aspiration, and frequent suctioning and chlorhexidine mouth rinses should be provided.
- While hyperglycemia has been associated with worsened neurologic outcomes in post-arrest patients, there is limited evidence for optimal glucose concentrations. Most institutions have protocols for maintaining normal glucose concentrations; the goal is to avoid either hypoglycemia or hyperglycemia.[23]

Q#4: What are the best ventilator settings in the post-arrest period?

Initial ventilator settings in the post-arrest period should be aimed at limiting acute lung injury. Maintaining a patient on volume assist-control with a tidal volume of 6–8 mL/kg of predicted body weight has been shown to minimize lung injury, decreasing the risk of development of ARDS. A lower tidal volume coupled with a higher PEEP (6–15cm H_2O) to encourage alveolar recruitment is preferred to maintain $PaCO_2$ 35–45mmHg and SpO_2 of 88–95%.[25,26]

What did the actual provider do?

Author comments (Weinstock):

An ECG is ordered, but while the leads are being placed, the sinus bradycardia changes to a sinus tachycardia with 1–2mm anterior ST depression on the monitor.

MDM (12:18): Given that he is young and this was reportedly a witnessed arrest and collapse, cardiology was consulted right away.

PE:

Vitals:

Time	Pulse	Resp	Syst	Diast	Sat	Pain
12:23	144	16	133	90	100% (vent)	9/10

MDM (12:25): Bedside ultrasound shows some apical wall motion abnormalities. I have spoken with cardiology and they will come to the ED and see the patient. No activation of cath lab at this time. Asked to expedite the lab results and to recall cardio when they return.

Labs:
WBC count = 7.1
Hb = 12.8gm/dL
Plt = 184thou/mcL

K+ = 2.7mmol/L (L)
Renal function – WNL
Glucose 324

ABG = 7.08/26/126

MDM (12:37): Patient does have an acidosis. Pt. is given bicarbonate and vent rate is increased to hyperventilate. Patient blood work shows a hypokalemia we'll replace. Hypothermia protocol will be initiated given his GCS is 3T without any sedation. Family has arrived and I did discuss with them and patient has been complaining of heartburn for 2 days. Patient went to urgent care today and was given medicine for that. Patient does have Flexeril on his possessions. They denied any smoking alcohol or recreational drug use.

DECISION POINT C – YOU ARE FACED WITH 2 QUESTIONS:

1. **Should hyperventilation be used with an acidotic patient post-arrest?**
2. **When should I consider ECMO?**

What does the data say?

Q#1: Should hyperventilation be used with an acidotic patient post-arrest?

With a primary goal of minimizing lung injury and maintaining normocarbia, a goal $PaCO_2$ of 35–45mmHg can be maintained via respiratory rate. Respiratory rates should not exceed 34 breaths per minute and additional strategies, such as hemodialysis, should be considered if the acidosis remains persistent or is severe. Upper limits of ventilator respiratory rates are due to potential for air trapping as lung compliance worsens.

Q#2: When should I consider ECMO?

If available, extracorporeal membrane oxygenation (ECMO) can be considered in the setting of cardiac arrest or in patients who are post-arrest and require further stabilization. Venoarterial ECMO allows for cardiac bypass and can be initiated during cardiac arrest. Our would have been a reasonable candidate for VA-ECMO in the setting of continued refractory ventricular fibrillation or with cardiogenic shock post-arrest as a bridge to cardiac catheterization and PCI. Venovenous ECMO allows for oxygen-carbon dioxide to exchange via extracorporeal membrane, as the name implies, and can be initiated for respiratory failure. Another candidate is the critically ill patient that has developed acute respiratory distress syndrome (ARDS) and is not able to be adequately ventilated or oxygenated until respiratory status improves. ECMO is not currently available in most institutions, and as such can only be feasibly considered in institutions with availability of the appropriate staff. If available, younger patients with normal neurologic function prior to arrest, short transport time (< 10 minutes), initial ventricular rhythms with minimal time prior to initiation of compression, and an arrest time of less than 1 hour might be reasonable candidates for ECMO, but further evidence regarding mortality from ECMO is required.[27]

MDM: Critical Care Time: 48 minutes of critical care time. This included multiple rounds of epinephrine for cardiac arrest. We are starting an epi drip. This included multiple tests including blood gas. This included talking to the family. Talking the cardiology ICU admitting team. This also included hyperventilation and bicarbonate for patient's respiratory metabolic acidosis.

ED impression and plan:

1. Cardiac Arrest
2. Comatose
3. Acute MI

Cardiology consult:

HPI: 44 yo AA male presents via squad after being found down in parking lot. He had just picked up medications at the local pharmacy and was (witnessed?) to collapse. CPR was performed and 911 arrival to find VF and unresponsive. Multiple shocks were performed to establish sinus rhythm and transported to the ED. Here initial echo revealed preserved LV function with no obvious valvular lesions. This rapidly deteriorated to a profound bradycardia and global severe hypokinesia. Bicarb and epi were administered along with quality CPR with restoration of LV function and sinus tachycardia. ABG revealed acidosis and hypercapnia. No other medical history available although he is reported to have use of heroin.

Immediate post-procedure note:

Cardiac catheterization:

***Acuity:** Salvage

***Pre-diagnosis:** Cardiac arrest (found down, multiple DC cardioversion, hypotensive)

***Post-diagnosis:** Occluded LAD

***Access:** Radial – Rt

Coronary arteries

Left main: no angiographic stenosis identified

Left anterior descending: proximal 100% occlusion/rescue PCI with placement of DES

Circumflex : no angiographic stenosis identified
Ramus: no angiographic stenosis identified
Right : 60% mid vessel, non-dominate
Ventriculography
Wall motion: apical hypokinesia (severe)
Ejection Fraction: 45
***Plan:** Hypothermia protocol/Ticagrelor/ASA/Vent management/

Echo:
The left ventricular systolic function is severely decreased.
The left ventricular ejection fraction is 15% per visual estimation.
The anteroseptal wall segment is dyskinetic.
*After resuscitation, the LV function is improved with akinesis of the anteroseptal wall.

A/P: Status post-proximal LAD occlusion with rescue PCI and placement of drug-eluting stent. Hemodynamically on pressor support. Rhythm has been stable. Very significant concern at this point of anoxic injury. Neurology following.

Critical care/ICU intensivist:*
Death notice: The patient was terminally extubated because of brain death. He had no pulse as well as no spontaneous respirations. His family was all present. The patient had no reflexes. His rhythm strip was flat with no electrical activity. The patient never took a single breath after extubation. He did not require any medication.

Active/Final diagnosis(es):
Anoxic brain damage, not elsewhere classified
Cardiac arrest, cause unspecified
Personal history of other specified conditions
Syncope and collapse
Unspecified coma

What happened?
Usually back pain is due to musculoskeletal causes, but in this case, the initial clinician missed a big red flag; the complaint of "heart burn." Be wary of symptoms that begin simultaneously (heartburn and back pain), as they are often related. From additional history, it was later learned from the family, both were present for 2 days. A more detailed history of present illness, physical exam, and ECG may have changed our patient's outcome.

The cardiac arrest was a ventricular arrest which resolved after ACLS algorithmic care. It was prudent of the emergency physician to discuss the case with the cardiologist for early cardiac catheterization. Many patients suffering OHCA will not have ECGs that meet STEMI criteria, even if their arrest was due to coronary disease. Bedside echocardiography and the early involvement of interventional cardiology can facilitate excellence in post-arrest care.

The emergency department physician in this case appropriately addressed the most important aspects by beginning a therapeutic hypothermia protocol and making note of electrolyte abnormalities that were to be managed at the time of induction as well as noting hemodynamic abnormalities that required intervention and commented on ventilator management. Having an awareness of the pathophysiological changes post-arrest and addressing in a timely fashion remain the responsibility of the ED physician and should not be delayed until transfer to the ICU.

Summary of teaching points:

1. Back pain is a common and often benign ED complaint, but it is our responsibility to consider life-threatening diagnoses.
2. Focused ultrasound during cardiac arrest can help identify reversible causes of arrest and assist in management.
3. High-quality CPR with minimal interruptions improves the chance for ROSC.
4. There are no antiarrhythmic medications that have been shown to improve mortality.
5. Epinephrine may exacerbate issues associated with the post-arrest syndrome.
6. Post-cardiac arrest syndrome is a disease state that causes myocardial dysfunction, cerebral injury, and multiorgan reperfusion injury. Post-arrest care is aimed at minimizing these effects.
7. Targeted temperature management, ventilator management, and hemodynamic monitoring and control should be started in the ED.
8. Early cardiac catheterization improves mortality post-arrest in STEMI patients.

References:

1. Rui P, Kang K, Ashman JJ. National hospital ambulatory medical care survey: 2016 emergency department summary tables. 2016; Available at: https://www.cdc.gov/nchs/data/ahcd/nhamcs_emergency/2016_ed_web_tables.pdf
2. Hernandez C, Shuler K, Hannan H, et al. C.A.U.S.E.: Cardiac arrest ultra-sound exam—A better approach to managing patients in primary non-arrhythmogenic cardiac arrest. Resuscitation 2008;76(2):198-06.
3. Huis In t Veld MA, Allison MG, Bostick DS, et al. Ultrasound use during cardiopulmonary resuscitation is associated with delays in chest compressions. Resuscitation 2017;119:95-8.
4. Martins HS, Silva RV, Bugano D, et al. Should naloxone be prescribed in the ED management of patients with cardiac arrest? A case report and review of literature. Am J Emerg Med 2008;26(1): 113 e5-8.
5. Neumar RW, Otto CW, Link MS, et al. Part 8: Adult advanced cardiovascular life Support: 2010 American Heart Association guidelines for cardiopulmonary resuscitation and emergency cardiovascular care. Circulation 2010;122(18 Suppl 3):S729-67.
6. Meaney PA, Bobrow BJ, Mancini ME, et al. Cardiopulmonary resuscitation quality: Improving cardiac resuscitation outcomes both inside and outside the hospital: A consensus statement from the American Heart Association. Circulation 2013;128(4):417-35.
7. Rubertsson S, Lindgren E, Smekal D, et al. Mechanical compressions and simultaneous defibrillation vs conventional cardiopulmonary resuscitation out-of-hospital cardiac arrest. JAMA 2014;311(1):53-61. doi:10.1001/jama.2013.282538
8. Cortez E, Krebs W, Davis J, et al. Use of double sequential external defibrillation for refractory ventricular fibrillation during out-of-hospital cardiac arrest. Resuscitation 2016;108:82–6.
9. Lee YH, Lee KJ, Min YH, et al. Refractory ventricular fibrillation treated with esmolol. Resuscitation. 2016;107:150-5.

10. Driver BE, Debaty G, Plummer DW, et al. Use of esmolol after failure of standard cardiopulmonary resuscitation to treat patients with refractory ventricular fibrillation. Resuscitation 2014;85(10):1337–341.
11. Boehm K, Keyes D, Mader L, et al . First report of survival in refractory ventricular fibrillation after dual-axis defibrillation and esmolol administration. West J Emerg Med 2016;17(6):762-65.
12. Kudenchuk PJ, Brown SP, Mohamud D, et al. Amiodarone, lidocaine, or placebo in out-of-hospital cardiac arrest. N Engl J Med 2016;374:1711-22.
13. Dumas F, Bougouin W, Geri G, et al. Is epinephrine during cardiac arrest associated with worse outcomes in resuscitated patients? J Am Coll Cardiol 2014;6.22 2014:2360-367.
14. Ranola, Merchant RM, Perman SM, et al. How long is long enough, and have we done everything we should? Ethics of calling codes. J Med Ethics 2014;41(8):663-6.
15. Pellis T, Sanfilippo F, Ristagno G. The optimal hemodynamics management of post-cardiac arrest shock. Best Pract Res Clin Anaesthesiol 2015;29(4):485-95.
16. Camuglia AC, Randhawa VK, Lavi S, et al. Cardiac catheterization is associated with superior outcomes for survivors of out of hospital cardiac arrest: Review and meta-analysis. Resuscitation 2014;85(11):1533-540.
17. Lemkes JS, Janssens GN, van der Hoeven NW, et al. Coronary angiography after cardiac arrest without ST-segment elevation. N Engl J Med 2019;380:1397-407.
18. Rab T, Kern KB, Tamis-Holland JG, et al. Cardiac arrest: A treatment algorithm for emergent invasive cardiac procedures in the resuscitated comatose patient. J Am Coll Cardiol 2015;66(1):62-73.
19. Cronberg T. Neurologic function and health-related quality of life in patients following targeted temperature management at 33°C vs 36°C after out-of-hospital cardiac arrest. JAMA Neurology 2015;72(6):634-41.
20. Mark DG, Vinson DR, Hung YY, et al. Lack of improved outcomes with increased use of targeted temperature management following out-of-hospital cardiac arrest: A multicenter retrospective cohort study. Resuscitation 2014;85(11):1549-56.
21. Bray JE, Stub D, Bloom JE, et al. Changing target temperature from 33° C to 36° C in the ICU management of out-of-hospital cardiac arrest: a before and after study. Resuscitation 2017;113:39-43.
22. Schenone AL, Cohen A, Patarroyo G, et al. Therapeutic hypothermia after cardiac arrest: A systematic review/meta-analysis exploring the impact of expanded criteria and targeted temperature. Resuscitation 2016;108:102-10.
23. Callaway CW, Donnino MW, Fink EL. Part 8: Post-cardiac arrest care. 2015 American Heart Association guidelines update for cardiopulmonary resuscitation and emergency cardiovascular care. Circulation 2015;132:S465–S482.
24. Roberts BW, Kilgannon JH, Chansky ME, et al. Association between postresuscitation partial pressure of arterial carbon dioxide and neurological outcome in patients with post-cardiac arrest syndrome. Circulation 2013;127(21):2107–113.
25. Weingart SD. Managing initial mechanical ventilation in the emergency department. Ann Emerg Med 2016;68(5):614-17.
26. Sutherasan Y, Vargas, Pelosi P. Protective mechanical ventilation in the non-injured lung: Review and meta-analysis. Crit Care 2014;18(2):211.
27. Winters ME, ed. Emergency department resuscitation of the critically ill. 2nd ed. Dallas, TX: American College of Emergency Physicians, 2011.

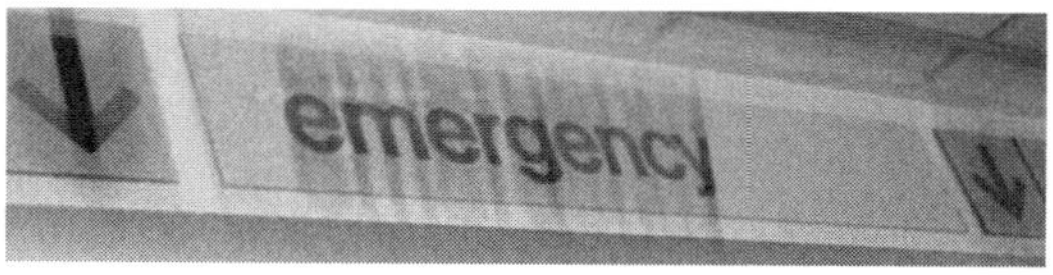

SECTION A – AIRWAY/ARREST

Chapter 2: A 53-year-old man with a tracheostomy and shortness of breath

Eric J. Adkins, MD, MSc, FACEP

Associate Chief Clinical Information Officer
Vice Chair of Clinical Affairs
Associate Professor of Emergency Medicine & Pulmonary/Critical Care Medicine
Department of Emergency Medicine
The Ohio State University Wexner Medical Center
Columbus, OH

Patrick Sylvester, MD

Fellow, Pulmonary & Critical Care Medicine
The Ohio State University Wexner Medical Center
Columbus, OH

Section editor:

Lillian L. Emlet, MD, MS, FACEP, FCCM

Clinical Associate Professor
Depts. of Critical Care Medicine & Emergency Medicine
Associate Program Director
IMCCM Fellowship of the MCCTP
Interim Associate Chief of Staff of Education, VA
University of Pittsburgh School of Medicine
Pittsburgh, PA

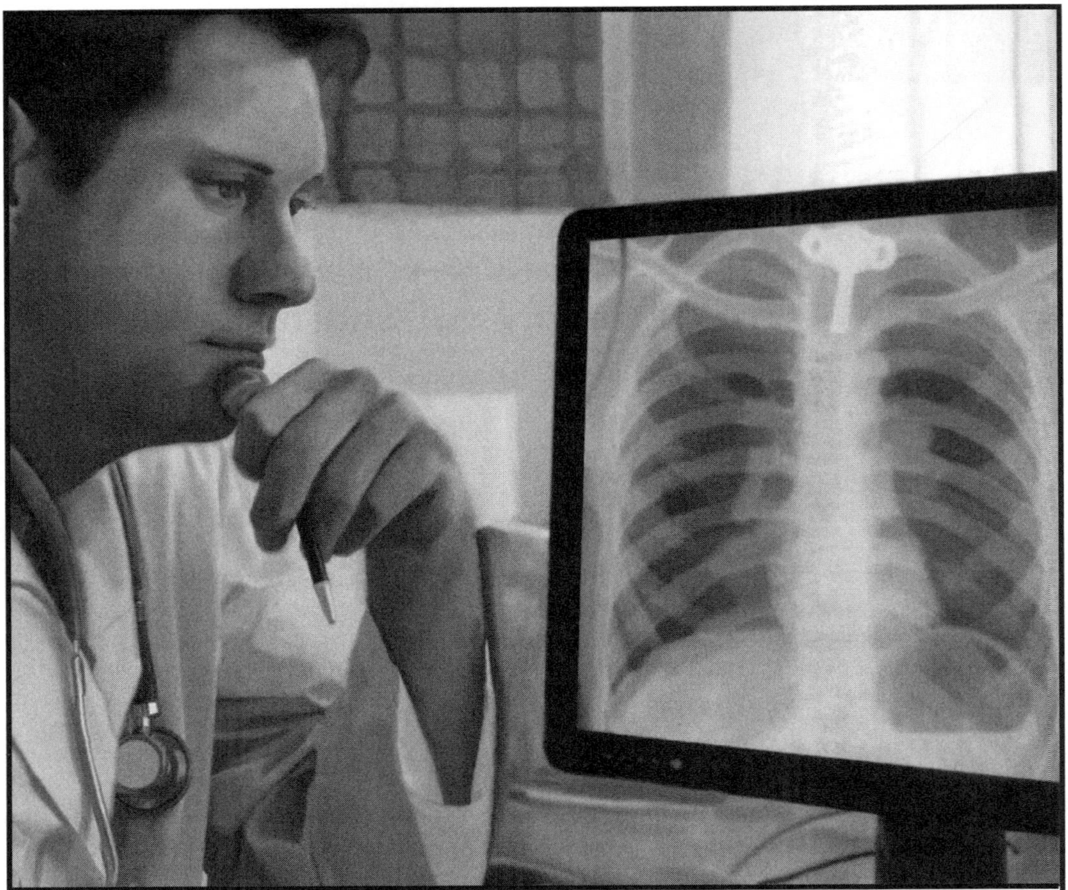

"HE SEEMS FINE TO SEND HOME."

SECTION A/CHAPTER 2

A 53-year-old man with a tracheostomy and shortness of breath

INITIAL ED VISIT

CC (13:16): Difficulty breathing

Vitals:

Time	Temp	RT	Pulse	Resp	Syst	Diast	Pos	O2	O2%
13:20	98.2	0	98	23	133	54	L 97	10 L track mask	
13:37			98	23	99	52	L 95	10 L track mask	

Triage/RN: Pt unable to speak but can shake head for yes and no. Difficulty breathing at ECF [extended care facility] improved. RN performed suction with Trach using a/an 14F. The patient tolerated the procedure well.

Past Medical History: NKDA
Medications: ASA, plavix, folic acid, quetiapine, warfarin, lisinopril, lopressor, zocor, cardizem, nexium, insulin, atarax, keppra, atrovent and albuterol aerosol, bactroban to sacral ulcer daily, tobramycin with each dialysis, jevity feeds through PEG
PMH: COPD, CHF, renal disease, CVA, alcohol and cocaine abuse, HTN, CAD, colon CA, MRSA, pneumonia, encephalopathy, anemia
PSH: Abdominal surgery

HPI (15:23): Transported to ED from ECF for eval of SOB. Pt cannot provide any substantial history. I spoke with the transporting ambulance crew who said the patient was very dyspneic upon arrival with sat of 60% range. He vigorously suctioned his tracheostomy tube and a large amount of mucus returned with the rapid improvement in his respiratory effort and oxygen saturations. I contacted the clinic and spoke with the nurse who had not been present at the time of transport but received report from the nurse present at that time. Apparently his symptoms developed abruptly this morning and appeared dyspneic to the staff. No complaints of chest pain. No recent fever. Staff had noted his respiratory secretions have recently been thick.

ROS: Unable to complete review of systems because patient unable to answer questions.

Exam (15:25)
CONSTITUTIONAL: Chronically ill-appearing male who appears much older than his stated age; in no acute respiratory distress-- he is on blow by oxygen with a respiratory rate of 22 per minute; no retractions or labored respirations.

NEURO: GCS=E3VtrachM6 Cranial nerves II-XII intact. Motor strength and sensation grossly intact.
ENT: Mucous membranes are moist.
NECK: Supple; non-tender; no cervical lymphadenopathy; no masses or thyromegaly, no JVD.
CARDIO: RRR; normal S1,S2,: no S3 or S4; no murmurs, rubs, or gallops. The pulses equal bilaterally and brisk capillary refill. There is no peripheral edema of the extremities.
RESP: Breath sounds distant bilaterally; no wheezes, rhonchi, or rales.
ABD: Normal bowel sounds; non-distended; non-tender; no palpable organomegaly.

Results:
EKG: Non specific changes

ABG:

Test	Flag	Value	Units	Ref. Range
pH		7.413		7.350-7.450
PCO_2	**H**	**49.9**	**MMHG**	**32.0-48.0**
PO_2	**L**	**60.1**	**MMHG**	**83.0-108.0**
HCO_3	**H**	**31.2**	**MMOL/L**	**21.0-28.0**
WB NA		139	MEQ/L	136-146
WB K		3.9	MEQ/L	3.5-5.0
WB LAC		0.8	MMOL/L	0.5-1.6
WB CL		99	MEQ/L	98-106
TCO_2		28.5	MMOL/L	22.0-29.0
SITE		LT.FEMOR		
O_2 SAT	**L**	**92.6 %**		**95.0-99.0**
FI O_2		35.00		

CXR (EP interpretation): Chest x-ray did not show any changes from previous studies.

Vitals:

Time	Temp	Pulse	Resp	Syst	Diast	Pos	O2	O2%
16:13		104	19	112	70	L	100	10 L track mask

Progress notes (15:36): During ER stay the rate at effort remained nl. Sats remained in the mid 90% range with blow by O_2 as he receives at the ECF. ABG was drawn while the mask was poorly fitting and essentially represents a RA blood gas. No signs of CO_2 retention. I felt he could return to the ECF.

Diagnosis (15:36): Acute respiratory distress – resolved
RN (16:24): Patient discharged home to nursing home, condition – stable

Initial visit discussion points:

Trach complications: Patients with tracheostomies can be challenging; difficulty in verbal communication creates a barrier to history-taking and the presence of a tracheostomy tube often implies a commensurate degree of medical complexity.

There are multiple categories of complications that might be considered a "trach problem."

- Simple dislodgement of the tracheostomy tube may have occurred, particularly in those with placement within the last 7 days, which may pose a challenge for replacement given the lack of a mature tract. Attempts at replacing may result in the tube being placed in the subcutaneous pre-tracheal space creating a false tract.[1]
- Complete or partial obstruction from normal or abnormal secretions may occur, which may be too difficult to clear with suction at home.
- The presence of a tracheostomy tube provides a nidus of infection and subsequently a source for more distal infection of the lower respiratory tract.
- Bleeding from a tracheostomy site is fairly common and can range from mild, due to crusting from a lack of humidified air or overzealous suctioning, to the life threatening—including a tracheoinominate fistula.[2]

What causes SOB in trach patients?

Shortness of breath in a patient with a tracheostomy should prompt a broad differential with the primary focus on the aforementioned complications of the tracheostomy device itself, but should also include consideration of other lower respiratory causes including pneumonia, pulmonary edema, pulmonary embolism (PE), myocardial infarction (MI), COPD exacerbation and other causes which would occur in a patient without a trach.

In our patient, the presence of thick secretions associated with dyspnea that resolved with suctioning seems fairly convincing for a secretion-related cause. Lack of fever documented on serial vital signs, as well as the lack of infiltrate or air-bronchograms on chest x-ray would be suggestive of a non-infectious etiology. We should differentiate between tracheitis (more appropriately known as "artificial airway-associated tracheobronchitis") from a pneumonic etiology of secretions. The former is characterized by the presence of increased sputum production and fever without the development of consolidative changes on exam or focal infiltrate on chest imaging and can be due to viral or bacterial cause. Unfortunately, tracheostomy tubes can be a fertile ground for bacterial colonization, frequently with highly resistant species, so management typically requires broad antibiotics directed towards nosocomial pathogens.

Section editor comments (Emlet):

The latter is characterized by purulent secretions, fever, elevated WBC count, increased inspired oxygen requirement, and findings on physical exam (wheeze, rhonchi, interstitial breath sounds) or radiologic exam (B lines on lung ultrasound or air bronchograms on chest x-ray).

Considerations for discharge:

In this case, the patient is subjectively improved and vital signs appear to be normalizing. It seems expected that a patient with a tracheostomy lives with a certain degree of secretions; if this is the only therapy necessary in the emergency department, why not send them back to the care facility?

There need to be some checkpoints in this patient's discharge, mostly dealing with the questions:

- Is the patient going to be able to receive the same degree of respiratory support when they leave the ED?
- Do they have suction equipment and tracheostomy supplies at home or at the ECF?
- What was their baseline oxygen requirement?

There are a fair number of patients who receive oxygen support via trach collar, but there are others that receive only humidified air. In this particular case, the ABG shows what seems to be adequate oxygenation on supplemental oxygen, but we do not know if the patient is normally on home oxygen. These values may be tolerable for a patient whose baseline oxygenation is room air, but in this case, the chart has documented these values on supplemental O_2.

Should he have been prescribed antibiotics?

Unfortunately, there is not a wealth of data; the use of procalcitonin levels to differentiate bacterial vs. other causes of infection has been examined, but routine use is not yet standard. In theory, the goal behind treating patients with suspected tracheitis would be to reduce the incidence of progression to pneumonia. One of the best studies to date examined tracheostomy-dependent patients admitted to ICU level care who developed the combination of fever, purulent sputum, and had a positive culture from tracheal aspirate.[3] Patients were randomized to either 8 days of broad spectrum antibiotics or placebo, with resultant decrease in mortality and ventilator-free days in the antibiotic group. This study may not be readily applicable to the ED population, given the inability to establish a positive tracheal culture and the differences in microflora between hospitalized and community-dwelling patients.

Consulting editor comments (Weingart):

If you start antibiotics on every single patient who has increased tracheal secretions, we're going to be building bugs that are indomitable. If we are going to start antibiotics, we need some other evidence that this is a bacterial infection as they're also going to have increased mucus with a viral infection. We need more, such as an actual infiltrate, a fever, or if they are hemodynamically unstable, and if so, then the balance goes to empirically starting antibiotics.

Chapter author summary:

The patient has a significant oxygen requirement with decreased PaO_2 on blood gas, we recommend admission for a course of empiric antibiotics and observation. If he improves in 24–48 hours with improved vitals and decreased oxygen requirement, antibiotics can be de-escalated.

Section editor comments (Emlet):

Additional questions which could have been asked at the initial visit include: When was the trach placed? Why was the trach placed? What is his neurologic baseline?

Consulting editor comments (Weingart):

Should these patients be admitted? Much of it comes down to ability to care for the patient after discharge; are they from home or from a skilled nursing facility? It's perfectly acceptable to send the patient back to their nursing facility if they are able to administer medications and monitor and address secretions. Home is a little tougher; do they have skilled nurses who can see if the secretions are getting better or worse? If they are just being cared for by an untrained family member, then it may be better to do a 24-hour observation. It's a big deal to admit a trach patient; it's not just a regular medicine bed, you're taking up either an ICU or step-down bed. And, those are often in short supply.

ED RETURN (2 hours and 32 minutes later)

CC/quote: patient arrived to ED in full arrest [which was a] witnessed arrest at ECF wife reports patient C/O chest pain prior to arrest. given 3 epi 2 atropine and 1 amp bicarb by ems. patient is trach dependent.

HPI (Physician – documented later): This is a 55-year-old who had a witnessed arrest at the ECF. He has history of stroke, tracheostomy and PEG and chronic renal failure. He was discharged from here 2 days ago with sepsis and was here briefly in the ED earlier today and was discharged back after his respiratory distress cleared with suctioning. Shortly after returning back to the ECF, he had a witnessed arrest and was pulseless. The medics did insert an endotracheal tube through his tracheostomy and bagged him and gave several routes of I/O ACLS medications with brief return of spontaneous circulation but it had again disappeared and he was pulseless for approximately 10 minutes prior to arrival. His wife is here at bedside and confirms that he is a full code.

PE:
CONSTITUTIONAL: he arrived pulseless and unresponsive in PEA
HEAD: Normocephalic; atraumatic
EYES: pupils non reactive
NECK: ETT thru his tracheostomy
RESP: Normal chest excursion with respiration; breath sounds bilateral rhonchi with bagging
CARDIO: no heart sounds
ABD: Non-distended; non-tender, soft with PEG tube noted
EXT: No pulses

Author comments (Weinstock):

We are at the bedside of a patient recently discharged from *the same ED* who is now in pulseless electrical activity (PEA). We are at:

DECISION POINT A – YOU ARE FACED WITH 4 QUESTIONS:

1. **What unique issues should be addressed in the PEA trach patient in full arrest?**
2. **If the patient is not able to be ventilated through the trach, what is the next step?**
3. **How should a trach be exchanged?**
4. **The paramedics placed an endotracheal tube into the trach site, how should you confirm it was placed correctly?**

Q#1: What unique issues should be addressed in the PEA trach patient in full arrest?

The management of the critically ill patient with tracheostomy is similar to others, in this case, the absence of pulses clearly takes precedence for employing the appropriate ACLS pathway and maintaining high quality chest compressions. However, there is special attention that should be paid to the assessment of airway.

- One should establish the age of the tracheostomy site and what type of appliance is present including the size and length of the tracheostomy.
- The presence or absence of a cuff to the tracheostomy should be confirmed by the presence of a pilot balloon.
- Extraneous devices connected to the tracheostomy circuit should be removed (e.g., speaking valves).
- The tracheostomy should be connected to a BVM (either directly or after removal of an inner cannula, if present).

Difficulty in bagging the patient may be the result of a proximal occlusion, dislodgement, or mucus plugging of the lower airways, which in its worst form can result in obstructive atelectasis and ipsilateral mediastinal shift due to volume loss and seen as a "white-out" of the hemithorax on chest x-ray.

Historically, many tracheostomies were placed due to tracheal obstruction, failed airways, or prolonged hospital stays on a ventilator. In current practice, many patients are trached early in the ICU stay to allow for liberation from the ventilator and reduce risk of nosocomial infection. If there is concern about proper function or placement of tube in the existing tracheostomy, consider attempting oral tracheal ETT placement via traditional airway tools.

Section editor comments (Emlet):

Determination of an obligate neck-breathing patient with prior history of total laryngectomy is vitally important, as patients with tracheostomy and total laryngectomy will NOT have a method of securing the airway from above (oral or nasal) as the larynx has been removed, separating the oral cavity from the trachea.

Q#2: If the patient is not able to be ventilated through the trach, what is the next step?

Our patient was "intubated" through the trach site by the paramedics. What if he still had a trach in place but was not able to be ventilated?

1. If there is concern for obstruction, the inner cannula of the tracheostomy can be removed, and a small-bore suction catheter placed within the tracheostomy. If there is significant resistance to the passage of a suction catheter, there should be immediate concern for the patency of the

tracheostomy and consideration should be made for replacement with an endotracheal tube. The ability of the catheter to pass smoothly with return of secretions argues for patency.

2. Further suctioning can be undertaken to remove an obstruction/secretions.

Section editor comments (Emlet):

Bronchoscopy should be performed urgently to prevent barotrauma and ensure clearance of tracheal obstruction. Begin the process to obtain additional alternative methods to replace the tracheostomy tube if end tidal CO_2 and/or bronchoscopy suggest occlusion (i.e. new endotracheal tube or replacement tracheostomy tube).

Q#3: How should a trach be exchanged?

The process for exchanging an obstructed tube or replacing a displaced tube have a similar set of principles. Firstly, it is imperative to know the age of the tracheostomy site, as tracheostomies placed within the last 7 days have a high rate of closure and creation of false tracts. In those cases, assistance should be sought from ENT or other experienced surgical consultants. The safety of these exchanges may be maximized by using adjuncts such as fiberoptic bronchoscope or a bougie exchange catheter to enter the existing tracheostomy tube or tract first. The presence of hang-up or palpation of tracheal rings using the bougie can be identified before placing the tracheostomy tube or ETT over top. Caution that the removal of an existing tracheostomy tube may result in fairly rapid edema and narrowing of the stoma site, so be prepared to replace the prior tracheostomy with one a size smaller.

If there is concern that replacement of a tracheostomy tube is not possible or too high-risk, consider deflating the patient's cuff to allow whatever residual ventilatory ability remains to occur around the tube, with subsequent intubation using the orotracheal route. Of note, prior to such attempts, confirm that the airway device in question is in fact a tracheostomy, and not a device within a stoma after laryngectomy. In the latter, the oropharynx will be completely disconnected from the trachea and thus the only way to gain access to the airway would be through the tracheal stoma.

Q#4: The paramedics placed an endotracheal tube into the trach site, how should we confirm it was placed correctly?

At the end of the day, both a cuffed ETT and a cuffed tracheostomy device serve the same function—which is to provide a secure pathway for the delivery of a given tidal volume with minimal leak. As it was documented, the patient's airway sounds to be sufficient for ongoing resuscitation. Further confirmation of ETT positioning could be determined by color-change or wave-form capnography and chest radiography. If available, the placement of a bronchoscope or nasopharyngoscope within the ETT should yield visualization of the carina, definitively confirming tracheal positioning.

(Figure on next page...)

Figure 1. Emergency Tracheostomy Management

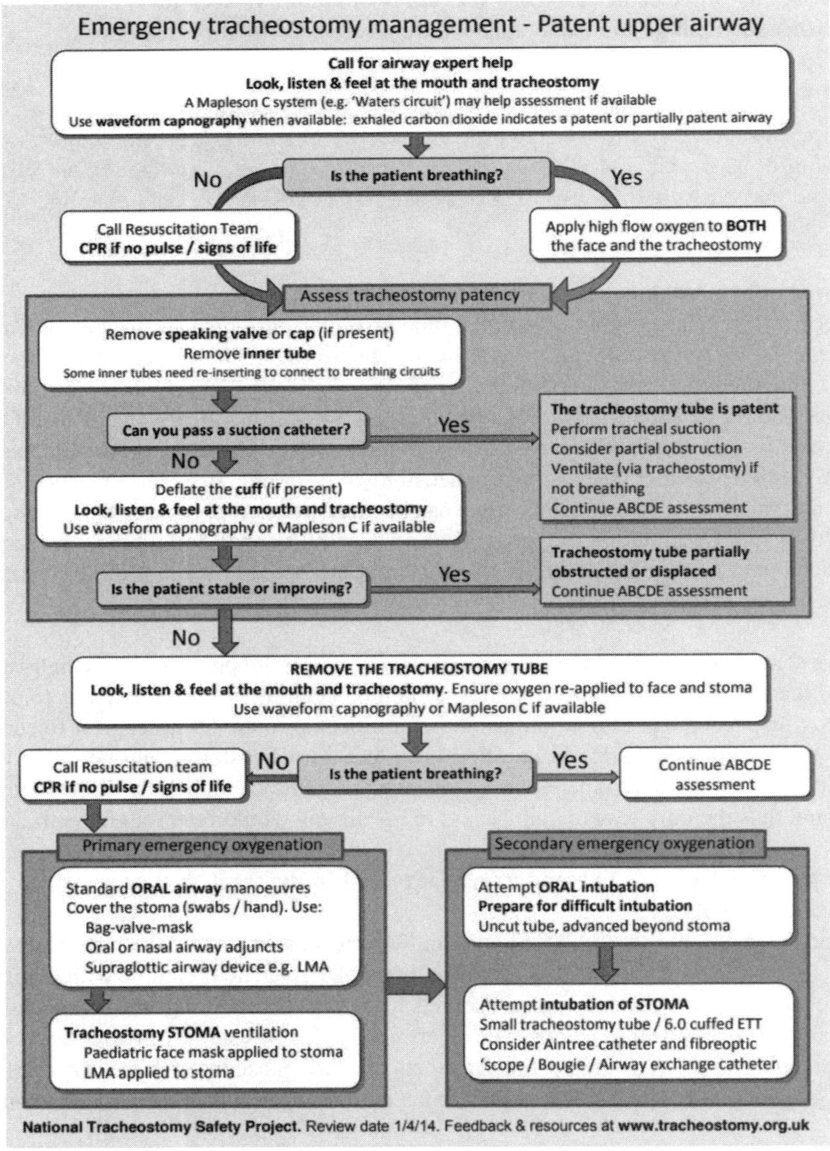

McGrath BA, Bates L, Atkinson D, Moore JA. National tracheostomy safety project. Multidisciplinary guidelines for the management of tracheostomy and laryngectomy airway emergencies. Anaesthesia. 2012;67(9):1025-41. Copyright © 2012 John Wiley & Sons. Used with permission.

* *For those seeking additional information, please see: www.tracheostomy.org/uk/resources*

What did the actual provider do?

- Leaves endotracheal tube (ETT) in place
- Continues chest compressions
- Pulse check after the patient was attached to monitor shows a tachycardia
- 12-lead ECG shows atrial flutter

Vitals:
Pulse 151
Respirations – bagging ET tube
BP 63/palp
Sat 94% on 100% FiO_2

Author comments (Weinstock):

Congratulations! With compressions and bagging, our patient now has a pulse, with a rate of 151 and a rhythm of atrial flutter, but he remains profoundly hypotensive with a sat of 94% on 100% FiO_2. We are at the bedside in the ED. We are at decision point B:

DECISION POINT B – YOU ARE FACED WITH 3 QUESTIONS:

1. **Our patient is tachycardic and profoundly hypotensive—what is the initial approach?**
2. **What is the differential diagnosis for underlying etiology of arrest?**
3. **Are antibiotics indicated?**

Q#1: Our patient is tachycardic and profoundly hypotensive—what is the initial approach?

This patient is clearly unstable, so we recommend synchronized cardioversion of the atrial flutter in an attempt to establish normal sinus rhythm. Rate control with agents such as diltiazem or an IV beta-blocker have no role in the management of this patient. Adenosine could have been considered as a diagnostic modality to clarify the presence of flutter waves; however, we would not expect this to abate this atrial tachycardia.

Q#2: What is the differential diagnosis for underlying etiology of arrest?

The documentation by EMS on the prior ED visit of profound hypoxia, coupled with the patient's presenting rhythm of PEA makes a compelling case for hypoxia as the primary mechanism of the arrest. Mucus-plugging seems highly plausible given his prior presentation with increased tracheal secretions. Pulmonary embolism would be a reasonable consideration given the conversion to a new onset atrial tachyarrhythmia after return of spontaneous circulation (ROSC). Profound acidosis seems less likely given the fairly normal ABG at the initial visit. We do not have information from the initial visit to suggest hyperkalemia, but the patient has a history of ESRD and is on dialysis.

Section editor comments (Emlet):

After we consider mechanical reasons for airway occlusion, malfunction, hypoxia, and re-expansion pulmonary edema, then look for the usual things that cause arrest including pulmonary embolism (PE) and myocardial infarction (MI) as well as tension pneumothorax (PTX) and pneumomediastinum as complications of aggressive bagging of occluded tracheostomy.

Q#3: Are antibiotics indicated?

The priority in management is targeted towards airway patency, adequate ventilation and oxygenation, and hemodynamics. However, in this still undifferentiated patient, it would be acceptable to start empiric antibiotics if thick or purulent mucus plugs were obtained, especially in the context of his prior ED visit which demonstrated significant issues with increased tracheal secretions. Such antibiotic coverage should be broad and target possibly resistant organisms such as MRSA, *Pseudomonas*, as well as other healthcare/ventilator–acquired pathogens.

Section editor comments (Emlet):

Prior to initiating antibiotics, respiratory therapy should obtain appropriate cultures by deep suctioning (blind bronchoalveolar lavage) to ensure later culture and sensitivities.

What the EP did:

18:58: The patient undergoes synchronized cardioversion with 100J with successful conversion to sinus tachycardia
19:12: A right femoral central line is placed. Confirmation is by return of blood
19:16: Piperacillin/tazobactam (Zosyn) and vancomycin are ordered
19:39: MDM: The BP 46/25 so I have started a dopamine drip at 10mcg/kg/min

Labs:

WBC count = 23.6
Hb = 10.9
Plt = 365
Lytes normal with bicarb 29. Creatinine 4.4, troponin 0.23

CXR (radiology interpretation): Congestive heart failure

DECISION POINT C – YOU ARE FACED WITH 3 QUESTIONS:

1. **Patient remains hypotensive after dopamine, what is the next step?**
2. **With the CXR showing congestive heart failure (CHF), how much intravenous fluid (IVF) should be given?**
3. **Does our patient have a diagnosis of septic shock?**

Q#1: Patient remains hypotensive after dopamine, what is the next step?

Of the vasoactive drips used in critical illness, dopamine is widely considered to be one of the most pro-arrhythmic. In fact, this has been well studied and borne out when comparing dopamine to norepinephrine. It seems curious that this would be chosen as a first-line agent given the presence of an atrial tachyarrhythmias that required synchronized cardioversion just a few moments prior. To be fair, however, head-to-head studies comparing norepinephrine to dopamine have largely shown similar effects on mortality in shock.[4] This is not surprising as the manner in which dopamine exerts its effect is by conversion to norepinephrine and epinephrine. It is the dopamine-induced arrhythmias which ultimately resulted in the adoption of norepinephrine as the vasopressor of choice by many large consensus groups including the Surviving Sepsis Campaign (SSC).

In the setting of bradycardia with hypotension, dopamine would be an appropriate choice, but that is not the case in the patient's clinical course. If there is need for a second vasopressor agent, consider one with a relatively pure vasomotor effect as opposed to additional inotropy. Vasopressin at a fixed dose would be a good option and is endorsed by the Surviving Sepsis Campaign.[5]

Author comments (Weinstock):

Norepinephrine may have been a better choice as the initial vasopressor of choice.

Q#2: With the CXR showing congestive heart failure (CHF), how much intravenous fluid (IVF) should be given?

Post-intubation hypotension should prompt consideration of a select number of complications including pneumothorax as well as an excessively high positive intrathoracic pressure compromising venous return. From what is described in this case, it doesn't sound like these are likely, given the presence of bilateral breath sounds. Chest radiography or bedside ultrasound for lung sliding should be considered as additional diagnostic modalities for pneumothorax.

With post-intubation/resuscitation hypotension, consider sedation or induction agents, but in our patient there's no documentation of any induction agents utilized by EMS or ongoing continuous sedation. Classic teaching would dictate a 30mL/kg fluid bolus up front for a patient in suspected septic shock, but we often are caught in a dilemma as to whether the patient will tolerate this large amount of fluid in the setting of heart failure or renal insufficiency. Hypotensive patients with co-existing CHF that are believed to have sepsis or septic shock that is volume responsive, should receive IV fluids.[6] Data regarding this issue is conflicting, and there is likely a role for tailoring fluid resuscitation to the needs of the patient. One method of achieving this may be through more frequent, smaller fluid boluses, with re-assessment of the hemodynamic response (HR, BP, and respiratory status) after each bolus. More sophisticated strategies for fluid responsiveness or fluid tolerance might include ultrasound measurement of IVC collapse, carotid Doppler or invasive hemodynamic monitoring including CVP (via central line), or passive leg raising.[7,8,9]

Consulting editor comments (Weingart):

When you say heart failure, people think CHF and that's clearly not what is going on here. Our patient is hypotensive, with the consideration of *cardiogenic shock*. Now, can you diagnose cardiogenic shock from a chest x-ray? No, and definitely not in a septic patient, because it's just as likely if you see an infiltrate in an undifferentiated septic patient that seems like CHF, it's the beginning of acute lung injury from their systemic inflammatory response.

So, the next thing you obviously do is you throw on an echo probe. Now if the heart is slamming away hyper-dynamically with those CHF-like infiltrates on the CXR, then what you have is acute lung injury. So that's easy. If on the other hand you do have signs of heart failure, specifically in this case left-sided heart failure, then you have some form of cardiomyopathy. It could be ischemic cardiomyopathy, but in this case, it's probably more likely sepsis-induced cardiomyopathy. These patients need some form of ionotropic bolstering which could be dobutamine; my preference is ionotropic dose epinephrine. Only after the inotropy is fixed should you consider giving fluids. It does not make any sense to give a patient with a failing heart, from whatever reason, additional fluids at that stage of the game.

Q#3: Does our patient have a diagnosis of septic shock?

Whether you're still holding on to SIRS criteria or have adopted Sepsis 3's qSOFA score, it's clear to see that the patient meets criteria for sepsis based on the presence of altered mentation, tachycardia, hypotension, and leukocytosis.[10] Our patient has ongoing inadequate tissue oxygenation and perfusion (aka shock) with signs of end-organ dysfunction and need for vasoactive agents to support mean arterial pressure. With acute respiratory failure, the most likely infectious foci is a pulmonary source, such as pneumonia.

Many patients with sepsis develop early ARDS from capillary leak that occurs at the alveolar level from the inflammatory state—this may be interpreted as pulmonary edema/CHF on chest x-ray. Antibiotic coverage directed towards this source should provide sufficient coverage towards health-care associated pneumonia given the patient's long-term residence in a skilled nursing facility. The antibiotics chosen by this provider (vancomycin and piperacillin-tazobactam) seem appropriate with good coverage for MRSA and *Pseudomonas*. A brief review of prior respiratory cultures might be helpful in establishing if there have been more extended-spectrum resistant organisms in the past. If there is any question, double-coverage of *Pseudomonas* with an aminoglycoside would be appropriate. Atypical coverage would also be appropriate with the addition of a macrolide or fluoroquinolone.

What happened with the patient?

19:50: Progress note (EP): Pt. remains hypotensive despite fluids and Dopamine—will add Levophed
20:20: Blood pressure increases to 108/80 and pulse decreases to 126

Diagnosis:
1. Cardiac arrest
2. Sepsis
3. Acute on chronic renal failure

Hospital course (actual documentation):
- Consults are placed to Cardiology, Renal, ID, and Pulmonary/critical care.
- **ID note:** This is a very unfortunate 55-year-old male with multiple medical problems, including end-stage renal disease, severe right-sided CVA with left hemiparesis, history of polysubstance abuse, chronic respiratory failure with tracheostomy who was recently hospitalized with pneumonia. His sputum had grown resistant *Pseudomonas* and *Acinetobacter,* both sensitive to tobramycin.
- **Plan:**
    1. Will follow-up on the pan culture which includes sputum, urine, blood and *C-diff* toxin.
    2. Would discontinue the Zosyn because his previous gram-negative rods have all been resistant to it.
    3. Continue the vancomycin, tobramycin and Flagyl until more data is back.

- **Renal note:** The patient does need dialysis. We should try to get EEGs and see what his mental status and recovery possibilities are before reinstituting dialysis.
- **Intensivist note (problem list):**
    1. Status post-cardiac arrest
    2. Respiratory failure, acute
    3. Chronic renal failure, hemodialysis dependent
    4. History of recurrent *Pseudomonas* and *Acinetobacter* pneumonia
    5. Coma
    6. Extensive stroke

Impression and recommendations: The patient presents status post-cardiac arrest, now without neurologic function. An EEG is pending. The rest may have been precipitated by hypoxia from a mucous plug, but this is speculative. The primary team is discussing code status and direction of care with the family; currently the patient is full code. Subcutaneous heparin will be added for DVT prophylaxis until the INR is therapeutic. The patient is currently tolerating tube feeds. Overall, outlook is extremely poor, and a palliative approach would be reasonable.

Chapter author summary and commentary:
Like most of the cases in this book, this patient's story provides a clear example of how quickly a patient's condition can change. The approach to a patient with a tracheostomy requires providers to have a thorough understanding of airway anatomy and the ability to apply that knowledge in a methodical fashion for patients in extremis. Take home points:

- The approach to the dyspneic patient with a tracheostomy involves a differential diagnosis and work-up similar to the general population, with a focus on potential mechanical obstructions, dislodgement and bleeding complications.
- An attempt at orotracheal intubation should be considered if there is uncertainty about the ability to safely replace or re-insert a tracheostomy tube, but remember that patients with tracheostomy and total laryngectomy will NOT have a method of securing the airway from above.
- Atrial tachyarrhythmias in sepsis are fairly common secondary to high adrenergic tone. Consideration should be taken towards vasopressor choice, with the understanding that atrial tachyarrhythmias are more frequently associated with dopamine compared to norepinephrine.

References:

1. Engels PT, Bagshaw SM, Meier M, et al. Tracheostomy: From insertion to decannulation. Can J Surg 2009;52(5):427-33.
2. Epstein SK. Late complications of tracheostomy. Respir Care 2005;50(4):542-9.
3. Nseir S, Favory R, Jozefowicz E, et al. Antimicrobial treatment for ventilator-associated tracheobronchitis: a randomized, controlled, multicenter study. Crit Care 2008;12(3):R62.
4. De Backer D, Biston P, Devriendt J, et al. Comparison of dopamine and norepinephrine in the treatment of shock. N Engl J Med 2010;362(9):779-89.
5. Dellinger RP, Levy MM, Rhodes A, et al. Surviving sepsis campaign: international guidelines for management of severe sepsis and septic shock: 2012. Crit Care Med 2013;41(2):580-637.
6. Ouellette DR, Shah SZ. Comparison of outcomes from sepsis between patients with and without pre-existing left ventricular dysfunction: a case-control analysis. Crit Care 2014;18(2):R79.
7. Préau S, Saulnier F, Dewavrin F, et al. Passive leg raising is predictive of fluid responsiveness

in spontaneously breathing patients with severe sepsis or acute pancreatitis. Crit Care Med 2010;38(3):819-25.

8. Sawe HR, Haeffele C, Mfinanga JA, et al. Predicting fluid responsiveness using bedside ultrasound measurements of the inferior vena cava and physician gestalt in the emergency department of an urban public hospital in sub-saharan africa. PLoS ONE 2016;11(9):e0162772.
9. Shokoohi H, Berry GW, Shahkolahi M, et al. The diagnostic utility of sonographic carotid flow time in determining volume responsiveness. J Crit Care 2017;38:231-35.
10. Marik PE, Taeb AM. SIRS, qSOFA and new sepsis definition. J Thorac Dis 2017;9(4):943-45.

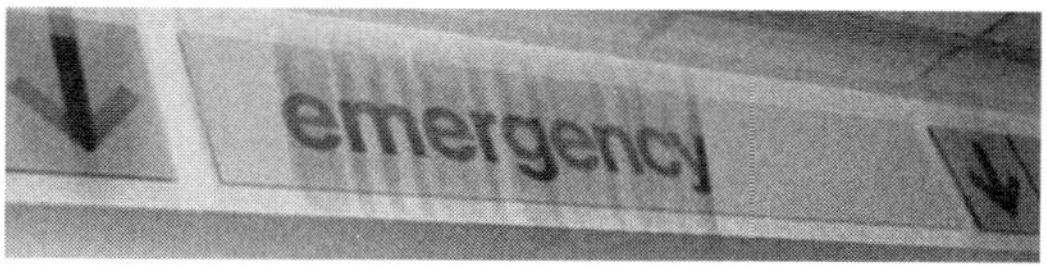

SECTION A – AIRWAY/ARREST

Chapter 3: A 41-year-old woman with chest pain

David A. Farcy, MD, FAAEM, FACEP, FCCM
Chairman, Department of Emergency Medicine
Director, Emergency Medicine Critical Care
Mount Sinai Medical Center, Miami Beach, FL
Clinical Associate Professor
Department of Emergency Medicine & Critical Care
Herbert Wertheim College of Medicine
Florida International University, Miami, FL
President, American Academy of Emergency Medicine

Ramin Vejdani, DO
Emergency Medicine Attending Physician
Director, Informatics
Mount Sinai Medical Center, Miami, FL

Legal commentary:
Gregory L. Henry, MD
Former President of The American College of Emergency Physicians (ACEP)
Former Professor of Emergency Medicine at the University of Michigan
Former CEO of Medical Practice Risk Assessment, Ann Arbor, MI

Section editor:
Lillian L. Emlet, MD, MS, FACEP, FCCM
Clinical Associate Professor
Depts. of Critical Care Medicine & Emergency Medicine
Associate Program Director, IMCCM Fellowship of the MCCTP
Interim Associate Chief of Staff of Education, VA
University of Pittsburgh School of Medicine, Pittsburgh, PA

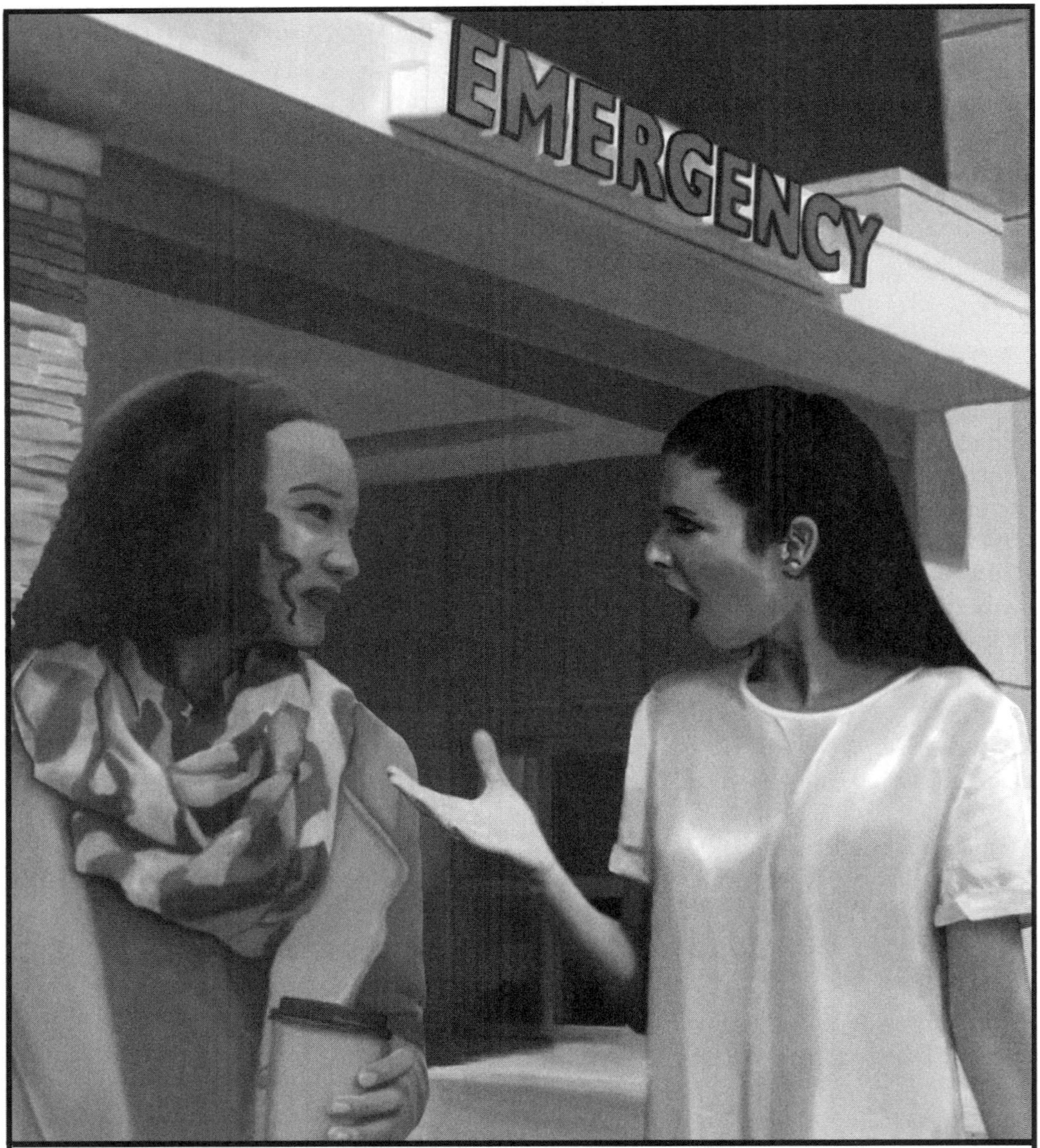

"THEY *NEVER* ANSWERED MY QUESTION!"

SECTION A/CHAPTER 3

A 41-year-old woman with chest pain

In the United States, 130.4 million patients visited an emergency department in 2013 and chest pain was the second most common chief complaint, accounting for about 6% of all visits. Chest pain is a complaint with a wide array of differential etiologies, ranging from benign, such as muscle strain, to life threatening, such as Acute Myocardial Infarction (AMI), Pulmonary Embolism (PE) and Thoracic Aortic Dissection (TAD). If missed or not diagnosed in a timely fashion, there may be catastrophic outcomes. The highest frequency of malpractice cases are missed AMI, acute appendicitis, and missed fracture, while missed AMI is the diagnosis associated with the highest paid verdicts.[1,2,3]

Diagnostic errors may occur from cognitive errors, perception, failure in fact finding, and/or bias. Thus, performing a good history of present illness (HPI), family history, risk factor stratification, physical exam, and then proceeding to appropriate usage of diagnostic testing will be essential to properly diagnosing patients with chest pain.

Lifetime risk factors include:

- Age
- Gender
- Hyperlipidemia
- Hypertension (HTN)
- Diabetes
- Smoking
- Race

While recognition of presence of these risk factors is important, they have little value in predicting acute disease. When none of these risk factors are present, the lifetime risk of CAD for a 45-year-old is estimated to be $< 5\%$, whereas with ≥ 2 major risk factors, it is 50% for men and 31% for women respectively."[4]

To make the evaluation even more difficult, patients do not read textbooks and commonly present with atypical ischemic complaints. Whereas the most typical complaints with ischemia are chest pain, chest pressure radiating down the left upper extremities, to the shoulders or jaw, associated with shortness of breath (SOB) and diaphoresis, atypical complaints, also referred to as "anginal equivalents," are dyspnea followed by nausea, dizziness, diaphoresis, malaise, back pain and/or unexplained weakness. Atypical presentations occur more commonly in elderly, female, African-American, Hispanic and diabetic patients.

Author comments (Weinstock):

This case has another dimension; after her bounceback and adverse outcome, the case proceeds to legal action. Actual trial testimony, as well as commentary by medical-legal emergency physician expert Greg Henry, follows. Before we jump to the case, please meet Stacy:

A 41-year-old woman with pain from her waist to her head

(extracted and summarized from trial testimony)

The patient's story:

Stacy is a hard worker, at one point working 3 jobs: cleaning the credit union and Mr. Payroll during the day and working at UPS at night. According to her mother, "She never stopped working. She did whatever anybody needed her to do."

At the age of 26, Stacy delivers a healthy baby girl, Celina. During the delivery, Stacy suffered a "diabetic stroke" and is told to have a tubal ligation. At this time, she is married to Leo, but the marriage ended badly, and she was left to raise Celina on her own—Leo does not provide assistance. Though she does not have much money, Stacy is a wonderful mother, supporting her daughter's interest in gymnastics and taking her to the beach. Through the years, Celina becomes her "best friend."

When Stacy sees others in need, she rises to the occasion; opening her home to two children of a father who hung himself after the mother disappeared, as well as taking in a little girl who is having problems with her stepmother.

In her early 30's Stacy starts dating a man named Robert. At one point, she walks upstairs after doing laundry and overhears Robert saying, "I don't want the baby. You might as well do something with it. I don't want it." When confronted he denies the conversation, so Stacy calls the woman back and says, "I'll take the baby. I'll raise him as my own." She borrows money for the adoption papers and brings the baby home from the hospital, calling him Matthew.

On the evening of October 2, 2007, Stacy calls her mother and tells her she is having pains in her chest. "Do you think its indigestion?" her mother asks.

"No." Stacy replies. "I've been taking something for indigestion and it's not working."

Stacy decides to go to the emergency department.

INITIAL ED VISIT

CC (RN AT 18:13): Chest pain - pain from above waist to head, neck and arms

Vitals:

Time	Temp (F) Rt.	Pulse	Resp	Syst	Diast	O2%	Pain
18:28	97.9	97	20	186	96	nl	8/10

NKDA
PMH: HTN, CVA, DM
PSH: Choly
SH: Smoker
Meds: Glucophage, Avandia, Norvasc, Accupril – pt out of meds last 3 months

HPI (18:55 - MD note): Pt is a 46-year-old woman with chief complaint of chest pain for the last 1 day or so. Pain is a tightness across the chest and upper arms which is worsened by deep breaths. Radiates to the left arm. PMH of high blood pressure and diabetes. No nausea and vomiting, coughing blood, syncope, feeling of doom, shortness of breath, sweating and palpitations. Nursing notes reviewed. SH Smoker. FH: Hx cardiac disease after the age of 55.

PE:
GENERAL: A&OX3, appears very uncomfortable
EYES: PERRL
CV: RRR without m/r/g. Normal heart sounds. Good capillary refill. No peripheral edema
RESP: No resp distress. Prolonged splinting and decreased air movement and wheezing.
ABD: Soft and NT throughout, without r/r/g
BACK: No CVAT
SKIN: Normal without petechiae, vesicles, erythema

CXR (19:11): WNL. Fingerstick BS= 255

Vitals:

Time	Temp (F) Rt.	Pulse	Resp	Syst	Diast	O2%	Pain
19:20		87	16			97	

ECG#1 @ 19:20

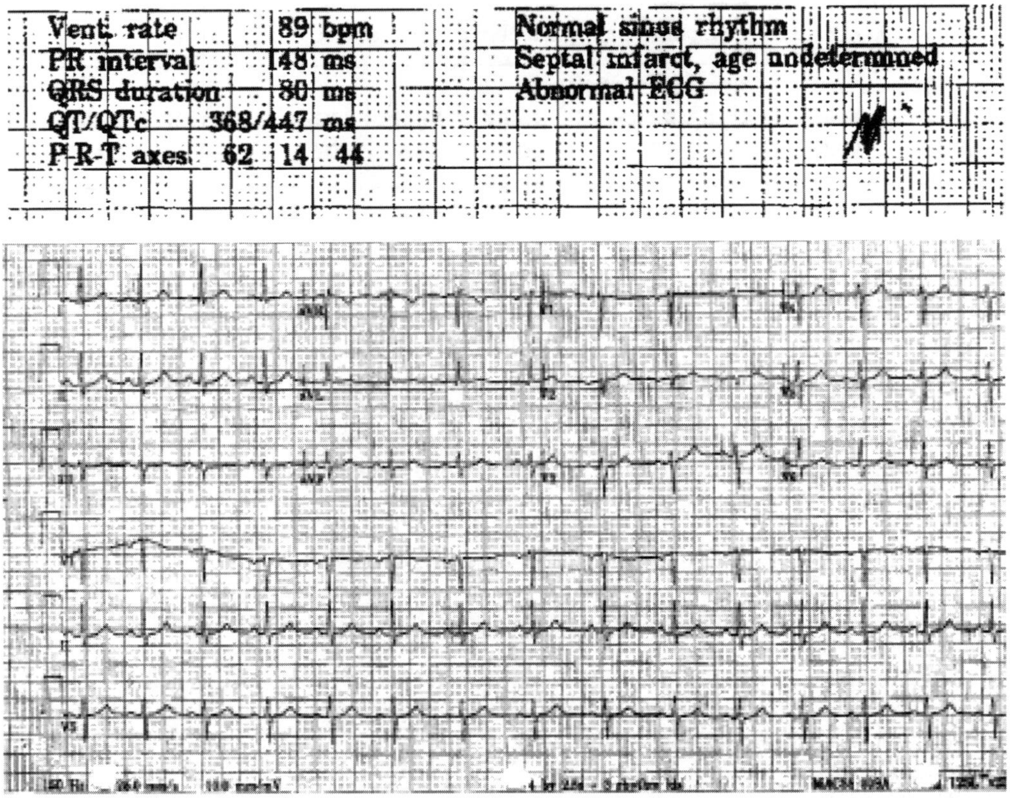

MDM:
Albuterol aerosol #1 (19:20)
Albuterol aerosol#2 (19:31)

Vitals:

Time	Temp (F) Rt.	Pulse	Resp	Syst	Diast	O2%	Pain
20:25		71	16	130	82	100	3/10

ECG#2 @20:55

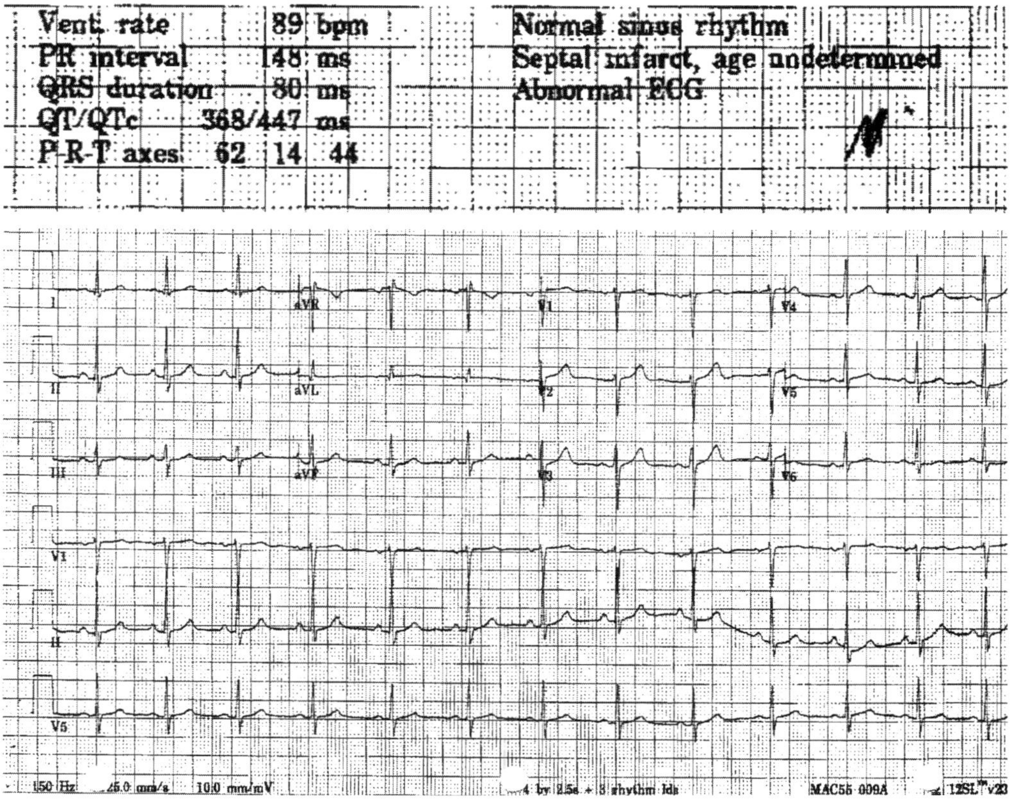

MDM/ED course: "CXR and ECG's reviewed. Albuterol aerosol, captopril 25mg PO"

Diagnosis: HTN, bronchospasm

Condition: Stable
Disposition: Home
RN: d/c home with driver. Pt states pain much better. Verbalizes understanding

Discussion of the initial visit—evaluation of chest pain, medical decision-making, documentation and patient safety:

Seems a straightforward case of "typical" angina with risk factors that include, DM (non-compliant), smoker, history of coagulopathy with TIA, and a potential positive family history. Certainly, a more thorough history and work-up could have been performed, as well as better documentation of the medical decision-making process. We believe the initial physician on the diagnosis of "bronchospasm," even though the patient did not have a history of asthma or COPD, but she is a smoker.

1. **Lack of correlation between chief complaint and final diagnosis:**

Let's start with the biggest problem with this evaluation; the final diagnosis of HTN, bronchospasm; this has no correlation with the presenting chief complaint (chest pain)! Bronchospasm typically presents with an intractable cough and wheezing, though as the bronchospasm worsens, an increased obstruction to air entry might limit the auscultation of audible wheezing secondary to lack of poor air exchange. The patient's chief complaint is chest pain with a respiratory rate of 20 and normal oxygen saturation, a focused review of systems stated no shortness of breath and the physical exam showed: *"no respiratory distress. Prolonged splinting and decreased air movement and wheezing."*

In short, nothing in the history or physical exam supports a diagnosis of bronchospasm. There is no cough, accessory muscle use, tachypnea, hx of asthma or COPD, or previous history of respiratory problems. The chart does point out chest pain: "Pain is a tightness across the chest and upper arms which is worsened by deep breaths. Radiates to the left arm." In a prospective analysis of 893 patients, investigators performed a multivariant analysis in AMI and Acute Coronary Syndrome (ACS) patients, finding that the most commonly associated symptom for both entities was chest pain that radiated to the shoulder or radiates to both arms.[5] Is a physician's gestalt good at predicting the diagnosis and outcome in patients with ACS? Several trials showed that gestalt alone had little to moderate diagnostic value compared to gestalt plus electrocardiogram (ECG) and troponin.[5]

2. **The ECG:**

Can an ECG aid in ruling out ACS? The initial ECG has a sensitivity of 20–60% for AMI, similar to flipping a coin.[6] If the ECG has ST-segment depressions greater than 0.05 mV with or without T-wave inversions, sensitivity increases to about 75%.[7] Unfortunately, the 12-lead has geography limitation, leaving the right ventricle and posterior wall untraced. Is there an approach to improving sensitivity? Though not commonly done, the addition of leads V3r, V4r, V5r, V7, V8, and V9, increases diagnostic sensitivity for ACS by 18%. The use of a 15-lead ECG containing V4r, V8, and V9 leads in addition to the 12 standard leads increases the diagnostic rate of AMI by 22% compared to standard 12-lead ECG.[8]

3. **Risk factors:**

Since gestalt combined with an ECG is not much help in ruling out ACS, what should we do? An assessment of risk factors originally came from the Framingham study group, which looked at the risk of developing cardiovascular disease over 10 years. Although they predict the long-term probability of a coronary event, cardiac risk factors are usually not helpful in identification of ACS in patients presenting with *acute* chest pain. A patient with no risk factors does not eliminate the possibility of ACS but does bring it to less than 5%. However, in patients less than 40 years of age, one study showed that in patients with a very high risk factor burden (4 to 5 risk factors) the likelihood of ACS was increased by > 20-fold.[9] Risk stratification tools have been developed, such as the HEART score and the Thrombolysis in Myocardial Infarction (TIMI) score; both incorporate risk factors.[10]

Now let's go back and look at our patient; just her age and past medical history gives her 4 factors, which puts her in a high-risk category. To add to the complexity, women experience significant differences in their presentation of ACS, leading to higher morbidity and delay in diagnosis of ischemic heart disease compared to men.[11,12]

Author comments (Weinstock):

Spoiler alert— the *actual* diagnosis was not: "HTN, bronchospasm." Something big was missed. At trial, the plaintiff's attorney focused on inadequate gathering of data, specifically risk factors. Though there is some controversy as to the utility of risk factors in the assessment of acute chest pain, we can all agree that it would be uncomfortable to sit on the stand and answer the following questions. The plaintiff's attorney was clever, not leaving anything to chance; there is only one way to answer these questions:

Plaintiff's attorney questioning physician testifying for the defense:

Q. Let's count the risk factors. One, diabetes, right?

A. Yes, sir.

Q. Two, smoking, correct?

A. Yes, sir.

Q. Three, hypertension or blood pressure, correct?

A. Yes, sir.

Q. Four, stroke?

A. Yes, sir.

Q. Correct? Five, age over 40, correct?

A. Yes, sir.

Q. Six, family history?

A. Yes, sir.

Q. It's a bunch, isn't it?

A. Yes, sir.

Poor history:

History taking is an art. We are asking questions not just to meet the billing standard but to also show consideration of "worst first." All non-traumatic chest pain patients need to be risk stratified as either low or high risk. In a 46-year-woman with chest pain; our differential includes:

- Acute coronary syndrome (ACS)
- Pulmonary embolism (PE)
- Thoracic aortic dissection (TAD)
- Pneumothorax

Because there is essentially no medical decision-making (MDM) section, we need to default to the history, exam and evaluation to determine what this provider actually considered in the differential. Unfortunately, the chart points only to consideration of ACS (2 ECGs were done). One could argue that pneumothorax was considered because a chest x-ray was ordered, though there was not a preliminary EP interpretation specifically addressing pneumothorax. It would have been nice to see an interpretation which stated that "there is no evidence of PTX or a widened mediastinum." Even during the cross-examination, the physician cannot defend his own actions.

Author comments (Weinstock):

The plaintiff's attorney hammers it home about the poor data gathering (history of present illness) obtained on this patient:

Plaintiff's attorney questioning physician testifying for the defense:
The importance of history:

Q. Now, in order to put the pieces of the puzzle together for what is causing chest pain, you need to get an accurate history, don't you?

A. Yes, sir.

Q. You don't just take the patient's words for it. There are criteria for doctors to probe into what exactly the nature of the pain is, isn't that correct? Those questions should have been asked, correct?

A. Yes, sir, they typically would be asked.

Q. And the reason they need to be asked is because we're dealing with something that could be missed and you need as much information to put the puzzle together?

A. Yes sir.

4. Tips for evaluating a multiple-complaint patient:

Unfortunately, multiple-complaint patients take longer, but it is essential to maintain an appropriate differential and that our evaluation is logical. Instead of viewing the patient as difficult, try to determine their underlying reason for presentation. This approach will provide insight into their *main* concern. Our patient had a chief complaint and many associated complaints. There was a poorly obtained history and an inadequate attempt to correlate the complaints into a cohesive story. Just considering her history of non-compliance puts her in a higher risk category.

Author comments (Weinstock):

Even if their concern seems unlikely to us, patient anxiety over a serious perceived diagnosis can be disabling. Though not as "emergent" as resuscitating an unrestrained MVA victim, understanding the reason for the patient's visit can focus the evaluation and guide the management and provide an opportunity; reassurance that a serious illness is not occurring is also a part of healing.

5. Poor documentation of MDM:

This is where everything should come together. Historically, EM physicians will over-document the catastrophic case, thinking they may be involved in a lawsuit; however, it is rarely those cases that come back to haunt us, but rather the cursory evaluation and discharge. In our case, there is no MDM, just a statement: CXR and ECG's reviewed. Albuterol aerosol, captopril 25mg PO.

The MDM is also a chance to address the key points on your initial differential. An example of a better MDM might have been to explain that the x-ray AP/Lat showed no pneumothorax, widen mediastinum, or aortic knob blunting. We all know that an x-ray lacks sensitivity but this screams to anyone reading your chart that you considered pneumothorax and aortic dissection.

A common error is ignoring or not following through on abnormal test results. In our patient, chest pain is referenced twice, 2 ECGs are done, but there is no mention of ACS. Imagine how things may have played out differently at trial if the documentation contained this discussion; "46 y/o with CP, TIMI score of 1 due to risk factors, initial ECG and repeat ECG without ST changes, no T wave inversion, no ischemic patterns. Pain is reproducible and more likely musculoskeletal. Follow-up care discussed with her PCP." Now this is only an example, since a troponin was not done, and in this case a TIMI score is not applicable, but this is an example of a reasonable discussion of consideration of ACS. We may disagree on the disposition, but this "example" MDM is clear, you considered ACS, you looked at the ECG, and you planned close follow-up. "Experts" can argue at your disposition, but not against your *thinking*; even if there is a bad outcome, your decision-making process is well-described and sound, which is defensible.

Of note, the considerations of PE (in a patient with pleuritic pain who is over the age of 35 and who is a smoker on oral contraceptives) and TAD (in a patient where there is no specific exclusion of pain radiating to the back) have still not been appropriately explored or excluded. Unfortunately, during the initial visit, the physician seems to have come to premature closure and anchored on a diagnosis of bronchospasm.

Authors comments (Weinstock):

"Hard stop" your MDM! Before the patient leaves, ask if you would be comfortable explaining your care to the patient's family or friends; if not, reassess and obtain additional data.

The story continues:
(information extracted from trial testimony):

When Stacy returns home from the hospital, she tells her daughter she is feeling better. As everything seems fine, Celina goes to bed around 10:00, but she is awoken around 2:00 with the sounds of her mother moving around the kitchen. According to Celina, "I went in there to see what was going on and [my mom] went outside to smoke a cigarette, so I went out there and sat [down on the front steps] with her. She told me that she loved me and that everything was going to be OK and she was sorry if she ever did anything to hurt me or my brother, [Matthew]."

"I told her I loved her too and that it was OK. She gave me a hug and kiss and then I went back to bed. [The next thing I remember] my mother's boyfriend Steve waking me up screaming and crying because my mom is on the floor and she is not talking to him. I called 911 and they told me to give CPR. I tried it but nothing helped."

ED RETURN (early the next morning)

CC: Cardiac arrest

EMS (summary-time of arrival on scene 4:21): 41 yo F apneic and pulseless according to family. Pt was up making coffee and collapsed. They stated she has been c/o chest pain for a couple of days. Pt unresponsive CPR and BVM assist with 100% O2. ET tube 7.5 25cm @ lip. Tube secured. BX X4 clear. IV. Epi 1:10000 1mg ivp. Pt rhythm changed to v-fib. Pt shocked 200 biphasic. Vasopressin 40 units IVP. Rhythm still v-fib. 300J shock biphasic. Amiodarone 300mg ivp. No change. CPR continues. Pt transported to hospital without incident or change. Report given to staff. Pt placed in hospital bed. The actual EMS sheet is reproduced below:

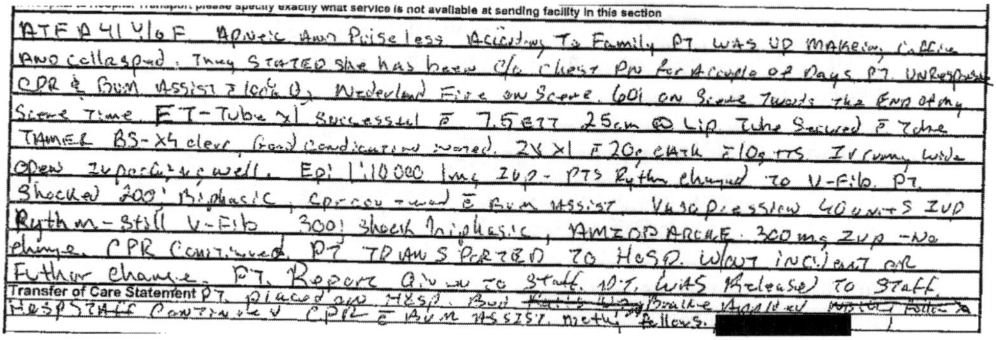
...please specify exactly what service is not available at sending facility in this section

ATF A 41 Y/o F Apneic And Pulseless According To Family PT WAS UP MAKEing Coffee
AND collasped. They STATED she has been c/o chest Pn for A couple of Days. PT UNRespons
CPR & BVM ASSIST c 100% O2 Wederland Fire on Scene. 601 on Scene Towards the END of my
Scene Time. ET-Tube x1 Successful c 7.5 ETT 25cm @ Lip Tube Secured c Tube
TAMER BS-X4 clear, Good condensation noted. 2X x1 c 20g cath c 10g tts IV running wide
open 2v positive well. Epi 1:10 000 1mg IVP - PTS Rythm changed to V-Fib. PT
Shocked 200 Biphasic, CPR continued c BVM ASSIST. Vasopressin 40 units IVP
Rythm - still V-Fib 300J shock biphasic, AMIODARONE 300mg IVP - No
change. CPR Continued. PT TRANSPORTED TO HOSP. W/OUT INCIDENT OR
Futher change. PT. Report Given to staff. PT. WAS Released TO STAFF.
Transfer of Care Statement PT. placed on HOSP. Bed ~~...~~ Brake Applied ... Follow
HOSP STAFF Continued CPR c BVM ASSIST. Nothing follows. [redacted]

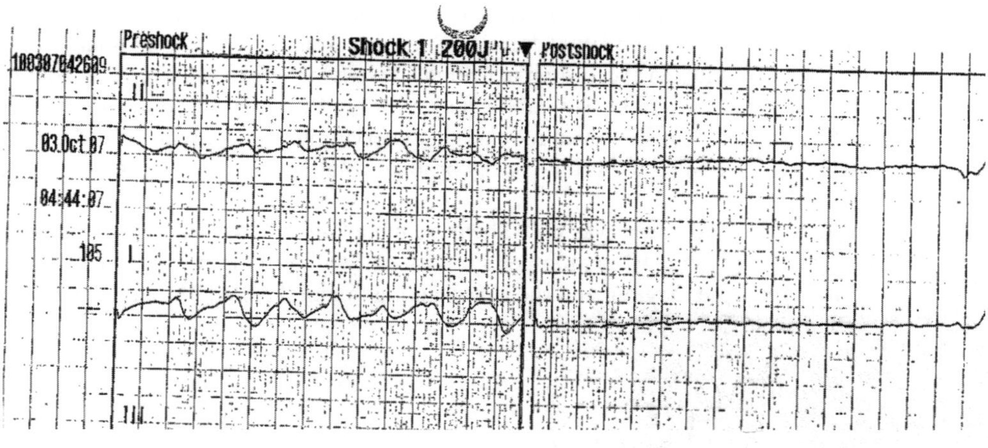

ED documentation:

HPI (physician): Presents via EMS w witnessed arrest by husband. Pt had complained of chest pain prior to arrival. EMS information reviewed. Pt is unable to give additional information secondary to medical condition of cardiac arrest.

PE:
GA: Unresponsive, CPR in progress
EYES: Pupils dilated and unresponsive
Neck: Normal
CV: No spontaneous heart tones
LUNGS: Clear with equal breath sounds with bagging
ABD: Slightly distended
Ext: Normal

ED course:
EMS arrival on scene 04:21
Pt arrives in ED @ 0500 in full arrest

Author comments (Weinstock):

You are at the bedside of a patient seen and discharged less than 24 hours ago, now in cardiac arrest. You are at decision point A:

DECISION POINT A – YOU ARE FACED WITH 4 QUESTIONS:

1. **What are the important actions to take prior to a patient in full arrest arriving in the ED?**
2. **What are the important actions to take *when* a patient in full arrest arrives in the ED?**
3. **Are mechanical compressions better than CPR?**
4. **What is the role of end tidal CO_2 monitoring during CPR?**

Q#1: What are the important actions to take prior to a patient in full arrest arriving in the ED?
EMS pre-arrival notification serves one main purpose; it is to give you time to prepare and anticipate what resources and equipment will be needed. In the case of impending arrival of cardiac arrest, ensure:

- The availability of end tidal CO_2, intubation equipment including difficult airway supplies, suction, IO and code cart.
- Review and establish each team member's specific roles including specifying the team leader, the procedure and airway person, and chest compression team as well as pharmacy and radiology and a unit clerk who will be able to contact additional help, such as a vascular surgeon for diagnosis of a ruptured abdominal aortic aneurysm (AAA) or interventional cardiology for a STEMI.

Q#2: What are the important actions to take *when* a patient in full arrest arrives in the ED?
EMS personnel provide invaluable information, including:

- Circumstances/discussions with family or bystanders
- Down time
- Location
- Initial rhythm
- Interventions
- Impending arrival of family/friends

Ask EMS to stick around if possible, should further questions arise. An initial rhythm of ventricular fibrillation or ventricular tachycardia points more to a cardiac origin, most commonly associated with a coronary artery obstruction. In contrast, an initial rhythm of Pulseless Electrical Activity (PEA) warrants a review of potentially reversible causes including:

1. Hypovolemia
2. Hypoxia
3. Hydrogen ion (acidosis)
4. Hypo-/hyperkalemia
5. Hypothermia
6. Tension pneumothorax
7. Cardiac tamponade
8. Toxins
9. Pulmonary or coronary thrombosis

For example, getting a history that a patient was found down in a park known to be frequented by "drug users" points to overdose with emergent oxygenation and naloxone. A history of mental illness or an empty pill bottle found near the patient points to a suicide attempt.

Q#3: Are mechanical compressions better than CPR?

Chest compression is the most important procedure in cardiopulmonary resuscitation. The rate should be 100–120 compressions per minute. Depth of chest compressions should be between 2in (5cm) and 2.4in (6cm), allowing full chest recoil after each compression with minimized interruptions. Over the years, several commercial mechanical devices have surfaced with the impetus being that rescuer fatigue is directly proportional to the quality of chest compression. One study found that during the first minutes of a resuscitation, CPR was performed correctly 92% of the time, but that number dropped to 39.2% after 3 minutes of chest compressions.[13] With limited pre-hospital personnel, mechanical chest compression makes, but does it improve survival in the ED? In two systematic reviews and meta-analysis, looking at survival to hospital discharged with Cerebral Performance Category score of 1 and 2 (both considered a good neurologic outcome), neither trial provided sufficient evidence of an advantage of mechanical chest compressions. They concluded that mechanical chest compression should not replace high quality manual chest compression, but rather serve as a supplemental therapy in the overall care off cardiac arrest patients.[14,15]

Q#4: What is the role of end tidal CO_2 monitoring during CPR?

The end tidal CO_2 ($ETCO_2$) monitor can serve as a surrogate for cardiac output during chest compressions, with the 2015 AHA guidelines stating that $ETCO_2$ should be maintained above 10mmHg after the patient is successfully intubated but does not recommend a specific cutoff value as a predictor of mortality or as a decision to stop resuscitation efforts. If there is a drop, this may suggest inadequate chest compressions, most likely related to fatigue, with an indication for replacement. Conversely, an abrupt increase in $ETCO_2$ could suggest return of spontaneous circulation (ROSC) even before a pulse check. Lack of an increase in $ETCO_2$ could help to limit interruptions for pulse checks. An $ETCO_2$ of 20mmHg has some correlation with a better outcomes, but the opposite is not true.[16]

DECISION POINT A – ***What did the actual provider do?***

Below is an image of the actual document in the ED recorded on the code sheet:

EMS stated they arrived and found pt pulseless and apneic @ 0421.
EMS arrived at ER at 0500.
0500 Arrival and attached to cardiac monitor
BS checked and confirmed
ETT 7.5 @ 22cm lip
0502 CPR continued
Epi 1mg
Atropine 1mg
Bicarbonate 50mEq
0508 Shock 150J
PEA, CPR continued
Lidocaine 100mg
0509 Epi 1mg
CPR held, Wide complex Bradycardia
2nd IV initiated at R AC (20ga), blood drawn
Dopamine @ 20mcg/kg/min (pt weight - 80kg)
BG - 343

Chapter author commentary: Were the provider's actions appropriate?

It is difficult to know what rhythm and specific algorithm was followed, as the patient received epinephrine and then atropine by the ED physician. Currently, atropine is only recommended for brady-arrhythmias that are symptomatic (altered mental status, ischemic pain, heart failure, shock) in nature and not for PEA or asystole. This recommendation was not reviewed or revised in the 2015 guidelines. The 2010 ACLS guidelines state that "Routine use of sodium bicarbonate (SB) is not recommended for patients in cardiac arrest;" however, ACLS guidelines recommend administration of SB for QRS widening in cases of severe cardiotoxicity or cardiac arrest from hyperkalemia or tricyclic antidepressant overdose. Bicarbonate has been de-emphasized as it makes the intracellular compartment more acidotic, resulting in cells which are more resistant to medication and electricity. Thus, SB is only indicated for a pH below 7.1 and in a prolonged arrest over 20 minutes.

Due to the prolonged down time, with our patient severely acidotic, the physician likely thought that would improve the pH… or it may have fallen under the "makes us feel better" doctrine—why not give it? It is understandable that we want to do more during a cardiac arrest, especially with previous ACLS protocols involving complex algorithms; however, there are serious limitations to our medications. Emphasizing high quality CPR, decreasing pulse checks, and consideration of underlying causes will provide the best chance for a positive outcome.

ED course: Vital signs are checked, showing:

Vitals:

Time	Temp	Pulse	Resp	Syst	Diast	Sat
05:09		77	bagged	82	18	82% vent

Author comments (Weinstock):

We have achieved ROSC, but our patient is still unconscious with an unknown etiology for her arrest and a sat of only 82% with100% vent oxygen. We are at decision point B:

DECISION POINT B – YOU ARE FACED WITH 4 QUESTIONS:

1. **The patient has a pulse—what are the initial steps after ROSC?**
2. **Was the initiation and choice of vasopressors appropriate?**
3. **Is rapid cooling indicated?**
4. **What are the best initial ventilator settings?**

What does the literature say?

Q#1: The patient has a pulse—what are the initial steps after ROSC?

Once a patient has ROSC, the highest priority should be (in this specific order):

1. Obtain a 12-lead ECG
2. Maintain perfusion by increasing the blood pressure
3. Address the respiratory status to prevent severe hypoxemia

In this case, at 5:09, the attending documented a wide complex bradycardia, so the differential diagnosis is fairly simple including an electrolyte abnormality including hyperkalemia, hypokalemia, and hypomagnesemia. Initiate suspected hyperkalemia management by administration of calcium chloride to stabilize the cardiac membrane. Calcium chloride is preferred, but if not available, then calcium gluconate is acceptable; however, a higher dose of gluconate will need to be administered as the dose of calcium chloride is 3 times the strength of gluconate.

ACLS guidelines have removed trans-venous and transthoracic pacing from their pulseless algorithm for complete AV dissociation. In a symptomatic bradycardia, such as hypotension in this case, one may consider transcutaneous pacing to see if capture is obtained and if the hemodynamic status is improved? Atropine in complete third-degree block has not been shown to improve outcome, but it often given since it has not been shown to cause harm.

Hypoxemia can also be a cause of bradycardia. In this case, the patient is saturating at 82%, while being ventilated by BVM. A patient who suffered complete cardiac arrest has lost their functional residual capacity. During daily activities, our lung volume never collapses to 0, thus making it easier to breath, but in cardiac arrest or trauma, patients lose those residual volumes. Bagging during the initial resuscitation causes inflation and deflation to a pressure of 0 and does not provide any recruitment of alveoli, thus providing a VQ mismatch.

There have been no studies that have shown any benefit of using BVM with a peep valve vs. no peep valve; however, those studies were conducted with animals and no human trials have been performed. It is the authors belief that adding a Peep valve to BVM at a minimum PEEP of 5, causes alveolar recruitment, thereby decreasing VQ mismatch and increasing alveolar oxygenation. The exact amount of PEEP is at the provider's discretion; however, a minimum of 5 is recommended.

It seems a common belief of EM physicians is that PEEP causes hypotension due to an increase in intrathoracic pressure resulting in decreased preload. This oftentimes results in the removal of PEEP in hypotensive patients. In an already hypovolemic patient, one would believe that the BP would drop; however, by providing fluids to a depleted tank and a vasopressor, preload will be increased.

Q#2: Was the initiation and choice of vasopressors appropriate?
What is the vasopressor "du jour?" There are two trials which help to clear up years of controversy. The first, published in 2010, which is a randomized double-blind controlled trial, demonstrated the superiority of norepinephrine over dopamine. Specifically, this trial demonstrated an increase in 28-day mortality among patients with cardiogenic shock who received dopamine as the first line agent when compared to those receiving norepinephrine. Also in this trial, the dopamine group was associated with a greater frequency of tachyarrhythmias including A-fib with RVR, V-tach and V-fib.[17] In the second trial, published in 2012, dopamine compared to norepinephrine had an increased mortality rate in septic shock, thus making norepinephrine the preferred initial pressor of choice. Now, one might argue, that in a symptomatic bradycardia, dopamine may be the preferred agent, secondary to the potential for tachyarrhythmia events. However, since it might increase mortality in cardiogenic shock, it is our belief at this time that norepinephrine is the preferred agent.[18]

Q#3: Is rapid cooling indicated?
To cool or not to cool—that is the question? Even after achieving ROSC, the chance of a full neurologic recovery is dismal. Nothing had been shown to either prevent or reverse anoxic encephalopathy associated with prolonged cardiac arrest until a landmark trial published in 2002 on targeted temperature management (TTM) as a neuroprotective therapy in post-arrest resuscitation. This trial was conducted in out of hospital V-tach/V-fib cardiac arrest patients. Patients were cooled within 6 hours post-ROSC if they were comatose, defined by a GCS or 8 or less for a period of 12–24 hours. Both groups who were cooled had a significant decrease in anoxic encephalopathy and better neurologic outcome based on a cerebral perfusion pressure (CPP) of 1–2. Several other trials have confirmed these neuroprotective benefits, but the optimal cooling temperature has varied. A 2013 prospective double-blind study, compared a cooling goal of 33° vs. 36° C, but there was no benefit in morbidity or mortality. The AHA 2015 guidelines strongly recommends TTM to be performed as soon as possible if no contraindications exist.

It is the belief of these authors that TTM should be an essential part of post-cardiac arrest resuscitation, since keeping a patient at 35°–36° C is only mild hypothermia and has few complications. It is our belief that the potential neurologic benefits far outweigh the minimal risks. We have noted that physician resistance to TTM is mainly due to a lack of understanding of that therapy and/or familiarity of its use. Some physicians mistakenly believe that 36° C is normothermic, thereby precluding the need to initiate cooling. However, the benefit of TTM may actually lie in the prevention of hyperthermia, which stimulates the inflammatory cascade that contributes to cell death. The exact understanding of this pathophysiology is still in its early understanding. TTM should be started immediately, even during the acute phase of resuscitation, with a goal of 36° C or less to be obtained as quickly as possible, but caution should be used to prevent a temperature < 35° C.[19,20,21]

Q#4: What are the best initial ventilator settings?

Patients in cardiac arrest will have complete collapse of their alveoli (de-recruitment), thus, the ventilator settings should be set to promote recruitment and decrease potential barotrauma which may be associated with high tidal volumes, as well as rapid opening and closing of alveoli. A tidal volume of 6–8mm of H_2O should be used as a lung protective strategy. Plateau pressures should be used to guide our tidal volume and should remain < 30mmHg. There has been much debate on the initial tidal volume secondary to the ARDS NDS net. In 2000, a decreased morbidity was shown with patients ventilated with a TV of 4–6mm to obtain a PP of < 30, but no benefit in non-ARDS has been reported in the literature. Thus, the exact tidal volume remains controversial, which is why we recommend 6–8mL per kg as the initial tidal volume.

The respiratory rate should be started anywhere between 12–16 and titrated to accommodate minute ventilation (a lower tidal volume would therefore require a higher respiratory rate since MV = TV x RR). The ventilator needs to be adjusted either by following oxygen saturation with a goal to maintain sat > 92% and/or based on an ABG.

FiO_2 should be started at 50–100%, based upon an understanding of the potential cause of the cardiac arrest. The AHA recommends starting at 100% FiO_2; however, recent data shows that hyperoxemia, defined as a PaO_2 > 300 is associated with increased cerebrotoxic effects. It is not clear if this hyperoxygenation injury is related to a prolonged vent setting at the higher FiO_2. We recommend starting the FiO_2 at 100% with a rapid titration of FiO_2 to maintain an oxygen sat of 92–95% by lowering FiO_2 by 10% in the first 1–2 hours post-resuscitation. If you are able to achieve normotension, then titration of the FiO_2 can be maintained by following end tidal CO_2 (titrating to 35–42mmHG) or by ABG PaO_2 < 300mmHg, but higher maintaining PaO_2 than 60mmHg.

Lastly, no mode of ventilation has been shown to be superior to another. Volume vs. pressure has also not been shown to be beneficial. We recommend using the mode with which you have greatest familiarity.

The ED course continues:

The patient is placed on the vent but with 4 minutes, again loses her pulse. The resus continues:
0512 – CPR is resumed and an additional epinephrine 1mg IVP is given. NS IVF bolus 500mg is started
0514 – Rhythm is PEA. Bicarb 50mEq IVP
0516 – Rhythm check shows wide complex PEA. Epi 1mg IVP
0518 – Rhythm check = V-fib
Shock 150J
Pulses present (femoral) – BP check recorded as 176/142. Pulse = 91. Pulse ox = 74%
V-fib
Shock 150J

The labs begin to return:

WBC = 14.5 (H)
Hb = 13.1gm/dL
Plt = 233thou/mcL (L)

Sodium = 141 mmol/L
Potassium = 3.0 mmol/L (L)
Chloride = 100 mmol/L
CO_2 = 17 mmol/L (L)

BUN = 10 mg/dL
Creatinine = 1.2 mg/dL
LFTs = WNL

Troponin = 1.09 ng/ml (H)
BNP = 53 pq/ml

The resus continues:
0519 – Pulse check reveals no pulses. CPR is continued
0520 – V-fib
Shock 150J
Atropine 1mg
0522 – CPR held – no pulse
0523 – CPR started
Epi 1mg IVP
Shock 150J
0526 – Epi 1mg IPV
0527 – Bicarbonate 50mEq
0531 – CPR held, pulses present.
0532 – Rhythm strip shows:

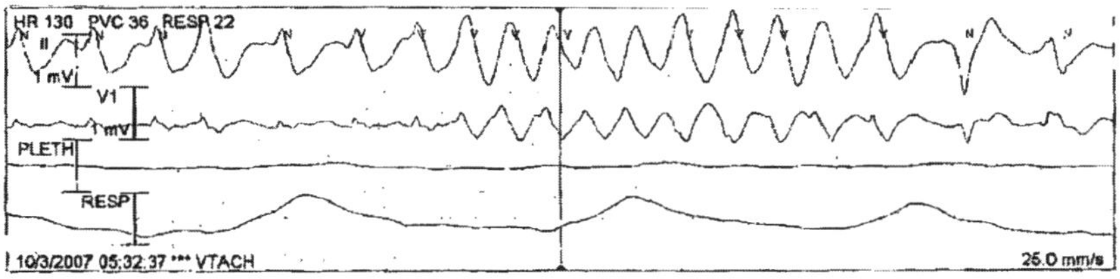

0534 –
Shock 150J
Shock 150J
Wide complex sinus rhythm – heart rate is 143. Pulse ox 72%
0537 – Amiodarone 150mg
Shock 150J
0538 – Levophed 4mg/250ml wide open

The patient is now is refractory V-tach with a pulse. How did the provider do?

DECISION POINT C – YOU ARE FACED WITH 5 QUESTIONS:

1. **How are refractory, V-fib and V-tach managed?**
2. **Our patient remains hypoxic, what can be done to optimize the oxygenation? Should the patient receive lytics for a suspected diagnosis of PE?**
3. **What is the role of cardiac US during a code?**
4. **When should the code be called?**
5. **What about ECMO?**

What does the literature say?

Q#1: How are refractory, V-fib and V-tach managed?

Meds: Refractory V-fib/V-tach is defined as persistence or re-occurrence of V-fib and or V-tach after 1 shock. The role of antiarrhythmics is to pharmacologically convert these non-perfusing rhythms into a perfusing one. Unfortunately, the evidence is troublesome; when amiodarone vs. lidocaine was used there was a trend for increase ROSC in the amiodarone group but no mortality difference. Similar trials with Procainamide showed some conversion and return of spontaneous circulation, but overall data did not show improved mortality. The AHA recommends the choice of antiarrhythmic agents be based on the morphology of the ventricular arrhythmia, with the 2015 AHA guidelines recommending amiodarone use initially.

Cutting edge defibrillation (single/multiple sequential): Let's first review the principles of defibrillation, specifically, the type of equipment available and their limitations. Monophasic uses a unidirectional form of electricity, while biphasic are bidirectional. Biphasic devices use one of 3 different designs: biphasic truncated exponential (BTE), rectilinear biphasic (RLB), and pulsed biphasic waveforms. They each have set joule protocols that are manufacturer directed, ranging from 120 joules to 200 joules, thus familiarity is critical.

In patients with refractory V-fib and V-tach, an emerging concept is double sequential defibrillation, performed by using 2 defibrillators by placing 1 set of pads posteriorly and anteriorly, while placing the other set at the apex and the sternum. Both defibrillators are charged at their maximum delivery of joules, while CPR is continued. When both defibrillators have fully charged, on the count of 3 (and after verifying that everyone is clear), both defibrillators are discharged together or within a second apart. The original data came from electrophysiologists who performed defibrillation and employed double sequential technique in the conversion of their patient and obtained conversion on their first defibrillation. Each shock was delivered between 0.4.–0.5 sec. None of these patients received pharmacological agents. The theory was that the sequential shock decreased the relative refractory period of the cardiac muscle and potentially decreased the transthoracic impedance by leading to more electrical delivery. Until recently, most of the trials were retrospective or case reports. Unfortunately, due to the patient population and conditions, it is very difficult to perform a double-blind, placebo-controlled trial. At this time, we can only say that adequate performance of CPR and delivery of early defibrillation is the standard. If the rhythm conversion is not successfully achieved after 3 defibrillations, double sequential defibrillation may be attempted. There is minimal potential for harm, falling into the category of a Hail Mary pass.

Whichever path is chosen, the primary emphasis is to only minimally interrupt chest compression.[19,20,21]

Q#2: Our patient remains hypoxic, what can be done to optimize the oxygenation? Should the patient receive lytics for a suspected diagnosis of PE?

Our patient had several episodes of PEA as well as ROSC but continued with severe hypoxemia. After careful consideration of the potential etiologies of the cardiac arrest, we must ask ourselves, what is the cause of this hypoxemia? Could it be a tension pneumothorax or PE? We can either intervene or do further diagnostic testing, such as performing a bedside ultrasound (which will be discussed in the next section) to evaluate for pneumothorax. If the suspicion of a PE remains high on the differential due to the clinical presentation, the use of tPA has shown some modest clinical benefit, without increased evidence of decreased morbidity and mortality, but the AHA in 2015 stated that no evidence is available to support or refute the effectiveness of empiric thrombolysis in suspected but unconfirmed PE.[21]

How about thrombolysis in ACS? The use of tPA in potential ACS as the etiology of the cardiac arrest is classified as not effective and potentially harmful. In summary, fibrinolytic therapy should not be routinely used in cardiac arrest. There have been multiple case reports where tPA was administered with a successful return of circulation and survival, but caution is warranted; these authors believe that it might be associated with timing of the thrombolytic. Currently, it is usually used as a last-ditch effort in prolonged arrest, but if administered early, could yield different results. Note that this is based on no evidence, but a single case study; no formal recommendations can be made at this time.

Our patient had 3 episodes of ROSC, lasting anywhere between 1 to 4 minutes, but no ECG was obtained—this should have been a priority. Placing ECG pads on the chest while CPR is performed, in the hope of ROSC, could have facilitated rapidly obtaining and ECG when ROSC was achieved; this could have been diagnostic and potentially lifesaving. In this case, from the initial visit to the second visit, this patient is screaming ACS.

Consulting editor comments (Weingart):

If you have a place that does not have ECMO and you highly suspect acute myocardial infarction, unless you're in that like one in a hundred place where they'll actually take the patient to the Cath lab with a mechanical CPR device (and those places are vanishingly small), then you pretty much have no chance except to push lytics. If I don't suspect PE or MI, then I will not empirically give lytics.

Q#3: What is the role of cardiac US during a code?

POCUS can be utilized during a code to evaluate for pneumothorax, cardiac tamponade, estimated cardiac EF, cardiac standstill, and to estimate the patient's volume status by looking at the IVC. Standstill is defined as no cardiac activity and can be used to terminate resuscitation efforts. Use caution as a prospective cohort study during cardiac arrest resuscitation comparing times between pulse check with ultrasound vs. pulse check alone found that the use of ultrasound was associated with nearly double the 10 second maximum duration recommended in 2015 current guideline.[19, 22]

Q#4: When should the code be called?

There are only several predictors in cardiac arrest including time from arrest to time of CPR initiation and a prolonged resuscitative effort. Much has been said on when to stop, but little is known. We recommend that family members or loved ones be given the opportunity to be present in the resuscitation efforts, as this serves multiple purposes.

- It will bring closure. They witness all the efforts that the team puts toward saving their loved one.
- There is opportunity for a discussion about advanced directives and quality of life while the resuscitation is being conducted.

We personally have experienced on several occasions family members asking to stop because of the futility of continuing the resuscitation. Note that patients in asystole or prolonged PEA over 30 minutes have little to no chance of a meaningful recovery.

Consulting editor comments (Weingart):

We have a tendency to run codes for a long time. Now that we are using ECMO, we begin to realize that our conceptions of how long we can perform CPR and still have neurologically intact survival are wrong. We've had ECMO patients an hour and 20 minutes with perfect neurologic outcome, and we've had patients without ECMO who had a code continue till the 45 minute mark who had a full recovery and walked out of the hospital. I have a tendency on young patients to run the codes a long time. After I've taken everything out of my arsenal and I have nothing at the 45 minute mark, what are you going to do? We don't have an end game at that point.

Q#5: What about ECMO?

E-CPR has recently had made a re-emergence in the medical literature. Even though the AHA in the 2015 guidelines does not recommend the use of E-CPR, several retrospective studies performed in Korea, Taiwan, and one in San Diego found an increased rate of survival with good neurological outcome defined by a CPP of 1 or 2. E-CPR is a costly, time-consuming maneuver that is best left to centers that are experienced and have dedicated ECMO resources. While we are excited about the future of E-CPR, it currently enjoys only limited availability; there is much to come from future research.[19]

What did the actual provider do?

ED course:

0538 – Vitals: Heart rate is 90. Sat is 72%. Summary: Dopamine and Levophed are running

0539 – Pulse check = no pulses. CPR is continued

0540 – V-fib

Shock 150J

Shock 150J

0541 – CPR held. The rhythm strip shows:

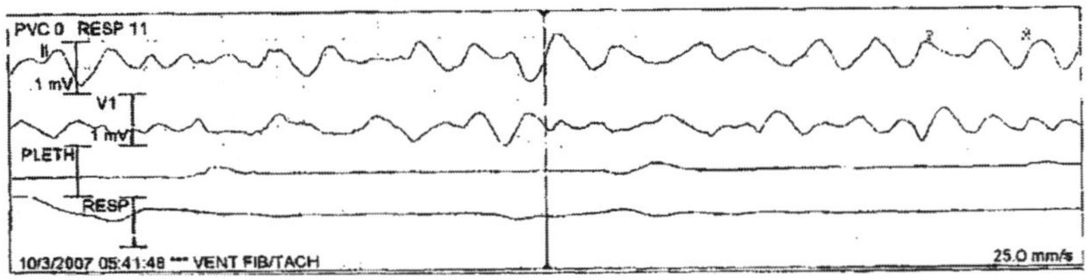

0542 – Pt. apneic and pulseless
0543 – Code called

Outcomes
Time CPR Stopped: 0543
Expired: 0543

0619 – Numerous family and friends arrive and are taken into the room by the chaplain to view the body

An autopsy reveals:

PATHOLOGICAL FINDINGS

1. **Acute myocardial infarction.**
2. **Severe atherosclerotic involvement of the circumflex and the right coronary artery.**
3. **Patchy fibrosis of the myocardium.**
4. **Medical history of hypertension, diabetes mellitis and prior cerebrovascular accident.**

CAUSE OF DEATH: Acute myocardial infarction due to severe atherosclerotic heart disease.

Summary: Patients in cardiac arrest benefit from:

- Early initiation of CPR.
- Adequate compressions at a rate of 100–120, and depth of 2–2.4 inches.
- Early defibrillation for V-fib/V-tach.
- Early ECG after ROSC to identify STEMI.
- Target Temperature Management should be obtained at 35–36° C for patients with ROSC and GCS of less than 8 without other contraindications.

THE LEGAL:

Shortly after Stacy's untimely death, a malpractice action was entered, proceeding to discovery, depositions and eventually a trial. Allegations of malpractice were entered not only against the initial treating physician, but against the hospital and nursing staff. As it turns out, the hospital had recently rewritten its procedure for triage with a recommendation to assign a triage category of 2 for chest pain patients, but Stacy had only been assigned a category of 3, in direct contradiction of the hospital's own policy.

This is one of the three cases in this book where we explore the legal issues. Following the testimony are comments by **Greg Henry, MD,** past president of ACEP and an expert in over 2,000 legal cases.

The plaintiff's strategy:
Stacy collapsed at her home just over seven hours after ED discharge. The pathologist who performed the autopsy testified that Stacy had severe atherosclerosis of the circumflex coronary artery and the right coronary artery. The left anterior descending artery had moderate atherosclerosis. A discolored region along the lateral side of the left ventricle indicated an acute MI. The plaintiff's expert on emergency medicine testified that St. Mary's nurses contributed to Stacy's death, partly because they assigned an incorrect triage category. They further opined that the proper treatment for unstable angina is to first make the diagnosis by assessing myocardial function, performing a cardiac perfusion study, or taking the patient directly to cardiac catheterization or CT angiography. Based on these findings, a decision would be made as to angioplasty and stenting or a bypass. The experts did not think that either the doctor or the nurses intentionally harmed Stacy, but Stacy presented with symptoms that were very consistent with unstable angina and myocardial infarction. In their opinion, with her significant risk factors of hypertension, smoking, and diabetes, the possibilities of myocardial infarction and unstable angina were not adequately evaluated.

The defense's strategy:
Though there was a delay in obtaining the ECG, there was no reason to believe that an earlier ECG would have changed the management. The chart reflects the presence of multiple risk factors for coronary artery disease, however, Stacy exhibited no associated symptoms—nausea and vomiting, coughing blood, syncope, feeling of doom, shortness of breath, sweating and palpitations—and a physical examination of her cardiovascular system—regular rate/rhythm, no murmur, no gallop, no friction rub, pulses full/equal—presented in normal range. She was not cyanotic, diaphoretic, or pallid. There were two "ECGs with a whole day of pain, not having acute changes." Because his impression was that Stacy's chest pain was of non-cardiac origin, the doctor did not order cardiac enzyme tests. According to the doctor, the level 3 triage assigned to Stacy provided more than enough time for him to make the correct decision.

The discharge nurse told Stacy to return to the emergency room if the pain returned or worsened. The doctor instructed Stacy to set up an appointment the following day with her doctor to address her high blood pressure. The nurse took Stacy's vital signs and assessed her pain. At 8:25 Stacy's blood pressure was "130/82," her pulse was "71," and her respirations were "16." Stacy would not have been discharged if those vital signs had been abnormal. The nurse acknowledged that a patient may have stable vital signs and still have unstable angina. The hospital's emergency admission record states that the doctor diagnosed Stacy with high blood pressure and prescribed lisinopril. Stacy was discharged at 8:45 p.m. The discharge instructions informed Stacy to call sooner if she thought it was necessary, and to return immediately if her symptoms worsened.

THE TRIAL:

Plaintiff's opening statement: Good morning, everybody. One of the major reasons people come to ED's in the U.S. is because of chest pain. Not all of it is fatal. And it's not always easy to diagnose. And the rule in ED's is that you treat chest pain as a heart attack until you rule it out. That's the rule. The evidence is going to show that when Stacy left the hospital with her friend Doreen, they were in shock. Doreen regrets to this day that she did not bar the door and say, "No, we're not leaving. We're not leaving." But they did.

It's going to be up to you to figure out whether the discharge of Stacy was wrong, was negligent—the failure to even get a basic history was a violation of the standard. We strongly believe that had these things been done, Stacy would be here today and she would be raising her children. Thank you.

1. Triage category:

Q. I want to get some clarity for the jury's sake. Your position is she shouldn't have been triage one.
A. Yes, sir.
Q. And you are going to stand by this statement?
A. Yes, sir.
Q. I want you to look at Exhibit #30, please. It says departmental procedure, correct?
A. Yes, sir.
Q. It was revised June of '07, that is 4 months prior to Stacy's presentation, correct?
A. Yes, sir.
Q. It is the emergency department policy. The purpose is to describe the steps to be taken when caring for patients over 18 with chest pain, correct?
A. Yes, sir.
Q. It says the SOC for all patients who present to the ED with a complaint of chest pain should be evaluated as soon as possible by the triage nurse to initiate appropriate steps to minimize mortality and morbidity, correct?
A. Yes sir.
Q. First, obtain a patient assessment. Next obtain a history including precipitating factors, duration of pain, quality, intensity of pain. She had at least 1, 2, 3, 4, 5, 6 risk factors. Read the department procedure to me.
A. Assign a triage category one or two.
Q. Didn't say 3, did it?
A. It does not.

2. Should the provider document that the ED is busy?

Author comments (Weinstock):

The physician alleged that it was very busy when Stacy presented... is this a good idea? Sounds like it... until, the attorney subpoenas the hospital for the patient logs for the day. They are reproduced below. Was it really too busy for good care? You be the judge...

Q. Now we agreed yesterday, doctor, that the most severe patient, the patient that was most urgent was triaged as a level one, correct?
A. Yes, sir.
Q. All right. Look on the log for October 2nd, is there a single triage 1 on there?
A. There does not appear to be.
Q. Okay. And we'll just go through it. What time did you come on duty that day?

A. Generally 6 p.m.

Q. Okay. And this is military time, so 6 p.m. would be?

A. That would be 1800.

The actual log from the chart is reproduced below:

Time In	LOS (Length of Stay)	Physician Time	Chief Complaint - Triage Level
13:29	6:05	15:04	right side flank pain-Level 4
16:42	5:59	16:45	Pneumonia Level 3
17:30	2:09	18:07	Fatigue Sore throat headache Level 3
17:35	3:21	17:59	Abdominal pain vomiting Level 3
17:58	1:25	18:22	Eye complaints (laceration) Level 3
18:01	1:42	18:15	leg hurts, chills, left leg giving out Level 3
18:13	2:37	18:28	[redacted] chest pain - Level 3
18:53	1:01	19:32	finger hurts - Level 4
19:27	3:32	19:34	attempted suicide - Level 3
19:59	1:32	20:52	shoulder pain - level 3
20:09	2:31	20:21	abdominal pain, chest pain - Level 3 (nurse practitioner)
20:17	1:36	20:37	Pediatric fever - Level 4
20:39	5:40	20:47	abdominal pain - Level 3 (nurse practitioner)
20:45	1:10	21:09	fell at Walmart, cut lip - Level 3
20:50	1:06	21:03	Left side hurts, Flank pain- Level 4

3. Plantiff goes a bit too far:

Q. Wouldn't it be nice to learn from a traumatic experience? Wouldn't it be nice to learn from somebody's death and be willing to say, "You know what? Maybe let's go back and let's retrace our steps, highlight granted, but do we want this to happen again?"

A. No sir, I think about this every day, I do not want it to happen again. This is very emotional for me. Do you know why I am a doctor? When I was 16—

Q. Your honor, can I have the witness instructed to…

A. I'm answering your question.

Q. Your honor, can I have the witness instructed to—

A. It's important for me to let this out. You asked me a question

Q. Your honor—

The court:

"Just a minute everybody, listen very carefully. Doctor, you will have a full opportunity to give your side of the story when counsel questions you. At the juncture, please answer the plaintiff's questions. I understand it's emotional for you and you want the jury to understand. You will have your opportunity, at this juncture, simply answer his question."

4. Emotional response: Defense attorney to physician:

Q. Doctor, you've been on the stand for a few hours. While you were giving testimony a few moments ago, you started to say something about why you became a physician and the plaintiff counsel stopped you. Would you like to share that with the jury?

A. Yes sir, he had asked if I understand what they're going through. When I was 16 I took a chemistry test and the secretary came and told me, "You're to go right home." I drove home. My mother had died of a heart attack at age 42. I understand what they're going through. This is a horrendous case for me. When they subpoenaed the documents, I mean, I literally sat down and sobbed, that—that I—all of those risk factors and everything is on there. And if the nurses mis-triaged it, it's my job to do that. And even there is enough information there, that I missed this. I don't know how I missed this. But I understand very well what they're going through. I go through it every day, I think about this case because it's almost an ironic mirror image of what happened. My mom had had some chest pains. Her doctor thought she was just an anxious housewife that drank too much sherry and it turns out she dropped dead of a heart attack at 42. So I'm very much aware of what they're going through. This is a very emotional case. And, again, I'm—I'm sorry that I am reacting this way, but this is—I understand what they're going through.

Q. Thank you for sharing that, doctor.

Author comments (Weinstock):

What follows next is truly astounding, the physician, besieged by genuine guilt and self-doubt, admits that they were wrong. On a side note, there were 2 legal actions, one against the physician, and the other against the hospital... read on....

5. I was wrong (Plaintiff's attorney to physician):

Q. You know what I'm getting at. At the hospital, worst case scenario, her chances are tremendously better than in a trailer park? You checked that she was stable when she left the hospital, correct?

A. I appear to be in error about her being stable.

Q. Whoa. Wait, wait. What did you just say?

A. I appear to be in error in checking she's stable. History has shown the fullness of time, she apparently had unstable angina, and so was not stable at discharge.

Q. So, you –

A. I was in error. I made a mistake. The nursing staff didn't make a mistake. The hospital didn't make a mistake. I made a mistake. I had a lady that had many risk factors. I thought I had answered her complaint with her BP and her bronchospasm and the 2 ECG's that didn't have evolving change. I thought she was stable. I was wrong. I failed her.

6. So, what happened?

The defense now starts calling witnesses, with the cardiologist undergoing direct examination by the defense counsel. He is being questioned about testimony we have just heard; that the doctor admitted wrongdoing to the jury. Then the [not adequately prepped] cardiologist admits that he knows the physician defendant has already settled his case. *At this point in the trial, this is *not* known by the jury:

Q. Did you learn that the doctor confessed to the jury that unstable angina caused her death?

A. When I did my report?

Q. No. Did you learn before you got on the witness stand?

A. I know that he—he has—he already settled his case with them and that he admitted he probably shouldn't have sent her home.

Q. He—he told the jury—and—

COURT: Why don't y'all approach [the bench].

Q. (Plaintiff): The cardiologist just blurted out that the [ED] doctor had settled. We have all been told by the court to instruct the witnesses not to mention that there was a settlement.

Author comments (Weinstock):

This is a *major* twist in our story. Why is it important? Because this trial was actually against the hospital, and in this trial, the physician was a witness for the defense! The concern for the plaintiff's attorney was that if the jury thought there was a big settlement which gave money to the family, they would be less likely to award additional money from the hospital to the family. Here is the plaintiff's attorney appealing to the judge:

Plaintiff's attorney: In my life, your honor, I have never moved for a mistrial, ever, in a civil case. But I think it is warranted here because you can't un-ring this bell. "Well the guilty party has already paid, and so, you know, the hospital should be exonerated." In this case, your honor, we are faced with a very high burden of willful and wanton behavior. The settlement amount [already paid] was $200,000, for a 46-year-old woman with 2 minor children, is insignificant and paltry.

The motion for mistrial is denied.

TRIAL OUTCOME:

Jury sides with plaintiff, according to the newspaper report "the jury hit the hospital with a $1.4 million verdict Thursday, concluding that the hospital nurses were negligent in their treatment of the late Stacy."

The hospital appeals, as in Texas there is a very high standard of malpractice saying the physician's actions need to be "Willful and Wanton."

VOTE ON APPEAL:

"We hold that the evidence of deviation from the standard of care by St. Mary's nursing staff is legally insufficient to support the jury's finding that the willful and wanton negligence of the hospital was a proximate cause of Stacy's death," the opinion states.

"Accordingly, we reverse the trial court's judgment and render a take-nothing judgment."

JURORS HEAR EMOTIONAL TESTIMONY FROM DOCTOR IN MALPRACTICE TRIAL!

January 13, 2010 1:43 PM
By David Yates
Reporter with the Southeast Texas Record, reprinted with permission.

The doctor who treated the late Stacy [________], recently testified during a malpractice trial that he could have done more to prevent her fatal heart attack.

Her family claims the nursing staff at Hospital violated nursing standards because they failed to assess her condition, failed to inquire and determine the nature of the chest pain and failed to discuss the case with the emergency room attending physician.

Nurses also failed to trigger the chain of command with a call to the nursing supervisor when no satisfactory resolution could be reached and failed to ask for orders from the ER physician for biochemical marker studies, according to the complaint.

MED-MAL TRIAL AGAINST LOCAL HOSPITAL ENDS WITH $1.4 M VERDICT

October 17, 2011 2:00 PM
By David Yates
Reporter with the Southeast Texas Record, reprinted with permission.

Last Thursday, the Texas Ninth Court of Appeals found the evidence "legally insufficient" for jurors to levy a $1.2 million verdict against the hospital

As previously reported, on Jan. 21, 2010, a Jefferson County jury concluded that nurses were negligent in their treatment of the late _____, levying a $1.4 million verdict against the hospital. Her mother, sued the hospital in November 2008, alleging nurses and [the initial doctor] incorrectly diagnosed and treated the patient.

Court records show she died of a heart attack a day after receiving treatment.

[The initial doctor] settled for $150,000 in August 2009, while the hospital opted to take its chances in court.

According to the charge of the court, jurors found [the initial doctor] was 20 percent responsible in his treatment and diagnosis, pushing the remaining 80 percent of the blame upon the hospital.

After the application of settlement credits, statutory damage caps and medical expenses, the judgment was reduced from $1,215,075 to $331,390, court papers say.

The following month, Christus filed an appeal questioning whether there was sufficient evidence of wanton negligence.

On Oct. 13 the Ninth Court issued an opinion, authored by Justice Charles Kreger, finding in favor of the hospital.

"We hold that the evidence of deviation from the standard of care by the nursing staff is legally insufficient to support the jury's finding that the willful and wanton negligence of the hospital was a proximate cause of death," the opinion states.

"Accordingly, we reverse the trial court's judgment and render a take-nothing judgment."

Gregory L. Henry, MD
Former President of The American College of Emergency Physicians (ACEP)
Former Professor of Emergency Medicine at the University of Michigan
Former CEO of Medical Practice Risk Assessment, Ann Arbor, MI

"First, there is no relationship in the documentation between the chief complaint and the diagnosis; this is a mountain which is difficult to climb."

Documentation and evaluation:
The approach to finding negligence with the initial doctor and hospital is simple, as our patient was a walking disaster when she entered the hospital. First, there is no relationship in the documentation between the chief complaint and the diagnosis; this is a mountain which is difficult to climb. Second, she is high-risk. She did not have a normal life expectancy. She a diabetic, she's a smoker, she's a this, she's a that. None of it is good. Third, the ECG was not normal. Exactly when her infarct took place is difficult to determine but considering all factors, this woman should be considered to have acute coronary syndrome. Confusing a jury with whether she should have been a category 1 or a category 2 is useless. She was in the department, she got her ECG, and she had a concerning presentation; that's enough! The triage category would not have changed the work-up. But the larger picture is clear. She has just about every risk factor, and we do not have another explanation for her chest pain. Defense of the first visit is difficult, and I would advise an insurance company to consider a reasonable settlement.

Insurance company payout:
The monetary expense from the insurance company falls into two parts:
1. The allocated loss adjustments which are the cost of running the case. This includes paying the attorneys, paying for analysis, paying the experts, etc. etc.
2. The second part is the award. This is then divided by the patient and the attorneys.

It is the combination of these two costs which determine the risk to the insurance company. Sometimes it is better when there are multiple problems to cap losses before a runaway jury does something untoward. I have been involved in discussion of settlements and believe the amount paid in this case was reasonable and probably could have been arrived at with early negotiations.

Defending the physician(s):
There is no question that being a defense expert for the first treating physician would be extremely difficult. It is a much different situation for the second physician. When a patient comes back and there had been a return of spontaneous circulation from an arrest, but no return of consciousness the prognosis of the patient is terrible. Comments are made about multiple defibrillations, using norepinephrine to support both heart rate and pressure, and when you're at this level, you're talking about minute numbers of patients saved. The real question is, are we saving patients who have a reasonable life? It is extremely rare that a patient who has gone down in the field without immediate ROSC is going to have a good outcome. The plaintiff would have been wise to strictly concentrate on the first visit. Juries like cases which are simple and easy to understand. They don't want to have to balance multiple people who have made multiple errors. Emphasis on the second visit would only serve to confuse the jury.

Hospital liability:

It is interesting to note that the 9th Circuit Court of Appeals found the evidence legally insufficient for juries to find against the hospital. This usually means the hospital personnel i.e. the nurses. Although the initial verdict included everyone, the court was essentially also focused on the first visit. It is also interesting that the initial EM doctor settled for $150, 000, while the hospital opted to take its chances in court. The attorney for the initial physician was very wise. The fact that the initial judgement was reduced from $1.2 million to $330,000 does say something about the legal system. It is also noted that the 9th Circuit Court issued an opinion finding in favor of the hospital, saying "We hold the evidence of deviation from the standard of care by nursing is legally insufficient to support the jury's finding that willful and wanton negligence of the hospital was a proximate cause of this death." The court therefore gave to the hospital essentially a "take nothing" judgment, meaning they got themselves out of the case.

Was it fair?

Is this fair? Well, it's difficult to say. The "willful and wanton" negligence standard in the state of Texas certainly had an impact on the results. Instead of coming away with $1.4 million the patient's family comes away with $150,000, a small amount to provide for parentless children, especially after attorney fees are deducted. Fairness is difficult to judge.

References:

1. Rui P, Kang K, Albert M. National hospital ambulatory medical care survey: 2013 emergency department summary tables. Available at: http://www.cdc.gov/nchs/data/ahcd/nhamcs_emergency/2013_ed_web_tables.pdf. Accessed on Sept 20, 2017.
2. Heart Disease Facts, Centers for Disease Control and Prevention. Available at: https://www.cdc.gov/heartdisease/facts.htm. Accessed on Sept 20, 2017.
3. Brown TW, McCarthy ML, Kelen GD, et al. An epidemiologic study of closed emergency department malpractice claims in a national database of physician malpractice insurers. Acad Emerg Med 2010;17(5):553-60.
4. Berry JD, Dyer A, Cai X, et al. Lifetime risks of cardiovascular disease. N Engl J Med 2012;366(4):321–9.
5. Goodacre S, Locker T, Morris F, et al. How useful are clinical features in the diagnosis of acute, undifferentiated chest pain? Acad Emerg Med 2002;9(3):203-8.
6. Speake D, Terry P. Best evidence topic report: First ECG in chest pain. Emerg Med J 2001;18:61-62.
7. Forberg JL, Green M, Björk J, et al. In search of the best method to predict acute coronary syndrome using only the electrocardiogram from the emergency department. J Electrocardiol 2009;42(1):58-63.
8. Ashida T, Tani S, Nagao K, et al. Usefulness of synthesized 18-lead electrocardiography in the diagnosis of ST-elevation myocardial infarction: A pilot study. Am J Emerg Med 2017;35(3):448-57.
9. Han JH, Lindsell CJ, Storrow AB, et al. The role of cardiac risk factor burden in diagnosing acute coronary syndromes in the emergency department setting. Ann Emerg Med 2007;49(2):145-52, 152.e1.

10. Backus BE, Six AJ, Kelder JC, et al. A prospective validation of the HEART score for chest pain patients at the emergency department. Int J Cardiol 2013;168(3):2153-58.
11. Pollack CV Jr, Sites FD, Shofer FS, et al. Application of the TIMI risk score for unstable angina and non-ST elevation acute coronary syndrome to an unselected emergency department chest pain population. Acad Emerg Med 2006;13(1):13-8.
12. Amsterdam EA, Wenger NK, Brindis RG, et al. 2014 AHA/ACC Guideline For The Management of Patients with Non ST-elevation Acute Coronary Syndrome: A Report of the American College of Cardiology/American Heart Association Task Force on Practice Guidelines. Circulation 2014;130:e344-426.
13. Crea F, Battipaglia I, Andreotti F. Sex differences in mechanisms, presentation and management of ischaemic heart disease. Atherosclerosis 2015;241(1):157-68. doi: 10.1016/j.atherosclerosis.2015.04.802. Epub 2015 Apr 27.
14. Li H, Wang D, Yu Y, Zhao X, et al. Mechanical versus manual chest compressions for cardiac arrest: a systematic review and meta-analysis. Scand J Trauma Resusc Emerg Med 2016;24:10. doi:10.1186/s13049-016-0202-y.
15. Bonnes JL, Brouwer MA, Navarese EP, et al. Manual cardiopulmonary resuscitation versus CPR including a mechanical chest compression device in out-of-hospital cardiac arrest: A comprehensive meta-analysis from randomized and observational studies. Ann Emerg Med 2016; 67(3):349-60. doi:10.1016/j.annemergmed.2015.09.023.
16. Hazinski MF, Nolan JP, Aickin R, et al. Part 1: Executive Summary 2015 International Consensus on Cardiopulmonary Resuscitation and Emergency Cardiovascular Care Science With Treatment Recommendations. Circulation 2015;132:S2-S39, originally published October 14, 2015.
17. Heradstveit BE, Sunde K, Sunde GA, et al. Factors complicating interpretation of capnography during advanced life support in cardiac arrest–a clinical retrospective study in 575 patients. Resuscitation 2012;83(7):813-8.
18. De Backer D, Biston P, Devriendt J, et al. Comparison of dopamine and norepinephrine in the treatment of shock. N Engl J Med 2010;362(9):779-89.
19. De Backer D, Aldecoa C, Njimi H, et al. Dopamine versus norepinephrine in the treatment of septic shock: A meta-analysis. Crit Care Med 2012;40(3):725-30.
20. Link MS, Berkow LC, Kudenchuk PJ, et al. Part 7: Adult Advanced Cardiovascular Life Support 2015 American Heart Association Guidelines Update for Cardiopulmonary Resuscitation and Emergency Cardiovascular Care. Circulation 2015(18 Suppl 2);132:S444-S464.
21. Callaway CW, Donnino MW, Fink EL, et al. Part 8: Post–cardiac Arrest Care 2015 American Heart Association Guidelines Update for Cardiopulmonary Resuscitation and Emergency Cardiovascular Care. Circulation 2015(18 Suppl 2);132:S465-S482.
22. Lavonas EJ, Drennan IR, Gabrielli A, et al. Part 10: Special Circumstances of Resuscitation 2015 American Heart Association Guidelines Update for Cardiopulmonary Resuscitation and Emergency Cardiovascular Care. Circulation 2015(18 Suppl 2);132:S501-S518.

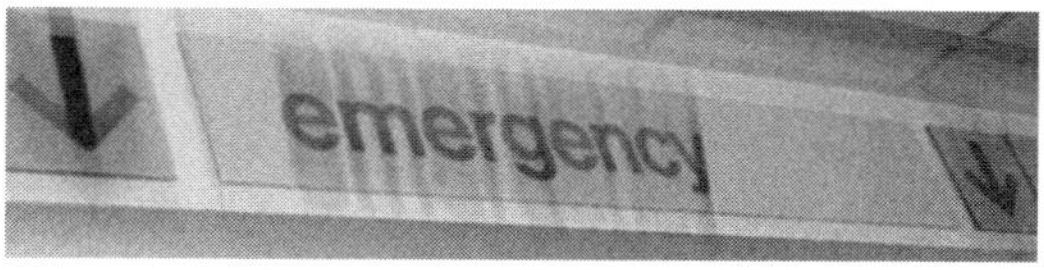

SECTION A – AIRWAY/ARREST

Chapter 4: A 47-year-old woman with anaphylaxis

Anand Swaminathan, MD, MPH

Assistant Professor of Emergency Medicine
St Joseph's Regional Medical Center, Paterson, NJ

Christina Chien, MD

Assistant Professor, Depts. of Emergency Medicine & Critical Care Medicine
Thomas Jefferson University, Philadelphia, PA

Legal commentary:

Gregory L. Henry, MD

Former President of The American College of Emergency Physicians (ACEP)
Former Professor of Emergency Medicine at the University of Michigan
Former CEO of Medical Practice Risk Assessment, Ann Arbor, MI

Mark Kitrick, Esq.

Kitrick, Lewis & Harris Co., LPA, Columbus, OH

Julia Turner, Esq.

The Ohio State University Wexner Medical Center, Columbus, OH

Section editor:

Lillian L. Emlet, MD, MS, FACEP, FCCM

Clinical Associate Professor
Depts. of Critical Care Medicine & Emergency Medicine
Associate Program Director, IMCCM Fellowship of the MCCTP
Interim Associate Chief of Staff of Education, VA
University of Pittsburgh School of Medicine, Pittsburgh, PA

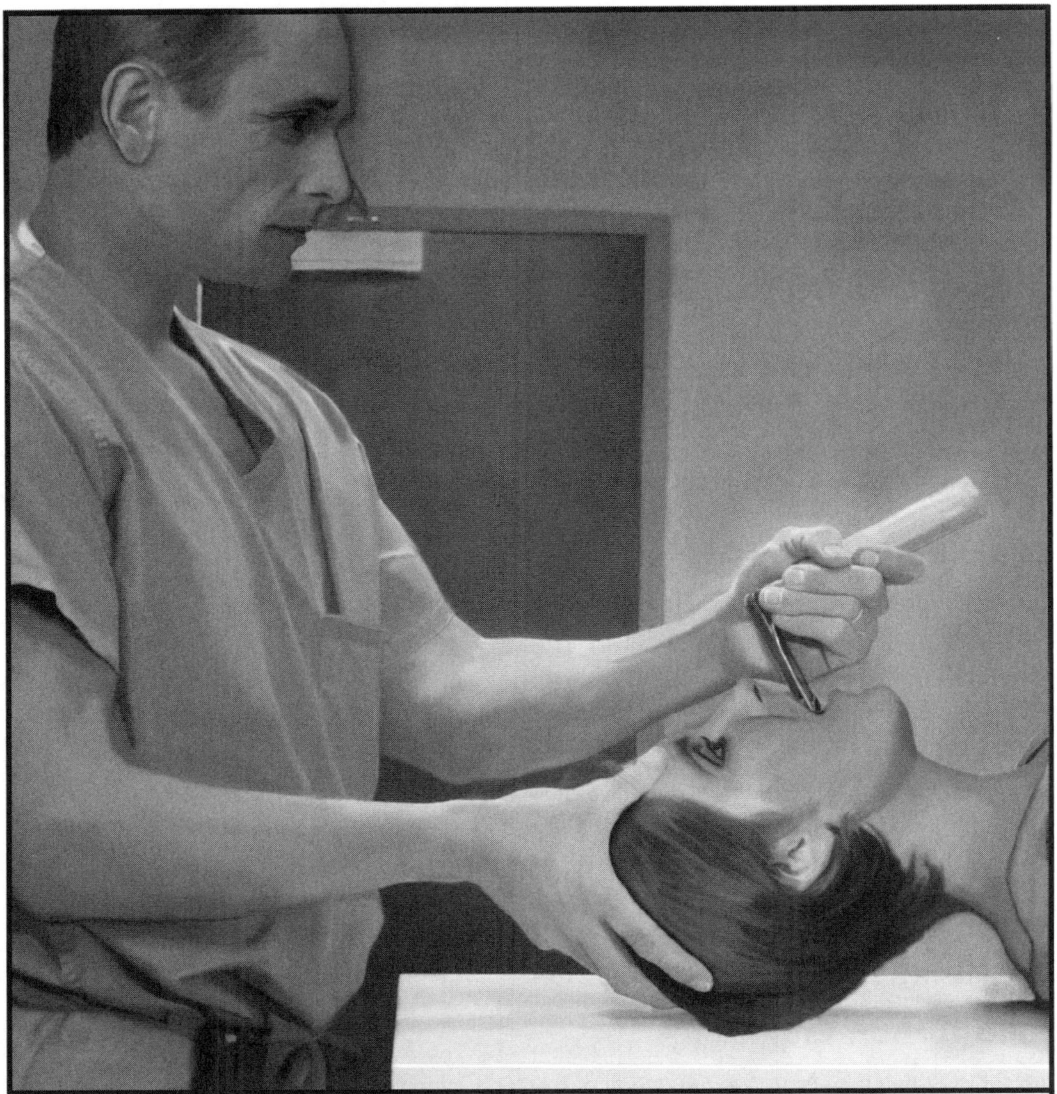

"I COULDN'T EVEN SEE THE CORDS."

SECTION A/CHAPTER 4

A 47-year-old woman with anaphylaxis

Anaphylaxis is a serious and generalized allergic reaction that can be potentially life-threatening. Overall mortality appears to be relatively rare, occurring in about 1% of all cases.[1] However, fatalities do occur and can progress rapidly and unexpectedly, from mild symptoms to respiratory arrest within minutes to hours.[2] Reducing mortality hinges on prompt diagnosis and immediate management. This can be difficult because presenting symptoms are variable and need to be distinguished from other conditions. As a result, anaphylaxis is frequently underdiagnosed and undertreated.[3] Multiple diagnostic criteria, including an update in 2015 by the Anaphylaxis Practice Parameter Workgroup, have been published to help make this clinical diagnosis easier to recognize. However, there remain difficulties in standardizing clinical practice, as there is no clinical test for diagnosis and no test that predicts severity.[2,4]

Questions which will be explored:

1. What is the gold standard for diagnosing anaphylaxis?
2. When and how should epinephrine be administered?
3. The nightmare scenario: What happens when patients with anaphylaxis lose their airway?

This case is real, including the documentation and medical decision-making. This case is a little different from other bounceback cases because the first visit was to the patient's primary care physician. However, the patient is still a bounceback, arriving at the ED a day later… and crashing soon after.

INITIAL VISIT

Initial visit summary: The patient is a 47-year-old woman who presents to her primary care physician with rhinorrhea, sinus pain, and cough for 2 days. She is prescribed Moxifloxacin for a diagnosis of acute sinusitis. She has additional symptoms of anxiety and intermittent sadness for the last several months and is also prescribed Sertraline (1/2 a pill a day for the first week, then 1 pill every day thereafter). On her way home, she drops the prescriptions off at the pharmacy and picks them up in the morning.

Author comments (Weinstock):

This primary care visit seems routine... in fact, likely occurring many thousands of times every day around the world. Whereas the full documentation of the visit to the primary care physician was not available, we don't know if the care was appropriate. We start with a brief discussion of the diagnosis and management of acute sinusitis.

Assessment of the case so far:
Since we do not have the full records of this visit to the primary medical doctor (PMD), it is difficult for us to follow the PMD's thought processes on treatment plans. Specifically, what were the patient's presenting symptoms that led to the diagnosis and treatment of acute sinusitis? Did she have a history of chronic sinusitis and this was an acute exacerbation, or was this a first-time diagnosis? There are also no vital signs available to help us determine if this patient was "sick vs. not sick."

How do we diagnose, treat, and manage acute sinusitis?
Rhinosinusitis, the symptomatic inflammation of the sinuses and nasal cavity, usually presents with symptoms of purulent nasal drainage, along with nasal obstruction, and/or facial pain or pressure. It can be classified as acute if it lasts less than 4 weeks, or chronic if it lasts more than 12 weeks.[6] Acute rhinosinusitis can be either bacterial or viral, and the distinction is important because the management is different for each.

Viral rhinosinusitis may be difficult to distinguish from bacterial rhinosinusitis, but most acute presentations of sinusitis with a short duration are due to a viral infection.[5] Antibiotics are not indicated in these cases, unless the patient is systemically ill. Otherwise, symptomatic relief, such as topical steroids and nasal saline irrigation, is appropriate.

Acute bacterial rhinosinusitis (ABRS) can be clinically diagnosed when a patient has symptoms of acute rhinosinusitis for at least 10 days without improving.[6] In these patients, either watchful waiting or antibiotics is appropriate. Amoxicillin or amoxicillin-clavulanic acid are the recommended first-line agents; in penicillin-allergic patients, fluoroquinolones, clindamycin, or cephalosporins are reasonable alternatives.

In our case, we do not have documentation of the presenting symptoms, but we do know that the duration of her symptoms was only 2 days. While it may be possible that her symptoms were severe enough to warrant treatment, the constellation of symptoms, rhinorrhea, cough and sinus pain, points more towards a viral cause. In addition, there is no documentation that the patient is allergic to penicillin or has a history of recent antibiotic use, and yet, she was started on Moxifloxacin, a fluoroquinolone that may not have been the most appropriate choice.

ED BOUNCEBACK

The next day the patient picks up her prescriptions on the way home from work and takes the medications after dinner (around 21:00). Soon after, she develops a rash and then a feeling of shortness of breath. The symptoms begin quickly, causing her anxiety to worsen. She calls EMS at 22:25.

When EMS arrives on scene at 22:33, the patient is lying on the floor, but is alert and oriented. A family member tells EMS that "she had an anxiety attack and took [Sertraline] for the first time today." The patient is transferred to the ED.

ED VISIT (1 day after initial PMD visit)

Triage (22:59): Patient arrivals vis EMS. Patient appears anxious. Per EMS, patient took ½ pill of Sertraline for the first time. Patient reports she took Moxifloxacin and Sertraline today, both new prescriptions. However, she had taken Moxifloxacin before without difficulties. Patient has hives all over body. Patient reports not being able to "catch her breath." SaO_2 is 89% on room air. Patient moved…to be placed on the monitor. The doctor is notified.

HPI (23:22): 47-year-old white female with a history of hypertension and hypercholesterolemia, otherwise in good general health, she does not smoke cigarettes. She was recently diagnosed with sinusitis. This evening at approximately 9 p.m. (two hours ago), she took her initial dose of the Moxifloxacin and Sertraline, these are two new drugs for her which she has never taken before. Approximately 1 hour later, she noted lightheadedness and lay down the floor, subsequent associated tightness in her throat and a global red rash migrating from her feet. Minimal shortness of breath, denies nausea or vomiting. Denies any chest pain, palpitations, diaphoresis, fever, bruising, abdominal pain. She has never had a reaction like this before.

PMH: HTN, HLD, depression, anxiety
PSH: Cholecystectomy, total abdominal hysterectomy, tonsillectomy
Allergies: Phenobarbital, Paroxetine, Naproxen
Medications: Bupropion, Propranolol, Atorvastatin

Vitals:

Time	Temp (F)	Pulse	Resp	Syst	Diast	O_2	Sat O_2%
23:20	96.9	75	16	73	27	99	4L NC (89% on RA)

CONSTITUTIONAL: Well-appearing; well nourished; A&O X 3, she is drowsy but responds appropriately and will sit up for lung sounds without assistance.
EYES: PERRL
NOSE: Normal nose; no rhinorrhea.
THROAT: Normal pharynx with no tonsillar hypertrophy.
NECK: Supple; non-tender; no cervical lymphadenopathy.
CARDIO: Regular rate and rhythm, no murmurs, rubs or gallops.
RESP: Normal chest excursion with respiration; breath sounds clear and equal bilaterally; no wheezes, rhonchi, or rales.
ABD: Non-distended; non-tender, without rigidity, rebound or guarding.
SKIN: Normal for age and race; warm and dry; diffuse global red rash non-raised, blanching consistent with an allergic reaction.

MDM (23:30): Patient with likely allergic reaction to Sertraline and will treat.

Author comments (Weinstock):

She doesn't look *too* bad... documented as "well-appearing and A&OX3." However, there is also documentation as to her being "drowsy." She is initially placed in a low acuity room, but moved quickly to a trauma/major medical room. Review of the vitals reveals two extremely concerning findings: room air hypoxemia and significant hypotension. We are standing in the footsteps of the emergency physician at the bedside. We are at decision point A:

DECISION POINT A – YOU ARE FACED WITH 4 QUESTIONS:

1. **What are the differential diagnosis considerations in this patient? What is the gold standard for diagnosing anaphylaxis?**
2. **What is the most likely medication to have caused the anaphylaxis?**
3. **What are the initial therapeutic medication options for anaphylaxis?**
4. **Should we proceed with intubation at this time?**

What does the literature say?

Q#1: What are the differential diagnosis considerations in this patient? What is the gold standard for diagnosing anaphylaxis?

Now that we have pieces of information from the initial PMD visit as well as the initial ED evaluation, we can start to put the pieces together and develop a differential. Though the diagnosis seems obvious, it is still important to start with a wide differential and then to narrow as we receive more information in order to minimize cognitive biases.

In this case, we are limited by the lack of information from the initial PMD visit, but we do know that the patient presented with cough, rhinorrhea, and sinus pain for 2 days. Although we do not have vital signs or the physical examination, important diagnoses to consider at that visit include headaches, orbital cellulitis, pneumonia, or influenza.

Upon the patient's arrival to the ED, we notice that the patient is hypotensive, hypoxic, short of breath, and mildly tachypneic. The differential is wide, including anaphylaxis, pulmonary embolism, sepsis secondary to an infection like pneumonia or sinusitis, acute coronary syndrome, pneumothorax, pericardial tamponade, anemia, foreign body aspiration, hereditary angioedema, carcinoid reaction, asthma, or even anxiety. The job of the ED physician facing a critically ill patient is to narrow the list down quickly.

In this patient, the diagnosis seems to be pretty obvious. The patient took 2 pills, and about an hour later, she developed a rash and shortness of breath. Classic story for an allergic reaction. Is it enough to make the diagnosis and start management?

The signs and symptoms of allergic reaction and anaphylaxis are extremely varied, making it difficult to clinically diagnose, and difficult to differentiate from other diagnoses. Symptoms that we classically consider "pathognomonic" for allergic reactions or anaphylaxis, such as urticaria and angioedema, only occur in 60–90% of patients.[2] The absence of cutaneous findings, therefore, does not rule out anaphylaxis. In fact, in some studies, the presence of cutaneous findings appears to be inversely proportional to the severity of the anaphylaxis.[1]

Because of the difficulties in diagnosis and resultant undertreatment, a multidisciplinary group published diagnostic criteria for anaphylaxis in 2005, which were then updated in 2015 by the Anaphylaxis Practice Parameter Workgroup, part of the Joint Task Force on Practice Parameters. Even with these diagnostic criteria, the diagnosis of anaphylaxis is still difficult to make, especially in atypical presentations.

Anaphylaxis is considered highly likely in the following patients where symptoms occur rapidly (minutes to hours) following exposure to an allergen:[4]

1. Cutaneous (e.g., urticaria or pruritus) or mucosal (e.g., swollen lips or tongue) involvement AND at least one of the following:
    a. Respiratory compromise (e.g., wheezing, hypoxemia, dyspnea or stridor)
    b. Hypotension or signs of end-organ dysfunction (e.g., syncope or incontinence)
2. Two or more of the following after a likely allergen:
    a. Cutaneous or mucosal involvement
    b. Respiratory compromise
    c. Hypotension or signs of end-organ dysfunction
    d. Persistent GI symptoms (e.g., vomiting or abdominal cramps)
3. Hypotension in patients after exposure to known allergens.

It is best to keep things simple. As it is hard to recall the exact diagnostic criteria when caring for a crashing patient, instead, just remember that patients with compromise to airway, breathing, or circulation, after a known exposure, should be considered to have anaphylaxis and be treated accordingly.

Our patient took 2 pills (it is unclear if these are likely or known allergens for her), and within hours, developed cutaneous symptoms (urticarial rash), respiratory compromise (shortness of breath, hypoxia), and hypotension. This constellation of symptoms should prompt the diagnosis of anaphylactic shock.

Q#2: What is the most likely medication to have caused the anaphylaxis?

Classic anaphylaxis requires a prior exposure for the patient to develop sensitization, and the subsequent reaction is mediated through immunoglobulin (IgE) antibodies. However, many anaphylactic-like reactions occur without prior sensitization and without IgE antibodies; these occur secondary to direct mast cell releasers and were termed anaphylactoid reactions. In 2003, the World Allergy Organization (WAO) removed this term, because regardless of the mechanism, the treatment for anaphylactic reactions is the same.[2] Instead, the WAO came up with immunologic anaphylactic reactions (patients develop anaphylaxis to medications they were previously exposed to) and non-immunologic anaphylactic reactions (patients develop anaphylaxis to medications they have never taken).

It is often difficult to determine the specific trigger leading to anaphylaxis. For our patient, it seems that Moxifloxacin and Sertraline were new medications for the patient; there was inconsistent documentation about previous medication exposure.

Anaphylaxis to fluoroquinolones can occur due to both immunologic and non-immunologic responses.[7] Moxifloxacin is chemically different from other quinolones, but there may be a high degree of cross-reactivity.[8] It is possible that our patient took a different fluoroquinolone in the past, become sensitized, and subsequently developed an immune-mediated anaphylactic response after taking Moxifloxacin this time. There have also been multiple case reports of patients with non-immunologic anaphylactic reactions to taking fluoroquinolones, including Moxifloxacin, after a single dose; this is noted in the package insert.

There is limited data looking at anaphylaxis to Sertraline; the packaging insert states that allergic reactions are extremely rare. Anaphylaxis to Sertraline is likely to be secondary to a delayed immunologic response, as it takes a few weeks for the body to develop antibodies to it. However, there was one case report that found possible cross-reactivity between Sertraline and Paroxetine.[9] Our patient had an unknown allergic reaction to Paroxetine in the past. It is therefore possible that she developed antibodies to Paroxetine and then had an immune-mediated anaphylactic response after taking Sertraline this time.

While we may never discover which medication triggered this anaphylactic reaction, clinically, it does not affect the management. It does, however, highlight the importance of appropriately prescribing based on the diagnosis, interactions, and reactions to previous similar medications.

Q#3: What are the initial therapeutic medication options for anaphylaxis?

There are numerous guidelines regarding the treatment of anaphylaxis, but many provide conflicting data and are limited by lack of evidence and lack of high-quality studies.[10] Traditionally, we are taught that the treatment options for anaphylaxis are corticosteroids, antihistamines, and epinephrine, but in a crashing patient, epinephrine is the immediate "go-to" drug. Whereas corticosteroids and antihistamines can be considered, the onset of action is not fast enough to prevent respiratory or cardiovascular compromise.[2] Surprisingly, corticosteroids and antihistamines are more frequently administered than epinephrine.[11]

Epinephrine has maximal effect within minutes of administration and targets multiple receptors involved in anaphylaxis.[12] The alpha-effects of epinephrine cause peripheral vasoconstriction, thereby reducing hypotension and angioedema. The beta-effects increase bronchodilation and suppress mediator release from mast cells and basophils.[13]

Epinephrine can be administered a few different ways, from subcutaneous (SQ) to intramuscular (IM) to intravenous (IV). Simons, et al. found in a prospective, randomized study in 2001 that plasma epinephrine concentrations were significantly higher after IM administration into the thigh vs. SQ administration into the arm.[14] Therefore, the current guidelines recommend IM dosing every 5–15 minutes if the initial response is inadequate.[15] In the U.S., the recommended dose is 0.01mg/kg, with a maximum dose of 0.5mg. In Europe, the dosing may be as high as 1.0mg. However, no comparative trials have been conducted to establish optimal dosing.[16]

Epinephrine is available in multiple different concentrations. It can be given via different routes and is dosed differently based on the clinical context. IM epinephrine has been shown to be safe from cardiovascular complications for the elderly population.[17] When given at the correct doses, epinephrine is safe. Most dosing errors occur in emergent situations: for example, it can be under-dosed in cardiac arrest and overdosed in IV administration for treatment of anaphylaxis.[18]

Corticosteroids down-regulate the late-phase inflammatory response.[11] They help mitigate the symptoms in anaphylaxis and can prevent recurrence of symptoms in cases of biphasic anaphylactic reactions. In the case of an acute anaphylactic reaction, the onset of action for corticosteroids is too slow to have any beneficial effect on a patient's emergent clinical status. In addition, there are no high-quality studies to support the use of corticosteroids in the acute management of anaphylaxis.[11] Corticosteroids are frequently prescribed to prevent subsequent reactions, but their use is not associated with decreased recurrence.[19]

Antihistamines inhibit mediator release from mast cells and basophils. They may be useful for mild symptomatic relief, such as pruritus and urticaria, but they have no role in treating the respiratory or cardiovascular symptoms of anaphylaxis. The onset of action is too slow to have any beneficial effect in a crashing anaphylactic patient. There are no high-quality studies to support the use of antihistamines in the treatment of anaphylaxis.[10] An additional consideration is that they are sedating —do we really want to administer to a patient who is already drowsy?

Q#4: Should we proceed to intubation at this time?

Airway edema in anaphylaxis are often rapid and unexpected. In patients with stridor and/or tongue or uvular swelling, immediate airway protection is crucial. Our patient, on the other hand, is hypoxic and sleepy, but not stridulous. While these are concerning symptoms, it is reasonable to treat the patient with oxygen and epinephrine to see if she will improve. It is also critical to monitor closely for worsening symptoms, as there is dynamic airway obstruction in anaphylaxis, and she is still at high risk for impending airway compromise. This is not the time to grab a bite in the cafeteria—check back at the bedside within a few minutes to make sure she has received the epi and to monitor response to treatment and progression of symptoms.

Performance of an upper airway endoscopy may be beneficial in establishing the presence or absence of airway edema. Patients with anaphylaxis are high-risk intubations; not only do they decompensate rapidly, but the airway edema present may make the intubation exceedingly difficult. Mobilizing resources early is key; early airway protection may even be beneficial.[20] The two most common reasons for mortality in anaphylaxis are delays in intubation and delays in epinephrine administration.[20] You are more likely to be criticized for delaying airway management than intervening too early.

Consulting editor comments (Weingart):

When the patient has a huge obstructed airway but they're breathing fine, talking fine, and swallowing fine (this is your prototypical angioedema case), we usually watch them. We've had good success with that, but we are prepared to perform a surgical airway. If you're not prepared to perform a surgical airway, then you need to intubate these patients much sooner.

If you look at and feel the patient's neck and there's nothing there and that makes you tentative, maybe you should send this patient for an earlier operating room intubation, especially if you're not comfortable with doing fiberoptic video bronchoscopy; but most of these angioedema patients are benign. They have a huge swollen uvula or tongue and they do just fine. I think—and this is not standard of care, this is just me making some statement from my personal opinion—that you should not be managing airways in emergency medicine unless you can perform a surgical airway. You don't have to be comfortable with the idea, but you need to get the job done and can't wait for anyone. If you're waiting for someone to perform a surgical airway, then you shouldn't be intubating.

DECISION POINT A – ***What did the actual provider do?***

MDM (23:30): Patient with likely allergic reaction to Sertraline and will treat with IVF 2L NS bolus, Epinephrine 0.3mg IM, Diphenhydramine 50mg IVP, Famotidine 40mg IV, Glucagon 1mg, and Dexamethasone 10mg IV. The patient is on the cardiac monitor and pulse oximeter and is sleepy, but not confused and is able to follow commands. Her blood pressure is low, and I expect this to improve with the IV fluids.

Discussion: There is immediate recognition and concern for severe allergic reaction and initiation of treatment with appropriate medications. The diagnosis is recorded as allergic reaction, but identifying this as anaphylaxis may be key in highlighting the acuity of this patient and mobilizing more resources. There is no documentation of consideration of other potential diagnoses. The provider thought the allergic reaction/anaphylaxis was secondary to Sertraline. Moxifloxacin was not considered to have been the cause. The provider's management is directed to the patient's most likely diagnosis, with 2L NS boluses, epinephrine, diphenhydramine, famotidine, glucagon, dexamethasone.

The story continues (23:36): The nurse is unable to start the IV so finds a tech who is good with the ultrasound. While they are attempting to find the vein, the monitor alarms, as the pulse ox has dropped to 88%, even with 4L oxygen per nasal cannula. The nurse calls respiratory who places a non-rebreather mask with minimal improvement in the oxygen saturation to 91%. The nurse calls you into the room.

(23:38): Checking in on the patient, her mental status has now decreased; the patient is now able to answer only simple questions and is difficult to arouse. After multiple attempts, a left AC 18g IV is established. Heart rate transiently drops into the 40's, then improves. Her repeat vital signs are:

Vitals:							
Time	Temp (F)	Pulse	Resp	Syst	Diast	O2	Sat O2%
23:38		106	36	110	palp	91	NRB

Author comments (Weinstock):

Her condition is worsening. We are back in the shoes of the emergency physician. We are at decision point B.

DECISION POINT B – YOU ARE FACED WITH 4 QUESTIONS:

1. **With the declining mental status and severe tachypnea, are different medications indicated?**
2. **Which airway adjuncts should be considered? How would a CO_2 monitor benefit care? Is intubation indicated now?**
3. **If peripheral access is difficult to obtain, what other options are available?**
4. **Which medications should be used for induction and paralysis for intubation?**

What does the literature say?

Q#1: With the declining mental status and severe tachypnea, are different medications indicated?

It is unclear whether our patient received the initial order of IV medications as there was difficulty obtaining IV access. It is also unclear if she received further rounds of IM epinephrine. Her worsening clinical status may be due to inadequate treatment or due to overwhelming anaphylactic response. Regardless, the immediate treatment is the same as this patient is critically ill.

In refractory anaphylaxis, the guidelines support continued administration of crystalloids, administration of vasopressors, and airway management.[15] Large volume replacement with crystalloids should be administered in patients with distributive shock. Supplemental oxygen and inhaled beta-agonists may help combat hypoxia and bronchospasm.[21,22] In patients who remain hypotensive or are refractory to multiple rounds of IM epinephrine, IV epinephrine should be used.[18] Start with an infusion of 5–20mcg/min and titrate up as needed.

While setting up the IV epinephrine drip, consider using push-dose epinephrine. While push-dose epinephrine has not been well studied, it may be an important bridge to epinephrine infusion as the drip is being readied. Push-dose epinephrine can be created by adding 100mcg of cardiac epinephrine (1mL of the 1:10,000 crash cart epinephrine) to 9mL of saline, achieving a concentration of 10 mcg/mL. Administer 5–20mcg every 1–5 minutes and titrate to response.[23]

Additional vasopressors can be considered in refractory anaphylactic shock, especially when both epinephrine and fluids are not effective. Epinephrine should be at maximal dose prior to initiation of other vasopressors. There is no systematic review with evidence-based medicine to support the use of other vasopressors, but multiple international guidelines do support their use, specifically dopamine and vasopressin.[21]

In refractory cases of anaphylaxis not responsive to epinephrine, glucagon can also be given, especially in patients who are on beta-blockers. Glucagon was given by the provider in this case, likely because the patient was in refractory anaphylactic shock and because she was on propranolol at home. Glucagon has both inotropic and chronotropic effects, by directly activating adenyl cyclase and by bypassing the adrenergic receptors. However, the clinical evidence for the use of glucagon in anaphylaxis is limited to case reports only.[21]

Methylene blue has also been proposed as an adjunctive agent for the treatment of refractory anaphylaxis. Methylene blue is thought to work by increasing peripheral vascular resistance through inhibition of guanylyl cyclase and nitric oxidase synthase activity, thereby decreasing histamine-mediated vasodilation.[24] Data on methylene blue in anaphylactic shock is limited to case reports.

Q#2: Which airway adjuncts should be considered? How would a CO_2 monitor benefit care? Is intubation indicated now?

Continued deterioration in both respiratory and hemodynamic parameters clearly indicates the need for airway management. The patient has become more somnolent and hypoxic, and while there is no documentation of stridor or angioedema, it can be safe to assume that the patient's anaphylaxis is rapidly worsening. Airway obstruction in these patients is dynamic and further delays in controlling the airway are likely to complicate intubation.

Patients should be maximally resuscitated prior to intubation, as preceding hypoxia or hypotension can lead to peri-intubation arrests.[25] This requires pre-oxygenation and vascular access to provide medications like fluids and vasopressors. There is a balance between resuscitation prior to intubation and delaying intubation, as the dynamic airway obstruction in anaphylaxis can lead to decreased first-pass intubation success.

While setting up for definitive airway management, an adjunctive therapy to bridge this patient to endotracheal intubation is non-invasive positive pressure ventilation (NIPPV). Bilevel positive airway pressure (BiPAP) or continuous positive airway pressure (CPAP) are great tools, especially in patients who cannot achieve acceptable oxygen saturations with high FiO_2 alone.[26] Though dogma teaches that we should not place NIPPV in an altered patient for fear of vomiting and aspiration, it is a safe intervention during directly monitored pre-oxygenation for endotracheal intubation. Preoxygenating adequately is key to first-pass intubation success, especially in critically ill patients who are at high risk for hypoxemia.[26] Laryngeal mask airway (LMA), nasopharyngeal, or oropharyngeal airway can be considered but should be used cautiously as they may not help in patients with developing airway edema or obstruction.

What is the difference between pulse oximetry and capnography? Pulse oximetry determines the amount of oxygen-rich vs. oxygen-poor hemoglobin in the blood (oxygenation status). Capnography, on the other hand, measures the expired carbon dioxide levels (ventilation status). In multiple studies, capnography has been shown to be superior as it immediately reflects the presence of apnea, whereas pulse oximetry will show an elevated level of oxygen saturation for a few minutes even when the patient is apneic.

Section editor comments (Emlet):

I agree, except with anaphylaxis that desaturates. That suggests upper airway or glottic occlusion with impending airway complete closure necessitating subglottic access. I disagree that any trial of non-invasive ventilation should be used, except as an adjunct for preoxygenating while preparing to fiberoptic intubate or with video laryngoscopy (VL) or direct laryngoscopy (DL). Use the biggest airway adjuncts including fiberoptic awake intubation, gum bougie/intubating stylet, or VL, with cricothyroidotomy back-up.

Consulting editor comments (Weingart):

Refractory anaphylaxis is scary. Start by thinking about how they are refractory.

- Is it simply by blood pressure? If so, then consider adding in other agents. Vasopressin has been mentioned in the literature. There are also crazy agents like methylene blue, which has some putative help in potentiating the effects of epinephrine. Extracorporeal membrane oxygenation is an option if available.
- Now the airway side is the other part. The decision about when to pull the trigger for intubation is dependent on your comfort level once the patient becomes stridulous. At this point, if they don't turn around immediately with your epinephrine, they should probably get a tube.

Q#3: If peripheral access is difficult to obtain, what other options are available?

Obtaining access is an important step in management. However, there were multiple attempts at placing a peripheral IV which delayed the delivery of critical medications (i.e., IV epinephrine). Placing an ultrasound-guided IV takes time, and may cause unnecessary delay; in this case, our patient did not have peripheral access until almost 40 minutes after arrival. During resuscitation, peripheral intravenous access can be difficult to achieve due to vasoconstriction, and central venous access may be too time-consuming.[27] Alternatively, an intraosseous line (IO) should be considered in critically ill patients. Obtaining IO access is quick and any medication that can be given intravenously can also be given intraosseously;[21] it is an efficient bridging method to stabilizing patients during resuscitation prior to securing central venous access. These authors recommend at most 2 simultaneous attempts at peripheral IV placement. If these attempts are unsuccessful, placement of an IO should be performed.

Q#4: Which medications should be used for induction and paralysis for intubation?

In this patient, who is already hypoxic despite being on a non-rebreather and who likely has significant airway edema from anaphylaxis, we should consider options other than rapid sequence intubation (RSI). While this may seem like blasphemy, paralysis in this situation can be potentially harmful, with loss of airway tone turning partial airway obstruction into complete obstruction. An awake intubation, on the other hand, does not cause paralysis and can allow for reduction of apnea time.

The decision to proceed with an awake intubation is difficult, requiring insight that the airway will be difficult and asking for help. Awake intubation occurs while the patient is spontaneously breathing without removing spontaneous respirations or airway reflexes. It can be useful where a difficult airway is anticipated. Maintaining spontaneous breathing means the apneic time is eliminated and the patient may maintain their oxygen saturation longer. However, because the airway reflexes are present, vomiting and aspiration can occur in response to laryngoscopy.

Ketamine is an ideal medication to use in an awake intubation, as it allows for sedation and analgesia, without taking away spontaneous respirations. After giving Ketamine, the patient can be endotracheally intubated or fiberoptically intubated, and once the endotracheal tube is seen to pass the cords, a paralytic agent can then be given. Ketamine can begiven to achieve analgesia (0.1-0.3 mg/kg), partial dissociation (0.4-0.8 mg/kg), or full dissociation (>0.7 mg/kg) (Strayer). In awake intubations, the full dissociative dose should be given; this allows the patient to be awake, but not aware. Partial dissociation should be avoided as patients will still be aware of their surroundings, and become agitated and difficult to control. Ketamine should be given slowly (over at least a minute) as it can cause apnea if pushed too quickly as an IV bolus.

If a patient is unstable, or having rapidly worsening hypoxia where an awake intubation is not possible, then laryngoscopy and with a surgical airway back-up can be attempted. In this more emergent situation, traditional RSI may be used, optimizing the chances of first-pass success, but requiring preparation for an emergency cricothyroidotomy if the first attempt fails.

If RSI medications are necessary, a hemodynamically neutral induction agent, such as Etomidate or Ketamine, is best. In patients who are in shock, peri-intubation hypotension can lead to increased risk of cardiopulmonary arrest (Heffner). Multiple studies have shown that Etomidate results in hemodynamic stability, even in hypovolemic patients or patients with limited cardiac reserve (Oglesby). Regardless of the induction agent selected, many experts advocate for a half-dose, as critically ill patients may exhibit dramatic changes in their hemodynamics. Paralytics are output-dependent; in patients who are in shock, higher doses of the paralytic may be required.

DECISION POINT B – ***What did the actual provider do?***

(23:48): In addition to the initial meds, the physician also orders Lasix at 20mg IVP as well as a DuoNeb and an epinephrine drip starting at 1mcg/min. Additional glucagon 1mg is administered x 3 as well as sodium bicarbonate. She is started on antibiotics with levofloxacin (Levaquin) and azithromycin (Zithromax). The epinephrine drip is increased to 2mcg/min. BiPAP is ordered, but the oxygen saturation stays in the low 90's.

Chest x-ray: A stat portable CXR is ordered which shows "extensive density in the left lung and central right lung. Appearance is that of extensive pulmonary edema." Labs begin to return:

Lab		Result	Reference range
WBC		5.3 K/uL	4.6 -10.2
HGB	H	16.2 G/DL	12.0-16.0
PLT		331 K/uL	142-424

Repeat vitals show:

Vitals:

Time	Temp (F) Rt.	Pulse	Resp	Syst	Diast	O2	Sat O2%
23:48		102	24	54	palp	91	BiPAP

(23:48) The physician gowns and drapes and places a right femoral central line.

MDM (00:58): Upon presentation, the patient was in anaphylactic shock. She did not respond to subcutaneous epinephrine, likely because she is on a beta blocker, and she became more bradycardic and more hypotensive. She received IV epinephrine and was moved to the trauma bay. We gave IV glucagon and started an epinephrine drip. No response. She became increasingly short of breath and developed pulmonary edema. At this point, I did discuss with the intensivist and he agreed that intubation was needed.

MDM (01:12): Patient received etomidate 20mg and succinylcholine 100mg, and I made three attempts orally without success. Anesthesia called stat to the ED after the second attempt. They also tried several times, unsuccessfully. We tried blind nasotracheal without success and I also tried a blind attempt with the bougie, also unsuccessful.

Chaplain (01:05): "Provided support in trauma room to patient's husband. They have been married for ten years. There are no family members here in town. Patient's mother lives 1 1/2 hours away, but her husband has called her to inform her of the status of the patient. Husband states he has done medic work and understands her condition, but how difficult it is when it is someone close to you."

Additional tests return:
ABG: 7.24/40/43/16

Lab	**Result**	**Reference range**
NA L	134	MMOL/L 136-145
K L	3.3	MMOL/L 3.6-5.1
CL	102	MMOL/L 98-107
AGAP	7.0	MMOL/L 6.0-18.0
CO_2	25	MMOL/L 22-32
BUN	20	MG/DL 8-20
CREAT	0.9	MG/DL 0.6-1.3
GLUC H	166	MG/DL 70-110

Author comments (Weinstock):

This is not your typical case; much was handled well, but difficulties were encountered, specifically the lack of ability to intubate. Where do we go from here? We are at decision point C:

DECISION POINT C – YOU ARE FACED WITH 3 QUESTIONS:

1. **When initial intubation is unsuccessful, what are the next steps?**
2. **How should hypotension be managed?**
3. **Is cricothyroidotomy indicated?**

What does the literature say?

Q#1: When initial intubation is unsuccessful, what are the next steps?

In a patient with anticipated difficult airway, always have a plan, a back-up plan, another back-up plan, and verbalize these plans so that all providers are on the same page. When an initial intubation unsuccessful, it is important to use an alternative approach, such as switching from direct laryngoscopy to video laryngoscopy or from one operator to another.[30]

Multiple attempts at endotracheal intubation can lead to decreased success rates.[31] This may be due to a variety of reasons, including blood in the airway from direct trauma, increased stress of the operators, and patients who are less preoxygenated than before. In some cases, an emergent surgical airway may need to be obtained. Another option is to allow the RSI medications to wear off and allowing the patient to spontaneously breathe again, although this may be dangerous in patients who need an airway because they could not initially be oxygenated or ventilated.

Q#2: How should hypotension be managed?

In our patient with anaphylactic shock, the initial vasopressor selected should be properly dosed epinephrine. If a patient is still hypotensive despite optimal epinephrine dosing and aggressive fluid resuscitation, further vasopressors can be considered. In refractory anaphylaxis, many international guidelines support the use of vasopressors, with some recommending dopamine and others recommending vasopressin and others recommending norepinephrine.[21]

In 2010, De Backer performed a randomized, blinded trial comparing dopamine against norepinephrine in undifferentiated shock, and there was no statistically significant difference in the mortality rate,[32] but dopamine was associated with more dysrhythmic events than norepinephrine. A *Cochrane* review in 2016 found no statistically significant differences in mortality outcome in studies comparing different vasopressors.[33]

Q#3: Is cricothyroidotomy indicated?

In patients that cannot be adequately oxygenated or ventilated after multiple attempts at endotracheal intubation, and are already hypoxic, a cricothyroidotomy is necessary to prevent further hypoxia that may lead to cardiopulmonary arrest. In this life-threatening situation, any delay in recognizing the need for an emergent surgical airway may adversely affect the patient's outcome. That being said, it is difficult to make the mental decision to "cut the neck." It is impossible to predict how much hypoxemia a patient can tolerate, and for how long. Do you risk cutting too early when a successful endotracheal intubation is imminent, or do you wait too long, and find the patient in respiratory arrest? There is no algorithm applicable in all situations, the most important consideration is preparation and recognition of signs of impending airway compromise.[34] However, Scott Weingart has proposed CricCon2 as a mental preparation pathway for emergency cricothyroidotomy, with anaphylaxis recommendation at Set or About to Go:[35]

CricCon2

Simplified Cricothyrotomy Alert Posture

@emcrit

Ready (All Patients)	**Discuss/Feel/See Kit**
Set (Difficult Airway)	**Mark/Kit Bedside**
About to Go (Crashing/Hypoxemic)	**Inject/Prep/Open & Set Kit/ Scalpel in Hand**

CricCon2 Chart provided courtesy of Scott D. Weingart, MD, EMCrit Podcast – Critical Care and Resuscitation, https://emcrit.org/emcrit/surgical-airway/

DECISION POINT C – ***What did the actual provider do?***

(02:06): We did let the sedation wear off and her stats were up in the high 80s to low 90s. Anesthesia has been at the bedside and does not feel any further attempts are needed. I again discussed with the intensivist and we will discuss with ENT with the tracheostomy kit at the bedside.

Vitals:

Time	Temp (F) Rt.	Pulse	Resp	Syst	Diast	O2	Sat O2%
02:10		97	16	140	93	100	vent

(02:14): ENT at the bedside
(02:42): Patient is orally tubed with LMA by anesthesia. Patient is then intubated with fiberoptic laryngoscope through the LMA by ENT with a #7 endotracheal tube.
(02:06): Patient remains hypotensive and epinephrine drip is increased to 15mcg/min. Levophed (norepinephrine) has been started.

What was the patient outcome?
The patient was admitted for acute respiratory failure and anaphylactic shock. She remained hypotensive, hypoxic, and became anuric. She was continued on broad spectrum antibiotics for the possibility of aspiration. Patient expired 1 day after admission secondary to multi-system organ failure.

Final hospital impression:
1. Anaphylactic shock
2. Acute respiratory failure complicated by pulmonary edema and likely aspiration
3. Acute hypotension secondary to #1
4. Acute oliguric/acute renal failure secondary to #1 and #2
5. Death

THE LEGAL:

Author comments (Weinstock):

This case proceesed to legal action. It is one of the three cases in this book where we explore legal issues in emergency medicine.

1. Following are salient sections of the deposition of the physician defendant by the plaintiff's attorney and some final questions by the defense attorney. Though the actual deposition is longer, below is the exact documentation, except for a few minor line edits.
2. Next is a risk assessment as compiled by the defense team and presented to the insurance company (the insurance company needs this to assess their own risk in consideration of settlement vs. trial).
3. Commentary by Greg Henry, MD, Former President of The American College of Emergency Physicians (ACEP) Former Professor of Emergency Medicine at the University of Michigan, Former CEO of Medical Practice Risk Assessment, Ann Arbor, MI.
4. The chapter ends with commentary by the plaintiff and defense attorney who participated in a mock trial (a two hour mock trial at The Ohio State University 2018) which was featured on emcrit.org and can be viewed at: http://emcrit.org/emcrit/refractory-anaphylaxis-mock-trial/.

Deposition testimony (actual deposition testimony):

A. How did she present? Are the times documented correlated with when the events occurred?

Plaintiff's attorney to defendant-physician:

Q. Do you know whether or not there was any communication between the EMS people and the hospital?

A. Yes, they called ahead, a few minutes prior. Their phone call said they were bringing in a female that they thought was having a panic attack. She had called complaining of feeling anxious. Their vital signs were normal. She, by her complaints and stable vital signs, was triaged by telephone to our—to Room [xx], which is our psychiatric room, initially. So she started out as a low acuity patient that was felt to be having a panic attack.

Q. Now, do you recall a conversation or are you testifying based upon your review of a record about these conversations with EMS people?

A. What I remember is that I was told somebody took the phone call. The physicians don't answer the squad box. But I remember being told that someone having a panic attack was coming into Room 11. That was the report I was told.

Q. Can you tell me—and please feel free to use the record that's in front of you to tell me when she actually hit the door. When did she arrive at the hospital that night? For example, one of the first times that I saw was 10:58, or 2258. And I don't know if she was there before that.

A. No, she wasn't. I would say that that's within a minute or two. It has to be accurate. I can't find anywhere that says exactly time. The first vital sign reflects that. The EMS report says they're on scene at 2233, that they left their house at 2240, that they were pulling in outside at 2250. So sometime in that interval.

Q. And so do you know from your recall and/or your review of this chart when you first saw this patient?

A. When I first laid eyes on her it was less than 10 minutes after she had arrived. She initially —we were given a phone call saying, you know, again, she was coming in for a panic attack. At that time of day, I'm working with the mid-level provider. This was a patient—we both were very busy, and somebody with stable vital signs coming in complaining of anxiety and a panic attack is very commonly seen initially by a mid-level provider. He saw her very quickly and thought that there was a bit more going on. He notified me of that. And I would say between five and ten minutes later I was at her bedside and we were already starting some interventions.

Author comments (Weinstock):

This is not an unusual way to begin a deposition. After establishing training and employment, the attorney will attempt to clarify portions of the record which are unclear. Next, they look for clarification of the physician's thought process during the initial encounter, if not adequately described in the chart.

B. What was the working diagnosis?

Q. We'll get to this in hopefully a little more detail, but did you make a diagnosis of what it was that caused her to have the distress that brought her to the emergency room?

A. We felt shortly after she had arrived that it was anaphylaxis. She appeared flushed, she complained of shortness of breath, and she was hypotensive. And she had started a new medication, Zoloft, and we were worried about an allergic reaction.

Q. And what was initially ordered?

A. We ordered epinephrine, which is a standard medication for anaphylaxis; Decadron; and Benadryl, an antihistamine; as well as a fluid bolus to try to treat her hypotension.

Q. In her initial vitals, she was hypotensive?

A. Correct. For the—throughout her stay in the ER, she was hypotensive.

Q. Was her heart rate in the normal range?

A. It was. And my feeling from the start on that was a lot of that was probably the fact that she's on a beta-blocker, which prevents any tachycardia.

Q. All right. When you evaluated her, what did you conclude? I see that there's a history and physical note, but I don't know if you made other notes which would have been different from or predated the time that you would have dictate the HPI.

A. Well, you know, my first note was a very late entry, but, you know, it was pretty clear from the moment she got there that she was in anaphylactic shock. Again, she was hypotensive. She appeared a bit flushed. She was complaining of some shortness of breath. And I mean, she had the presentation that was consistent again with profound anaphylaxis.

Author comments (Weinstock):

Making contemporaneous notes, though desirable, is not always possible, especially during a critical care encounter. If making a note later, make sure that it is timed and reflects the events that occurred, and the management strategy of the provider. The provider's notes in this case were good, but some were entered later due to the critical nature of the encounter. The attorney cuts right to the "chase," with a question about an order for a quinolone in the ED–the same class of medication as the Avelox that she was prescribed, with Zoloft, by the primary care provider. Did the ED provider worsen the anaphylaxis with another dose of the offending medication... or was the allergic reaction to the Zoloft, then new medication that was prescribed?

C. What medication caused the anaphylaxis—did the IV levofloxacin ordered by the emergency physician worsen her anaphylaxis?

Q. One of the medications in question in this visit was a medicine she was prescribed the day prior to her emergency visit, Avelox. She had also been started on Zoloft that same visit.

A. Zoloft was an entirely new medication for her. The Avelox was actually a medication she had been on that class of at least three other times and tolerated without problems. But the Zoloft was a completely new medication for her.

Q. And what does that mean to you, looking [back] to the time that you cared for her?

A. During the time in the emergency department? It [didn't] mean a lot at that time, but in hindsight, I think it kind of makes it pretty clear the source of her presumed anaphylaxis.

Q. What was what?

A. The Zoloft.

D. What was done after the initial medications for anaphylaxis failed?

Q. All right. At what point—I'm trying to get a bit of a chronology here. At what point did you consult with other physicians or begin that process of consulting with other physicians?

A. After she had been given two doses of epinephrine and had not responded, she was becoming more short of breath, her blood pressure was not improving. We made a second move from the monitor room to our highest acuity trauma room. At this point, it was pretty clear that, you know, she was in refractory anaphylaxis.

Q. And what time would that have been that that move took place?

A. That was—she had her second dose of—her first dose of epinephrine was around 2312, I believe. And then her second dose was about 10 minutes later, roughly. And she did not respond to that. So at that point, we moved her to the trauma room, and I had asked pharmacy to come to the bedside to mix up an epinephrine drip. This was at around—I believe I called pharmacy to the bedside at around 2320. We started an epinephrine drip because oftentimes even without response to sub-Q epinephrine, an aggressive dosing of glucagon—if you start an epinephrine drip, it's very unusual that it wouldn't respond, although it does happen. So at around 2340 an epinephrine drip had been started. It was started at, I believe, two micrograms a minute. She continued to infuse with that. She was becoming—complaining of a bit more short of breath.

Her sats were dropping a bit. She was not responding to aggressive IV fluid boluses. At this point, I was worried that we may need to discuss the case with the pulmonary critical care specialist because, again, she had, you know, refractory anaphylaxis, although I'm not really sure at that point there were a lot of other interventions to recommend anyway, because it's—the treatment of choice for anaphylaxis is epinephrine, whether it's given sub-Q, IM or—IV titration even trumps both of those.

E. Airway: Why was the decision made to intubate and what difficulties were encountered?

Q. And then what was the conclusion that you and he reached about protecting the airway by the time that call was completed?

A. We did decide that she needed to be intubated. So within a few minutes we set up to do a rapid-sequence intubation.

Q. All right. Is there anything in the record that will tell me when the first attempt was made?

A. The first attempt was made at the time of the administration of etomidate and succinylcholine, which if I remember right, was around 0010, roughly. I'm sorry. 0013 she was given etomidate and succinylcholine.

Q. All right. So an attempt follows that?

A. Yes.

Q. And you were the one that—

A. Yes.

Q. —tried to intubate?

A. Yes. I made three attempts. My standard approach with the first attempt, after she's bagged to a hundred percent, is with a curved blade. I took an attempt with the curved blade. Unfortunately, she had a lot of airway edema. Her anatomy made her airway very challenging.

As we discussed earlier, she had—as we found out later, she had a difficult airway at baseline anyway, but also because of the swelling she had in her airway from her allergic reaction. And then she also at this point was becoming a bit more short of breath as well. So I made an attempt with the curved blade, then the straight blade attempt, and then again with the curved blade. So I tried three attempts with direct visualization with no success. She never became hypoxic through this, though. Her sats never dropped below 90 percent. What's standardly done is you make an attempt you bag up the patient. You make an attempt. When you see you're having difficulty, you have the respiratory therapist watching the pulse ox, and once the pulse ox starts to approach 88, 89, 90 percent, you stop and start bagging. Fortunately, she never had any hypoxia, so she didn't sustain any injury through that.

Q. All right. So present at the time these attempts were made was yourself, the respiratory therapist, correct?

A. Yes.

Q. Were there others?

A. A few nurses. I think there were two nurses there, maybe even three.

Q. And you've mentioned the edema. I don't want to try to limit this. I'm just trying to make sure I get everything here. The edema was one of the main reasons that you felt the intubation was difficult?

A. One of numerous reasons.

Q. All right. I want to get a list from you as to what you believe the [airway] problems were.

A. Her anatomy. I mean, she had a short neck, which makes that difficult. She also, as we found out later, had a big thyroid—or we found out at that time she had a thyroid goiter, and she also had—again, because of the airway edema from the allergic reaction, there was a lot of airway edema. It was difficult to visualize the cords from that.

Q. A short neck was something that's visible just when you look at someone, right? You can tell that I don't have a short neck, right?

A. Yeah.

Q. You knew that she had edema just by looking down her throat; you could see the edema?

A. She had laryngeal edema until I actually took a look with the laryngoscope. That wasn't anything that was known beforehand.

Q. So kind of give me an idea. I know you're in there trying to intubate. I've only seen that stuff on TV, but how long does it take to complete three attempts?

A. Well, she never needed resedated or reparalyzed.

Q. Was she bagged in between?

A. She bagged in between. Succinylcholine has a duration of action of less than 10 minutes, usually five to eight minutes. Some of the things that we found out later in terms of her difficult airway. She actually had had an elective surgery a few years prior and she had a tremendously difficult airway even in a controlled elective setting and that she had to have a semi-awake intubation as opposed to the more standard intubation that would oftentimes be used.

Q. What elective procedure was that, if you recall?

A. I think it may have been a cholecystectomy, but I'm not completely sure.

F. Send in the consultants…

Q. All right. So, obviously, you told someone to call anesthesia.

A. Yes, yes.

Q. Can you tell me what time someone from anesthesia arrived?

A. They were there—that's in the consult note. I don't know where that is in here. Yes. They may have gotten the call around the third attempt. [Around 00:20]. There may have been—I don't remember if they were called after the three attempts were unsuccessful or if I was in the process of the third one. I don't remember which of those two.

Q. Okay. So they were called. So you don't talk to anybody until that person gets there—

A. Correct.

Q.—literally?

A. Correct.

Q. And what, if anything, do you remember talking with [the anesthesiologist] about?

A. In that scenario, you give a brief to-the-point history of why you're asking for their consultation. I briefly told him that it was a patient that was in anaphylactic shock, was not responding to pressors and had increasing oxygen requirements, and then she had airway edema on top of a difficult airway to start with, and I was unsuccessful in getting her intubated.
Q. All right. Now, I understand that he recorded this consult at 02:45?
A. Yes.
Q. But he does record goiter. Do you know how he drew that conclusion?
A. Well, that was where I was going a little bit ago. As things progressed and he made his attempts and were unsuccessful, again, we were able to bag her. She never became hypoxic. She always was—her sats always hovered around 90 or higher. We were able to get a little bit more information from her husband afterwards of, you know, what else could have led to a difficult intubation, if there weren't enough things already, and he also discovered that she had a goiter.
Q. So he offered that to you when you asked?
A. Yes. Well, what I remember is the husband, myself, and the specialist discussing and conferring why we were having a difficult intubation, and that extra piece of information was discovered.
Q. Were you still there when he made his attempts?
A. Yes.
Q. Okay. Did you and he draw any conclusions about what alternatives there were before he started his work?
A. Before he tried to intubate?
Q. Yes.
A. No. It was clear that he still wanted to make an attempt to try to orally intubate the patient.
Q. All right. I'm not sure if he records how many times he tried. Do you have any idea?
A. From what I remember, it was two, but I don't know that he recorded it anywhere. And I'm not sure that that's—
Q. So he's essentially attempting with the same method that you had attempted; is that right?
A. Orally. Direct visualization orally.
Q. That's what you were doing.
A. Yes.
Q. So that was not successful. What do you remember happening when those attempts did not work?
A. The other attempt actually that I had also made during this time was another attempt with a bougie, which is a blind, stiff, rigid catheter that you sometimes can blindly advance into the airway. That catheter will bounce off the rings inside the trachea, if it's in the right spot, and then you can advance the tube. That also was unsuccessful. So that was another method I had tried as well.
Q. So is that a fourth attempt, quote, unquote, because you talked to me about three.
A. Well, that was a—that's not a direct visualization. That's a blind—that's a blind attempt. That one was also made before [the anesthesiologist] had come.
Q. So that was a separate attempt after you had tried the three with direct visualization?

A. Yes, yes.

Q. Go ahead. What else happened, then, between you and he as you were there and you started him watching his work?

A. Once he made the few attempts, she at this point was waking up. She was still hypotensive. She remained hypotensive through all of this.

Q. She is waking up from the succinylcholine?

A. Yes. She was still hypotensive, but she was still oxygenating okay. So it was still clear at this point that her hypotension was a major hurdle. I mean, it never—her blood pressure never came up. We discussed that she needed a crash airway now, which at that point would be a surgical airway. We both felt like she's oxygenating fine now. She was placed on a nonrebreather and then was eventually placed on BiPAP, and that did keep her oxygen level in the low 90s, which is tolerable for a short time, until we can get a definitive airway. In light of the goiter on top of her other difficult anatomy and edema, we felt that we needed to get an ENT involved to discuss a surgical airway. At this point, we called Dr. ENT, and the intensivist and I discussed the case with him.

Q. Okay. When you say it's okay for a short time, can you give me some parameter as to how — what the range would be?

A. As long as you've got someone at the bedside, which at this point we had three physicians at the bedside, watching her and watching her saturations hang in there, I mean, that could be tolerated for, you know, a long time until her airway is definitively controlled, because a saturation of 90, 91, 92 percent is tolerable as long as she's being closely observed.

Q. You said three physicians? I missed one?

A. At this point—the timing of when [the hospitalist] doctor got involved, I don't remember the specifics of, but he was also at this point involved, and the three of us at this point were at the bedside until Dr. ENT came. Dr. ENT got involved because, you know, she was clearly critically ill. He would be the admitting, managing physician, and I wanted him to be involved with what was going on in the emergency department as we were trying to stabilize her blood pressure.

Author comments (Weinstock):

One of the main allegations of the plaintiff is that the airway was not adequately controlled and that contributed to her ultimate demise. Though the issue of a surgical airway has been mentioned, the attorney decides to confront this issue head-on.

G. More on consideration of a surgical airway:

Q. Why wasn't a surgical airway attempted? What happened there? Did you speak with ENT?

A. I spoke with him at length, and we all agreed that her airway needed to be controlled. Again, she was not hypoxic at that point, so it was not anything that she needed a crash surgical airway at that moment. But I discussed with him that I thought that, you know, her airway needs controlled, that she may need a tracheostomy if nothing—if we can't get her intubated orally. Their conclusion was, with her hypotension on top of her goiter, avoiding a surgical airway is probably still the best thing, because with her hypotension, then you attempt a surgical airway on somebody that's still oxygenating well, you could run into big problems with bleeding. A goiter is tremendously vascular, and if we had decided to immediately do a surgical airway on somebody that's still tolerating BiPAP, is oxygenating, is ventilating, you're going to potentially get into more problems than not. Remember right at that point, because she was tolerating BiPAP and was oxygenating fairly [well, we] did not feel like yet another attempt at laying her down and orally intubating her without a surgeon with expertise in surgical airways at the bedside was not appropriate. So he wanted to wait, continue the BiPAP, watch her oxygen saturations closely until ENT got there, and then they would make another attempt.

Q. And you were in agreement with that?

A. Absolutely, because she was not hypoxic, she was ventilating, and her hypotension was still her biggest issue at this point.

Q. All right. Try to give me a little bit more as to the risk of the surgical airway with the goiter. You say the goiter is very vascular.

A. A goiter has—

Q. What are the risks to that procedure with a patient with a goiter?

A. With a goiter, the thyroid is enlarged and is right around the part of the airway that you would be cutting into. It would be very easy to cut into a vessel and you get some tremendous hemorrhage. And on someone that's already extremely hypotensive, the smallest amount of bleeding could put her into a full-blown arrest. It was not worth the risk of cutting into her neck on somebody that is still oxygenating and still ventilating. I would have been less hesitant to make another attempt at putting her down flat and trying to orally intubate her if she had not been so hypotensive. In someone that's that hypotensive and you again try to sedate them, it would be very easy to completely lose the airway, and at that point, then, it would be turned into a crash surgical airway, which, as we just discussed, was the last thing you wanted to do. So we all were in agreement that the hypotension needed to be stabilized because she was still tolerating BiPAP and she was still oxygenating. So, at this point, it was still a hypotension issue. It was not an airway issue.

Author comments (Weinstock):

It all sounds reasonable and this defendant-physician is doing an excellent job answering questions in a cool and logical manner. Still, I am sure they would rather be elsewhere...

H. Do you know what happened to the patient after she left the ED?

Q. Okay. Did you play any role in her care after 2:43 in the morning?

A. No.

Q. Did you have any discussion about what happened to her subsequently with any of the physicians caring for her?

A. No. I had just heard people saying that she wasn't doing well. She was in the ICU for a few days. But I had no direct involvement with anything after she left the ER.

Q. So did you form an opinion from looking at any of this in probability as to what caused her to die?

A. She had refractory anaphylaxis that did not respond to the usual medications. Her blood pressure finally improved near the end of her resuscitation, but it improved 30 minutes before the airway was secured with the intubating LMA. By that time, we had maxed out an epinephrine drip and then started a second vasopressor, which is quite unusual. But she ended up, from the way this looks, went into multi-organ system failure from her refractory and persistent hypotension from her anaphylaxis.

Author comments (Weinstock):

At the end of the deposition, the physician's defense attorney typically has an opportunity to ask questions or to clarify a few issues. Here is that exchange:

I. Did she die because of difficulties with her airway and hypoxemia?

Defense attorney to defendant-physician:

Q. Is it fair to conclude from your testimony—and you mentioned any number of times here today that during this entire process from her arrival until the time she was ultimately intubated that her O_2 sats stayed fine.

A. Absolutely. She also was oxygenating. Her blood gas showed that she was ventilating fine because her CO_2 was okay. She tolerated oxygen saturation of low 90s while everyone was closely tending to her. She tolerated that fine. Her hypotension was her issue. Whether she had been intubated by you on your first attempt, it [would not have mattered]

A. Yeah. [Her oxygenation] was tolerable throughout the entire resuscitation. The intubation was an airway protective issue, and that was the primary reason for it.

Q. Is it fair to conclude from your testimony—and you mentioned any number of times here today that during this entire process from her arrival until the time she was ultimately intubated that her O_2 sats stayed fine.

A. Absolutely. She also was oxygenating. Her blood gas showed that she was ventilating fine because her CO_2 was okay. She tolerated oxygen saturation of low 90s while everyone was closely tending to her constantly. She tolerated that fine. Her hypotension was her issue.

Author comments (Weinstock):

Following is a document commissioned by the insurance company and prepared by the defense firm assessing risk.

I. Theory of the case:

A. Plaintiff:

1. That this patient needed to be intubated by midnight, about an hour after her ED presentation, but was not intubated until almost 3 hours later.
2. That as a result of this, she sustained significant hypoxic damage to her heart and other bodily organs resulting in her death. Additionally, antibiotics (Levaquin and Unasyn) were given which have a known cross reactivity to the Avelox which may have been the cause of her anaphylaxis, thus potentiating or prolonging it.

B. Insured:

1. That this was a case of severe, refractory anaphylaxis, unresponsive to first- and second-line therapies.
2. That multiple onsite consultations were made, and the consensus was that the patient was oxygenating sufficiently such that an emergency surgical airway was not required. Given that the patient had received the antibiotic Avelox twice before, it is unlikely Avelox caused the anaphylactic reaction here, in which case the giving of Levaquin and Unasyn are meaningless.
3. That the patient' s cardiac damage was the result of massive histamine release with a directly injurious effect on the myocardium, compounded by necessary epinephrine administration. That the problem with the patient's blood pressure was not hypoxic myocardial failure, it was rather massive capillary dilation and changes in permeability, both of which, despite administration of fluid and pressors, resulted in vascular instability to the point of collapse which cannot be remedied by control of the airway.

II. Liability evaluation:

A. Overall:

Assume that the trial is one (1) week away and state whether liability against the insured is probable, questionable, doubtful or non-existent. Outline the strengths and weaknesses of all sides of the case. Provide an opinion as to whether the case should be tried against the Insured. Provide an evaluation of the venue, judge and anticipated jury panel. Please answer this hypothetical question: the jury has just returned a verdict against the Insured, why was the case lost?

Assuming, as you require, the trial is one week away, I would have to say liability against Dr. Defendant is questionable to doubtful.

Plaintiff's case is that positive airway control in this refractory anaphylaxis patient was not obtained until about 2:45 AM whereas plaintiff says it should have been obtained shortly after midnight. Plaintiff further alleges that antibiotics administered by Dr. Defendant against the possibility of aspiration pneumonia were potentially cross-reactive to the Avelox which the records document as being the drug thought responsible for the patient's severe anaphylaxis.

It is, in fact, true that intubation was decided upon shortly after midnight on 3-22-08, but was not physically accomplished until about 2 1/2 hours later. It is also true that antibiotics given during the prolonged resuscitation were probably not a great choice under the circumstances. Both of these points will have some jury appeal, at least initially.

On the other hand, it seems to me that the defense has the better side of the case. In the first place, following initial rounds of epinephrine, Benadryl, Glucagon, and Pepcid, including the establishment of an epinephrine drip, all of which happened in the first 55 minutes of treatment, Dr. Defendant appropriately determined that the patient should be intubated, shortly after midnight, on March 26th. This was likely in response to the patient's clinical deterioration and a blood gas result from 2 minutes earlier with a pO_2 of 43.9 and an oxygen saturation of 74%. Dr. Defendant immediately paged anesthesia anticipating a difficult intubation due not only to the patient's anaphylaxis, but also her goiter which, according to the ENT consult, obliterated normal airway landmarks.

The records document Dr. Defendant and Dr. Anesthesiologist making multiple attempts at intubation by various techniques. During this hour, from midnight to 1:00 AM or so, the patient is described as "becoming more pink" with saturations ranging from 89% to 92%. There is little evidence that she was hypoxic from lack of oxygen. There is, on the other hand, much evidence that there was great difficulty in maintaining her blood pressure. This is the story of refractory anaphylaxis which can cause widespread peripheral vasodilation and can also cause extensive third spacing, a condition where fluid from the blood vessels leaks through them into surrounding tissues resulting in edema and drops in blood pressure. That appears to be the primary culprit here as opposed to simple hypoxia.

Oxygen delivery depends upon oxygenation in the blood, but also depends on delivery of it to the tissues. That delivery is reflected by the blood pressure which, in this patient, was low and stayed low despite extensive volume replacement and pressors. Besides calling anesthesia, Dr. Defendant also consulted pulmonology/critical care specialist Dr. Intensivist and also otolaryngologist Dr. ENT who is recorded at the bedside at 2:15 AM. Dr. ENT was, finally, able to place a laryngeal mask airway through which the patient was intubated. This resulted in a change in her oxygen saturation to 97% whereas it had been at 93% on mask ventilation. This is a small improvement.

Plaintiff will suggest that a tracheostomy should have been created early on. This, however, was not the opinion of any of the physicians who emergently consulted on the case for the reason that the patient did not require it. We know the option was on Dr. Defendant's mind because, at 1:15 AM he entered a progress note documenting "anesthesia has been at the bedside and does not feel further attempts (at intubation) are needed.

I again discussed with Dr. Intensivist and we will discuss with ENT with the trach kit at the bedside." Reference to the tracheotomy kit at the bedside tells us that Dr. Defendant was well aware of the surgical option and was prepared to do it should the patient's airway deteriorate and was discussing the subject with his consultants. An additional factor which will have to be considered would include the patient's diffuse goiter and its effect on any attempted surgical procedure in the area. The evidence is that the patient died from acute cardiac and renal failure, with her troponin level going from normal to an impressive 84, hours after admission, with concurrent evidence of acute renal failure. Again, while this may well be hypoxic in origin, it is hypoxia due to failure of the vascular system, not failure to provide oxygen to the lungs.

On the issue of the giving of cross-reactive antibiotics late in the course, there is evidence that this patient had received Avelox in the past without a problem, according to her own history. If this is evidence that Avelox was likely not the problem drug here, then the giving of these antibiotics is irrelevant. If Avelox is the problem, there is no evidence that either of the antibiotics administered was followed by any profound decompensation of the patient.

I believe Dr. Defendant will be given credit for immediately involving anesthesia, then pulmonary critical care, then internal medicine, then ENT, all in an attempt to help this patient. In addition, the management of the patient's anaphylaxis appears to be very much in accordance with published standards calling for subcutaneous or intramuscular, then intravenous epinephrine, steroids, antihistamine, glucagon, gastric acid suppressants, aerosol bronchodilators, vasopressors, and vigorous fluid administration. This patient received all those. She was pretty much unresponsive to all of her treatment, perhaps, in part, because she was a long-term user of beta-blockers which render the body less sensitive to the effects of epinephrine. The only hint of criticism that I discerned from looking at the medical literature on the subject is a minor one. It comes from a small handful of case reports suggesting the use of the alpha-agonist drug Phenylephrine in patients with anaphylaxis who do not respond to multiple doses of epinephrine. This suggestion is not incorporated in either the American or British guidelines on the subject, however.

At this point I believe this is a case that should be tried.

B. Percentage chance for insured to prevail:
Assign a specific estimated percentage chance for the Insured to prevail at trial. Assignment of 50/50 is unacceptable. At this early date and admittedly without benefit of expert review, I would assign a 70% chance of winning.

C. Estimated verdict value:
Provide an estimation of the adverse verdict value for this case. Include an evaluation as to whether punitive or exemplary damages are recoverable for this case in this venue. $1,000,000. I do not believe punitive damages would be either requested or allowed on these facts.

Gregory L. Henry, MD
Former President of The American College of Emergency Physicians (ACEP)
Former Professor of Emergency Medicine at the University of Michigan
Former CEO of Medical Practice Risk Assessment, Ann Arbor, MI

"Saying I'm sorry is not the same as saying I'm guilty."

General:
It's easy being a Monday morning quarterback, but the facts are that we're all hesitant to intubate patients who seem to be functioning reasonably well. For us to say now, that we know exactly what to do and when it should be done, is a bald-face lie.

How the case will be tried:
The plaintiff will handle this case in only one manner and that is to emphasize the phrase. "Too little, too late." But that is a legal strategy, and not an approach which should have changed our approach at the bedside. We could have always done it sooner, we could have always made the decisions faster, but the care here was appropriate. The fact that the patient had taken a medication shortly prior to onset of symptoms, led the providers to believe that this was some sort of allergic or anaphylactic response, but this does not change the medications or approach—it is only the speed with which you act. If I was advising the defense on this case, my advice to the defending physician would be straightforward; use the double D defense: Dedicated Doctor. There is no suggestion here that they did not try their best with multiple and timely administration of medications, recognition of illness, and consultation of specialists. This doctor provided dedicated and excellent care to the patient.

The medicine:
What people forget is that the suffusion of fluid happens at the capillary level. Just because you have a tube in the throat, does not mean that there is not fluid pouring into the lungs. It is likely that even when the patient is sent to the ICU the full effect of the fluid in the lungs had not yet taken place. There's very little to suggest that earlier placement of the endotracheal tube would have changed the outcome.

The legal:
This is the kind of case, however, that places great stress in insurance company executives. You have a relatively young woman, an intact family, and a death. The plaintiff's arguments will tear at the heartstrings of a jury. One of the decisions about settling the case will be to determine the ability of the physician to appear caring and concerned to the jury. The fact that there are multiple physicians involved in the case always makes it more complex. It is helpful that the emergency physician sought advice from anesthesia and pulmonary medicine.

I would agree to be a defense expert on this case:
I would be pleased and proud to be an expert for the defense in this matter. There is little evidence that earlier intubation would have changed the outcome. One can always make up a story, and that's what many plaintiff's experts do. But to say that there is actual proof that there's a difference in the outcome is a lie. As I read the answers to the deposition questions, the physician seems to be honest and straightforward. Assuming that he keeps that demeanor at trial, I would expect that he could easily get a defense verdict. Plaintiffs prefer much simpler cases. When there are many reasonable physicians involved in the care, all trying to do the best they can, it presents a long row for the plaintiff to hoe. To prove that there were violations of the standard of care by the preponderance of the evidence would be very difficult in this case. Is this a bad disease in an otherwise wonderful patient? Yes. Did the physician cause this? No. Saying I'm sorry is not the same as saying I'm guilty.

Author comments (Weinstock):

In 2018, the emergency medicine residencies from Adena Health Systems and The Ohio State University commissioned a mock trial using the facts from this case. Following is an analysis of the legal points by the plaintiff's attorney and defense attorney who participated.

They were not the actual attorneys who were involved with this case. The mock trial can be seen at: https://emcrit.org/emcrit/refractory-anaphylaxis-mock-trial/

LEGAL IMPLICATIONS:

(Discussion by a plaintiff's and a defense attorney)

Defense:
In every medical malpractice case, it is imperative that the medical providers be perceived as credible, competent and compassionate. In most jurisdictions the court and jurors start the process with a favorable opinion of medical providers. The medical providers must take the steps to prove that opinion is well-founded. Jurors want the witnesses to confirm their initial opinion. Confirming the jury's favorable opinion of medical providers is accomplished by thorough preparation for both depositions and trial.

Preparation for depositions must include being prepared to address every potential issue in the case. A deposition is sworn testimony which will be used by the attorneys during the trial to either affirm the jury's favorable opinion or to diminish the credibility of the medical providers and undermine their competence and compassion. Credibility can be diminished if the medical provider testifies differently at trial than in the deposition. Competence can be bolstered or diminished depending on the medical provider's familiarity of relevant literature. Compassion can be bolstered or diminished by the medical provider's demeanor during both the deposition and trial. Medical providers must always "take the high road" in order to maintain the impression of being credible, competent and compassionate.

Julia Turner, Esq.
Medical defense attorney
The Ohio State University
Columbus, Ohio

Plaintiff:
This is a very complex medical malpractice claim for several salient reasons. First, there are many physicians involved and either separately or collectively, they could not save the patient's life even after they provided numerous opinions and attempted vis-à-vis a variety of appropriate procedures, tests, and drugs to alleviate her serious medical issues. A jury will have a difficult time believing that all the physicians/experts were negligent and wrong. Second, it is unclear that there truly was a breach of the appropriate standards of care. For the plaintiff to win, the jury tends to demand proof that the defendant doctors made egregious errors or major mistakes. In other words, a jury is told that the standard relates to professional negligence. However, juries want to be taught or be aware of medical bright lines as to what a physician should or should not do under the circumstances and whether that bright line was breached. That means providing books, treatises, rules, regulations, and other documents that set forth what a physician should or should not do.

If the plaintiff establishes that the defendants breaches a bright line standard, the plaintiff is more likely to win. If there are no bright lines or if the physicians do not violate standards in a significant or obvious way (which in practical terms is more than negligence), juries tend to give the benefit of a doubt to the defendants. Although the law is that the physicians must violate the relevant standards of care and the plaintiff must prove same by a preponderance of the evidence (or a similar standard), juries often conclude that "the doctor did not mean to hurt the patient" and therefore render a verdict for the physician when there are no evident breaches of standard of care. It is important to remember that the vast majority of jury verdicts in the U.S. favor hospitals and doctors.

Third, it also appears that the 47-year-old patient was very sick upon admission. While rare, the patient's problems were life threatening. Thus, even when the team of doctors engaged in aggressive measures, it seems unlikely she would have survived, sadly.

In terms of strategies and tactics, either by good practice or as state law requires most excellent trial attorneys do not or cannot file a Complaint until after consulting with the appropriate medical experts who must review the related chart/autopsy and provide Affidavits (usually Affidavits of Merit) setting forth that the target defendants breached the applicable standards of care and that this breach or those breaches was/were a direct and proximate cause of serious damage or death to the patient. In this case, finding such experts anywhere will not be easy.

Assuming plaintiff's counsel locates such experts, plaintiff's counsel should devise a theme that resonates with lay people/juries. Once counsel creates a theme, depositions of the defendants, nurses and other medical providers must be taken. Counsel should continuously evaluate the case merits as depositions progress.

I would not have taken this case due to the complex medical history, the heroic efforts the doctors made attempting to save the patient's life, and the massive costs (six figures) entailed with hiring experts to testify against a multitude of defendants and all the experts the defense will hire.

Mark Kitrick, Esq.
Plaintiff's attorney
Kitrick, Lewis & Harris Co., L.P.A.
Columbus, Ohio

Chapter summary:

- In anaphylaxis, IM epinephrine is first-line agent for treatment, and takes priority over corticosteroids and antihistamines.
- In refractory anaphylaxis, maximize IV epinephrine dosing and aggressively fluid resuscitate.
- Securing the airway early may increase the chances of first-pass success. Awake intubation should be considered.
- When a patient cannot be intubated, oxygenated, or ventilated, emergent cricothyroidotomy should be performed to minimize the chances of a hypoxic cardiopulmonary arrest.
- Death in anaphylaxis is caused by delay to epinephrine administration and delay to intubation.

References:

1. Bjornsson H, Graffeo C. Improving diagnostic accuracy of anaphylaxis in the acute care setting. West J Emerg Med 2010;9:456-61.
2. Lieberman P, Nicklas RA, Randolph C, et al. Anaphylaxis – A practice parameter update 2015. Ann Allergy Asthma Immunol 2015;115:341-84.
3. Sclar D, Lieberman P. Anaphylaxis: Underdiagnosed, underreported, and undertreated. Am J Med 2014;127:S1-S5.
4. Kim H, Fischer D. Anaphylaxis. All Asth Clin Immun 2011;7:6-S12.
5. Pynnonen MA, Lynn S, Kern HE, et al. Diagnosis and treatment of acute sinusitis in the primary care setting: A retrospective cohort study. Laryngoscope 2015;125(10):2266-72.
6. Rosenfeld RM, Piccirillo JF, Chandrasekhar SS, et al. Clinical practice guideline (update): Adult sinusitis. Amer Acad of Otolaryn 2015;152:S1-S39.
7. Thong B. Update on the management of antibiotic allergy. Allergy Asthma Immunol Res 2010;2(2):77-86.
8. Gonzalez I, Lobera T, Blasco A, et al. Immediate Hypersensitivity to quinolones: Moxifloxacin cross-reactivity. J Investig Allergol Clin Immunol 2005;15(2):146-49.
9. Khairkar PH, Bang GM, Singh AB, et al. Possible cross-sensitivity between sertraline and

paroxetine in a panic disorder patient. Indian J Pharmacol 2010;42(2):110-11.
10. Alrasbi M, Sheikh A. Comparison of international guidelines for the emergency medical management of anaphylaxis. Eur J Aller Clin Immunol 2007;62(8):838-41.
11. Choo K, Simons F, Sheikh A. Glucocorticoids for the treatment of anaphylaxis. Evid Based Child Health 2013;8(4):1276-94.
12. Song T, Lieberman P. Epinephrine in anaphylaxis: Doubt no more. Curr Opin Allergy and Clin Immunol 2015;15(4):323-28.
13. Kemp SF, Lockey RF, Simons FE. Epinephrine: The drug of choice for anaphylaxis. a statement of the World Allergy Organization. Eur J Aller Clin Immunol 2008;63(8):1061-70.
14. Simons FR, Gu X, Simons K. Epinephrine absorption in adults: Intramuscular versus subcutaneous Injection. J Allergy Clin Immun 2001;108(5):871-73.
15. Simons FE, Ardusso LR, Bilo MB, et al. International consensus on (ICON) anaphylaxis. World Allergy Organ J 2014;7(1):9-27.
16. McLean-Tooke, Bethune CA, Fay AC, et al. Adrenaline in the treatment of anaphylaxis: What is the evidence? BMJ 2003;27(7427):1332-35.
17. Kawano T, Scheuermeyer FX, Stenstrom R, et al. Epinephrine use in older patients with anaphylaxis: Clinical outcomes and cardiovascular complications. Resuscitation 2017;112:53-8.
18. Wood J, Traub S, Lipinski C. Safety of epinephrine for anaphylaxis in the emergency setting. World J Emerg Med 2013;4(4):245-51.
19. Grunau BE, Wiens MO, Rowe BH, et al. Emergency department corticosteroid use for allergy or anaphylaxis is not associated with decreased relapses. Ann Emerg Med 2015;66(4):381-89.
20. Tupper J. Anaphylaxis: A review and update. Can Fam Physician 2010;56(10):1009-11.
21. Kemp A, Kemp S. Pharmacotherapy in refractory anaphylaxis: When Intramuscular Epinephrine Fails. Curr Opin Allergy and Clin Immunol 2014;14(4):371-78.
22. Muraro A, Roberts G, Worm M, et al. Anaphylaxis: Guidelines from the European Academy of Allergy and Clinical Immunology. Eur J Aller Clin Immunol 2014;69(8):1026-45.
23. Weingart S. Push-dose pressors for immediate blood pressure control. Clin Exp Emerg Med 2015;2(2):131-32.
24. Lo J, Darracq M, Clark R. A review of methylene blue treatment for cardiovascular collapse. J Emer Med 2014;46(5):670-79.
25. Heffner AC, Swords DS, Neale MN, et al. Incidence and factors associated with cardiac arrest complicating emergency airway management. Resuscitation 2013;84(11):1500-04.
26. Weingart S, Levitan R. Preoxygenation and prevention of desaturation during emergency airway management. Ann Emerg Med 2012;59(3):165-75.
27. Anson J. Vascular access in resuscitation: Is there a role for the intraosseous route? J Amer Soc Anesth 2014;120:1015-31.
28. Strayer R. Strayerisms: Anaphylaxis rebuttal. EM: RAP 2016. Available from: https://www.emrap.org/episode/snakebitesand/strayerisms.
29. Oglesby A. Should etomidate be the induction agent of choice for rapid sequence intubation in the emergency department? Emerg Med J 2004;21:655-59.
30. Apfelbaum JL, Hagberg CA, Caplan RA, et al. Practice guidelines for management of the difficult airway: An updated report by the American Society of Anesthesiologists Task Force on Management of the Difficult Airway. J Amer Soc Anesth 2013;118(2):251-70.
31. Goto T, Gibo K, Hagiwara Y, et al. Multiple failed intubation attempts are associated with decreased success rates on first rescue intubation in the emergency department: a retrospective

analysis of multicentre observational data. Scan J Trauma Resusc Emerg Med 2015;23:5-14.
32. De Backer, Biston P, Devriendt J, et al. Comparison of dopamine and norepinephrine in the treatment of shock. N Engl J Med 2010;362(9):779-89.
33. Gamper G, Havel C, Arrich J, et al. Vasopressors for hypotensive shock. Cochrane Database Syst Rev 2016;2:CD003709.
34. Bonanno F. The critical airway in adults: The facts. J Emerg Trauma Shock 2012;5(2):152-59.
35. Weingart, S. EMCrit Podcast 131 – Cricothyrotomy – Cut to air: Emergency surgical airway. Available from: https://emcrit.org/racc/surgical-airway/.
36. Bloom BM, Grundlingh J, Bestwick JP, et al. The role of venous blood gas in the emergency department: a systematic review and meta-analysis. Eur J Emer Med. 2014;21(2):81-88.
37. Pongdee T. Medications and drug allergic reactions. American Academy of Allergy, Asthma and Immunology. 2017. Available from: https://www.aaaai.org/conditions-and-treatments/library/at-a-glance/medications-and-drug-allergic-reactions.

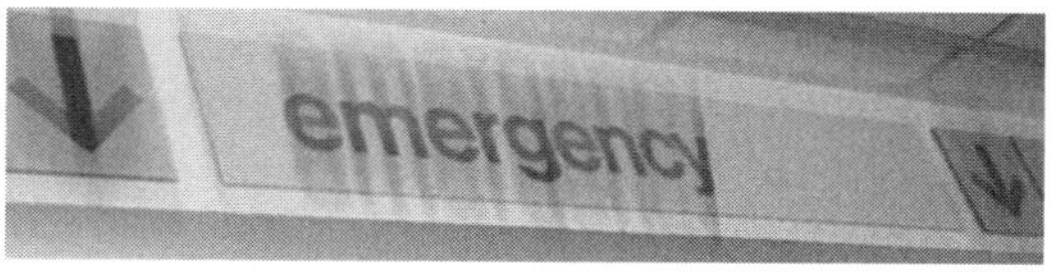

SECTION A – AIRWAY/ARREST

Chapter 5: An 11-month-old child with thrush and lethargy

Ilene Claudius, MD

Associate Professor Clinical Emergency Medicine
David Geffen School of Medicine at UCLA
Los Angeles, CA

Section editor:

Lillian L. Emlet, MD, MS, FACEP, FCCM

Clinical Associate Professor
Depts. of Critical Care Medicine & Emergency Medicine
Associate Program Director
IMCCM Fellowship of the MCCTP
Interim Associate Chief of Staff of Education, VA
University of Pittsburgh School of Medicine
Pittsburgh, PA

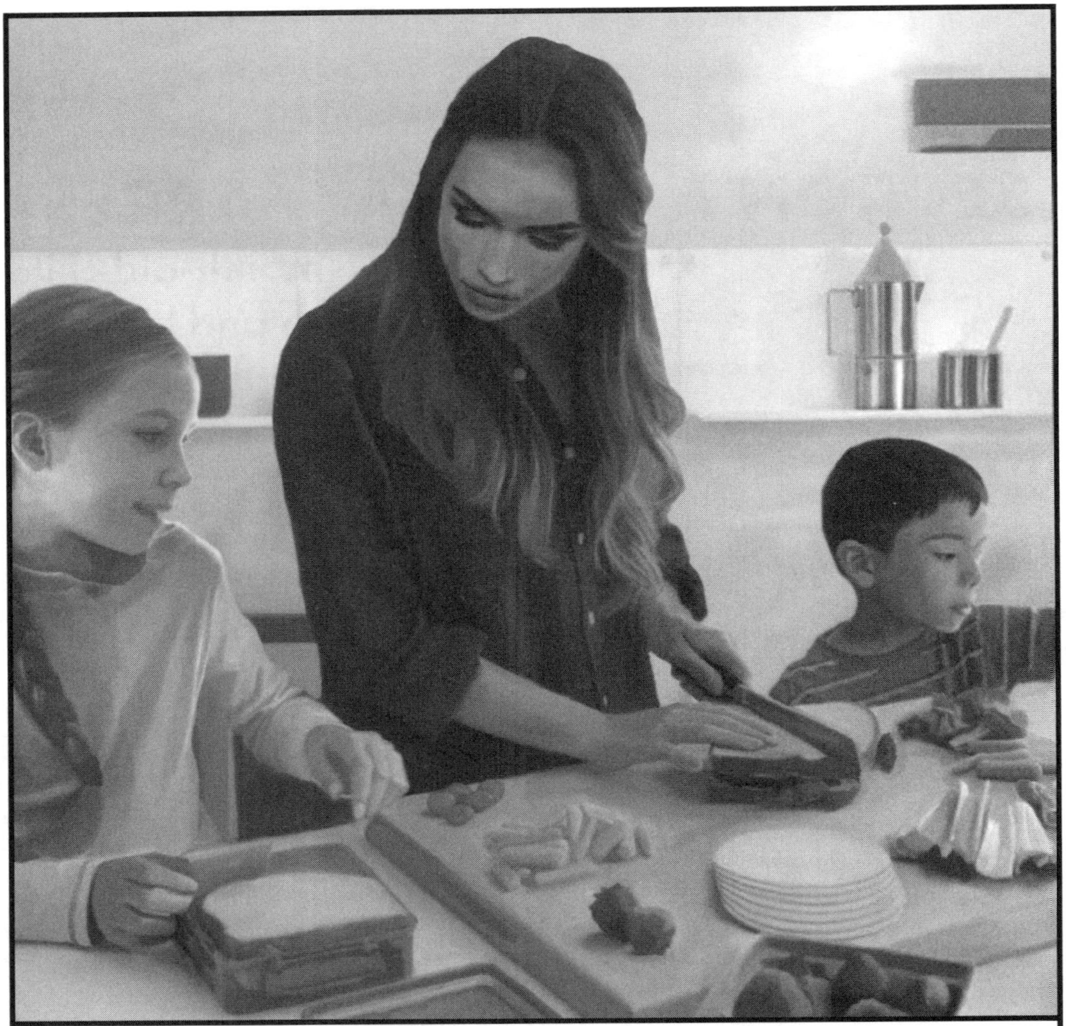

"WHERE'S CODY?"

"I THINK HE'S STILL SLEEPING."

SECTION A/CHAPTER 5

An 11-month-old child with thrush and lethargy

"Lethargy" is one of those inflammatory words in pediatric emergency medicine. I have heard trainees scornfully silenced for merely suggesting that a patient might be lethargic. We've become so focused on not overusing the term "lethargic" that we occasionally lose sight of the fact that some ill children are, in fact, lethargic!

Lethargy can signify many things, but front-line providers must consider sepsis, meningitis, toxins, neuromuscular disorders, severe dehydration, intracranial pathology, derangements of glucose and electrolytes, and intussusception. Sometimes, children with nothing more than a fever or a brief seizure can transiently appear lethargic and recover before any testing is performed, but children with enduring or relapsing lethargy demand evaluation. And, speaking of lethargy, let me introduce you to Cody.

PRIMARY CARE VISIT

Cody is an 11-month-old boy, the youngest of 6 children, being raised by a single mother. Cody was a term vaginal delivery without complications and cared for by the grandmother and other siblings. The family does not have much, subsisting on government aid, but the siblings are close, each pitching in to help with household responsibilities.

On a rare overcast Los Angeles afternoon, the grandmother notices that Cody is less active than usual. The mother is at work, so she calls the primary care clinic and gets an appointment for the same afternoon. Cody's vitals are normal, as is his exam, with the exception that he has bright white bumps on his tongue and buccal mucosa. He is diagnosed with thrush and is placed on nystatin, 4 times a day.

The next morning, with some children on the way to school and the others getting ready, Cody's mother realizes that he is not yet up, and asks his sister to wake him; she finds him still asleep, noticing that a dry diaper and that he does not cry out when moved. Concerned, Cody's sister and mother call to the grandmother, who is helping pack the last school lunch. "Maybe he's just extra tired. Let's try and give him a bottle." The approach is unsuccessful, and after the last child is off to school, they head for the emergency department.

INITIAL ED VISIT

CC (nursing): AMS-fever

HPI: 11-month-old male is brought to the ER by the family for lethargy. The family has noted that the patient was lethargic for 2 days now. Yesterday the patient was lethargic however able to drink and slept throughout most of the day. Today the patient has not woken up at all. Have not noticed any fevers, chills, nausea, vomiting, cough, congestion or shortness of breath. They report 3 days ago as far as they can tell he was healthy. They did report he was diagnosed with thrush yesterday and placed on nystatin. They have not noted any trauma. No fever, rash, additional systems unable to be obtained. I reviewed the nurse's notes.

NKDA
Meds: Nystatin
PMH: Neg
PSH: Neg
FH: No items selected
SH: No items selected

PE:

Vitals:

Time	Temp (F)	Pulse	Resp	Syst	Diast	Sat
18:43	101.2	146	28			97% (RA)

GA: Ill-appearing, Lethargic, not alert, not responsive.
SKIN: Warm, dry, pink, intact.
HEAD: Normocephalic.
NECK: Supple, trachea midline, there is bruising noted on the left anterior neck/chin.
EYE: Sclera anicteric.
CARDIO: Regular rate and rhythm, No murmur, Normal peripheral perfusion, No edema.
RESP: Lungs are clear to auscultation, breath sounds are equal, Respirations: Bradypneic.
CHEST WALL: No tenderness.
GASTRO: Soft, Nontender, Non distended.
NEURO: Posturing noted on the left side of the body. No response to pain on the left arm and leg. The patient did withdraw on the right arm and right leg. Right pupil is blown and nonreactive. Approximately 7 mm. Left pupil is 3 mm, nonreactive.

Author comments (Weinstock):

What is more critical than an unresponsive 11-month-old? Rapid action while concurrently considering possible etiologies is required of the team leader. You are in the footsteps of the EP, at the beside; you are at Decision Point A:

DECISION POINT A – YOU ARE FACED WITH 3 QUESTIONS:

1. **What is the differential diagnosis?**
2. **Is immediate intubation warranted?**
3. **What are other initial steps for the ED physician to take?**

What does the literature say?

Q#1: What is the differential diagnosis?

Short of an eye surgery, direct eye injury, or accidental eye exposure to an anticholinergic or sympathomimetic substance (e.g. ipratropium splash during asthma treatment), a unilaterally blown pupil typically means uncal herniation with resultant traction on the 3rd cranial nerve. The cause of this herniation, however, will require further investigation to guide management.

- Meningitis and encephalitis are leading causes of stroke in childhood; resultant edema from cortical ischemia can lead to herniation.
- Brain tumors peak at 7–8 years, but there are some which occur in infants.
- AV malformations can bleed and cause rapid neurologic decompensation.
- While there is no history of trauma, non-accidental trauma could cause a space-occupying bleed or edema.

While these 4 entities might all require similar initial evaluation (CT scan) and management (intubation and hyperosmolar therapy), the secondary management could include antibiotics, surgery, interventional radiology, or children's services consultation.

To round out the list, there are certainly other causes including diabetic ketoacidosis (associated with cerebral edema), but the findings would typically be more diffuse. A seizure (with resultant Todd's paralysis) would be low on the differential for our patient but checking a glucose and electrolytes should be quickly accomplished.

Q#2: Is immediate intubation warranted?

Whereas equally competent providers might make different decisions regarding the timing of intubation and degree of pre-intubation resuscitation required, with our patient, lethargic with a blown pupil, immediate intubation for airway protection is reasonable. Aspiration is less likely in children compared with adults, but Cody may have elevated intracranial pressure which would increase the risk of emesis and may require a subsequent invasive procedure. Though there are a number of non-invasive alternatives for ventilatory support in children, securing the airway early while he is still stable, at least from a cardiovascular standpoint, is wise.

Q#3: What are other initial steps for the ED physician to take?

Given the pupil exam in the setting of an altered patient, rapid treatment for elevated intracranial pressure is also warranted. Hyperosmolar therapy, mannitol or hypertonic saline, should be administered urgently. The Brain Trauma Foundation recommends 3% saline to be given as 6.5–10mL/kg bolus.[1] Other concentrations, most commonly 7.5% and 23.4% saline, have been investigated with similar effectiveness. There does not seem to be a statistically significant mortality or ICP reduction difference between mannitol compared to hypertonic saline; in fact, several pediatric studies indicate superiority of hypertonic saline for lowering ICP at 30, 60 and 120 minutes.

If mannitol is given without adequate response, using hypertonic saline as a rescue medication has been shown effective.[2,3]

Steroids may be helpful if the etiology of the cerebral edema is a malignancy or in the case of meningitis but would be unlikely to benefit our patient. A brain CT should be able to be obtained quickly, and if intracranial hemorrhage is not apparent and a higher suspicion for meningitis or brain mass is entertained, they could be started at that time. Children with traumatic brain injury and GCS < 8 typical undergo placement of an ICP monitor. While monitor placement is out of the purview of most ED physicians, mobilizing appropriate services should be done early.

A coagulopathy is common in head trauma, thus checking and correcting these issues is required if the CT indicates intracranial hemorrhage. Finally, as non-accidental trauma is on our differential diagnosis, the extent of the trauma is unknown. Fatal head injury is most common in infants, but assessing for abdominal injury via FAST, point-of-care hemoglobin, and other laboratories should be done.

What did the actual provider do?

MDM: Patient is presenting with a blown pupil and lethargy. The patient also has a fever while here. I suspect there is an intracerebral injury based on my exam. I suspect the fever is likely related to the intracerebral injury. This could also be potentially meningitis. The findings on exam do indicate a CNS injury of some sort. The patient was brought into our trauma room immediately. My initial exam demonstrates a blown pupil and poor protective reflexes of the airway. His blood glucose initially was low. BL IVs were placed by ancillary staff. We did give him D 25, 2 mL. In addition, we gave him D10, 20 mL. His blood glucose responded without any improve in mental status. We subsequently decided to intubate the patient.

Labs begin to return (19:22):

WBC Count	**20.1 thou/mcL HI**
Hemoglobin	11.3 gm/dL
Platelet Count	291 thou/mcL
Sodium Level	144 mMol/L
Potassium Level	5.0 mMol/L
Chloride Level	**110 mMol/L HI**
Carbon Dioxide Level	**16 mMol/L LOW**
Anion Gap	18.0 mMol/L
Glucose Level	99 mg/dL
BUN	11 mg/dL
Creatinine	0.39 mg/dL
Calcium Total	10.3 mg/dL
Alkaline Phosphatase	149 Units/L

ALT/SGPT	**364 Units/L HI**
AST/SGOT	**89 Units/L HI**
Bilirubin Total	1.2 mg/dL
Bilirubin Direct	0.2 mg/dL
Protein	7.2 gm/dL
Albumin Level	3.8 gm/dL
Bilirubin Indirect	1.0 mg/dL
Prothrombin Time (PT)	**13.9 Sec HI**
INR	1.26
Partial Thromboplastin (aPTT)	33.0 Sec
Lactic Acid Level	1.5 mMol/L
Blood Type ABO and Rh(D)	OPOS

DECISION POINT B – YOU ARE FACED WITH 5 QUESTIONS:

1. **Why is the WBC count so high? Is it because of an intracranial injury as the EP suspects, or should an evaluation for sepsis be pursued?**
2. **What is the approach to pediatric head injury intubation?**
3. **What are common reasons for airway management failure and solutions?**
4. **What should be used for sedation after intubation?**
5. **Was this an acceptable miss by the primary care provider the day prior?**

What does the literature say?

Q#1: Why is the WBC count so high? Is it because of an intracranial injury as the EP suspects, or should an evaluation for sepsis be pursued?

Patients with even minor head injuries can have an elevation in their WBC counts,[4] and greater leukocytosis predicts worse outcomes.[5] However, the literature on the link between trauma and leukocytosis is not robust. In patients with blunt abdominal trauma, several studies have correlated solid organ injury with elevated serum WBCs.[6] As the extent of trauma to Cody is unknown, it may be wise to send liver enzymes (looking for AST or ALT > 80 IU/L) to determine if an abdominal CT is warranted. If clinical suspicion for infection existed, antibiotics would be prudent, but the suspicion shouldn't rest exclusively on the WBC count.

Q#2: What is the approach to pediatric head injury intubation?

Intubating a pediatric patient is comparable to intubating a small adult. The tube size can be calculated using the formula 4+ (age in years/4). This calculates the uncuffed tube size, with a cuffed tube requiring a decrease in size of 0.5–1 to accommodate the cuff. Both straight and curved blades used seem comparable, at least for airway visualization,[7] and a good rule of thumb for blade sizing is to switch from a 1 to a 2 at age 2 years and from a 2 to a 3 in 3rd grade (age 8). There is also a 1.5 size blade (Wis-Hipple®) that is particularly useful in the intubation of toddlers. For this 11-month-old, a size 4 tube and size 1 blade should suffice.

The oral, laryngeal, and pharyngeal axes should be aligned as closely as possible, as in adults, which often requires placement of a thin bolster under the shoulders to accommodate for the large head size of an infant.

Etomidate is an ideal sedative for head injured patients at a dose of 0.3mg/kg. The decision between succinyl choline (1.5–2mg/kg) and rocuronium (0.6-1.2mg/kg) as the paralytic is difficult. In children under 5 years of age, particularly boys, there is the small possibility that an undiagnosed patient with muscular dystrophy or another myopathy may have excess release of potassium with administration of succinylcholine, thus, rocuronium is more frequently used, as it avoids the potential for hyperkalemia. Unlike in adults, there is no difference between succinylcholine and rocuronium in achievement of optimal intubating conditions in the pediatric population. Rocuronium will paralyze a child for substantially longer than succinylcholine (21–63 minutes). Atropine prior to intubation is no longer considered mandatory per the 2015 AHA guidelines but should be considered when there is a high risk of bradycardia.[8]

Q#3: What are common reasons for airway management failure and solutions?

Most pediatric airways are not difficult, and even when they are, use of a bag valve mask is typically able to oxygenate. When an airway is challenging, it is typically predictable, such as children with craniofacial anomalies such as bilateral cleft lip, cleft palate, macroglossia, and micrognathia.[9]

Neonates can be difficult, as can children who have had challenging intubations in the past. In any of these cases, if there is any elective nature to the intubation, it should be delayed until back-up is available. When complications occur, they are often desaturations or episodes of hypotension.[10]

One of the biggest differences between infants and adults is the rapidity of desaturation, with infants desaturating in 96 seconds. Getting all needed materials prepared and using a nasal cannula to provide apneic oxygenation may help to avoid desaturations. Most studies of video laryngoscopy (VL) specifically for children indicate a longer time to intubation, with some actually showing a higher failure rate, so beginning with direct laryngoscopy (DL) is appropriate.[11] Other rescue options for infants include a pediatric Bougie (or tube changer), and needle cricothyrotomy and transtracheal jet ventilation.

Author comments (Weinstock):

Please see comments at the end of the chapter on Scott Weingart's thoughts regarding resident education and use of DL vs. VL.

Q#4: What should be used for sedation after intubation?

Propofol is most commonly used following pediatric intubation. However, hypotension may occur initially and "propofol infusion syndrome" can occur after several days of use. While not typically an issue in the first several hours after intubation, other options may be preferable for patients requiring prolonged sedation. Dexmedetomidine has been studied in children with respiratory failure. While there is little literature specific to the head injured patient, its stable hemodynamic profile would make it a reasonable choice. Additionally, remifentanil as a single agent at a median dose of 0.25mcg/kg/min has been shown effective in pediatric patients with head injury.[12]

Q#5: Was this an acceptable miss by the primary care provider the day prior?

Backing up a little, we can't help but wonder if he was appropriately discharged from the primary care physician's office? It sounds like he looked well the day prior, and hopefully most of us would not have jumped to a diagnosis of child abuse in a well-appearing child with mild thrush. However, there are some concerning features of this visit:

- **Thrush:** Though thrush is quite common in young infants, and a 2-week-old with red-rimmed white plaques on their tongue and buccal mucosa shouldn't trigger the search for an immunodeficiency, a new diagnosis of thrush in a previously unaffected 11-month-old is unusual.
- **Lethargy:** I have a sense of unease when diagnosing a condition that fails to explain the chief complaint. Isolated thrush causes no systemic symptoms; it certainly doesn't cause lethargy. Is it possible that the chief complaint of lethargy was not adequately evaluated by the primary care provider, and that thrush was incidentally noted? Of course. Is it equally possible that the physician found a diagnosis and anchored on it, not taking a step back to recognize that the diagnosis is not a reasonable explanation for the chief complaint? It is impossible to say if the initial miss was acceptable; it is fair to say that the charting should clearly explain the thought process when a child presents with lethargy and leaves with a diagnosis and treatment for isolated thrush without systemic candidemia.
- **Child abuse:** Child abuse is frequently missed by both emergency and primary care providers who either fail to consider the possibility or talk themselves out of reporting for fear of being wrong. In the U.S., the abuse rate is 0.92/100 children. If you have seen 100 children and not reported abuse, you have likely missed it as well.[13] There are about 1.5/1000 unrecognized serious inflicted injuries per year in the U.S.[14] and 31% of infants diagnosed with abusive head injury have been previously seen by a provider who failed to recognize the abuse.[15] There are clinical prediction tools for inflicted head injury available, but they suffer from either a low sensitivity (PredAHT, sensitivity 72.3%) or a low specificity leading to over-reporting and untoward social implications for the family (Pediatric Brain Injury Research Network, specificity 43%).[16]

What did the actual provider do?

MDM (19:07): Pt was intubated with versed and succinylcholine. Initial chest x-ray demonstrated a right mainstem on my read. There was an episode of bradycardia which resolved with withdrawing the ET tube. Patient had normal O2 saturation and good response of his heart rate. I did note emesis in the airway.

Radiology interpretation CXR:
EXAMINATION TYPE: Portable XR Chest 1 View
IMPRESSION: Endotracheal chest into the right main bronchus. Total opacification of the left hemithorax with possible underlying lung consolidation. Right upper lobe atelectasis. Air distended stomach.

MDM: He was sent to CT scan immediately after intubation and stabilization. Upon my review of the CT scan, I was able to ascertain a right hemispheric infarct. The infarct involved the entire right hemisphere. Mild subdural [blood] as well as blood in the sinus. He was subsequently brought back to the trauma bay.

Official radiology interpretation:

1. Extensive abnormalities with low-attenuation throughout the right hemisphere and portions of left frontal lobe. Findings likely reflect edema from either infarct or trauma. Trauma is favored given the extensive additional abnormalities. Small areas of subdural blood are seen on the right. Hemorrhage along the falx is also noted. In addition, there is a nondisplaced right calvarial fracture.
2. Severe mass effect with midline shift to the left, dilatation of left lateral ventricle effacement of the right lateral ventricle. Subfalcine and transtentorial herniation are likely present.
3. I discussed the findings with the emergency physician at the time of exam.

Vitals (19:37):

Pulse Rate	Syst BP	Diast BP
186 BPM >HHI	106 mm Hg HI	0 mm Hg <LLOW

DECISION POINT C – YOU ARE FACED WITH 3 QUESTIONS:

1. **How is an altered child post-intubation with intracranial pathology managed?**
2. **If the child needs to be transferred, what is the safest and most expedient strategy?**
3. **With suspicion for abuse, is there information that the ED physician needs to obtain or should this all be left to the police?**

What does the literature say?

Q#1: How is an altered child post-intubation with intracranial pathology managed?

Not only does vent management of the head injured patient require attention to neuroprotection, but consideration of neurogenic pulmonary edema which can occur children as well as up to 20% of adults. These considerations may place us between a rock and a hard place, as some ventilator modalities which can be advantageous in the management of pulmonary edema (e.g. PEEP) might elevate ICP and be deleterious from a neurologic standpoint.

The initial settings should target a lung-protective strategy with low tidal volumes (6mL/kg) and plateau pressures (< 30cm H_2O). Reduced oxygen levels have been correlated with poor outcomes in severe pediatric TBI; thus, adherence to the adult Brain Trauma Foundation guidelines of maintaining the PaO_2 above 60mmHg (oxygen saturation > 90%) is advised. Permissive hypercapnia, often used as a lung protective strategy in intubated patients, has been shown to have a detrimental effect in a brain injured population in a few small studies. If permissive hypercapnia is required, maintain a pH > 7.32 and a pCO_2 < 45mmHg.[17]

Q#2: If the child needs to be transferred, what is the safest and most expedient strategy?

In the absence of a pediatric neurosurgeon and PICU, our patient will require transfer. While the consideration of child abuse should be discussed with the receiving physician, the onus for reporting to social services is typically on the initial physician. Plain and simple, the law requires a licensed provider suspicious of child abuse to report the abuse to Child Protective Services or to law enforcement. Legally, if the receiving physician fails not to report, the transferring physician could be held responsible for not initiating a report.

Practically, allowing Child Protective Services to speak to the initial treating physician is valuable, and allows for optimal and rapid transfer of information. Early reporting will facilitate safer transport of the patient. In our case, it is unlikely the family will ask to leave AMA or elope with their intubated infant. However, in the case of a more stable child, the physician cannot legally prevent the family from leaving and taking the baby until a "protective hold" is placed. While the physician may be able to justify a "medical hold" briefly, initiating a Child Protective Services hold early minimizes the risk of elopement in transfer.

Q#3: With suspicion for abuse, is there information that the ED physician needs to obtain or should this all be left to the police?

It's important for those of us in emergency medicine to remember that the world doesn't always think like we do when treating cases of non-accidental trauma. Our patient has intracranial hemorrhages and a skull fracture with no trauma history—obviously this is an abuse case. But in court, the experts (and perhaps the treating physician as well) will be grilled on why the child couldn't have a coagulopathy and a bone mineralization disorder. Vague stories of trauma never mentioned until long after the visit will be presented for feasibility. As ridiculous as this sounds, these cases are tough to prosecute, and every bit of information helps. Were there bruises, bite marks or burns? What was the size, location, and pattern of the injuries? What was the story offered by each family member present (or were they asked, and no story was offered)? Grossly, what is the child doing developmentally? There is an old adage, "kids who don't cruise rarely bruise."[18]

Finding out if the child is walking, even "cruising" with the support of holding onto furniture, is helpful if possible. Undoubtedly a CBC and coagulation labs would have been ordered for medical reasons, and it will also be helpful in demonstrating lack of a coagulopathy.[19] The police will also obtain a history, but one of the red flags for abuse is a changing history. Each provider's contemporaneous documentation can be used to trace the history. Finally, a skeletal survey to identify other fractures and a retinal exam for hemorrhages need to be done, but this can be deferred to the inpatient team.

What did the actual provider do?

MDM: We attempted to hyperventilate the patient. I did order Decadron, mannitol, vancomycin, Rocephin, Keppra. However, the pharmacy was unable to make these formulations in time as we did initially call the transport team from Children's Hospital upon the child's arrival. The transfer team arrived as a patient was coming back from CT. Medications were not ready at this time.

We opted to transport the child as we felt neurosurgical evaluation was critical. The antibiotics did arrive; however, given the findings on exam, we opted to hold them until he was evaluated in the ER at [Children's Hospital].

Impression and plan:
DIAGNOSIS: Anoxic brain injury, occipital skull fracture, intracerebral hemorrhage

Plan
Condition: Critical
Disposition: Admit: Transferred
Counseled: Family, Regarding diagnosis, Regarding diagnostic results, Regarding treatment plan, Regarding prescription, Family agreeable to plan

Re-examination/Re-evaluation:
Time: 19:52
Notes: Updated [Children's Hospital] on skull fx as I was just called by the radiologist. Social worker will contact the social worker at [Children's Hospital] as given the findings on CT as well as the bruising, an investigation will have to be performed by the police. The patient has had a couple of episodes of bradycardia but has subsequently responded. Prognosis appears to be poor based on the CT head. Family was updated on the findings of the CT scan. In addition, I did give them a heads up in regard to the process at [Children's Hospital] as well as the likelihood of a CPS case being filed.

Bonus "nightmare scenarios" (chapter author): It is difficult to imagine this getting worse. We already have an intubated infant with a poor prognosis, police involvement, and likely abuse. The poor ED provider likely has their shift to complete, without time for decompression. Could this have gotten worse?

- *What if* our patient had developed status epilepticus? The 2012 Brain Trauma Foundation Guidelines[1] recommend phenytoin prophylaxis for children with severe TBI. There is some equipoise as to the impact of this prophylaxis on ICU outcomes. A recent study indicated that about 80% of qualifying children receive seizure prophylaxis, and that fosphenytoin and phenytoin were the most commonly used. Phenobarbital and levetiracetam were given less often, although there is research indicating that levetiracetam is as effective as phenytoin.[20]
- *What if* a full cardiopulmonary arrest occurred? In many pediatric patients with systemic illness, even mild hypotension portends arrest. In this author's experience, hypotension is such a late finding that in patients with sepsis, cardiogenic shock, asthma, or status epilepticus, that the onset of hypotension often portends arrest within 5–10 minutes. However, patients aged 0–4 years with isolated serious head injury have a relative risk of hypotension of 2.5, comparable to age-matched patients with hemorrhagic traumatic injuries. Therefore, hypotension can be seen from head injury alone, and does not necessarily portend arrest.[21,22] Careful observation and a trial of fluids is reasonable initial therapy.

Teaching points:

- Major causes of altered consciousness and a "blown pupil" include meningitis, encephalitis, brain tumors, AV malformations, and intracranial hemorrhage from accidental or non-accidental trauma.
- Treatment for elevated intracranial pressure includes hyperosmolar therapy with mannitol or hypertonic saline.
- Etomidate is an ideal sedative for head injured patients at a dose of 0.3mg/kg. Either rocuronium (0.6–1.2mg/kg) or succinyl choline (1.5–2mg/kg) may be used as a paralytic (use rocuronium if there is a concern for possible hyperkalemia).

- Propofol is commonly used for sedation after pediatric intubation but use over 24 hours may cause propofol infusion syndrome.
- Ventilator management should be initiated with a lung protective strategy with an eye toward balance the risk of neuroprotection with the risk of neurogenic pulmonary edema.

Consulting editor Scott Weingart's recommendations regarding resident education with intubation:

Direct laryngoscopy (DL) vs. video laryngoscopy (VL):
We have a problem with the terms; saying VL is a useless turn of phrase. It doesn't mean anything. It needs to be specified if this is the standard geometry video laryngoscope blade or the hyperangulated video laryngoscope blade. Standard geometry blades are identical to a Macintosh blade, in every way... except they have the addition of a camera.

In any learning program—whether you're teaching PAs or residents, or anywhere that is an academic situation—the only acceptable way that is fair to your patients and fair to your learners, is to use standard geometry video laryngoscopy for all intubations initially. There is no reason to ever use DL if you have standard geometry video laryngoscopy available. If your learners want to learn how to intubate without the camera, and that is a valid concern, then they just should not look at the screen.

The advantage for learners is that it allows whoever is supervising to actually teach; otherwise, we have no idea what they're doing wrong. The advantage for patients is that they will not undergo multiple attempts in the face of a failing learner; that's not fair to the patients. Intubation's too high risk to have 1–2 failed attempts, and then only have their airway secured after edema and trauma has been induced.

On the other hand, if the standard geometry VL is being done, you could correct that first attempt; your learner learns, your patients benefit, and they've actually taken some knowledge from the encounter. What happens quite often is they fail twice, you take over as the attending, and then not only did they not learn, but they've reinforced bad habits because there was no explanation to them of what they were doing wrong in the first place.

Now they could look at the screen—which I think is actually more beneficial to their learning curve. But if they ask, "I want to learn DL. What if I don't have a camera when I start practice?" It's my thought, as well as many people who teach airway, that if you did 20 intubations looking at the screen and then were handed a direct laryngoscope, you would perform much better than someone who did 20 direct laryngoscopies not looking at the screen, because it's exponentially more beneficial for your technique to be able to see with better visualization the anatomy and what you're doing right and wrong.

Finally, when does hyperangulated come in? That is a rescue technique, or it is used for specific circumstances. For instance, a patient in C-spine immobilization. And that is an entirely separate technique; building skill there will actually not help your direct laryngoscopy skills much.

References:

1. Kochanek PM, Carney N, Adelson PD, et al. Guidelines for the acute medical management of severe traumatic brain injury in infants, children, and adolescents-second edition. Pediatr Crit Care Med 2012;13(Suppl 1):S1-82.
2. Rallis D, Poulos P, Kazantzi M, et al. Effectiveness of 7.5% hypertonic saline in children with severe traumatic brain injury. J Crit Care 2016;38:52-6.
3. Burgess S, Abu-Laban RB, Slavik RS, et al. A systematic review of randomized controlled trials comparing hypertonic sodium solutions and mannitol for traumatic brain injury: Implications for emergency department management. Ann Pharmacother 2016;50(4):291-300.
4. Alioglu B, Ozyurek E, Avci Z, et al. Peripheral blood picture following mild head trauma in children. Pediatr Int 2008;50(3):281-3.
5. Rovlias A, Kotsou S. The blood leukocyte count and its prognostic significance in severe head injury. Surg Neurol 2001;55(4):190-6.
6. Lee WC, Kuo LC, Cheng YC, et al. Combination of white blood cell count with liver enzymes in the diagnosis of blunt liver laceration. Am J of Emerg Med 2010;28(9):1024-9.
7. Varghese E, Kundu R. Does the Miller blade truly provide a better laryngoscopic view and intubating conditions that the Macintosh blade in small children? Paediatr Anaesth 2014;24(8):825-9.
8. de Caen AR, Berg MD, Chameides L, et al. Part 12: Pediatric advanced life support: 2015 American Heart Association guidelines update for cardiopulmonary resuscitation and emergency cardiovascular care. Circulation 2015;132(18 Suppl 2):S526-42.
9. Bai W, Golmirzaie K, Burke C, et al. Evaluation of emergency pediatric tracheal intubation by pediatric anesthesiologists on inpatient units and the emergency department. Paediatr Anaesth 2016;26(4):384-91.
10. Long E, Sabato S, Babl FE. Endotracheal intubation in the pediatric emergency department. Paediatr Anaesth 2014;24(12):1204-11.
11. Abdelgadir IS, Phillips RS, Singh D, et al. Videolaryngoscopy versus direct laryngoscopy for tracheal intubation in children (excluding neonates). Cochrane Database Syst Rev 2017;24(5):CD011413.
12. Hungerford JL, O'Brian N, Moore-Clingerpeel MM, et al. Remifentanil for sedation of children with traumatic brain injury. J Intensive Care Med 2019;34(7):557-62.
13. Ross AH, Juarez CA. A brief history of fatal child maltreatment and neglect. Forensic Sci Med Pathol 2014;10(3):413-22.
14. Chadwick DL, Castillo EM, Kuelbs C, et al. Missed and missing cases of abusive injuries: The magnitude and the measurement of the problem. Child Abuse Negl 2010;34(12):943-50.
15. Jenny C, Hymel KP, Ritzen A, et al. Analysis of missed cases of abusive head injury. JAMA 1999;281(7):621-6.
16. Cowley LE, Morris CB, Maguire SA, et al. Validation of a prediction tool for abusive head trauma. Pediatrics 2015;136(2):290-8.
17. Rettig JS, Duncan ED, Tasker RC. Mechanical ventilation during acute brain-injury in children. Paediatr Respir Rev 2016;20(9):17-23.
18. Sugar N, Taylor J, Feldman K. Bruises in infants and toddlers: Those who don't cruise rarely bruise. Arch Pediatr Adolesc Med 1999;153:399-03.

19. Horsley L. AAP guidelines on evaluating suspected child physical abuse. Am Fam Physician 2008;77(10):1461-4.
20. Ostahowski PJ, Kannan N, Wainwright MS, et al. Variation in seizure prophylaxis in severe pediatric traumatic brain injury. J Neurosurg Pediatr 2016;18(4):499-506.
21. Gardner AR, Diz DI, Tooze JA, et al. Injury patterns associated with hypotension in pediatric trauma patients: A national trauma database review. J Trauma Acute Care Surg 2015;78(6):1143-8.
22. Gardner A, Poehling KA, Miller CD, et al. Isolated head injury is a cause of shock in pediatric trauma patients. Pediatr Emerg Care 2013;29(8):879-83.

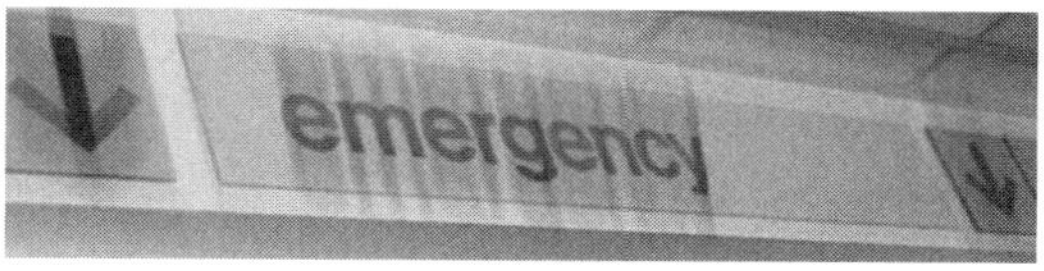

SECTION B – BREATHING/ PULMONARY

Chapter 6: A 36-year-old healthy woman with tachycardia and leg pain

Erica Simon, DO, MPH, MHA
Attending Physician
Emergency Medicine
Military Emergency Medical Services Disaster Medicine Fellow
San Antonio Uniformed Services Health Education Consortium, Ft. Sam Houston, TX

Brit Long, MD
Assistant Professor
Emergency Medicine
San Antonio Uniformed Services Health Education Consortium, Ft. Sam Houston, TX

Alex Koyfman, MD
Assistant Program Director
Clinical Assistant Professor
Emergency Medicine
University of Texas Southwestern Medical Center, Dallas, TX

Section editor:
Donald M. Yealy, MD
Chair, Department of Emergency Medicine
University of Pittsburgh/University of Pittsburgh Physicians
Vice President, Emergency and Urgent Care Services, Physician Services
UPMC Professor of Emergency Medicine, Medicine and Clinical and Translational Sciences
University of Pittsburgh School of Medicine, Pittsburgh, PA

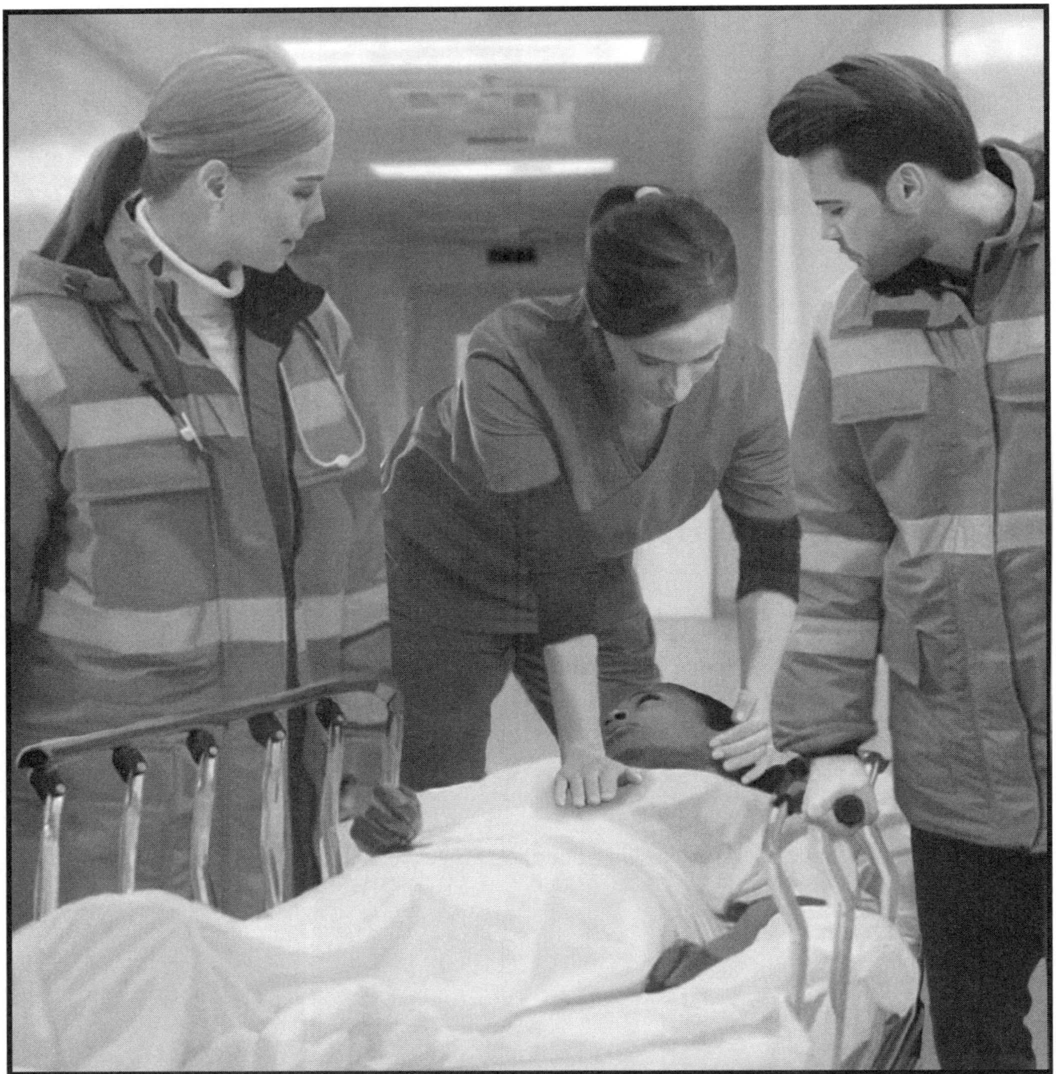

"WE JUST LOST THE PULSE!"

SECTION B/CHAPTER 6

A 36-year-old healthy woman with tachycardia and leg pain

"Vital signs are vital"—A simple phrase possessing profound meaning for individuals practicing emergency medicine. Research has identified pre-hospital, emergency department (ED), and discharge vital sign abnormalities as predictors of hospital admission, in-patient mortality, and unanticipated death following ED departure.

OB/GYN visit

MR#XXXXX

20 May 2010
Time Stamp: 09:45

HPI: The patient is a 36-year-old female with a previous medical history of human papilloma virus infection, cervical dysplasia, and insomnia who presents for an annual women's health examination. The patient is currently without female genitourinary complaints.

Allergies: NKDA

Social history:
Occupation: Lawyer
Marital Status: Divorced
Living Situation: Lives at home with fiancé and 2 children

Family history:
Mother: Lupus
Father: Hyperlipidemia

Sexual history: G2P2002, sexually active with fiancé. Oral contraceptives. LMP: 2 weeks prior. Colposcopy performed secondary to cervical dysplasia x2 (low-grade squamous intraepithelial lesion), most recent: 2 years ago. PAP smear 06/19/09: WNL.

ROS: Patient reports lower extremity pain; plans to follow-up with PCM. Insomnia manageable with zolpidem, reports 30-45 minutes of physical activity six days a week, utilizes a diet plan low in saturated fats and refined sugar. AOSN
PMH: As above
PSH: None

Vitals:

Temp	Pulse	Respir	Syst	Diast	Sat	Pain
98.4	118	16	126	86	99% (RA)	0/10

GA: Alert and oriented x3, pleasant, conversant.
EYES: Pupils equal, round, and reactive to light an accommodation (PERRLA).
CARDIO: Tachycardic, regular rhythm, without m/r/g. Normal heart sounds.
RESP: CTAB, no wheezes, rales, rhonchi. Good chest excursion.
BREAST: Bilateral examination: absent nipple discharge, no palpable masses, no superficial skin irregularities or discoloration. No axillary, infraclavicular or supraclavicular lymphadenopathy.
ABDOMINAL: Soft and non-tender throughout, Murphy's sign negative, without rebound or guarding.
BACK: No costovertebral angle tenderness to palpation (TTP).
FEMALE GENITAL EXAM: No inguinal lymphadenopathy. No vulvar erythema, edema, or lesions. Vaginal vault: normal mucosa; absent edema, erythema, and lesions. Cervix: Internal and external os closed. Cervical ectropion. No cervical discharge. Bimanual examination: no adnexal TTP, no palpable adnexal masses.

TESTING: PAP smear, urine β-hCG

MDM: Well-appearing 36-year-old G2P2002 presents for annual women's health exam. History of HPV and cervical dysplasia. No complaints. Physical exam unremarkable. Refill for OCPs - will check U preg and call in Rx if neg. PAP smear done: ok to leave voicemail on patient's cell phone.

IMPRESSION: Well-appearing 36-year-old female, HPV positive, continuing to monitor.

PLAN: Follow-up PAP smear and urine β-hCG.

MR#1234567 **22 May 2010**

TELEPHONE CONSULT: PAP smear WNL, urine preg neg. Discussed results w pt. Phoned pharmacy OCP refill. F/u 1 yr.

Discussion: Seems to be a straightforward representation of a well-exam, right? But if we look closely, the patient is tachycardic at 118bpm. The increased pulse is recognized in the PE cardiovascular exam stating "Tachycardic, regular rhythm, without m/r/g," but despite this finding, the remainder of the note lacks exploration of an underlying etiology. Though not discussed further, there is mention of lower extremity pain.

Should we give the OB/GYN a pass? There is no great data on an elevated heart rate during a scheduled gynecology visit! But we do know two things which are pertinent to *all* providers: an evaluation needs to consider and address abnormal findings, and abnormal vital signs may be the lone finding of a serious condition in a well-appearing patient.

In contrast to individuals experiencing supraventricular tachycardias (who often report palpitations), patients with sinus tachycardia are frequently asymptomatic as this response is compensatory and often adequate—for a while (or until it's not).[1] Could this be an accelerated junctional rhythm? Junctional tachycardia is most frequently encountered in digoxin toxicity, myocardial ischemia, myocarditis, or following cardiac procedures,[2] making it unlikely in our patient. What's the point? Tachycardia is abnormal and should be explored—and the first step is seeing what the rhythm is by getting an ECG—rather than to speculate or ignore.

ECG characteristics of sinus tachycardia include a narrow-complex (QRS duration of $\leq$ 0.12 seconds) tachycardia (HR $\geq$ 100bpm) with normal p waves preceding every QRS complex. The heart rate of sinus tachycardia should vary, rather than staying at 1 particular value; rarely is specific rhythm therapy indicated. However, detecting and treating the cause is the key—a step omitted here.

Differential Diagnoses of Tachycardia[1,2]	
Anxiety	Infection/Sepsis
Pain	Pulmonary Embolism
Hypovolemia	Chronic Pulmonary Disease
Hyperthyroidism	Hypoxia
Pheochromocytoma	Anemia
Stimulants (caffeine, amphetamines, etc.)	Pericarditis/Myocarditis
Medication withdrawal (B-blockers)	Left Ventricular (LV) Failure
Atrial Infarction	Myocardial Infarction (anterior infarct with LV dysfunction)

The bottom line: The patient was sent home with an unaddressed VS abnormality. For EMS providers, abnormal vital signs predict admission; in hospital patients, abnormal vitals predict ICU admission and mortality; and for ED providers, abnormal vitals are associated with increased death after discharge.

- **Burstein, et al. 1995:**[3] Prospective observational cohort study of 1,238 patients in one Emergency Medical Service (EMS) system in Suffolk County, New York finding that factors associated with an increased likelihood of admission were bradycardia (90%), hypertension (89%), hypotension (80%), and tachycardia (72%).
- **Barfod, et al. 2012:**[4] Retrospective review of ED admissions from September 2009 to February

2010 at Hillerød hospital (level-2 acute care facility), North Zealand, Denmark which found an association between the number of abnormal vital signs and ICU admission, as well as in-hospital mortality.

- **Sklar, et al. 2007:**[5] Retrospective cohort study of 387,334 ED discharges from February 1994 to November 2004 at the University of New Mexico Health Sciences Center showing that in patients with death with 7 days of discharge possibly related to a medical error, 71% had unexplained tachycardia, and 85% had abnormal vital signs.

ED BOUNCEBACK (3 weeks later)

6 June 2010

18:55: MEDCOM personnel dispatch an ambulance to the residence of a 36-year-old female complaining of a rapid heart rate and shortness of breath.

19:22: A paramedic radios MEDCOM requesting immediate transfer to the nearest ED (on diversion) for the unstable 36-year-old patient with chest pain, a rapid heart rate, and hypoxemia.

19:25: The ED charge nurse accepts the patient but reports that all current beds are occupied.

19:40: As paramedics burst through the double bay doors, accompanied by the patient's fiancé, cardiopulmonary resuscitation (CPR) is in progress: "She lost pulses as soon as we pulled up." While one medic performs chest compressions, the other delivers bre aths with the bag-valve-mask (BVM) and gives you the report:

"36-year-old female, unknown medical history. We were called to the residence for the complaint of rapid heartbeat and shortness of breath. Upon arrival she was tachycardic and tachypneic. VS: BP 132/89, HR 155, RR 28, SpO_2 96% RA. Initial 12-lead showed SVT. We transferred her to the rig, got IV access, and gave 6mg of adenosine with no change. At that point she started to complain of chest pain. We gave 12mg of adenosine with no change. Then her lips turned blue and her pulse ox was 79%. We put her on non-rebreather, and as we pulled in she arrested."

19:43: A patient occupying the nearest trauma bay is hurriedly rolled into the hallway, and the patient is wheeled in.

Author comments (Weinstock):

At this point, for the purpose of discussion, we will reproduce the ED physician's note which was recorded later.

ED PRESENTATION

MR#XXXXX

6 June 2010
Time Stamp: 19:40

CC (at 19:40): Tachycardia (Per medics)

HPI (documented at 20:36): The patient presents per paramedics and is not able to give any medical history secondary to being unresponsive. The history is from the paramedics, the patient's boyfriend, and her mother. She reportedly has had two weeks of left lower extremity pain and swelling, and then this afternoon, while at work, she suddenly developed shortness of breath and called 911. During transport the patient became cyanotic and also complained of sharp chest pain. The paramedics gave adenosine times two which was not effective. I did review the monitor strip, and she did appear to be in sinus tachycardia with a rate over 150 beats per minute. The patient did, according to paramedics, go into cardiopulmonary arrest just prior to entry into the emergency department, and chest compressions were initiated immediately.

EMS Interventions prior to arrival:
Peripheral IV access
Adenosine: 6 mg IV, 12 mg IV
Oxygen therapy via non-rebreather
Initiation of CPR

EMS 12-lead ECG and rhythm strip reviewed: Prior to arrest: sinus tachycardia, 157–165bmp, right axis deviation, T wave inversions V1-V3.

Allergies: NKDA
PMH: Unable to obtain
PSH: Unable to obtain

Vitals:

Temp (F)	Pulse	Resp	Syst	Diast	Sat O2%	Pain
			10 (BVM)		88% (RA)	-/10

PE:
CONSTITUTIONAL: The patient does appear cyanotic and she is unresponsive without spontaneous heart tones or breathing.
HEAD: Normocephaulic; atraumatic
EYES: PER
NOSE: Normal in appearance without rhinorrhea
RESP: No spontaneous breath sounds
CARDIO: No spontaneous heart tones
ABD: Abdomen is minimally distended
SKIN: Mottled

Author Comments (Weinstock):

Like many ED patients, decompensation may occur quickly. This is not only a witnessed arrest... but witnessed in the squad bay! We have not had time to prepare. We are at decision point A:

DECISION POINT A – YOU ARE FACED WITH 5 QUESTIONS:

1. **What is the differential diagnosis of cardiac arrest?**
2. **Which life-threatening diagnosis may be found with an ECG?**
3. **Which reversible etiologies of cardiac arrest can be found with POCUS?**
4. **Does lack of cardiac activity on POCUS predict unsuccessful resuscitation?**
5. **Are there recommendations regarding termination of a code?**

Q#1: What is the differential diagnosis of cardiac arrest?

Though history is often unavailable, knowledge of past history of cardiac disease allows initial stratification. Additionally, there is often pre-arrest information available from bystanders, family, and EMS. Witnessed cardiac arrest should be differentiated from a patient who is "found down."

Differential Diagnoses of Sudden Cardiac Death[6,7]

Individuals With Known Cardiac Disease	Individuals Without Known Cardiac Disease
Coronary Disease	**Cardiac Etiologies**
Anomalous Coronary Circulation	Arrhythmogenic Right Ventricular Cardiomyopathy
Coronary Spasm	Brugada Syndrome
Ischemic Heart Disease	Catecholaminergic Polymorphic Ventricular Tachycardia
Cardiomyopathies	Coronary Spasm
Arrhythmogenic Right Ventricular Cardiomyopathy	Long-QT Syndrome
Dilated Cardiomyopathy	Myocarditis
Hypertrophic Cardiomyopathy	Sarcoidosis (VT arising from an arrhythmogenic granulomatous scar[8])
Infiltrative Cardiomyopathy (e.g., sarcoid, amyloid)	Short-QT Syndrome
Myocarditis	**Metabolic Derangements**
Takotsubo Cardiomyopathy	Acidosis
Other	Drug Toxicity (calcium channel blockers, beta blockers, digoxin, etc.)
Commotio Cordis	Hyperkalemia/hypokalemia
Wolff-Parkinson-White Syndrome	Hypocalcemia
	Hypomagnesemia
	Non-cardiac Etiologies
	Acute Intracranial Hemorrhage
	Epilepsy
	Massive Pulmonary Embolism
	Aortic Aneurysm Rupture
	Pacemaker Failure

Q#2: Which life-threatening diagnosis may be found with an ECG?

If performed prior to arrest, the ECG may demonstrate findings suggestive of the diagnosis. For example:

- Ischemic heart disease: Hyperacute T waves, ST segment elevation and/or depression, T wave inversion.
- Hypertrophic cardiomyopathy: Left ventricular hypertrophy and early repolarization abnormalities.[8]
- Arrhythmogenic Right Ventricular Cardiomyopathy: depolarization abnormalities (Epsilon wave) in V_1–V_3, right bundle branch block, and inverted T waves.[9]
- Wolff-Parkinson-White Syndrome (WPW): Shorte ned PR interval, delta wave, and widened QRS interval with possible secondary repolarization changes (inverted T waves).[10]
- Brugada Syndrome: Coved or saddleback ST segment elevation in V_1–V_3.
- Acute intracranial hemorrhage: Diffuse T wave inversions, prolonged QTc, shortened PR interval, U waves.[11]
- Massive pulmonary embolism: Sinus tachycardia, complete or incomplete right bundle branch block, S1Q3T3, and T wave inversions in V_1–V_4.[12,13]

Q#3: Which reversible etiologies of cardiac arrest can be found with POCUS?

In the hands of a skilled operator, point-of-care ultrasound (POCUS) can be used to rapidly assess for reversible etiologies of cardiac arrest, detect cardiac activity in the absence of a palpable pulse, and direct resuscitative efforts.[14-17]

A. Cardiac tamponade:

- If a pericardial effusion (an anechoic stripe of fluid between the parietal and visceral pericardium) is identified on POCUS, cardiac tamponade should be the presumed etiology of arrest until proven otherwise.
    - o Note: The parasternal long axis view allows for differentiation between pericardial and pleural effusions. Free fluid adjacent to the aorta is pleural fluid and not amenable to pericardiocentesis.[14,17]
    - o In the setting of cardiac arrest, a dilated IVC (> 2mm) measured 2–3cm from the right atrium, supports this diagnosis.[18]

B. Pulmonary embolism:

- Apical 4-chamber view demonstrates right ventricular dilation:
    - o Right-to-left ventricular area ratio > 0.66 is 85% specific for pulmonary embolism.[19]
    - o Bowing of the septum into the left ventricle may be visualized.[14,20]
- Flattening of the interventricular septum may also be observed secondary to volume and pressure overload of the right heart.[19,21]

C. Pacemaker failure secondary to myocardial perforation:

- Pacemaker lead(s) may violate the right ventricular (single-lead) or right atrial (dual-lead) wall; best seen in the apical 4-chamber view on POCUS.
    - o As many as 7% of transvenous electrodes perforate, usually within days after insertion, with the potential to cause pericardial effusion and tamponade.[22]

D. Hypovolemia:

- Severe hypovolemia is often apparent on POCUS as reduced filling of the left and right sides of the heart.
- Assessment of the size and collapsibility of the IVC is widely used as an indicator of volume status (requires a subxiphoid view with the prove indicator cephalad).[18] In the case of cardiac arrest, a flat IVC (< 5mm) should prompt aggressive fluid resuscitation.[18,20]

E. Ruptured aortic aneurysm:

- Ruptured aortic aneurysm represents a common cause of PEA secondary to hypovolemia.[14,18]
- Bedside ultrasound findings of a collapsed IVC should also prompt an assessment of the aorta.
    - o An aortic diameter > 5cm suggests vascular rupture as the etiology of hypovolemia.[14,15]

F. Tension pneumothorax:

- Visualization of a single, sagittal lung window through the upper lung fields, with the linear transducer, reliably detects pneumothoraces. Sensitivity is increased by scanning a number of areas along the anterior and lateral chest walls.[23-26]
- Signs of pneumothorax include (may be observed during BVM ventilation or following intubation of our patient):
    - o Absence of lung sliding: physiologic sliding of the lung surface, best visualized at the lung bases.[22,23] (M-mode may be utilized as an adjunct to identify the "seashore sign." M-mode demonstrates the "barcode sign" in pneumothorax.)
    - o Absence of B lines (comet-tail artifact): reverberation artifact arising from physiologic fluid; seen only where the visceral and parietal pleura are in contact.[22.23]

Negative POCUS examinations eliminate specific components of the differential diagnosis. For example, the negative predictive value for ultrasound evaluation of tension pneumothorax approaches 100% with high sensitivity.[23,25]

Q#4: Does lack of cardiac activity on POCUS predict unsuccessful resuscitation?

Cardiac activity on an initial ultrasound is associated with increased survival to hospital admission and discharge, whereas only 0.6% of patients without cardiac activity survive to hospital discharge.[27] An assessment for a palpable pulse is frequently inadequate in the setting of cardiopulmonary resuscitation, as 54% of patients with PEA have cardiac activity on ultrasound.[27]

- Gaspari R, et al. 2016:[27] The REASON Trial: A non-randomized, prospective, protocol-driven observational study at 20 hospitals across the United States and Canada of patients presenting with out-of-hospital or in-ED arrest with PEA or asystole:
    - o Total 793 patients—ultrasound performed at the beginning and end of ACLS. Primary outcome: survival to hospital admission. Secondary outcomes: ROSC, survival to hospital discharge:
        - – 263 patients with cardiac activity on initial ultrasound (note that 142 patients with presumed PEA demonstrated cardiac activity):
            - 134 (51%) achieved ROSC
            - 76 (28.9%) survived to hospital admission

    - 10 (3.8%) survived to hospital discharge
  - 530 patients without cardiac activity on initial ultrasound:
    - 76 (14.3%) achieved ROSC
    - 38 (7.2%) survived to hospital admission
    - 3 (0.6%) survived to hospital discharge
  - Additional findings: POCUS identifies conditions that respond to non-ACLS interventions:
    - Pericardial effusion: 34 patients (pericardiocentesis increased survival to discharge rates: 15.4% vs. 1.3%)
    - Pulmonary embolism: 15 patients received thrombolytics with survival to discharge 6.7%

Ultrasound demonstrated a positive predictive value of 83.7% for ROSC in patients initially presenting with cardiac activity.

- Bolvardi E, et al. 2016:[28] Non-randomized, prospective, observational study of patients (≥ 18 years of age) presenting to Imam Reza Training and Research Hospital, Iran: evaluation of bedside echocardiogram as a predictor of survival in cardiac arrest (ultrasound performed immediately prior to the initiation of ACLS):
  - o 159 patients:
    - 49 patients with cardiac activity: 41 (83.7%) with ROSC
    - 110 patients without cardiac activity: 15 (16.3%) with ROSC

Cardiac activity on bedside ultrasound demonstrated a positive likelihood ratio for ROSC of 4.26 (95% CI: 2.63– 6.92) and a negative likelihood ratio of 0.18 (95% CI: 0.10–0.31). Echocardiography performed during cardiac arrest that demonstrates an absence of cardiac activity harbors a significantly lower (but not 0) likelihood that a patient will experience ROSC.[29]

- Blyth L, et al. 2012:[29] Meta-analysis of studies utilizing transthoracic echocardiography during resuscitation to predict the outcome of cardiac arrest:
  - o 12 studies representing 568 patients for whom ultrasound was utilized to determine the presence or absence of kinetic cardiac activity with the primary outcome of ROSC: As a predictor of ROSC during cardiac arrest, echocardiogram demonstrated a pooled sensitivity of 91.6% (95% CI: 84.6–96.1) and a specificity of 80% (95% CI: 76.1–83.6).

Q#5: Are there recommendations regarding termination of a code?

The AHA and European Resuscitation Council guidelines assist the physician in determining the termination of resuscitative efforts:[30-32]

(Table on next page...)

Guidelines for Cardiopulmonary Resuscitation Termination[30-32]	
American Heart Association	**European Resuscitation Council**
Team leader makes determination based upon: Time to CPR Initiation Time to defibrillation Comorbidities Pre-arrest state Initial arrest rhythm	Presence of an advanced directive Asystole > 20 minutes in the absence of a reversible etiology Patients arresting out-of-hospital who require ongoing CPR without return of pulses during transport Team leader's clinical judgment

Summary of decision point A: US may assist in diagnosis and management of patients in arrest with identification of asystole, determination of cardiac activity without palpable pulses, and identification of reversible etiologies of cardiac arrest, but it remains an adjunct to clinical assessment in predicting patient outcome.[20]

What did the actual provider do?

MR#XXXXX **June 2010**
Time Stamp: 20:05

Progress Note: CPR continued by ED trauma team. Patient noted to have adequate bilateral breath sounds and equal chest rise with bagging; femoral pulses palpable with compressions. A definitive airway was obtained by direct laryngoscopy – first pass success with a 7.5 endotracheal tube (ETT). ETT position was confirmed by bilateral breath sounds and color capnography.

Author comments (Weinstock):

The physician has intubated the patient and is working on a central line. We are back at the bedside. We are at decision point B:

DECISION POINT B – YOU ARE FACED WITH 5 QUESTIONS:

1. **Does the patient require a central line at this point in her care?**
2. **Should she undergo thrombolysis?**
3. **How should thrombolysis be administered in massive PE?**
4. **How does systemic thrombolysis compare to surgical thrombectomy/embolectomy?**
5. **Branch point: Should all cardiac arrest patients get a thrombolytic?**

Q#1: Does the patient require a central line at this point in her care?

Recall that peripheral IV access had been established by EMS personnel for the administration of adenosine. Central venous catheterization is rarely required during resuscitation attempts if large bore peripheral access has been established.[32] Although time to systemic drug circulation and peak drug concentration are prolonged with peripheral vs. central administration, the establishment of peripheral access does not require interruption of CPR, and often creates a quicker time to effective drug delivery.[33] AHA guidelines recommend a 20mL bolus of IV fluids and elevation of the respective extremity for 10–20 seconds following the delivery of resuscitation medications to facilitate delivery to systemic circulation.[32,34]

IO cannulation is fairly easy to perform (especially using assembled kits) and offers similar pharmacokinetics as central venous access.[33] In adults and children, IO access during resuscitation is safe and effective for drug delivery, fluid resuscitation, and blood sampling.[35-38]

Note that ACLS medications including lidocaine, epinephrine, atropine, naloxone, and vasopressin can be delivered through the endotracheal tube as they are absorbed through the alveoli. However, there are decreased blood concentrations when compared to similar doses given by the IV or IO route.[39-41] Animal studies suggest that the lower concentrations of epinephrine achieved per ETT administration may result in transient beta-adrenergic effects resulting in hypotension, decreased coronary artery perfusion, and decreased potential for ROSC.[34,42,43]

Q#2: Should she undergo thrombolysis?

We will discuss four studies of thrombolysis in cardiac arrest or shock patients with a confirmed or suspected PE:

- Sharifi, et al. 2016:[44] Prospective cohort study of 23 patients experiencing PEA and cardiopulmonary arrest due to massive PE, treated with 50 milligrams of the tissue plasminogen activator, alteplase, administered over a 1-minute duration, during active CPR:
  - PE identified in 20 patients by CTPA prior to administration of alteplase.
  - PE identified following the administration of alteplase and CTPA in 3 patients.
  - ROSC achieved in 2–15 minutes in all but 1 patient.
  - At follow-up (22 ± 3 months): 20 patients (87%) alive.
  - No evidence of minor/major bleeding during CPR.
  - No recurrent venous thromboembolism or bleeding during hospitalization or at follow-up.
- Le Conte, et al. 2003:[45] Retrospective review of 21 patients experiencing shock or cardiopulmonary arrest due to a PE, treated with 0.6mg/kg alteplase (max 50milligrams) over 15 minutes followed by heparin:
  - 5 patients died (4 within the first 4 hours of hospital admission).
  - Systolic and diastolic BPs improved within the first 2 hours of after thrombolysis.
  - 5 minor bleeding events occurred.
- Newman, et al. 2000:[46] Literature review of 9 studies involving 67 patients who were treated with thrombolytic agents during CPR for suspected PE demonstrated an overall survival rate of 75%.
- Stein & Matta, 2012:[47] Retrospective review of the Nationwide Inpatient Sample utilizing International Classification of Disease billing data to identify patients who were deemed hemodynamically unstable due to PE:
  - 21,390 patients treated with thrombolysis vs. 50,840 who were not:
    - All-cause mortality in the thrombolytic group was significantly lower when compared to the group that did not receive thrombolytics (15% vs. 47%, $p < 0.001$).

In patients with confirmed or suspected PE, thrombolysis improves hemodynamics and has the *potential* for mortality benefit.[44-47] To date, there is no evidence supporting the routine use of thrombolytics for those with *submassive* PE who are hemodynamically stable.

Consulting editor comments (Weingart):

If you have a patient who has a diagnosis of PE and codes in front of you, definitely give lytics. If you have a patient you strongly suspect has a PE who codes in front of you, give lytics.

Q#3: How should thrombolysis be administered in massive PE?

Give the agent by whatever IV route exists—but if there is a choice, use central over peripheral, and at a compressible site versus a non-compressible site. Although exceedingly rare, tissue necrosis secondary to subcutaneous bleeding may occur after thrombolytic delivery via intraosseous catheter, therefore this method of delivery is not advised.[48]

In the U.S., the majority of trials on thrombolytic use during cardiac arrest assessed alteplase. While approved by the Food and Drug Administration for the treatment of PE as an infusion delivered over 2 hours, alteplase dosing in cardiac arrest is unclear. Currently, experts recommend giving alteplase as a 50mg bolus, followed by an additional 50mg if the first dose is unsuccessful.[48] Studies of tenecteplase, a third generation thrombolytic created by modifying alteplase to extend the plasma half-life, are ongoing (off-label use).[48]

What are relative and absolute contraindications to thrombolysis?

Contraindications to the Use of Alteplase[46]

Absolute	Relative
Internal bleeding	Age > 75 years
Previous intracranial hemorrhage	Current anticoagulation
History of cerebral vascular accident within the past 3 months	History of chronic, severe, poorly controlled hypertension (SBP > 180/110mmHg)
Recent intracranial/spinal surgery/ trauma	Traumatic or prolonged CPR (>10 min)
Intracranial Neoplasm	Recent internal bleeding (within 2–4 weeks)
Arteriovenous malformation or aneurysm	Non-compressible vascular punctures
History bleeding diathesis	Dementia
	Remote ischemic stroke (> 3 months)
	Major surgery within the preceding 3 weeks

Closed chest compressions are considered a relative contraindication to thrombolysis administration[48] due to conflicting trial results. While a number of studies have demonstrated no change in outcome with regarding to bleeding associated with thrombolytic administration during CPR with closed chest compressions,[49-51] the largest trial (Böttiger, et al. 2008) identified 10 of 525 patients treated with thrombolytics as experiencing intracranial hemorrhage after thrombolytic therapy.[52] Despite their increased risk of bleeding, patients receiving thrombolytics in the setting of cardiac arrest secondary to PE survived to the study's 30-day outcome endpoint—perhaps the tradeoff remains positive overall. Another vexing issue is recent surgery—both a relative contraindication for the administration of alteplase, and a risk factor for the development of venous thromboembolism. We see the tradeoff in cardiac arrest or near arrest as positive in this group and recommend thrombolysis. We also recommend continuing compressions after thrombolysis if the patient remains pulseless.

Chapter author note: In the majority of cases, we won't know all details regarding the patient's medical and surgical history. Based upon our review of the data, hemorrhage is a possibility, but death occurring secondary to hemorrhage is uncommon.[53] Our conclusions are that patients experiencing cardiac arrest secondary to PE may benefit from thrombolysis including increased survival to hospital discharge and improved 30-day mortality.

Q#4: How does systemic thrombolysis compare to surgical thrombectomy/embolectomy?

Survival occurs in a small number of patients with PE-induced cardiac arrest following percutaneous thromboembolectomy or surgical embolectomy with or without treatment with fibrinolysis:[54]

- Thromboembolectomy:
  - Fava, et al. 2005:[50] 7 patients with massive PE causing cardiac arrest underwent percutaneous mechanical thromboembolectomy. Pulmonary perfusion was restored in 6 patients (85.7%); 3 received a tissue plasminogen activator as an adjunct.
- Surgical embolectomy:
  - Konstantinov, et al. 2007:[51] 8 patients with massive PE causing cardiac arrest underwent pulmonary embolectomy: 2 intraoperative deaths (30-day mortality rate 28.5%), 1 patient required a right ventricular assist device post-procedure, and another patient died 8 months following the procedure due to long-term complications of cerebral damage which occurred during initial resuscitation.
  - Schmid, et al. 1991:[53] Retrospective review of 27 patients (ages 21–79) with cardiac arrest due to PE who underwent pulmonary embolectomy between January 1975–January 1991.
    - 11 patients did not require prolonged resuscitation: mortality rate after undergoing surgical embolectomy was 36%.
    - 5 patients required resuscitation without the need for cardiac massage: mortality rate after undergoing surgical embolectomy was 60%.
    - 11 patients were connected to ECMO devices during CPR: mortality rate after undergoing surgical embolectomy was 45%.
    - Ultimately, 12 patients died early postoperatively; 8 died in hospital secondary to right heart failure, 2 died in the hospital of brain death, and an additional 2 died of sepsis (3 patients survived to discharge).

Consultation with an interventional radiologist or cardiothoracic surgeon is warranted—but this is often not possible in the time-sensitive nature of cardiac arrest (or near cardiac arrest) care.[54] Failed thrombolysis does not preclude a patient from percutaneous or open surgical interventions.

Q#5: Branch point: Should all cardiac arrest patients get a thrombolytic?

Even with the minimal history available, there is a high likelihood that our patient is suffering from a massive PE. Current data suggests that massive PE accounts for 8–13% of unexplained cardiac arrests,[53,54] 65% of which are ultimately fatal.[55-57]

Let's consider undifferentiated cardiac arrest:

- Böttiger, et al. 2008:[52] Double-blind, multi-center trial that randomly assigned adult patients with witnessed out-of-hospital cardiac arrest to received tenecteplase or placebo during CPR:
  - No significant difference in the primary endpoint of 30-day survival between the treatment groups (525 placebo patients, 525 tenecteplase patients): 14.7% vs. 17.0% (p=0.36, relative risk 0.87; 95% CI: 0.65–1.15).
    - In the patient population with a presumed PE: 2 of 15 individuals given thrombolytics (13.3%) vs. 0 of 22 given placebo were alive 30 days following their arrest.
  - No significant difference in the secondary end points of hospital admission, ROSC, 24-hour survival, survival to hospital discharge, and neurologic outcome.
  - Patients receiving tenecteplase were more likely to experience intracranial hemorrhage (2.7% with thrombolytics vs. 0.4% with placebo, $p < 0.05$).
- Stadlbauer, et al. 2006:[58] Post hoc analysis of a double-blinded, prospective, multicenter, randomized, controlled clinical trial of 1,186 patients randomized to the receipt of thrombolysis or placebo (primary endpoint: hospital admission; secondary endpoint: hospital discharge).
  - Admission and discharge rates for patients who underwent thrombolysis (after logistic regression modeling for confounding variables) were not significantly different.

Bottom line: If given widely in all forms of cardiac arrest patients, thrombolytics demonstrate no mortality benefit and carry the risk of severe hemorrhage.[52-58]

What did the actual provider do?

Progress Note: The patient underwent a failed attempt at a right femoral central line. Central access was subsequently obtained through the left femoral vein, and epinephrine (1mg) was administered in addition to a 2L bolus of normal saline. Although initially presenting in PEA, after two rounds of CPR, the patient was noted to have a shockable rhythm (VF). The patient had a femoral central line placed by myself. This was accomplished with some difficulty and was initially attempted in the right femoral and then obtained in the left femoral. During this time, I did make the decision to thrombolyse as it did seem that this was probably secondary to a large saddle pulmonary embolus. While they were mixing the TPA, the central line was placed, and was immediately given with a bolus, and then a drip. In addition, the patient had multiple rounds of intravenous epinephrine, atropine, and one amp of sodium bicarbonate. She also was defibrillated several times for what appeared to be initially ventricular fibrillation, and then pulseless ventricular tachycardia. She had a prolonged course of chest compressions and did intermittently get back a pulse towards the end and then finally her pulse returned and remained and her blood pressure is currently 84. I did speak with the vascular surgeon who came to the ED. He will place a filter.

Vitals:

Pulse	Resp	Syst	Diast	Sat
128	12 (vent)	84	0	91

Ventilator Settings: AC/VC, TV 400, PEEP 5, RR 12, FiO_2 50

ECG Interpretation: Sinus tachycardia, right axis deviation, RBBB, T wave inversions V_1-V_3

Laboratory Studies:

Test	Flag	Value	Units	Ref. Range
WBC	H	22.7	K/uL	4.6-10.2
HGB		15.0	G/DL	12.0-16.0
PLT		194	K/uL	142-424

Test	Flag	Value	Units	Ref. Range
NA		140	MMOL/L	135-144
K		3.9	MMOL/L	3.5-5.1
CL		102	MMOL/L	98-107
AGAP	H	27.9	MMOL/L	6.0-18.0
CO_2	L	14	MMOL/L	22-29
BUN	H	22	MG/DL	7-18
CREAT	H	1.8	MG/DL	0.6-1.3

Test	Flag	Value	Units	
CKMB		1.8	NG/ML	0.0-5.0
TROPI		.10	NG/ML	.00-.27

DDIMERQUNT H 86.34 MG/L

Radiology: Portable CXR: The patient's endotracheal tube and nasogastric tube appear to be in satisfactory position. No acute cardiopulmonary disease is identified.

Author comments (Weinstock):

Seems as if the thrombolytic worked... but there are still decisions to be made. We are at:

DECISION POINT C – YOU ARE FACED WITH 2 QUESTIONS:

1. **After she regains a pulse, is a CT angiogram (CTA) advisable?**
2. **Now that the patient has achieved return of spontaneous circulation (ROSC), what other interventions should be considered?**

Q#1: After she regains a pulse, is a CT angiogram (CTA) advisable?

There is little data about advanced imaging post-administration of thrombolytics. US could aid by assessing RV function, and CT angiogram might confirm diagnosis but likely will not drive the immediate post-recovery phase.

Chapter author commentary: We agree the patient should have received a thrombolytic but feel it could have been given sooner.

Q#2: Now that the patient has achieved return of spontaneous circulation (ROSC), what other interventions should be considered?

The acute post-resuscitative phase (occurring within 72 hours post-ROSC) occurs secondary to prolonged whole-body ischemia experienced during cardiopulmonary resuscitation and tissue damage occurring during and after reperfusion.[59,60] Management of the post-cardiac arrest patient centers on addressing central nervous system injury, myocardial dysfunction, systemic hypoperfusion, multi-organ failure, and the precipitating cause of the cardiac arrest.

Interventions focus on the optimization of ventilation and oxygenation, and consideration of therapeutic temperature management:

- Post-cardiac arrest brain injury represents the cause of death in 68% of out-of-hospital cardiac arrests and 23% of in-hospital cardiac arrests.[61]
  - To improve neurologic outcomes, interventions should focus on continued monitoring to maintain cerebral perfusion pressure, attain and maintain euglycemia, and avoid hypoxia and hyperoxia.
- Global myocardial dysfunction, without impaired coronary perfusion, is frequent following ROSC. This occurs secondary to myocardial stunning in the setting of a transient increase in local and circulating catecholamines.[59]
  - Cardiac monitoring and treatment with inotropes allow for the rapid reversal of this condition (animal models demonstrate improved systolic and diastolic dysfunction after cardiac arrest following the administration of dobutamine).[62]
- Systemic hypoperfusion and multi-organ failure following cardiac arrest are manifestations of myocardial dysfunction and whole-body ischemia, triggering the activation of immunologic and coagulation pathways.[59]
  - Management in an ICU allows for directed evaluation and management of resultant intravascular volume depletion, impaired vasoregulation, impaired oxygen delivery and utilization, and increased susceptibility to infection.

The International Liaison Committee on Resuscitation; the AHA Emergency Cardiovascular Care Committee; the Council on Cardiovascular Surgery and Anesthesia; the Council on Cardiopulmonary, Perioperative, and Critical Care; the Council on Clinical Cardiology; and the Council on Stroke recommend the following in terms of patient management:[62]

1. Monitoring in an ICU setting.
2. Early hemodynamic optimization with goals of:
   a. MAP 65–100mmHg (taking into consideration the patient's normal blood pressure, cause of arrest, and severity of myocardial dysfunction).
   b. Central Venous Pressure 8–12mmHg.
   c. $ScVO_2 > 70\%$.
   d. Urine output > 1mL/kg/hr.
   e. A normal or decreasing serum or blood lactate level.
3. Maintenance of arterial oxygen saturation: 94–96%.
4. Optimized ventilation:
   a. Adjusted to achieve normocarbia as monitored by arterial blood gas.
   b. Avoidance of hyperventilation (increases intrathoracic pressure which decreases cardiac output).

5. Restoration and maintenance of end-organ perfusion through the use of volume expansion and vasoactive or inotropic drugs.
    a. Early echocardiography enables the extent of myocardial dysfunction to be estimated and may guide therapy.[62]
    b. Intra-aortic balloon pump, extracorporeal membrane oxygenation, or transthoracic assist devices may be considered in the setting of volume and inotrope failure.
6. Glucose control with a target of up to 8mmol/L (144mg/dL) with frequent monitoring to avoid hypo/hyperglycemia.
7. Prompt evaluation and treatment of seizure activity (seizures occur in 5–15% of adult patients achieving ROSC, and 10–40% of those remaining comatose secondary to anoxic injury).[63] Consider clonazepam, sodium valproate, or levetiracetam for myoclonus.
8. Therapeutic temperature control may be initiated in all comatose survivors of cardiac arrest, regardless of initial rhythm and location of arrest (out-of-hospital vs. in-hospital) as studies demonstrate increased survival and improved neurologic outcomes in patients presenting with ventricular fibrillation (VF), and the potential for increased neurological outcomes in patients with rhythms other than pulseless ventricular tachycardia (VT)/VF.[60,64-67]
    a. Guidelines currently recommend cooling for 24 hours at 32° C–36° C, though prior studies evaluated temperatures less than 36° C."[68-70]
    b. Adequate sedation and/or neuromuscular blockade to prevent shivering and support ventilation is key.
    c. Conventional thinking is that targeted temperature management (avoiding post-resuscitation hyperthermia) is a critical component of post-resuscitation management, and some experts believe this provides the primary benefit, previously attributed to therapeutic hypothermia.

What did the actual provider do?

Plan: Patient is hemodynamically improving following the administration of alteplase. Current SBP 91. Plan to hang a third liter of normal saline and discuss inotropic support with the intensivist. Patient currently in the radiology suite: CTPA to confirm diagnosis. Intubation and sedation: VBG pending—will titrate settings to avoid hypercarbia and trend lactate if results obtained prior to ICU admission.

Labs reviewed: ECG as documented. D-dimer elevated—coincides with presumed diagnosis of cardiac rest secondary to massive PE.
CXR independently reviewed: ETT and NGT in position, no acute cardiopulmonary pathology.

Consult placed to Intensivist: Discussed care at 2025—Admit to ICU
Consult placed to Vascular Surgeon: Discussed care at 2035—Will see patient.

Diagnosis: Cardiopulmonary Arrest, Hypotension, Hypoxemia.

MR#XXXXX **6 June 2010**
Time Stamp: 22:50

CT Pulmonary Angiography:

1. Bilateral large saddle emboli extending into bilateral lobar and segmental branches.
2. Multifocal pulmonary opacities and ground-glass opacities consistent with pulmonary infarctions.
3. Tip of endotracheal tube 3cm above carina.

Patient transported to the ICU at 23:26:

Vitals:						
Temp	Pulse	Resp	Syst	Diast	Sat	Pain
99.6	76	12 (vent)	98	65	97% (40% FiO_2)	- / 10

What was the patient's outcome?

MR#XXXXX **7 June 2010**
Time Stamp: 02:30

Vascular Surgery Consultation: This patient is an unfortunate 36-year-old, who apparently earlier today was complaining of shortness of breath, was brought into the emergency room by the rescue squad. Upon arrival to the ED, the patient had a full cardiopulmonary arrest, was promptly intubated, and CPR was done. Thought of pulmonary embolus was entertained, and the patient was then promptly given tPA. After approximately 20–30 minutes of CPR, and the tPA, apparently her pulse and rhythm returned with the assistance of vasoconstrictive agents. I then had the opportunity to interview the patient's mother and boyfriend, who stated that she has had a swollen, sore, left leg for approximately 2 weeks, and thought that she might have pulled a muscle. She denies significant past medical history, but does use birth control pills. Family history is positive for a grandmother with unprecipitated venous thrombosis in one of her legs at the age of 50. Given this information, I felt that she indeed had a pulmonary embolus and suggested that we do a CT angiogram. The CTA showed a large saddle embolus. I have therefore explained to the patient's family that we should proceed with the placement of a vena cava filter.

MR#XXXXX **8 June 2010**
Time Stamp: 05:38

Hospital Day: #1
ICU Provider Progress Note: US left lower extremity: DVT of the left common femoral vein.

MR#XXXXX **8 June 2010**
Time Stamp: 11:40

Hospital Day: #1
Neurology Consultation: The exam was limited. The patient was intubated; mildly agitated since

she has been off Diprivan for the past 10–15 minutes. Blood pressure 107/41, Temperature 99.2, Pulse 135 beats per minute. Her eyes were open. She had disconjugate gaze off and on, deviated to the left. Pupils were about 3mm bilaterally, both reactive to light. Corneal reflexes were hypoactive bilaterally. Gag present. Jaw jerk was normal. Fundoscopic exam was unremarkable – no evidence of papilledema; however, I did not note normal venous pulsations on either side. Oculocephalic maneuver was impaired; the left eye could not pass midline. Tone was within normal limits. I did not appreciate any myoclonus involver her face or limbs. She was moving her extremities randomly, predominately on the left side. There was no pathologic posturing. Hyporeflexia throughout. Toes do not move with plantar stimulation. No meningeal signs. No cranial tenderness. Carotid pulses 2+ bilaterally. Difficult to discern the presence or absence of carotid bruits given the sound of the ventilator.

Summary of Findings: Left disconjugate gaze and hyporeflexia – likely secondary to anoxic brain injury. Tachycardia.

MR#XXXXX **8 June 2010**
Time Stamp: 11:40

Hospital Day: #2
ICU Provider Summary: Hematology consulted. Patient noted as oliguric/anuric (creatinine 1.8 » 5.7). As laboratory data indicate improving CPK levels, this acute renal failure is likely due to systemic hypoxia and hypoperfusion. Nephrology consultation placed.

MR#XXXXX **8 June 2010**
Time Stamp: 14:40

Hospital Day: #2
ICU Provider Progress Note: Discussed case with nephrologist. Dialysis to be initiated this afternoon.

MR#XXXXX **9 June 2010**
Time Stamp: 08:11

Hospital Day: #3
Hematology Consultation: Acute pulmonary embolus. This 36-year-old non-smoking young female with no other medical problems presents with a new onset PE. The patient is on oral contraceptive pills which can increase the risk of blood clots. No known history of hypercoagulable state. Other than the grandmother, no known family history of hypercoagulable state. The patient has already been tested for dyscrasias: protein C, protein 2, antithrombin III, factor V Leiden mutation, prothrombin mutation, homocysteine level. As these labs are send-outs, I await the results; however, I am not sure as to whether or not the blood draws were performed prior to, or following, heparin administration. The results of these tests will not impact current patient management: anticoagulation for 1 year, and discontinuation of birth control containing estrogens. If the patient is found to have a blood dyscrasia pre-disposing to thrombosis, life-long anticoagulation will be warranted. Will continue to follow.

MR#XXXXX

9 June 2010
Time Stamp: 16:55

Hospital Day: #3
ICU Provider Summary: Patient successfully extubated. Neurologic exam: short-term memory impairment, myoclonus of the upper and lower extremities, and difficulty with rapid-alternating-movements. EEG revealing slowing of background activity consistent with diffuse encephalopathy. Discussed with Neurology provider: lorazepam for myoclonus; initiation of cognitive therapy.

MR#XXXXX **10 June 2010**
Time Stamp: 01:09

Hospital Day: #4
Vascular Surgery Progress Note: Patient doing well. IVC filter placed today without complication.

After 24 days of hospitalization, the patient's renal function normalized, she was transitioned to warfarin, her myoclonus was controlled with lorazepam, and she displayed improvement in cognitive function. An MRI was unable to be obtained secondary to the placement of the IVC. An extensive evaluation of inherited and autoimmune etiologies of hypercoagulability revealed no underlying etiology. On discharge, she was ambulatory and walked out of the hospital on her own.

Hospital discharge diagnoses: Pulmonary embolism/infarct, cardiac arrest, respiratory failure, hypotension, acute renal failure, anoxic brain damage, encephalopathy, deep venous thrombosis of the common femoral vein.

References:

1. Yealy DM, Kosowsky J. Dysrhythmias. In Rosen's Emergency Medicine. 8th ed. Philadelphia. Saunders Elsevier. 2014; 79:1034-1063.e1.
2. Mega J, Morrow D. ST-Elevation myocardial infarction: Management. In: Braunwald's heart disease: A textbook of cardiovascular medicine. 10th ed. Philadelphia: Elsevier, 2015;52:1095-154.
3. Burstein J, Hollander J, Henry M, et al. Association of out-of-hospital criteria with need for hospital admission. Acad Emerg Med 1995;2(10):863-6.
4. Barfod C, Lauritzen M, Danker J, et al. Abnormal vital signs are strong predictors for intensive care unit admission and in-hospital mortality in adults triaged in the emergency department – a prospective cohort study. Scand J Trauma Resusc Emerg Med 2012;20(1):28.
5. Sklar D, Crandall C, Loeliger, E, et al. Unanticipated death after discharge home from the emergency department. Ann Emerg Med 2007;49(6):735-45.
6. Modi S, Krahn A. Sudden cardiac arrest without overt heart disease. Circulation 2011;123(25):2994-3008.
7. Sauer W. American College of Cardiology: Cardiac sarcoidosis and sudden death risk: what is the "consensus" regarding the approach to management, diagnosis, and treatment? 2015: Available at http://www.acc.org/latest-in-cardiology/articles/2015/03/26/07/57/cardiac-

sarcoidosis-and-sudden-death-risk.
8. Agarwal S, Tuzcu E. Hypertrophic cardiomyopathy. In: Cardiovascular intervention: A companion to Braunwald's heart disease. 1st ed. Philadelphia: Elsevier, 2016;31;498-518.
9. Orgeron G, Calkins H. Advances in the diagnosis and management of arrhythmogenic right ventricular dysplasia/cardiomyopathy. Curr Cardiol Rep 2016;18(6):53.
10. Hoyt W, Snyder C. The asymptomatic Wolff-Parkinson-White syndrome. Prog Pediatr Cardiol 2013;35(1):17-24.
11. Ko N. Cardiac manifestations of acute neurologic lesions. In: Aminoff's neurology and general medicine. 5th ed. Philadelphia: Elsevier, 2014;10:183-98.
12. Casazza F, Pacchetti I, Rulli E, et al. Prognostic significance of electrocardiogram at presentation in patients with pulmonary embolism of different severity. Thromb Res 2018;163:123-7.
13. Carroll B, Heidinger B, Dabreo D, et al. Multimodality assessment of right ventricular strain in patients with acute pulmonary embolism. Am J Cardiol 2018;122(1):175-81.
14. Mallin M, Butts C. Emergency cardiac ultrasound: evaluation for pericardial effusion and cardiac activity In: Emergency Medicine: Clinical Essentials 2nd Ed. Philadelphia: Elsevier, 2013;5:43-9.
15. Shoenberger J, Massopust K, Henderson S. The use of bedside ultrasound in cardiac arrest. Cat J Emerg Med 2007;8(2):47-50.
16. Whitson M, Mayo P. Ultrasonography in the emergency department. Crit Care 2016; 20:227
17. American College of Emergency Physicians. Policy Statement. Ultrasound Guidelines: Emergency Point-of-care, and Clinical Ultrasound Guidelines in Medicine. 2016. Available at: https://www.acep.org/globalassets/new-pdfs/policy-statements/ultrasound-guidelines—emergency-point-of-care-and-clinical-ultrasound-guidelines-in-medicine.pdf
18. Hernandez C, Shuler K, Hannan H, et al. C.A.U.S.E.: Cardiac arrest ultra-sound exam—a better approach to managing patients in primary non-arrhythmogenic cardiac arrest. Resuscitation 2007;76(2):198-06.
19. Littmann L, Bustin D, Haley M. A simplified and structured teaching tool for the evaluation and management of pulseless electrical activity. Med Princ Pract 2014;23(1):1-6.
20. Volpicelli G. Usefulness of emergency ultrasound in nontraumatic cardiac arrest. Am J Emerg Med 2011;136(9): 691-700.
21. Budhram G, Reardon R, Plummer D. Critical care. In: Ma & Mateer's Emergency Ultrasound. 3rd ed. New York: McGraw-Hill, 2014;8;191-224.
22. Goldhaber S. Echocardiography in the management of pulmonary embolism. Ann Intern Med 2002;136(9):691-700.
23. Steiner R, Tegtmeyer C, Morse D, et al. The Radiologic Society of North America: The Radiology of Cardiac Pacemakers. Radiographics. Available from: http://pubs.rsna.org/doi/pdf/10.1148/radiographics.6.3.3317544.
24. Blaivas M, Lyon M, Duggal S. A prospective comparison of supine chest radiography and bedside ultrasound for the diagnosis of traumatic pneumothorax. Acad Emerg Med 2005;12(9):844-9.
25. Garofalo G, Busso M, Perotto F, et al. Ultrasound diagnosis of pneumothorax. Radiol Med 2006;111(4):516-25.
26. Knudtson J, Dort J, Helmer S, et al. Surgeon-performed ultrasound for pneumothorax in the trauma suite. J Trauma 2004;56(3):527-30.

27. Gaspari R, Weekes A, Adhikari S, et al. Emergency department point-of-care ultrasound in out-of-hospital and in-ED cardiac arrest. Resuscitation 2016;109:33-9.
28. Bolvardi E, Pouryaghobi S, Farzane R, et al. The prognostic value of using ultrasonography in cardiac resuscitation of patients with cardiac arrest. Int J Biomed Sci 2016;12(3):110-4.
29. Blyth L, Atkinson P, Gadd K, et al. Bedside focused echocardiography as predictor of survival in cardiac arrest patients: a systematic review. Acad Emerg Med 2012;19(10):1119-26.
30. ECC Committee. 2005 American Heart Association guidelines for cardiopulmonary resuscitation and emergency cardiovascular care. Circulation 2005;112(24 Suppl): IV1-203.
31. Baskett P, Steen P, Bossaert L. European Resuscitation Council guidelines for resuscitation 2005. Section 8. The ethics of resuscitation and end-of-life decisions. Resuscitation 2005;67(Suppl 1):S171-80.
32. American Heart Association. Part 7.2: Management of cardiac arrest. Circulation. 2005;112:IV-58-IV-66.
33. Barsan W, Levy R, Weir H. Lidocaine levels during CPR: differences after peripheral venous, central venous, and intracardiac injections. Ann Emerg Med 1981;10(2):73-8.
34. Emerman C, Pinchak A, Hancock D, et al. Effect of injection site on circulation times during cardiac arrest. Crit Care Med 1988;16(11):1138-41.
35. Banerjee S, Singhi S, Singh S, et al. The intraosseous route is a suitable alternative to intravenous route for fluid resuscitation in severely dehydrated children. Indian Pediatr 1995; 31(12):1511-20.
36. Brickman K, Krupp K, Rega P, et al. Typing and screening of blood from intraosseous access. Ann Emerg Med 1992;21(4):414-7.
37. Fisher T, Walker W, Seibert J, et al. Tibial length following intraosseous infusion: a prospective, radiographic analysis. Pediatr Emerg Care 1997;13(3):186-8.
38. Ummenhofer W, Frei F, Urwyler A, et al. Are laboratory values in bone marrow aspirate predictable for venous blood in paediatric patients? Resuscitation 1994;27(2):123-8.
39. Wenzel V, Linkner K, Prengel A, et al. Endobronchial vasopressin improves survival during cardiopulmonary resuscitation in pigs. Anesthesiology 1997;86(6):1375-81.
40. Prengel A, Rembecki M, Wenzel V, et al. A comparison of the endotracheal tube and the laryngeal mask airway as a route for endobronchial lidocaine administration. Anesth Analg 2001;92(6):1505-9.
41. Jassani M, Nadkarni V, Finkelstein M, et al. Effects of different techniques of endotracheal epinephrine administration in pediatric porcine hypoxic-hyperbaric cardiopulmonary arrest. Crit Care Med 1994;22(7):1174-80.
42. Vaknin Z, Manisterski Y, Ben-Abraham R, et al. Is endotracheal adrenaline deleterious because of the beta adrenergic effect? Anesth Analg 2001;92(6):1037-41.
43. Manisterski Y, Vaknin Z, Ben-Abraham R, et al. Endotracheal epinephrine: a call for larger doses. Anesth Analg 2002;95(4):1037-41.
44. Sharifi M, Berger J, Beeston P, et al. Pulseless electrical activity in pulmonary embolism treated with thrombolysis (from the PEAPETT study). Am J Emerg Med 2016;34(10):1963-7.
45. Le Conte P, Hutchet L, Trewick D, et al. Efficacy of alteplase thrombolysis for ED treatment of pulmonary embolism with shock. Am J Emerg Med 2003;21(5):438-40.
46. Newman D, Greenwald I, Callaway C. Cardiac arrest and the role of thrombolytic agents. Ann Emerg Med 2000;35(5):472-80.

47. Stein P, Matta F. Thrombolytic therapy in unstable patients with acute pulmonary embolism: saves lives but underused. Am J Med 2012;125(5):465-70.
48. Logan J, Pantle H, Huiras P, et al. Evidence-based diagnosis and thrombolytic treatment of cardiac arrest and periarrest due to suspected pulmonary embolism. Am J Emerg Med 2014;32(7):789-96.
49. Jaff M, McMurtry M, Archer S, et al. American Heart Association Council on Cardiopulmonary Critical Care, Perioperative and Resuscitation; American Heart Association Council on Peripheral Vascular Disease; American Heart Association Council on Arteriosclerosis, Thrombosis and Vascular Biology. Management of massive and submassive pulmonary embolism, iliofemoral deep vein thrombosis, and chronic thromboembolic pulmonary hypertension: a scientific statement from the American Heart Association. Circulation. 2011;123(16):1788-830.
50. Fava M, Loyola S, Bertoni H, et al. Massive pulmonary embolism: percutaneous mechanical thrombectomy during cardiopulmonary resuscitation. J Vasc Interv Radiol 2005;16(1):119-23.
51. Konstantinov I, Saxena P, Koniuszko M, et al. Acute massive pulmonary embolism with cardiopulmonary resuscitation: management and results. Tex Heart Inst J 2007;34(1):41-6.
52. Böttiger B, Arntz H, Chamberlain D, et al. Thrombolysis during resuscitation for out-of-hospital cardiac arrest. N Engl J Med 2008;359(25):2651-62.
53. Schmid C, Zietlow S, Wagner T, et al. Fulminant pulmonary embolism: symptoms, diagnostics, operative technique, and results. Ann Thorac Surg 1991;52(5):1102-7.
54. Vanden Hoek T, Morrison L, Shuster M, et al. Part 12: cardiac arrest in special situations: 2010 American Heart Association Guidelines for cardiopulmonary resuscitation and emergency. Circulation 2010;122(18 Suppl 3):S829-61.
55. Konstantinov I, Saxena P, Koniuszko M, et al. Acute massive pulmonary embolism with cardiopulmonary resuscitation: management and results. Tex Heart Inst J 2007;34(1):41-6.
56. Hess E, Campbell R, White R. Epidemiology, trends, and outcome of out-of-hospital cardiac arrest of non-cardiac origin. Resuscitation 2007;72(2):200-6.
57. Deasy C, Bray J, Smith K, et al. Out-of-hospital cardiac arrests in young adults in Melbourne, Australia—adding coronial data to a cardiac arrest registry. Resuscitation 2011;82(10):1302-6.
58. Stadlbauer K, Krismer A, Arntz H, et al. Effects of thrombolysis during out-of-hospital cardiopulmonary resuscitation. Am J Cardiol 2006;97(3):305-8.
59. Brady W, Monteleone P, Sochor M, et al. Management of cardiac arrest and post-cardiac arrest syndrome. In: Emergency Medicine: Clinical Essentials. 2nd Ed. Philadelphia: Elsevier, 2013;7:55-71.
60. Nolan J, Neumar R, Adrie C, et al. Post-cardiac arrest syndrome: epidemiology, pathophysiology, treatment, and prognostication. A Scientific Statement from the International Liaison Committee on Resuscitation; the American Heart Association Emergency Cardiovascular Care Committee; the Council on Cardiovascular Surgery and Anesthesia; the Council on Cardiopulmonary, Perioperative, and Critical Care; the Council on Clinical Cardiology; the Council on Stroke. Resuscitation 2008;79(3):350-79.
61. Laver S, Farrow C, Turner D, et al. Mode of death after admission to an intensive care unit following cardiac arrest. Intensive Care Med 2004;30(11):2126-8.
62. Kern K, Hilwig R, Berg R, et al. Postresuscitation left ventricular systolic and diastolic dysfunction. Treatment with dobutamine. Circulation 1997;95(12):2610-3.

63. Daviness J, Brown P. Myoclonus: current concepts and recent advances. Lancet Neurol 2003;3(10):598-607.
64. Hypothermia after Cardiac Arrest Study Group. Mild therapeutic hypothermia to improve the neurologic outcome after cardiac arrest [published correction appears in N Engl J Med. 2002;346:1756]. N Engl J Med 2002;346(8):549–56.
65. Bernard S, Gray T, Buist M, et al. Treatment of comatose survivors of out-of-hospital cardiac arrest with induced hypothermia. N Engl J Med 2002;346(8):557-63.
66. Oddo M, Schaller M, Feihl F, et al. From evidence to clinical practice: effective implementation of therapeutic hypothermia to improve patient outcome after cardiac arrest. Crit Care Med 2006;34(7):1865-73.
67. Sunde K, Pytte M, Jacobsen D, et al. Implementation of a standardized treatment protocol for post resuscitation care after out-of-hospital cardiac arrest. Resuscitation 2007;73(1):29-39.
68. Holzer M, Bernard S, Hachimi-Idrissi S, et al. Collaborative Group on Induced Hypothermia for Neuroprotection After Cardiac Arrest. Hypothermia for neuroprotection after cardiac arrest: systematic review and individual patient data meta-analysis. Crit Care Med 2005;33(2):414-8.
69. Nolan J, Morley P, Hoek T, et al. Advancement Life Support Task Force of the International Liaison Committee on Resuscitation. Therapeutic hypothermia after cardiac arrest: an advisory statement by the Advanced Life Support Task Force of the International Liaison Committee on Resuscitation. Resuscitation 2003;57(3):231-5.
70. Nielsen N, Wetterslev J, Cronbert T, et al. Targeted temperature management at 33°C versus 36°C after cardiac arrest. N Engl J Med 2013;369(23):2197-206.

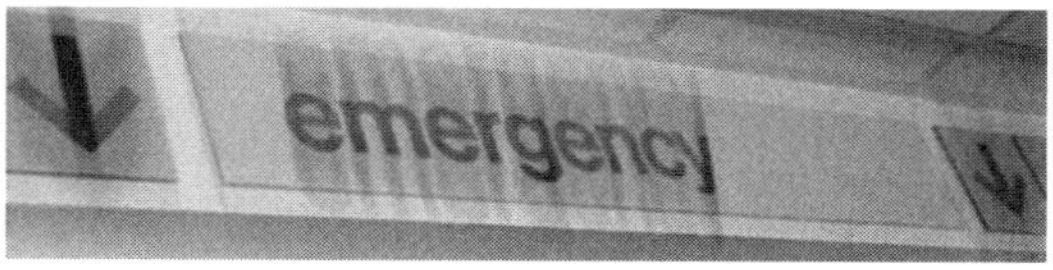

SECTION B – BREATHING/ PULMONARY

Chapter 7: A 56-year-old healthy man with bronchitis and shortness of breath

Michael Pallaci, DO, FACEP

Clinical Professor
Emergency Medicine
Ohio University Heritage College of Osteopathic Medicine
Athens, OH

Brent Arnold, DO

Emergency Medicine Attending
Envision Healthcare
St. Petersburg, FL

Section editor:

Donald M. Yealy, MD

Chair, Department of Emergency Medicine
University of Pittsburgh/University of Pittsburgh Physicians
Vice President, Emergency and Urgent Care Services, Physician Services
UPMC Professor of Emergency Medicine, Medicine and Clinical and Translational Sciences
University of Pittsburgh School of Medicine
Pittsburgh, PA

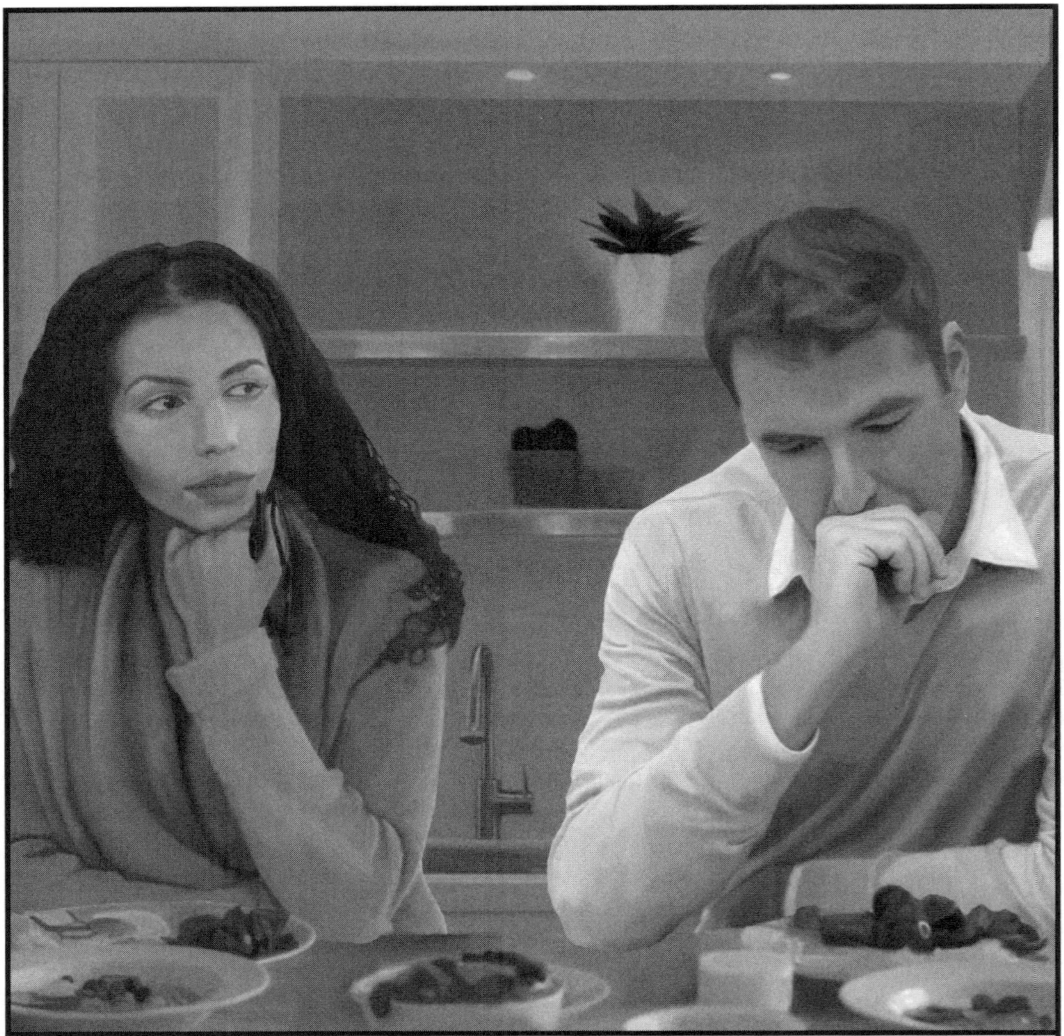

"I JUST CAN'T CATCH MY BREATH..."

SECTION B/CHAPTER 7

A 56-year-old healthy man with bronchitis and shortness of breath

The patient's story:
Doug Panchin is a middle-aged man who visits his primary care physician for a 5-day history of cough and is prescribed an antibiotic and a cough syrup. His symptoms minimally improve. A week later, his cough worsens and he develops shortness of breath, even with minimal exertion. He ignores the symptoms, but when his wife sees him in the kitchen, an elbow on the table as he struggles to catch his breath, she dials 911.

EMS arrive to find him diaphoretic with an ambient oxygen saturation of 71%. They place him on a facemask with minimal saturation improvement, so they convert to CPAP. His blood pressure is 85/palp, and 2 IVs are started; he is taken to the Emergency Department.

ED VISIT

CC-Triage RN (16:52): Respiratory Distress

HPI: I have reviewed the nurse's notes. This is a 56-year-old former smoker with history of hypertension who presents for evaluation of shortness of breath and mild chest pain. Patient was treated a week and half ago with bronchitis and last Thursday started on Levaquin for pneumonia. Patient reports over the last couple days his symptoms got worse with the dyspnea with exertion and then chest pain and cough. Wife called EMS due to shortness of breath. EMS found the patient in respiratory distress breathing 30-40 times a minute and severely hypoxic satting 71% on room air. Patient was put on CPAP. Patient is talking but does report shortness of breath. No history of family history of blood clots. No leg swelling recent long travel. No history of heart attack or strokes. Patient quit smoking in 1989 and never been diagnosed with lung problems like asthma or COPD. No recent hospitalizations. No allergies same medicines. She denies any fever, bleeding disorders, blood in the urine or stool, edema, abd pain, rash, immunocompromise.

Health Status:
NKDA
Meds: None
PMH/PSH: None

PE:

Vitals:

Time	Temp	Pulse	Resp	Syst	Diast	Sat (NRB mask)
16:64		105	36	89	54	81%

CONSTITUTIONAL: Alert, is able to speak in 1-2 word sentences only, mildly diaphoretic, color good
HEAD: Normocephalic; atraumatic
NECK: No JVD or distended neck veins
RESP: Normal chest excursion with respiration; tachypneic, breath sounds coarse with bibasilar rales
CARDIO: Regular rhythm, without murmurs, rub or gallop
ABD: Non-distended; good bowel sounds; soft and non-tender; without rigidity, rebound or guarding, no pulsatile mass
EXTREMITIES: Pulses are 2 plus and equal times 4 extremities, no peripheral edema or calf muscle pain

Author comments (Weinstock):

You are at the bedside of a patient who is diaphoretic, hypoxemic on CPAP, and in obvious acute respiratory distress. You are in the footsteps of the EP at decision point A:

DECISION POINT A – YOU ARE FACED WITH 4 QUESTIONS:

1. **What is the differential diagnosis?**
2. **Which diagnostic tests should be ordered?**
3. **What is the initial approach to evaluation of a tachypneic, alert patient with profound hypoxemia?**
4. **Is intubation indicated?**

What does the literature say?

Q#1: What is the differential diagnosis?

Chest pain (CP) and shortness of breath (SOB) are common complaints, but there is a big difference between subjective SOB and acute respiratory distress. A logical way to organize the potential causes of our patient's presentation is to use a systems-based approach that assesses **airway, respiratory, cardiac, systemic, and central findings.** As is true with any presentation, no matter how emergent (even cardiac arrest), the evaluation starts with an H&P and focuses on life-threatening etiologies:

- **Airway:** Foreign body, angioedema/anaphylaxis, epiglottitis, croup, mass, mucus plug.
- **Respiratory:** Pneumonia, pneumothorax (including tension), ARDS, pulmonary embolism (PE), COPD/asthma, lung cancer, pulmonary hypertension, pulmonary fibrosis.
- **Cardiac:** Acute coronary syndrome (ACS), heart failure, cardiac tamponade, valvular heart disease, pericarditis/myocarditis, endocarditis, arrhythmia.
- **Systemic/Vascular:** Aortic dissection, Boerhaave's syndrome, anemia, metabolic acidosis, diabetic ketoacidosis (DKA), thyroid abnormality.

- **Central:** Psychological, myasthenia gravis, Guillain-Barre syndrome, botulism, Cheyne-stoke respirations (from intracranial pathology).

Q#2: Which diagnostic tests should be ordered?

An ECG will identify STEMI, dysrhythmia, some signs of PE (tachycardia, right heart strain), low-voltage or electrical alternans in effusion with tamponade, pericarditis, or electrolyte abnormalities. The CXR can identify pneumonia, pleural effusions, pulmonary edema, pneumothorax or pneumomediastinum and masses; it can point us in the direction of dissection, although with poor specificity and inadequate sensitivity. Still, we get lots of information from two cheap, non-invasive, easy-to-interpret, tests.

Section editor comments (Yealy):

Small abnormalities are easy to miss on plain chest radiography—including infiltrates or air collections—but those subtleties rarely cause profound symptoms or hypoxemia alone. In someone has a truly normal chest radiograph and profound symptoms or an oxygenation deficit, think PE, hemoglobinopathy, or a non-chest cause.

Consulting editor comments (Weingart):

I have found profound multi-lobar pneumonias that were not apparent on CXR, even retrospectively. If there is hypoxemia without obvious cause, it should prompt a chest CT, and a CTA if the patient milieu allows. It is acceptable to perform a non-con chest CT first if there is a concern about contrast.

A targeted laboratory evaluation can also be helpful:

- CBC/BMP: These two simple tests identify significant anemia, leukocytosis, oncologic emergencies such as acute blast crisis, and platelet abnormalities, while the metabolic panel will identify serious electrolyte abnormalities, renal failure, and hyper or hypoglycemia.
- Troponin: Troponin elevation occurs in MI, but it is also predictive of a poor prognosis in patients with heart failure, sepsis and PE (one of the criteria for submassive PE), and can also be elevated in myocarditis.

Section editor comments (Yealy):

Newer high sensitivity troponin assays are excellent markers for myocardial injury (though the reason the injury exists requires other testing and clinical information).

- D-dimer: This is a poor screening test due to its low specificity and is not sensitive enough to rule out PE in high-risk patients but is useful in patients who are low to moderate risk. Our clinical suspicion for PE is low in this case but likely not low enough to rule out PE on clinical grounds alone. We do recommend a D-dimer for our patient.
- Brain Natriuretic Peptide (BNP) assays have the ability to assess for heart failure, mostly by ruling out the diagnosis with a very low level. BNP elevation can occur in numerous conditions, both chronic (renal failure, heart failure, COPD) and acute (heart failure, submassive PE), with a negative predictive value of the BNP for heart failure of 94–98%. Schwam, et al. summarized that when the pretest probability of HF was thought to be 95–100%, then the actual rate of HF was 95%. When the pretest probability was thought to be 0–4%, the actual rate of HF

was 7%. In these 2 situations, the clinical judgment was better than the BNP levels. But for the pretest probabilities in the middle (5–94%), clinical judgment alone was not adequate and other testing was necessary. In these patients, a BNP level lower than 50–80pg/mL basically rules out HF, a level of 400–1,000 has a moderate ability to rule in HF, and if the BNP level is > 1,000, there is a high likelihood of HF. They concluded that BNP levels between 80 and 400 are not helpful in the diagnosis of acute HF.[1,2]

- ABG: Burri, et al. concluded that "ABGs on presentation did not help to identify a specific cause, nor to differentiate a pulmonary from non-pulmonary cause, in unselected patients presenting to the ED with acute dyspnea."[3] If acidemia or hypercarbia is a concern, a VBG, especially when combined with a pulse ox, will provide information that is just as useful at a lower cost and with less discomfort to the patient.[4]

Section editor comments (Yealy):

In the patient with any concern of chronic and superimposed acute respiratory failure, an ABG remains preferred over VBG—when "you need to know pH and CO2 together," the ABG remains the best test.

Author comments (Weingart):

I have a different viewpoint as I can't imagine a scenario where the discrepancy between venous pH and PaCO2 and arterial would make a difference, especially since the venous indices are probably more representative of tissue values.

- Lactic acid: An easy tool that helps identify less obvious gaps in tissue perfusion and fluid resuscitation in sepsis.
- Blood cultures: These usually add little, especially in early care. In a systematic review, blood cultures in CAP were found to lead to a broadening of antibiotic therapy in 0–1% of cases and to a narrowing of antibiotic therapy in 0–3%, a cost of up to a whopping $8000 per change in therapy.[5] Another study found that blood cultures would need to be performed in 125 patients with pneumonia to identify 1 patient with a resistant infection.[6] ACEP issued a Level B recommendation in their 2009 clinical policy against routine blood cultures in patients with CAP.[7] However, cultures may help direct antibiotic therapy in patients who are immunocompromised, septic, in respiratory failure, who are otherwise critically ill, or who have failed outpatient treatment. We do recommend blood cultures for our patient in this case.
- Other laboratory tests, such as thyroid testing, coagulation studies and fibrinogen (DIC) are based on the clinical situation but are not recommended for our patient.

We agree that the decision to hold on intubation for now is reasonable as long as resources are at the bedside and immediately accessible.

Summary: For our patient, we would initially order a CBC, BMP, BNP, Troponin, D-Dimer, Lactate and blood cultures as well as an ECG, CXR and place the patient on a pulse ox and cardiac monitor.

Q#3: What is the initial approach to evaluation of a tachypneic, alert patient with profound hypoxemia?

Patients with tachypnea, tachycardia, accessory/abdominal muscle use, fatigue, agitation, changes in mental status, and conversational dyspnea are at high risk for deterioration. The obvious first step is oxygen; if that alone is inadequate, the next choices (aside from underlying disease therapies) are non-invasive positive pressure ventilation (NIPPV–CPAP, BiPAP) and intubation.

Choosing the next step is easier in the extremes: Respiratory distress + altered mental status = intubation and mechanical ventilation. No respiratory distress + normal vitals = other support while completing the history, exam and testing, and closely monitoring for changes. What makes our patient difficult is that his parameters are terrible, i.e., hypoxemia on a non-rebreather mask then CPAP, but he is alert and talking to us.

What are our options?

- Replace CPAP with BIPAP. The benefit of BiPAP over CPAP is improved ventilation, not improved oxygenation. Considering that our patient lacks any evidence of hypercarbia, changing CPAP to BiPAP wouldn't offer much benefit.
- Humidified oxygen via a high flow nasal cannula (HFNC). HFNC can improve respiratory status in patients with hypoxemic respiratory failure [8,9] when compared to facemask oxygen delivery systems in adults. A follow-up study concluded that while HFNC did not decrease the need for intubation, it did improve oxygenation and was associated with a significant reduction in mortality [9] when compared to BiPAP.
- Beyond oxygenation, decisions regarding other disease-specific interventions are directed by clinical suspicion for the underlying cause. While these therapies are started, prepare for intubation.

Consulting editor comments (Weingart):

I think most of the benefits of the HFNC devices come from compliance; if your patient can tolerate NIPPV masks without a leak, I doubt HFNC is any better and may be worse. A potential benefit comes when they are on the floor with less intense observation—emesis will not be as much of a concern compared to an NIPPV mask.

Should the CPAP mask have been removed in the ED? Though there is some utility in checking oxygen saturation (assuming CPAP improved it) off positive pressure, usually other clues including respiratory rate and effort and blood gas analysis will be helpful. While resuscitation and stabilization are still ongoing, we recommend uninterrupted use of NIPPV, barring vomiting or a change in status.

Q#4: Is intubation indicated?

Brown and Walls divided the reasons to intubate into 3 categories:

- *Failure to maintain or protect the airway:* There is no issue with the airway in our patient.
- *Failure of ventilation or oxygenation:* This is a clinical judgment that can be made at the bedside with a combination of physical exam findings and bedside monitoring equipment. ABG and VBG are equivalent in assessment of pH and ventilation (CO_2), and neither are superior to clinical judgment. Our patient is awake and coherent, and the decision to intubate should be made clinically, regardless of the pH or $PaCO_2$. Assuming a working pulse oximeter with a

good waveform, the PaO_2 does not add anything to the clinical assessment. He is persistently hypoxemic despite NIPPV with CPAP, which would justify intubation.

- *The patient's anticipated clinical course and likelihood of deterioration:* While he is in respiratory distress, nothing yet suggests that he is tiring out. If CT is being considered, he may not tolerate lying supine on the table for the study, and this would need to be taken into consideration when deciding whether or not to intubate.

So, should he be intubated? While it would be hard to argue against a decision to intubate based on his persistent hypoxemia, these authors recommend close observation and a trial of HFNC first.

What did the actual provider do?

Results: CXR: Worsening airspace opacities which may be progressive pulmonary edema or widespread pneumonia.

MDM: Physician Medical Decision Making (17:03): 57-year-old male presents with respiratory distress. Patient is talking but in severe respiratory distress, breathing up to 40 times a minute. We got a stat arterial blood gas which shows he is not acidotic. ECG with sinus tachycardia and nonspecific changes. Chest x-ray shows bilateral infiltrates. Differential includes pneumonia, ARDS, acute CHF, PE. We'll get CT angios chest rule out PE. We'll check blood work including a screening lactate for sepsis. Pneumonia is high in the differential as he has just been on Levaquin and he is acutely ill. We'll put him on broad-spectrum antibiotics for Pneumonia. We'll get blood cultures. We'll give IV fluids.

Were the provider's actions appropriate?

First things first; the missing temperature is a problem. We've heard the "vital signs are vital" mantra; making decisions without basic information invites poor choices, especially in a critically ill patient.

Consulting editor comments (Weingart):

The first recorded temperature is 2 days later at 0800 and was 99 (route not documented).

Perhaps the most important information would come from a bedside ultrasound. While septic shock is the most likely explanation for his hypotension, it is far from certain. Using the RUSH protocol (or other established bedside protocols) for undifferentiated hypotension will give information that is available within minutes and can often determine the etiology of the patient's shock. This would include an assessment of volume status and LV function, and check RV strain which would be present with a massive or submassive PE. Further, lung ultrasonography can quickly identify the cause of dyspnea in the ED. [10-14]

We agree that the decision to hold on intubation for now is reasonable as long as resources are at the bedside and immediately accessible.

Labs return (17:45):

WBC Count: 7.9thou/mcL	
Hemoglobin: 12.3gm/dL	**(Low)**
Platelet Count: 271thou/mcL	
Sodium Level: 130mMol/L	**(Low)**
Potassium Level: 3.7mMol/L	
Chloride Level: 100mMol/L	
Carbon Dioxide Level: 20mMol/L	**(Low)**
BUN: 29mg/dL	**(High)**
Creatinine: 1.21mg/dL	
Glucose Level: 165mg/dL	**(High) (18:07:26)**
Troponin 0.06 (neg)	
Lactic acid 2.6mmol/L	

Author comments (Weinstock):

The nurse tells you that the wife has now arrived. The patient has BiPAP started and is maintaining a sat of 89–91%, but is mildly diaphoretic. She asks if he is going to be OK. There is an uncomfortable silence as she looks toward her husband. You look over her shoulder and see him sitting up in the bed, breathing fast—he appears to be tiring out. We are at:

DECISION POINT B – WE ARE FACED WITH 5 QUESTIONS:

1. **Has the differential diagnosis changed?**
2. **Which physical exam and test findings are helpful to differentiate the etiology?**
3. **Should antibiotics be given at this time?**
4. **Should additional studies be ordered?**
5. **Is intubation indicated *now*?**

What does the literature say?

Q#1: Has the differential diagnosis changed?

At this point, he likely has acute respiratory distress syndrome (ARDS) with hypoxemic respiratory failure secondary to a diffuse bilateral community acquired pneumonia refractory to outpatient therapy, complicated by septic shock. The differential includes:

- *Aspiration:* Unlikely in this case (not an alcoholic, not debilitated, hasn't been vomiting).
- *Legionella: Legionella* has a high rate of treatment failure [15] and is one of the common causes of drug-resistant pneumonia. Other than his age and a distant history of smoking, he does not have risk factors typically associated with *Legionella*, but evaluation for this entity is recommended by the CDC [16] in patients with CAP who fail outpatient therapy or who are severely ill.
- *Viral pneumonia:* Viral pneumonias can be difficult to diagnose and treat. Influenza is the most common, but treatment with oseltamivir, amantadine or rimantadine remains controversial, despite the current CDC recommendations for treatment. RSV is the most common cause of viral pneumonia in children and the second most common cause in adults. Other less common causes include adenoviruses, coronaviruses (MERS, SARS), arboviruses, rotavirus, parainfluenza virus and hantavirus (rats). Viral pneumonia remains a consideration in our patient.

- *Tuberculosis:* Classic CXR findings in tuberculosis include upper lobe infiltrates, cavitary lesions or a miliary pattern. While the absence of these findings doesn't rule out TB, their absence in combination with the absence of risk factors and other typical symptoms (hemoptysis, night sweats, exposure to others with TB, weight loss) make this diagnosis unlikely.
- *Bacterial pneumonia resistant to Levofloxacin: Pneumococcus,* MSSA/MRSA, and *Pseudomonas* are relatively common causes of treatment failure in community acquired pneumonia (CAP), although MRSA and *Pseudomonas* are more common in nursing home patients or from nosocomial infections. Drug-resistant pneumococcus has become increasingly common. Less common bacterial causes of drug-resistant pneumonia include *Coxiella* (cats, goats, sheep, cattle), *Tularemia* (rabbits, ticks), *Leptospirosis* (rats), *Psittacosis* (birds), and *Nocardia* (steroid treatment).[15] A drug-resistant bacterial pneumonia remains high on the differential for our patient.
- *Fungi:* While uncommon, fungal pneumonias need to be considered if the history raises red flags. Possibilities include histoplasmosis (Ohio River Valley, Mississippi River Valley), coccidiomycosis (southwestern US), blastomycosis (Ohio River Valley, Mississippi River Valley, upper Midwest, southeastern Canada), *Pneumocystis jiroveci* (formerly known as *Pneumocystis carinii* pneumonia/PCP as seen in immunocompromised patients, especially those with AIDS), and *sporotrichiosis* (tropical regions). While our patient is not immunocompromised, a detailed travel history is advisable.
- *Right-sided endocarditis with septic pulmonary emboli:* Given the absence of murmur and the absence of risk factors such as IV drug abuse, endocarditis is unlikely.
- *Non-infectious causes:* Examples include acute chest syndrome in patients with sickle cell disease, silicosis, bronchiolitis obliterans with organizing pneumonia (BOOP), farmer's lung, hypersensitivity pneumonitis, acute eosinophilic pneumonia, oncologic causes (lymphangitic spread of lung cancer), and immunologic causes (Wegener's granulomatosis, sarcoidosis, Goodpasture's syndrome).

Q#2: Which physical exam and test findings are helpful to differentiate the etiology?

Physical exam and CXR findings are unreliable in identifying the causative organism in pneumonia, but some patterns can provide clues to the diagnosis. For example,

- *Klebsiella* (more common in alcoholics or patients from nursing homes) is a consideration in patients with relative bradycardia.
- Extra-pulmonary (especially GI) symptoms should raise suspicion for *Legionella* or *Mycoplasma.*
- Cavitary lung lesions have a broad differential diagnosis that includes *Staphylococcci, Klebsiella* and tuberculosis.
- A miliary pattern on CXR suggests miliary TB or carcinomatous lymphangitis.
- Calcified mediastinal adenopathy is suggestive of sarcoidosis.

WBC, C-reactive protein and other inflammatory markers are unhelpful in the acute evaluation of pneumonia.

Q#3: Should antibiotics be given at this time?

For patients with community-acquired pneumonia being admitted to the ICU, the IDSA/ATS guidelines [17] recommend a beta-lactam (cefotaxime, ceftriaxone or ampicillin-sulbactam) plus either azithromycin or a fluoroquinolone. An antipneumococcal, antipseudomonal beta-lactam (piperacillin-tazobactam, cefepime, imipenem, or meropenem) is recommended if *Pseudomonas* is suspected, and either vancomycin or linezolid is recommended for community-acquired MRSA.

Section editor comments (Yealy):

For the most sick patients like this one described, choose broad coverage and give it fast — stewardship and narrow selection are not high concerns with respiratory failure and shock!

Q#4: Should additional studies be ordered?

Yes. Though blood cultures are not recommended for most immunocompetent patients being admitted with CAP, they should be obtained in critically ill patients going to the ICU and for patients who have failed outpatient therapy. Sputum[18] cultures on expectorated sputum are notoriously low-yield, but in intubated patients, tracheal aspirates have an excellent diagnostic yield. This is the method of choice for diagnosis of *Legionella*, tuberculosis, and other important causes of CAP with treatment failure. Urinary antigens for *Legionella* are not part of the routine work-up for CAP but are recommended by the IDSA and others in patients who are intubated or who have failed outpatient treatment.[19] Echocardiography should be performed if pulmonary edema, pulmonary embolism or endocarditis are still being considered.

Q#5: Is intubation indicated *now*?

We still are not concerned about airway protection. He is not acidemic or hypercarbic, but he is persistently hypoxemic despite BiPAP, and he is now showing signs of tiring out. Based on the description provided, these authors feel that it is time for intubation.

What did the actual provider do?

The provider requested a chest CT; later, the tech calls stating that the patient cannot lie flat for the CT. The physician orders Ativan 1mg IVP and asks the tech to tell the patient that the test needs to be done as soon as possible.

Section editor comments (Yealy):

Giving a sedative absent mechanical ventilation for an enclosed procedure is a dangerous gamble in someone with shock and partially compensated respiratory failure. Avoid this path!

CT chest (radiology read): Study is very limited for the evaluation of pulmonary emboli due to motion and technical factors. No central pulmonary embolism. The segmental and subsegmental vessels are not well assessed. Extensive lung opacification likely representing pneumonia although pulmonary edema may appear similar. Mild nonspecific mediastinal lymphadenopathy, likely reactive.

Physician MDM: Pt. does not show any obvious PE. Bilateral infiltrate concern for ARDS. Adding flu swab. Pt. has severe hypoxia with repeat blood gas was PO_2 of 63 on 100% FiO_2 BiPAP. I will intubate for severe hypoxia ARDS and respiratory distress. Patient was given 15 etomidate and 100mg Succinylcholine for the intubation. An 8-0 ET tube was placed at 22cm at the teeth. Post-intubation patient remained hypoxic despite aggressive ventilation. Given his sats were as low as 20% after the intubation with bagging a code was called and ICU and anesthesia came down. Patient never lost pulses and never had an arrest.

Author comments (Weinstock):

Being prepared is key; though mnemonics can be difficult to remember, here are 2 worth the effort: post-intubation hypoxemia and hypotension. We are at:

DECISION POINT C – YOU ARE FACED WITH 4 QUESTIONS:

1. **Which medication(s) should be used for intubation and sedation?**
2. **What is the differential diagnosis for post-intubation hypoxemia?**
3. **What is the differential diagnosis for post-intubation hypotension?**
4. **What initial ventilation settings are appropriate for a patient with suspected ARDS?**

What does the literature say?

Q#1: Which medication(s) should be used for intubation and sedation?

To optimize intubating conditions together with a neuromuscular blocking agent—usually succinylcholine or rocuronium—we need an induction agent. The ideal induction drug has:

- Rapid onset and short duration of action.
- Minimal side-effects, minimal drug interactions, and no contraindications.
- Is hemodynamically neutral (i.e., does not cause a drop in blood pressure or cardiac performance), and that does not increase intracranial pressure.
- A reliable dose-response curve.
- Is readily available to us in the ED.

Etomidate:

Etomidate is a mainstay sedative/induction agent used for rapid intubation in U.S. EDs. Onset of action is approximately 20 seconds and duration of action is brief, giving it ideal pharmacokinetics for RSI. It has no analgesic properties, so co-administration of an analgesic such as fentanyl is suggested. It is hemodynamically neutral and decreases ICP (therefore improving CPP) and also decreases cerebral metabolic rate. Though there is a known association between etomidate and adrenal suppression, even with a single dose [20, 21] (two meta-analyses [22, 23] have shown increased rates of adrenal suppression and death, while a subsequent meta-analysis [24] showed an association with adrenal suppression but no statistically significant increase in mortality), most agree that single dose etomidate is acceptable, even in sepsis. If in doubt, give a stress dose of hydrocortisone after etomidate; the dose for intubation is 0.3mg/kg IV, although some advocate using a lower dose (0.15–0.2mg/kg) in hypotensive patients.

Propofol:

Propofol is commonly used both for intubation and for procedural sedation. It is highly lipophilic and crosses the blood brain barrier quickly, leading to a rapid onset of action, about 30 seconds, and short duration of action, 3–10 minutes after a bolus of 1mg/kg. Like etomidate, it has no analgesic properties, but it is not hemodynamically neutral—it can cause hypotension, especially with bolus dosing. When used for prolonged sedation in the ICU, the rate of recovery in patients sedated > 72 hours is faster with propofol [25] when compared to midazolam. It is an ideal agent for post-intubation sedation.

Midazolam:
Midazolam, as with all benzodiazepines, works on the post-synaptic GABA receptor. GABA is the major inhibitory neurotransmitter, so binding to those receptors allows more GABA to be present, leading to sedation. It is not an ideal agent for intubation, as at doses required for induction (0.1-0.3mg/kg) it has significant hemodynamic effects. It is an option post-intubation, although its longer duration of action makes it a less popular choice than propofol. Dose adjustments are needed for renal impairment. The recommended starting dose is 20–100mcg/kg/hr as an IV drip, titrated to effect.

Fentanyl:
Fentanyl is an opioid and is frequently used as a rapid-on, rapid-off analgesic, as well as an adjunct for procedural sedation, intubation and post-intubation sedation and analgesia. Most recommend co-administering fentanyl if using a non-analgesic induction agent prior to intubation.

Ketamine:
Ketamine is a dissociative agent acting as a NMDA receptor antagonist, which blocks glutamate. Onset is within 30–60 seconds when administered intravenously. One effect of clinical importance is hypertension which is created through a central mechanism, causing increased catecholamine release, useful in patients who are already hypotensive. However, since many of these patients have already depleted their endogenous catecholamines, this increase in blood pressure is not always seen, and some patients actually have a drop in blood pressure due to the negative inotropic effect.

Ketamine has intrinsic analgesic properties, so no additional analgesic agent is required. It also is a bronchodilator, which makes it a popular choice in asthmatics and in patients with COPD. Previous concerns about increases in ICP have been disproven, but it does lead to an increase in intraocular pressure, and should be avoided in patients with known glaucoma. It can have neuropsychiatric side effects in higher doses, so should be used with caution in patients with underlying psychiatric disease.

The dose for intubation is 1–2mg/kg IV. There is anecdotal evidence and case series to support its use as a post-intubation agent, but the evidence is not as robust as for procedural sedation or induction.

Another potential use for ketamine was described by Weingart and colleagues in *Annals of Emergency Medicine* in 2015. Delayed sequence intubation[26] (DSI) is essentially procedural sedation, with the procedure being pre-oxygenation. This was accomplished by giving a dissociative dose of ketamine to patients on NIPPV that were altered or unable to tolerate traditional pre-oxygenation or peri-intubation procedures. They observed no complications and suggest DSI as an "alternative to RSI in patients requiring emergency airway management who will not tolerate pre-oxygenation or peri-intubation procedures."

Q#2: What is the differential diagnosis for post-intubation hypoxemia?

The DOPES mnemonic details the life-threatening causes of post-intubation hypoxemia:

D – Displacement of the ETT
O – Obstructed ETT (kinked, mucus plugging)
P – Patient related (PTX, PE, pulmonary edema, ARDS, etc)
E – Equipment (torn cuff, ventilator problems, power, oxygen source disconnected or depleted)
S – Stacked breaths—need to be familiar with vent settings

Q#3: What is the differential diagnosis for post-intubation hypotension?

Though there are many possible etiologies of post-intubation hypotension, consider "AAHH SHIT(E)", a crowd sourced mnemonic developed by R.E.B.E.L. EM's[27] Dr. Rob Bryant.

A–Acidosis, with concomitant tachypnea in an attempt for respiratory compensation, is common in patients prior to intubation. When the patient is sedated and paralyzed with RSI, the respiratory compensation is suppressed, and the pH can plummet. If the minute volume is set too low, the acidosis will worsen. A classic case is patients with Kussmaul respirations intubated for DKA. Therefore, the respiratory rate should be set high enough (30s) to compensate. A post-intubation ABG/VBG can be useful.

A–Anaphylaxis to induction agents or paralytics is rare but does occur, with reported rates of approximately 1/2,000 for Succinylcholine and 1/2,500 for Rocuronium.[28] Treatment for anaphylactic shock: epi, epi, epi…

H–Heart (Tamponade) Even if previously compensated, patients can rapidly decompensate and become hypotensive when positive pressure is applied after intubation. If a pericardial effusion is present, prepare for immediate relief of tamponade with an ultrasound-guided pericardiocentesis

H–Heart (Pulm HTN) Patients with pulmonary hypertension can pose a real challenge as they tend to desaturate quickly, and fluid boluses can lead to worsened right-sided heart failure. With development of hypotension, treatment is vasopressor support with norepinephrine and inotropes until the cause of the worsening pulmonary hypertension can be identified and treated. Early pulmonary consultation is critical.

S–Stacked breathing (a.k.a., auto-PEEPing) occurs when there is inadequate time for the intubated patient to exhale before the next breath is delivered. This is common in chronic obstructive lung disease (COPD) patients leading to hypotension through IVC compression due to the increase in intra-thoracic pressure and resultant decreased venous return. If breath stacking is suspected, disconnect the patient from the vent and allow full exhalation (assisting by manually compressing the chest); this is essentially diagnostic if effective. When the patient is put back on the vent, the I:E ratio should be adjusted to allow for a longer exhalation time.[29]

H–Hypovolemia is the first consideration in post-intubation hypotension secondary to true hypovolemia from inadequate resuscitation, hemorrhage, or diabetes insipidus, or from decreased venous return (increased ICP due to breath stacking, PEEP).

I–Induction agents, as well as analgesics in the pre-and post-intubation setting and sedatives post-intubation, may cause hypotension. Choosing the right drug at the right dose while adjusting for renal/hepatic dysfunction, and closely monitoring during and after intubation can mitigate these effects.

T–Tension pneumothorax can develop secondary to the positive pressure from ventilation, particularly in those with COPD and poor lung compliance. Treatment is with needle decompression followed by emergent tube thoracostomy. Bedside US or post-intubation CXR may be useful if the diagnosis is in question, but this is usually a clinical diagnosis.

E–Electrolyte abnormalities, specifically hyperkalemia, are an uncommon but potentially important potential cause of post-intubation hypotension. The classic concern is when succinylcholine is used for paralysis in a patient who is in renal failure and already hyperkalemic, or with an unrecognized pre-existing contraindication such as muscular dystrophy. But there is significant momentum in the recent anesthesia literature to suggest that these risks are exaggerated. Schow, et.al. retrospectively reviewed 40,000 cases over 6 years and found 38 with a pre-operative $K+ \geq 5.6$. No dysrhythmias or other major morbidity occurred, although the small sample size led to a 95% confidence interval of 0–7.9%.[30] A review by Thapa and colleagues found sufficient evidence to support "the current consensus" that succinylcholine can be safely given to patients with renal failure,[31] and a prospective ICU trial by Blanie, et.al. found only prolonged ICU stay (> 16 days) to be associated with hyperkalemia, let alone cardiac events.[32] Treatment with calcium should be initiated if there is strong suspicion based on the clinical presentation and ECG findings.

Q#4: What initial ventilation settings are appropriate for a patient with suspected ARDS?

This is an important question because even with "perfect" treatment, the mortality for severe ARDS is over 45%.[33] Lung-protective ventilation uses tidal volume of 6mL/Kg predicted or ideal body mass (and peak pressures below 30cm H_2O) to avoid barotrauma; this targeted volume was once infrequent in the ED, but as awareness has increased in recent years, it has become more common. Too much oxygen can cause harm; do not target a saturation of 100% sat as 95% is a better choice for most patients.

Section editor comments (Yealy):

Prone positioning can aid respiratory support in those on mechanical ventilation that is failing—but requires help to achieve as well as close bedside monitoring. It is often overlooked in the ED.

We will mention the "open lung approach," which uses recruitment maneuvers to reverse atelectasis, followed by application of high levels of PEEP to keep recruited alveoli open. As of 2017, four large randomized clinical trials failed to demonstrate improved mortality, with the ART trial showing higher mortality rates.[34]

The key points to remember about lung protective ventilation:

- Low (6mL/kg) tidal volumes of ideal body weight, whether or not the patient is in ARDS
- Low/constant PEEP (5–10 range)
- Titrate FiO_2 as low as possible (40–60%) without causing a drop in PaO_2 (trend P/F ratios)
- Keep plateau pressures < 30cm H_2O

Back to our case: Our patient is in shock, likely septic. Working on this assumption, the choice of low-dose etomidate was reasonable; however, the use of ketamine would be at least as good a choice.

What did the actual provider do?

MDM: Patient was bagged aggressively and FiO_2 came up to 85%. Chest x-ray shows ET tube placement and worsening bilateral pulmonary edema. I am adding a flu swab and patient will go immediately to the ICU.

Hospital course: The admitting diagnosis was ARDS and acute respiratory failure secondary to multi-lobar pneumonia. Once admitted to the ICU he was started on ARDS net protocol and was sedated. Treatment for CAP was continued, and he required vasopressor support for septic shock secondary to pneumonia. His course was prolonged due to an extended period of intubation. He was eventually discharged to an extended care facility with a PEG tube due to dysphagia from the prolonged intubation.

ARDS review: ARDS is, per the 2012 Berlin definition, an "acute diffuse, inflammatory lung injury, leading to increased pulmonary vascular permeability, increased lung weight, and loss of aerated lung tissue...[with] hypoxemia and bilateral radiographic opacities, associated with increased venous admixture, increased physiological dead space, and decreased lung compliance." ARDS is classified as mild, moderate, or severe based on the PaO_2/FiO_2 ratio. This is obtained by taking the PaO_2 value from the ABG and dividing it by the FiO_2 that the patient is receiving. For those of us who are mathematically challenged, yes, there's an app for that! For example, a PaO_2 of 65 on a FiO_2 of 70% would result in a P/F ratio of 65/0.70 = 93, indicating severe ARDS. The table below lists the 2012 diagnostic criteria for ARDS with their associated mortalities.

ARDS Severity	PaO2/FiO2*	Mortality**
Mild	200 - 300	27%
Moderate	100 - 200	32%
Severe	< 100	45%
*on PEEP 5+; **observed in cohort		

Adapted from Ranieri VM, Rubenfeld GD, Thompson BT, et al. The ARDS Definition Task Force. Acute respiratory distress syndrome: The Berlin Definition. JAMA. 2012;307(23):2526-33.

Chapter author comments/debrief: For a condition with such a high mortality, there is little margin for error in our management. Although his initial evaluation could use a few tweaks, it was mostly reasonable. We never want to ignore a missing vital sign, and his temperature ended up not being documented until more than 36 hours after arrival. The lack of a bedside ultrasound delayed the process of ruling in or out several important diagnoses. In the absence of an ultrasound, a BNP, if low, would have removed heart failure from the differential.

- Antibiotics were administered in a relatively quick timeframe. He had a reasonable differential diagnosis, and his choice of broad spectrum antibiotics (Vancomycin and Piperacillin-Tazobactam) were appropriate.
- Early resuscitation with fluids (starting 30cc/kg isotonic), with use of vasopressors based on response, is the current approach for septic shock, using a mean pressure of 60mmHg or above. Following lactate levels can also guide resuscitation.
- The decision to delay intubation after the initial assessment (Decision Point A) is justifiable, but the decision to delay again at Decision Point B was an opportunity for improvement.
- The choice of etomidate for induction is acceptable, but fentanyl or another analgesic should be added. Ketamine would be another attractive alternative as it can be given as a single agent due

to its intrinsic analgesic properties and lacks the theoretical downside of worsening hypotension.

- We are not told what ventilator settings were initiated in the ED, although the charting from the ICU indicates that the ARDS net protocol for LPV was initiated in the unit. While documenting that the patient's SaO_2 (mis-documented as FiO_2) only came up to 85% with aggressive bagging, he does not tell us what he considered as possible causes of his post-intubation hypoxia, or if he did anything to try to improve oxygenation other than "aggressive bagging." Did he consider the possibilities in the DOPES mnemonic? Did he consider placing the patient prone? We do know that the patient was sent "immediately" to the ICU, which seems appropriate.

Chapter summary:

- The differential diagnosis of CAP with treatment failure is broad and includes both infectious causes (drug-resistant bacteria, viruses, fungi, right-sided endocarditis with septic pulmonary emboli) and non-infectious causes (Acute Chest Syndrome, lymphangitic carcinomatosis, BOOP and others).
- Use lung protective ventilation (Vt. 6cc/kg ideal body weight, plateau pressures < 30cm H_2O) in all intubated patients in order to prevent ARDS, not just those already meeting the criteria.
- The DOPES mnemonic lists causes of post-intubation hypoxemia and the AH SHITE mnemonic lists causes of post-intubation hypotension.
- Humidified oxygen by high-flow nasal canula (HFNC) is an option in severe hypoxemia.
- Bedside ultrasound is useful in the setting of unexplained hypotension and is at least as good as CXR in identifying pneumonia.
- The choice of drugs for induction and for post-intubation sedation need to be individualized; in septic shock, etomidate is controversial but acceptable, while ketamine is effective and lacks the theoretical downside of worsened hypotension.

References:

1. Schwam, E. B-type natriuretic peptide for diagnosis of heart failure in emergency department patients: A critical appraisal. Acad Emerg Med 2004;11(6):686-91.
2. Yealy DM, Hsieh M. BNP is not a value-added routine test in the ED. Ann Emerg Med 2009;53(3):387-9.
3. Burri E, Potocki M, Drexler B, et al. Value of arterial blood gas analysis in patients with acute dyspnea: an observational study. Crit Care 2011;15(3):R145.
4. Zeserson E, Goodgame B, Hess JD, et al. Correlation of venous blood gas and pulse oximetry with arterial blood gas in the undifferentiated critically ill patient. J Intensive Care Med 2016;33(3):176-81.
5. Afshar N, Tabas J, Afshar A, et.al. Blood cultures for community-acquired pneumonia: are they worthy of two quality measures? A systematic review. Hosp Med 2009;4(2):112-23.
6. Kennedy M, Wright SB, Bates DW, et.al. Do emergency department blood cultures change practice in patients with pneumonia? Ann Emerg Med 2005;46(5):393-400.
7. Nazarian DJ, Eddy OL, Lukens TW, et.al. Clinical Policy: Critical issues in the management of adult patients presenting to the emergency department with community-acquired pneumonia. Ann Emerg Med 2009;54(5):704-31.
8. Lenglet H, Stzyrmf B, Leroy C, et.al. Humidified high flow nasal oxygen during respiratory failure in the Emergency Department: feasibility and efficacy. Resp Care 2012;57(11):1873-8.

9. Frat J-P, Thille AW, Mercat A, et. al. High-flow oxygen through nasal cannula in acute hypoxemic respiratory failure. N Engl J Med 2015;372(23):2185-96.
10. Bourcier JE, Paquet J, Seinger M, et al. Performance comparison of lung ultrasound and chest x-ray for the diagnosis of pneumonia in the ED. Am J Emerg Med 2014;32(2):115-18.
11. Laursen CB, Sloth E, Lassen AT, et al. Point-of-care ultrasonography in patients admitted with respiratory symptoms: a single-blind, randomized controlled trial. Lancet Resp Med 2014;2(8):638-46.
12. Nazerian P, Volpicelli G, Vanni S, et al. Accuracy of lung ultrasound for the diagnosis of consolidations when compared to chest computed tomography. Am J Emerg Med 2015;33(5):620-25.
13. Zanobetti M, Poggione C, Pini et.al. Can chest ultrasonography replace standard chest radiography for evaluation of acute dyspnea in the ED? Chest 2011;139(5):1140-47.
14. Zanobetti M, Scorpiniti M, Gigli C, et al. Point-of-care ultrasonography for evaluation of acute dyspnea in the Emergency Department. Chest 2017;151(6):1295-01.
15. Menendez R, Torres L. Treatment failure in community-acquired pneumonia. Chest 2007;132(4):1348-55.
16. Centers for Disease Control and Prevention, Legionella (Legionnaires' disease and Pontiac fever) diagnosis, treatment, and prevention. https://www.cdc.gov/legionella/clinicians/diagnostic-testing.html.
17. Mandell LA, Wunderkink RG, Anzueto A, et.al. Infectious Diseases Society of America/American Thoracic Society guidelines on the management of community-acquired pneumonia in adults. Clin Infect Dis 2007;44:S27-S72.
18. Wu CL, Yang DI, Wang NY, et al. Quantitative culture of endotracheal aspirates in the diagnosis of ventilator-associated pneumonia in patients with treatment failure. Chest 2002;122(2):662-68.
19. Falguera M, Ruiz-Gonzalez A, Schoenenberger JA, et al. Prospective, randomised study to compare empirical treatment versus targeted treatment on the basis of the urine antigen results in hospitalised patients with community-acquired pneumonia. Thorax 2010;65(2):101-06.
20. den Brinker M, Hokken-Koelega ACS, Hazelzet JA, et.al. One single dose of etomidate negatively influences adrenocortical performance for at least 24h in children with meningococcal sepsis. Intensive Care Med 2008;34(1):163-68.
21. Vinclair M, Broux C, Faure P. Duration of adrenal inhibition following a single dose of etomidate in critically ill patients. Intensive Care Med 2008;34:714-719.
22. Albert SG, Ariyan S, Rather A. The effect of etomidate on adrenal function in critical illness: a systematic review. Intensive Care Med 2011;37:901-10.
23. Chan CM, Mitchell AL, Shorr AF. Etomidate is associated with mortality and adrenal insufficiency in sepsis: a meta-analysis. Crit Care Med 2012;40:2945-53.
24. Gu WJ, Wang F, Tang L, et.al. Single-dose etomidate does not increase mortality in patients with sepsis: a systematic review and meta-analysis of randomized controlled trials and observational studies. Chest 2015;147:335-46.
25. McKeage K, Perry C. Propofol: a review of its use in intensive care sedation of adults. CNS Drugs. 2003;17(4):235-72.
26. Weingart DS, Trueger NS, Wong N, et al. Delayed sequence intubation: A prospective observational trial. Ann Emerg Med 2015; 65:349-55.

27. Bryant R. Post intubation hypotension: The AH SHITE mnemonic. 2017. http://rebelem.com/post-intubation-hypotension-the-ah-shite-mnemonic/.
28. Reddy JI, Cooke PJ, van Schalkwyk JM, et al. Anaphylaxis is more common with rocuronium and succinylcholine than with atracurium. Anesthesiology 2015 Jan;122(1):39-45.
29. Brochard L, Mancebo J, Tobin M. Searching for evidence: don't forget the foundations. Am Rev Respir Dis 1982 Jul;126(1):166-70.
30. Schow AJ, Lubarsky DA, Olson RP, et.al. Can succinylcholine be used safely in hyperkalemic patients? Anesth Analg 2002;95:119-22.
31. Thapa S, Brull SJ. Succ etc. Succinylcholine-induced hyperkalemia in patients with renal failure: an old question revisited. Anesth Analg 2000;91:237-241.
32. Blanie A, Ract C, Leblanc PE, et.al. The limits of succinylcholine for critically ill patients. Anesth Analg 2012;115:873-9.
33. Santos RS, Silva PL, Rocco JR, et al. A mortality score for acute respiratory distress syndrome: predicting the future without a crystal ball. J Thorac Dis 2016;8(8):1872-6.
34. Cavalcanti AB, Suzumura EA, Laranjeira LN, et al. Writing Group for the Alveolar Recruitment for Acute Respiratory Distress Syndrome Trial (ART) Investigators. Effect of lung recruitment and titrated positive end-expiratory pressure (PEEP) vs low PEEP on mortality in patients with acute respiratory distress syndrome: a randomized clinical trial.

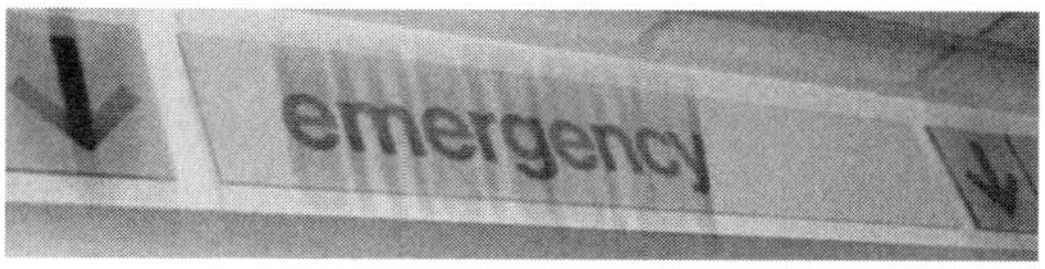

SECTION B – BREATHING/ PULMONARY

Chapter 8: A 78-year-old man with end-stage renal disease (ESRD) and shortness of breath

Brit Long, MD

Assistant Professor
Emergency Medicine
San Antonio Uniformed Services Health Education Consortium
Ft. Sam Houston, TX

Alex Koyfman, MD

Assistant Program Director
Clinical Assistant Professor
Emergency Medicine
University of Texas Southwestern Medical Center
Dallas, TX

Section editor:

Donald M. Yealy, MD

Chair, Department of Emergency Medicine
University of Pittsburgh/University of Pittsburgh Physicians
Vice President, Emergency and Urgent Care Services, Physician Services
UPMC Professor of Emergency Medicine, Medicine and Clinical and Translational Sciences
University of Pittsburgh School of Medicine
Pittsburgh, PA

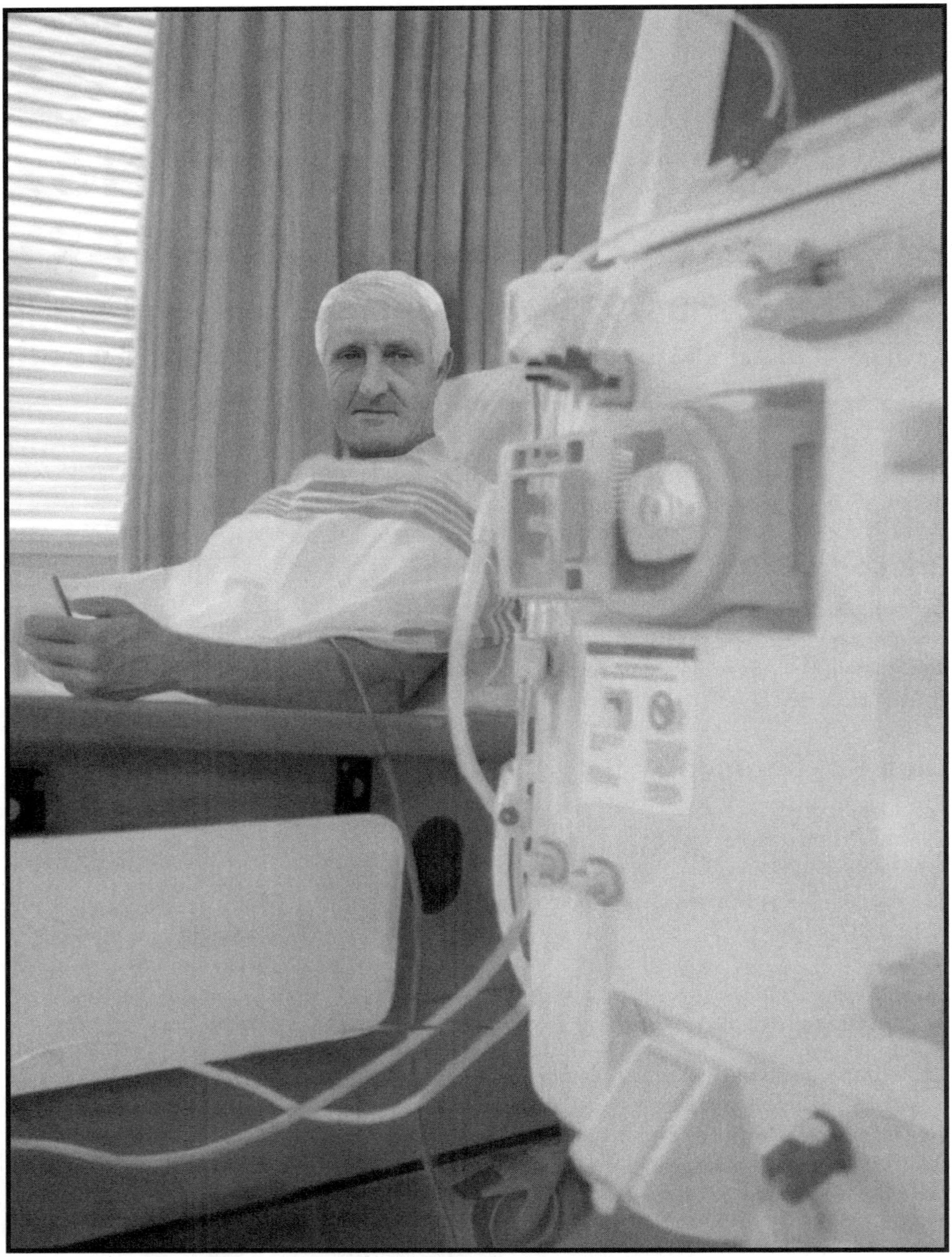

SECTION B/CHAPTER 8

A 78-year-old man with end-stage renal disease (ESRD) and shortness of breath

In the U.S., 354 patients per million require dialysis, and patients may present to the ED with a diverse set of issues.[1-5] ESRD is defined by glomerular filtration rate less than 15mL/min and often affects organs other than the kidney.[5-7] When compared to patients with normal renal function, ESRD patients demonstrate a relative risk (RR) of 5.9, 3.4, and 3.1 for all-cause mortality, cardiovascular events, and hospitalization, respectively.[8,4]

Management of ESRD may include hemodialysis (HD) or peritoneal dialysis (in some, until return of adequate functioning), or renal transplantation in appropriate candidates.[3] Hemodialysis access site complications are common, and ESRD patients on HD are at high risk of mortality. Only 50% of patients are alive 3 years after starting HD,[7-9] with cardiovascular events accounting for the majority of deaths. However, death may also occur from involvement of the neurologic, immune, gastrointestinal, and hematologic systems.[5-7, 9]

With this background, let's get to our case.

The patient's story:
Alan Higgins has struggled for years with hypertension, unsuccessfully dealing with side-effects including weakness, dizziness, and angioedema. He eventually decided to forgo therapy with medications and initially felt much better, but a routine outpatient blood test revealed an elevated creatinine.

Over the next several years, his renal function continued to decline, culminating with the recommendation for dialysis. Though he initially refused, progressive edema and fatigue convinced him otherwise. In addition to dialysis, he was also diagnosed with heart disease resulting in stent placement and then heart failure.

On a September evening, he becomes progressively short of breath (SOB), prompting his daughter to say, "enough is enough."After dinner, despite his continued protests, she dials 911. Upon arrival, EMS find the patient tachypneic and hypoxemic, but alert. En route to the ED, he becomes confused and combative. The paramedics start continuous positive airway pressure (CPAP) support.

ED VISIT

CC per RN (21:22): Shortness of Breath/Dyspnea
Mode of arrival: EMS
Limitations: altered mental status

HPI (documented @ 21:45): The patient is a 79-year-old male who was brought in via EMS for shortness of breath and was placed on CPAP by EMS en route. Patient had dialysis earlier today but had shortness of breath before dialysis and continued to have shortness of breath with steady decline. Patient received midazolam by EMS to help calm the patient on CPAP. Patient also has a history of CHF and COPD.

Medical history: Arthritis, cardiomyopathy, CHF, coronary artery disease, GERD, hyperlipidemia, hypertension, myocardial infarction, renal disease
Surgical history: angioplasty/stent, cataract, knee replacement, orthopedic, other, pacemaker/AICD
Psychiatric history: anxiety
Medications: Simvastatin, Lexapro, Flomax, Imdur, metoprolol, zyloprim, asa, Plavix, Proscar, ammonium lactate, Flonase, Lasix
Social History: No smoking, alcohol, drugs

Vitals:

Time	Temp	Pulse	Syst	Diast	Sat
21:08		71	102	70	100% (CPAP)

PE:
GA: Thin, frail, altered level of consciousness, on CPAP machine.
EYE: Normal appearance, PERRL.
ENT: Normal exam, normal oropharynx, mucous membranes very dry.
NECK: Normal inspection, full ROM, trachea midline, negative JVD.
CHEST: Patient has bilateral equal rise and fall of chest wall. Non-tender to palpation.
RESP: Clear to auscultation bilaterally without wheezes, rales, or rhonchi.
CARDIO: Regular rate, normal rhythm, normal heart sounds, without murmurs, rubs, or gallops.
ABDOMINAL: Soft, nondistended, Non-tender light and deep palpation in all quadrants. Bowel sounds normoactive throughout all 4 quadrants. Negative for hypo or hyperresonance.
EXTREMITIES: Normal inspection, full ROM.
BACK: Normal inspection, full ROM. Absent: tenderness, CVA tenderness (R), CVA tenderness (L).
SKIN: Warm, dry, intact, normal color.

Author comments (Weinstock):

Our patient has end-stage renal disease (ESRD), a difficult diagnosis to begin with, now tachypneic and altered. We are at:

DECISION POINT A – WE ARE FACED WITH 4 QUESTIONS:

1. **He was SOB *before* the dialysis—what is the differential diagnosis?**
2. **The patient has altered sensorium—is this because of the hypoxemia, CO_2 retention, or the midazolam?**
3. **Upon ED arrival the patient is hypotensive—what are the possibilities?**
4. **Our patient is altered, SOB, and hypotensive—should he be intubated?**

Q#1: He was SOB *before* the dialysis—what is the differential diagnosis?

Shortness of breath is common in patients on dialysis. Missed sessions can result in fluid overload with resultant pulmonary edema, one of the most common causes of dyspnea.[5-7, 9] Establishing a timeline of recent dialysis is important. If the patient has received dialysis, or the dyspnea started before dialysis, fluid overload is less likely, and another etiology must be considered. Failure to consider other conditions can delay care or cause harm.[6,7]

With the initial evaluation, maintain a broad differential but focus on imminently life-threatening problems including other cardiopulmonary etiologies, not simply pulmonary fluid overload.[5,7,9,10] The differential of dyspnea in patients with ESRD includes:

1. Cardiopulmonary disease:
    a. Congestive heart failure (CHF)
    b. Acute coronary syndrome (ACS)
    c. Pericardial effusion or tamponade
    d. Pleural effusion
    e. Chronic obstructive pulmonary disease (COPD)
    f. Pulmonary embolism (PE)
    g. Pulmonary edema
    h. Arrhythmia (due to ischemia or electrolyte abnormalities)
2. Neurologic disease
3. Metabolic disorders (acidosis, diabetic ketoacidosis (DKA))
4. Hematologic disorders (anemia)
5. Toxins (carbon monoxide toxicity or ingestion such as salicylates)
6. Airway obstruction
7. Psychiatric disease (a diagnosis of exclusion, such as anxiety)

The differential diagnosis(es) list is quickly narrowed by a combination of history, physical exam, and rapidly performed diagnostic tests. Obtain information on the dialysis schedule, recent missed sessions, baseline blood pressure, prior complications, average dry weight, and average amount of fluid removed during the session. The exam should first focus on the ABCs, including patient hemodynamics and mental status. If the patient does not require immediate intubation, evaluate the cardiopulmonary system (signs of heart failure including wheezes/rales, edema), vascular access site (erythema, warmth, discharge, bleeding, swelling), and neurologic status (mental status, focal deficits, and asterixis).[6,7,11]

Initial orders depend on the clinical presentation, but include CBC, renal function/electrolytes, chest x-ray, cardiac markers, and venous blood gas (VBG). A bedside ED focus ultrasound (US) can reliably and rapidly provide vital information. For example, the presence of greater than 3 "B lines" in multiple lung fields bilaterally suggests pulmonary edema;[12,13] air bronchograms suggest pneumonia; and cardiac windows can show global heart function, effusion, and focal wall abnormalities.[13]

Our patient has a history of COPD, MI, cardiomyopathy, and CHF, making a focused history and exam with US valuable. With this presentation, we think the most likely reason for his decompensation (which started before dialysis) is likely associated with a primary cardiopulmonary pathology.

Rapid IV access and use of noninvasive positive pressure ventilation, as occurred here, is potentially life-saving.

Consulting editor comments (Weingart):

For patients who have shortness of breath after dialysis (as was initially thought), I would just treat this as the normal evaluation for a dyspneic patient, just treat them and don't get confused that this is a dialysis problem, with the exception being the consideration of potentiation of heart failure. The patient who is short of breath before dialysis presents a different differential, which has been discussed.

Q#2: The patient has altered sensorium—is this because of the hypoxemia, CO_2 retention, or the midazolam?

An agitated patient—any agitated patient, including one with long-standing renal failure and cardiovascular disease—requires careful consideration of choosing a sedation path and potential adverse medication effects. Commonly, benzodiazepines, such as Versed (midazolam) are utilized. Other options include ketamine and first and second generation antipsychotics. All choices are hampered by different pharmacokinetic and pharmacodynamic effects in patients with ESRD.

Section editor comments (Yealy):

Before sedating, ask "Why am I doing this? Is it treating the trigger?" *If not, intubate with caution or not at all.* Secondly, I personally *abhor using antipsychotics for non-psychosis*—we are depending on those agents' side-effects to be our desired benefit, and those side-effects are irreversible.

Benzodiazepines should be used with caution. Midazolam is hepatically metabolized and renally excreted. In ESRD, the metabolites' circulation is prolonged, and due to decreased protein binding in renal failure, free levels of the medication are increased. If used, decrease the dose by half, to 1–4mg IV, or 2–5mg IM. Lorazepam is not recommended in ESRD due to the renal elimination needs. Diazepam may be used in doses of 2–10mg IM or IV.[6,14,15]

Antipsychotics include first and second-generation agents. Haloperidol undergoes hepatic metabolism, and doses of 2–5mg IM can be used in ESRD (no dose adjustment is needed).

Droperidol is another first-generation antipsychotic that can be used in doses of 5–10mg IM, with no change in dosing. Risperidone is a second-generation antipsychotic, but its use in ESRD patients is limited due to more complex metabolism and excretion in patients with ESRD. Ziprasidone requires similar considerations in ESRD with IM administration due to renal excretion of metabolites. Olanzapine is another second generation medication, given in doses of 10mg IM, and no dose change is needed in ESRD. Aripiprazole also does not need adjustment and can be used in agitated patients with ESRD at doses of 5.25–15mg IM.[16-18]

Ketamine, an NMDA antagonist, is a popular choice in the ED.[15,19-21] Past uses included procedural sedation and induction in intubation. Ketamine is now commonly used for pain and care of an agitated patient. Ketamine 4–5mg/kg IM or 1–2mg/kg IV can be used for rapid control, with no change in dose in ESRD. On occasion, you will need to intubate after using this agent,[19-21] though usually ketamine preserves airway reflexes and respiratory drive.

What are options with our patient?

Our patient received midazolam (Versed) en route to assist with CPAP. It could have contributed to his declining mental status.

Of course, there are many causes of confusion in the patient with ESRD. Uremia is a clinical syndrome, with complications mainly occurring when GFR < 15mL/min. Unfortunately, BUN and creatinine cannot be relied on to assess the severity of current symptoms, though a BUN over 60mmol/L is associated with greater risk of complications.[22-26]

Other causes for AMS in someone with ESRD are structural or metabolic. These include:

1. Structural: Ischemic stroke, intracerebral hemorrhage, abscess, tumor.
2. Metabolic: Uremia, dialysis disequilibrium, dialysis dementia, medication effects, meningitis, hypertensive encephalopathy, hypoglycemia, hyperglycemia, hypercalcemia, hypotension, hypoxia, thyroid disease, among others.
3. Uremic encephalopathy is due to imbalance of over 70 toxins and neurotransmitters and affects older patients and those with comorbidities most severely. It parallels the severity of the renal failure. Presentations include tremor, myoclonus, confusion, and asterixis (especially in earlier stages). More severe stages include lethargy, hallucinations, and coma. Focal deficit may be present, and the deficit may change.[22-26] Uremic encephalopathy is a clinical diagnosis and requires dialysis.
4. Dialysis disequilibrium syndrome (DDS) occurs when dialysis results in changes in serum osmolality due to urea removal, followed by diffusion of water into the brain and ensuing cerebral edema. Risks for DDS include the first HD session, BUN > 60mmol/L, CKD, metabolic acidosis, older age, and prior stroke or hemorrhage.[6,7,22,23,27,28]
5. Intracerebral hemorrhage is a significant complication in ESRD. ESRD patients are at high risk for bleeding due to uremic platelet dysfunction and anticoagulation, with subdural hematoma occurring 10–20 times more frequently than the general population, even without trauma.[6,29-32] Presentations range from confusion to focal deficits, and the bleed may be unilateral or bilateral. If intracranial pressure is elevated (evidenced by pupil asymmetry, posturing, focal neurologic deficit, decline in mental status), measures to decrease ICP are needed and anticoagulation should be reversed.[6,11,33,34]

6. Ischemic stroke occurs more commonly in patients with chronic kidney disease than patients with diabetes, HTN, hyperlipidemia, and obesity. Renal disease is a predictor of poor outcome in stroke.[6,32,35] Head CT should be performed without delay, and thrombolytics should be considered as in patients without renal failure.[35,36]

Though our patient may have uremic encephalopathy, this is a diagnosis of exclusion, and we have to first consider other, life-threatening causes of altered mental status (AMS). Focused assessment of the neurologic exam (seeking lateralization) and mental state, coupled with fingerstick glucose check are required. Obtain a basic metabolic panel (BMP), complete blood cell count (CBC), coagulation panel, phosphate and calcium levels, and ECG. Consider a toxicology screen and thyroid assessment, as thyroid abnormalities can present with a wide range of signs and symptoms. Head CT is needed, especially with any lateralization, profound alteration, or absent another clear cause.[6,7,9,23]

Q#3: Upon ED arrival the patient is hypotensive—what are the possibilities?

Not only is our patient dyspneic and hypoxemic, but also hypotensive, a dangerous combination. Hypotension occurring before or early in a dialysis session is often due to volume loss or low intravascular volume, occurring in up to 50% of patients.[6,7,9] Removal averages 1–3L during a session (which typically last 4 hours),[37] and sometimes the removal interval does not allow enough time for transcellular fluid shift to replace lost intravascular fluid. Most of the cases of hypotension during dialysis respond to a decrease in hemodialysis blood flow rate or small amounts of IV fluids. In patients with post-dialytic hypotension, consider hemorrhage or blood loss from the access site.[7,9,12]

What about other causes?

Differential:

- Pre-dialytic (Volume loss => think GI losses, decreased intake, cardiac dysfunction, arrhythmia, tamponade, medications, sepsis).
- Intra-dialytic (Usually excess filtration, but consider air embolism or hemorrhage).
- Post-dialytic (Vascular access blood loss, medications, sepsis, cardiac dysfunction, pericardial disease, arrhythmia, air embolism).

Other factors include medication effects (antihypertensives, analgesics), decreased vascular tone due to sepsis, and cardiac dysfunction (myocardial infarction, arrhythmia, tamponade, cardiac failure/shock), which is the number one cause of mortality in ESRD patients.[38-40] Pulmonary or air embolism can cause hypotension if severe/massive, though these are not as common as other causes. Cardiac tamponade is life-threatening and may occur suddenly with hypotension and/or dyspnea.[6,7,41-43]

US again is invaluable to assess cardiac function, lungs, and for the presence of cardiac and/or pleural effusion.[6,13] Patients may have a cardiac effusion at bedside, but right ventricular diastolic collapse is highly suggestive of tamponade, especially with a plethoric inferior vena cava (IVC).

Another cause of hypotension is hyperkalemia and dysrhythmia or pump malfunction. Though this is rare in patients who have recently completed dialysis, hyperkalemia can occur with missed sessions, or in prolonged hypotension or low flow states. ECG and a VBG (which measures potassium) are essential. If there is a concern for hyperkalemia, give empiric IV calcium for cardiac membrane stabilization.[44,45]

Q#4: The patient is altered, SOB, and hypotensive—should he be intubated?

Classically, intubation and mechanical ventilation are needed in several circumstances when other interventions fail or conditions are severe: 1) maintaining airway patency, 2) preventing aspiration (or airway protection), 3) oxygenation and/or ventilation, and 4) expected clinical course. Newer recommendations expand the ABCs to the ABCDEFs:[46]

A. Airway: If a mouth or neck pathology such as cancer, foreign body, Ludwig's angina, or epiglottitis is present, with stridor, voice changes, difficulty with secretions, or patient posturing, consider emergent intubation by the most experienced provider.
B. Breathing: Failure to oxygenate or ventilate is the most common reason we intubate in the ED. The airway itself is typically normal, but the patient has a high oxygenation deficit. Note potential for rapid desaturation once sedatives and paralytics are administered.
C. Circulation: Critically ill patients (such as severe sepsis) may require intubation to decrease the metabolic demand of the pulmonary system/respiratory muscles. Resuscitation before intubation and use of small induction doses are recommended.
D. Disability, including neurologic disease or inability to protect the airway, may require intubation due to risk for aspiration. Do not rely on the gag reflex, as it is not present in over 20% of the population.
E. Expected clinical course: With transport or a patient leaving the department for imaging, if there is consideration for reasons A–D above, intubation may be necessary. A difficult airway while inflight is a nightmare!
F. Feral: The feral patient may require intubation to control agitation, allowing further evaluation and treatment.

This patient meets several criteria for intubation: early stages of respiratory fatigue, hypotension, disability (altered mental status), and clinical course. Do we have another option? Noninvasive positive pressure ventilation (NIPPV) can decrease mortality and the need for intubation in patients with pulmonary edema, CHF, and COPD.[47-51] A trial of NIPPV with close bedside monitoring may result in significant improvement. If the patient can tolerate the mask, oxygenation can also improve, decreasing the risk for desaturation if an intubation attempt later occurs.[52] NIPPV requires patient cooperation and close monitoring. In patients with altered mental status who will not cooperate, consider delayed sequence intubation using ketamine (see below).

Chapter author comments: We tried NIPPV, but the patient decompensated. This could be due to a variety of reasons, including decreased preload and end organ perfusion due to NIPPV, respiratory failure, or a combination. At this point, endotracheal intubation is needed due to failure to ventilate, disability and unresponsiveness, and clinical course.

Section editor comments (Yealy):

The "definitive airway" is the one that meets patient demands safely; endotracheal intubation is valuable when respiratory failure is profound or unabated after other interventions.

ED COURSE

MDM (21:24): The patient is switched over to BiPAP but began to increase his rate and work of breathing. He is now unresponsive.

The patient is worsening and now unresponsive. Repeat vitals show the BP has worsened. A decision is made to intubate, but this is not your typical intubation – our patient has multiple comorbidities and is hypotensive – truly a high-risk intubation.

Vitals:

Time	Temp	Pulse	Respir	Syst	Diast	Sat
21:27		82	12	95	61	100% (BiPAP)

Procedure note (21:30):
Time: 21:21
Sedative: Etomidate
Mg Given: 20
Paralytic: Rocuronium
Mg Given: 60
Laryngoscope: Macintosh
ET Tube Size: 7.5
ET Tube Uncuffed: No
Tube Secured Depth (cm): 24
Tube Secured Location: teeth
Tube Placement Confirmation: visualized tube passing through cords, equal breath sounds bilaterally, no breath sounds over epigastrium, confirmation by capnometry

DECISION POINT B – WE ARE FACED WITH 4 QUESTIONS:

1. **Which approaches will confirm tube placement?**
2. **Which ventilator settings should be used post-intubation?**
3. **Which medications should be used for sedation after intubation for our patient with ESRD and hypotension?**
4. **What is an approach to fluid resuscitation in a hypotensive ESRD patient? Is there a concern for fluid overload?**

What does the literature say?

Q#1: Which approaches will confirm tube placement?

Unrecognized misplacement of an ETT can be disastrous and can happen in up to 25% in patients intubated in the field.[53,54]

Section editor comments (Yealy):

The best advice is to use 2–3 methods to confirm, with at least one being direct visualization or detecting appropriate CO_2 exhalation (if not both.) Any one method might fool you! When in doubt, check oxygenation and remove/use a bag valve device to restore adequacy. Don't "hope or assume."

In confirming endotracheal placement, bedside observation alone may be misleading. Be wary—fogging or condensation of the ETT occurs in up to 83% of esophageal intubations.[55,56] Chest wall movement may occur with intubation of the esophagus as well, and breath sounds incorrectly identify at least 16% of esophageal intubations.[55-57]

While no technique is 100% definitive,[53,54,57-61] the most reliable confirmation is to see the tube pass through the vocal cords. Direct visualization is not always possible, such as in the airway obscured with blood or emesis, as well as the anatomically difficult airway.

Esophageal detector devices are easy to use and are inexpensive, but they do not demonstrate reliable accuracy in obese patients, those with large amounts of air in the esophagus or stomach, and those with pulmonary secretions. These devices do not allow continued monitoring of tube position.[53,57,58]

One of the most reliable methods is using capnometry, either qualitative or quantitative. Capnometry measures the end-tidal carbon dioxide ($EtCO_2$) with a device attached to the ventilator tubing to measure CO_2 concentration in exhaled gases. Qualitative markers will turn yellow when exposed to carbon dioxide. Quantitative $EtCO_2$ capnometry provides a dynamic waveform with numeric values.[62-65] Accuracy approaches 100%, though in cardiac arrest, sensitivity decreases.[66-68] Lack of any $EtCO_2$ reading is suggestive of tube misplacement. Capnometry is not reliable in patients with poor perfusion.[62-65]

A radiograph can aid placement determinations—whether the ETT is a placed too deep, such as in a right mainstem intubation, or to evaluate for complications including aspiration, tracheal injury, pneumothorax, or pneumomediastinum. However, radiograph is unreliable for confirming tube placement in the trachea vs. esophagus.

Ultrasound by a trained user can confirm ETT placement with high sensitivity and specificity.[69,70] Use a high frequency linear US transducer, with the probe oriented horizontally at the suprasternal notch level.[69,70] If the ETT is in correct position in the trachea, the US will show shadowing of the ETT without esophageal visualization. If the esophagus is intubated, the esophagus will appear to the left of the trachea with posterior shadowing due to the ETT. Another method uses a similar probe at the level of the cricothyroid membrane, with the probe oriented longitudinally. A "snowstorm" appearance between the hyperechoic anterior and posterior laryngeal walls suggests appropriate ETT placement.[69,70] Ultrasound can also evaluate for lung sliding bilaterally, which assists in confirming tracheal placement, as well as detection of right mainstem intubation. If right mainstem intubation occurs, no lung sliding will be found on the left.

Q#2: Which ventilator settings should be used post-intubation?

Mechanical ventilation changes respiratory physiology, and one size does not fit all.
Mechanical ventilation comes in two types of cycles: volume or pressure.

- In the ED, we most commonly utilize volume cycle or volume controlled ventilation.[52,71,72]
- Pressure cycled ventilation is useful if you do not want to exceed a specified lung pressure.

For volume cycled ventilation, assist-control (AC), continuous mechanical ventilation (CMV), and synchronized intermittent mandatory ventilation (SIMV) are the primary modes. Assist-control is the most common mode utilized in the ED, which allows inspiration triggered by patient intrinsic effort or after an elapsed time interval, providing a predetermined tidal volume. Continuous mechanical ventilation is most commonly used in the OR. SIMV provides a predetermined number of ventilator breaths, synchronized to patient effort. If the patient's rate is below the set rate, this mode functions as AC ventilation. If the patient breathes above the set rate, these further breaths are not assisted, which increases patient work of breathing.[52,71,72]

For our patient, we recommend using AC volume cycle. When picking the initial settings, both the patient and pathology need to be considered. A lung protective strategy focuses on low tidal volume breaths to reduce lung injury such as volutrauma and barotrauma.[73,74] This can be used for patients with lung injury or any patient requiring ventilation in the ED. The other strategy is an obstructive strategy, used in patients with obstructive disease (asthma, chronic obstructive pulmonary disease).

Settings include:

- Mode
- Rate
- Fraction of inspired oxygen
- Positive end-expiratory pressure (PEEP)
- Minute ventilation

Initial ventilator settings should focus on optimizing oxygen, plateau pressures, and hemodynamics.

For lung protective strategy, we recommend:

Mode: AC mode

Respiratory Rate: This varies based on patient physiology and disease with a goal $PaCO_2$ as the target. A rate of 14–16bpm commonly provides normocapnia.

Tidal Volume: The volume of breath provided is for alveolar protection; start with 6mL/kg of ideal body weight (not actual body weight). These tidal volumes may prevent further lung injury.

FiO_2 and PEEP: These should be used for titrating oxygenation. FiO_2 is the fraction of oxygen provided during ventilation. Start with 100% and titrate down to FiO_2 30–40%. PEEP is the positive pressure provided at the end of each breath with a typical initial setting of 5cm H_2O. Hyperoxia and hypoxia are both associated with worse outcomes. The ARDS NET ARMA Table should be used for titration of PEEP and FiO_2 to target oxygenation 88–96%.[52,74]

Inspiratory flow rate: When a patient begins to breathe, a large amount of gas is inspired in the immediate part of the breath, which tapers towards the end in a decelerating pattern. This flow is associated with patient comfort, and an initial setting of 60L/minute is usually adequate.

Once these settings are in place, check a plateau pressure every 30 minutes. The peak pressure combines alveolar pressure, large airway resistance, and equipment resistance, while the plateau pressure approximates the pressure found in the alveoli. The plateau pressure can be measured by pressing the inspiratory hold button on the ventilator at the end of a breath. Target a level less than 30cm H_2O; if above, decrease the tidal volume by 1mL/kg. Tidal volumes as low as 4mL/kg are acceptable. The respiratory rate may need to be increased to ensure $PaCO_2$ goals are met, though some elevation is permissible.[52,73,74]

Q#3: Which medicationss should be used for sedation after intubation of our patient with ESRD and hypotension?

Post-intubation analgesia and sedation are necessary in any patient mechanically ventilated. ESRD patients demonstrate challenging pharmacokinetics and pharmacodynamics that complicate decisions, especially in the presence of hemodynamic instability and drug interactions.[5,15,75,76]

Section editor comments (Yealy):

While post-intubation sedation aids many patients mechanically ventilated, it can also prolong ventilation needs and raise complication frequency—a delicate balance. The latter are usually seen with more prolonged sedation protocols, not in the ED care setting, prompting sedation "holidays" to lessen the impact. Think carefully about using a specific agent and have a conversation with the next treating physician—usually, short-term sedation with a rapidly excreted agent is a good starting point.

Analgesia: Inadequate pain relief worsens the physiologic stress response and increases delirium and anxiety. Assessment of pain and agitation (RASS) and patient vital signs can provide clues to pain management. Opioids are the most common medications administered for rapid, reliable analgesia; however, they may result in respiratory depression, hypotension, urinary retention, flushing, pruritis, and worsening delirium. There are several types of opioids available, discussed in Table 1. Fentanyl has a short half-life and time of serum distribution, with minimal (if any) renal metabolism and is reliable with a rapid onset of action. We recommend this agent as the primary analgesic.[5,15,76]

(Table on next page...)

Table 1. Analgesics in ESRD

Medication	Dosing	Metabolism and Excretion	Considerations
Morphine	2-5 mg every 5-15 min IV until pain controlled, then scheduled every 2-4 hours	Hepatic metabolism and renal excretion	- Prolonged effect in ESRD and liver disease - Results in histamine release, with several CNS side effects
Hydromorphone	0.2-1.0 mg IV every 10-20 minutes until pain controlled, then scheduled every 2-4 hours	Metabolites inactive, but the metabolites are renally excreted	- Metabolites can accumulate in ESRD, prolonging medication effect - No histamine release
Fentanyl	Titratable with loading dose 25-100 micrograms every 5-10 minutes, followed by 25-250 microgram/hr infusion	Large volume of distribution due to lipophilicity Does not undergo renal elimination	- Synthetic Opioid with rapid onset and short duration - Titratable with rapid onset - First line agent in hemodynamically unstable patients or ESRD
Remifentanil	Infusion 0.05-2.00 micrograms/kg/min	- Esterase dependent clearance mechanism, not associated with renal physiology - Half-life less than 10 minutes	- Dosing based on ideal body weight - Bradycardia and hypotension can occur with administration

Sedative agents include ketamine, propofol, benzodiazepines, and dexmedetomidine.[5,15,75] Benzodiazepines are not recommended for prolonged infusions (sedation in the intubated patient) due to poor patient outcomes including increased ventilator time, increased length of stay, and increased cognitive dysfunction/post-traumatic stress disorder[75] (Table 2). Our patient received dexmedetomidine, which is appropriate.

Table 2. Sedatives in ESRD

Medication	Dosing	Metabolism and Excretion	Considerations
Propofol - Diisopropylphenol anesthetic and GABA agonist	Bolus 0.5-2 mg/kg IV, infusion 25-75 mcg/kg/min (lower dosing in hypotension and elderly patients)	Hepatic metabolism and clearance with glucuronidation, though kidneys account for 1/3 of clearance	- Infusions > 48 hrs at doses > 75 mcg/kg/min associated with propofol infusion syndrome
Dexmedetomidine – Alpha-2-agonist	Bolus 1 mcg/kg over 10-20 minutes, with infusion 0.2-0.7 mcg/kg/hour (lower bolus in hypotension)	Hepatic metabolism, with no renal involvement	- No dose adjustment needed in ESRD - Rapid bolus or high dose infusions can result in bradycardia and hypotension
Ketamine – NMDA antagonist	Bolus 1-2 mg/kg IV, followed by infusion 5-20 mcg/kg/minute (lower bolus in hypotension)	Hepatic metabolism, with urine excretion	- No dose change needed in patients with ESRD - Possesses analgesic properties - Can be neuroprotective - May increase HR and BP
Benzodiazepines – GABA agonist Include midazolam, lorazepam, and diazepam	Midazolam: Loading dose 0.2 mg/kg IV, followed by 0.05-2 mg/kg/hr Diazepam: Loading dose 0.1-0.3 mg/kg IV Lorazepam: Loading dose 0.1 mg/kg IV	Lorazepam undergoes hepatic metabolism and urine excretion Midazolam and metabolites demonstrate prolonged half-lives in ESRD Diazepam undergoes hepatic metabolism	- Use for sedation associated with poor patient outcomes, including increased time on ventilator, ICU length of stay, and brain dysfunction - No dose change needed for lorazepam - Midazolam is not recommended in ESRD

Q#4: What is an approach to fluid resuscitation in a hypotensive ESRD patient? Is there a concern for fluid overload?

During the initial evaluation of hypotensive patients, we often anchor on a diagnosis of hypovolemia, but sepsis is a possibility. Patients with ESRD on HD are at increased risk for bacteremia and sepsis due to several factors.[5,7] Access sites are common sources of infection, with catheter-related bloodstream infections possessing an incidence of 5.5 episodes every 1000 catheter days.[77-81]

Pneumonia, cellulitis, bacteremia, pyocystitis and *Clostridium difficile* colitis are other common infections. As renal function decreases, risk of infection increases due to poor leukocyte function and T-cell activity, with patients with chronic kidney disease on HD possessing 100–300 times the risk for mortality from sepsis.[82] This same study finds that sepsis was most commonly due to an indwelling catheter, followed by lower respiratory tract infection, with *Escherichia coli* and *Staphylococcus epidermidis* the most common organisms with mortality reaching 40%.[78,82]

The standard treatments for sepsis include source control, IV antimicrobials, and IV fluid resuscitation. What about the patient on hemodialysis—can we use the same approach? Aren't they prone to fluid overload? Studies demonstrate time to antimicrobials and time to fluid resuscitation can affect outcome,[83] and current data suggest patients with ESRD and sepsis are not given enough IV fluid.[78] The Surviving Sepsis Campaign and the federal CMS guidelines recommend 30cc/kg bolus of isotonic IV fluids within the first 3 hours of resuscitation.[83] While ESRD patients may appear fluid overloaded on exam, they are can be truly intravascularly depleted.

We recommend providing a 1L bolus in patients with sepsis even if on hemodialysis, with frequent reassessment with bedside evaluation and US. Provide further boluses if needed. If excess fluid is given, the patient can be dialyzed later once improved. Early vasopressors such as norepinephrine should also be considered.

What did the actual provider do?

BACK TO THE CASE

ED course – test results begin to return:

Labs (21:42):	**Result**	**Range/Units**
WBC	4.4	(4.3-11.1)K/mcL
Hgb	6.8 L	(12.9-16.9)g/dL
Plt Count	137 L	(140-400)K/mcL
Sodium	143	(136-145)mEq/L
Potassium	2.4 L*	(3.5-4.5)mEq/L
Chloride	114 H	(98-109)mEq/L
Carbon Dioxide	21	(19-29)mEq/L
BUN	114	(8-26)mg/dL
Creatinine	4.78 H	(0.72-1.25)mg/dL
Glucose	117 H	(70-99)mg/dL
Calcium	6.3 L	(8.6-10.8)mg/dL
Troponin I	0.04 H*	(0-0.03)ng/mL
Total Bilirubin	0.6	(0.2-1.2)mg/dL
Direct Bilirubin	0.4	(0.0-0.5)mg/dL
AST	13	(5-34)Units/L
ALT	9	(0-55)Units/L
Alk phos	117	(38-126)Units/L
Albumin	2.0 L	(3.5-5.0)g/dL

Chest x-ray 08/14/17 (21:23)—(per radiology)—Cardiomegaly with mild pulmonary edema. Moderate asymmetric left perihilar airspace disease could represent superimposed aspiration or pneumonia.

ECG taken at 2112hrs shows a paced rhythm at a rate of 60bpm wide irregular complexes. Old ECG shows QRS complexes that appear similar to new ECG, rate 95bpm.

MDM (22:11): Patient presents in respiratory distress unconscious and unresponsive on BiPAP, was intubated in the ED, and placed on mechanical ventilation. Post intubation chest x-ray showed possible superimposed pneumonia in the left lower lung. Sepsis workup initiated, cultures ordered, and antibiotics ordered. Patient is also anemic with a Hb of 6.8, and 2 units PRBCs have been ordered. Patient was found to be hypokalemic at 2.4, so 40 mEq of potassium IV ordered. Fecal occult blood test was negative.

Patient currently stabilized on mechanical ventilation and sedated with dexmedetomidine.

The patient's family members and POA have been briefed and updated on patient's status and why it was necessary to intubate. Patient's POA stated that they went through the same thing with their grandmother, the patient's wife, around the time she passed. They were just really surprised that the patient left their home alert and oriented, and by the time they saw him in the room, he was intubated. This brought back memories from when the patient's wife was admitted for her last time. They stated patient is full code. I let them know that we are doing everything possible for him right now. I also let them know that the patient's condition is very serious and the interventions were necessary given his rapid decline. They do understand the patient outcome is poor at this time.

DECISION POINT C – YOU ARE FACED WITH 4 QUESTIONS:

1. **The patient is profoundly hypokalemic. What are your next steps?**
2. **What are possible causes of anemia in a patient with ESRD, and what should be done?**
3. **How should we manage someone with an infiltrate and ESRD, and how can we be fooled?**
4. **Which antibiotics should be given to ESRD patients with pneumonia?**

What does the literature say?

Q#1: The patient is profoundly hypokalemic. What are your next steps?

Hypokalemia most commonly occurs due to GI losses (vomiting or diarrhea) or urinary losses (diuretics). Like every electrolyte issue, it may present with a variety of symptoms dependent on the duration and severity of potassium reduction. Serum levels ranging from 3–3.4meq/L are defined as mild to moderate. Symptoms tend to exist with levels less than 3.0meq/L, with weakness beginning in the lower extremities and then moving upward when levels hit 2.5 meq/L.[84,85] Levels less than 2.5meq/L are severe, especially if symptomatic. As levels continue to decrease, rhabdomyolysis can occur, as well as nausea, vomiting, and ileus.[85-87] Finally, respiratory muscle weakness may occur, resulting in respiratory failure. Hypokalemia may have contributed to our patient's respiratory failure.

On the ECG, U waves are one of the classic findings, most common in precordial leads V_4–V_6. T waves may decrease in amplitude or appear as a down-up T wave. T wave flattening may result in sagging ST segments and ST depression. The QT interval appears prolonged, though this is due to a fusion of the T and U wave. PVCs, PACs, AV blocks, and ventricular dysrhythmias may also occur.[88,89]

Focus initial treatment on preventing life-threatening dysrhythmias and complications such as respiratory failure—completed by increasing potassium to a safe level, followed by replacing the deficit at a slower rate over days. Monitoring is necessary to prevent rebound hyperkalemia.[90,91] Patients most at risk from problems due to hypokalemia include older patients, those with comorbidities like heart disease, and patients on antidysrhythmics.[85] These are present in the current patient.

There are multiple preparations for potassium including potassium chloride, potassium phosphate, potassium bicarbonate, and potassium gluconate. For patients with acidosis, potassium bicarbonate is a great choice.[85,92-94] Potassium phosphate can be used if phosphate is also low (such as in renal tubular acidosis). Potassium chloride is the most commonly preferred preparation, as patients with hypokalemia and metabolic alkalosis often have decreased chloride. As it turns out, correction of potassium and chloride may enhance potassium retention.[85,94,95] Potassium chloride also increases serum levels faster than other preparations. Oral forms of KCl can be given as liquid, tablet, or capsule. Salt substitutes contain approximately 50–65meq per teaspoon and are safe and better tasting. Liquid forms taste poorly, and tablets can cause GI ulcers and bleeding, though this risk is low. An IV formulation of KCl is available for severe hypokalemia or if the patient is unable to take PO. If you're thinking of giving the patient a banana, please reconsider, as it takes 2–3 bananas to provide 40meq.[85,95,96]

Section editor comments (Yealy):

Unless a barrier exists—such as the patient cannot tolerate oral intake or is unstable—oral replenishment is fast, effective, and cheap. A dose of 40–60meq by mouth is safe and usually readily absorbed; getting that much delivered safely IV requires much time and often a central catheter. *Think oral replenishment,* in a solution form, if your patient is willing and able.

Hypokalemia is often associated with hypomagnesemia, especially in the setting of diarrhea or diuretics. Unless elevated serum levels exist, give oral or IV magnesium 1g, recognizing that serum magnesium is not reliable in predicting total body magnesium levels.[84,91]

For mild–moderate hypokalemia, or levels 3.0–3.4meq/L, patients rarely present with symptoms. The easiest approach is oral potassium chloride given in doses of 10–20meq 2–4 times per day. For severe hypokalemia (or moderate with symptoms), IV potassium chloride in saline solution is commonly used, though it must be given slowly and diluted. Pain with infusion and phlebitis can occur if the medication is given through a peripheral vein at rates greater than 10meq/hr. A large peripheral IV or central line should be used for faster infusion rates. If hypokalemia is life-threatening, potassium 40meq/hr through a central line is recommended.[84,85,95,96]

Q#2: What are possible causes of anemia in a patient with ESRD, and what should be done?

Normochromic, normocytic anemia is common in chronic kidney disease patients, with hematocrit levels ranging from 18–25%.[3,7,9,97,98] Normocytic anemia is defined by mean corpuscular volume (MCV) of 80–100, with decrease in hemoglobin and hematocrit.

Causes of normocytic anemia include decreased production of normal-sized RBCs (ESRD, chronic disease, aplastic anemia), increased production of HbS in sickle cell disease, increased destruction of RBCs, increased loss of RBCs, increase in plasma volume, vitamin deficiency (B6, B12), or a mixture of microcytic and macrocytic anemia.[3,7,9]

As GFR and renal function decrease, the incidence of anemia increases. In patients with ESRD and no bleeding, over time Hgb levels will often stabilize at 8g/dL.[3,7,99] Several mechanisms account for anemia in these patients, including decreased production of erythropoietin (which stimulates RBC production), increased RBC destruction (intra and extravascular), blood loss (multiple blood draws), increased RBC hemolysis, blood loss from dialysis, and nutritional deficiencies.[7,97,98]

Anemia is treated with recombinant erythropoietin infusions, which are associated with improved quality of life, and/or iron infusions (need for iron based on ferritin levels). Most patients with ESRD receive erythropoiesis-stimulating agents, including epoetin alfa and darbepoetin alfa, which results in hemoglobin production. Low ferritin levels require iron infusion. Target hemoglobin levels are 11–12g/dL, which result in fewer hospitalizations and lower mortality. Levels above 13g/dL are not recommended.[3,7,9]

Anemia can trigger nonspecific symptoms including fatigue, generalized weakness, syncope/near-syncope, chest pain, palpitations, cold intolerance, and nausea. Physical exam may show pallor, decreased cognition, pale conjunctivae, tachypnea, orthostatic hypotension, and tachycardia. Anemia due to the ESRD is a diagnosis of exclusion unless it is known to previously exist and has not changed.

The etiology of the anemia can be further differentiated through RBC indices, peripheral blood smear, and a reticulocyte count. If new anemia is found, bleeding is the first consideration.[6,7,9,11]

If anemia is chronic, limit RBC transfusions; if acute or changed from baseline, transfusion based on symptoms, rather than a number (Table 3), is recommended. Syncope, chest pain, severe shortness of breath, and hemodynamic instability warrant RBC transfusion. Severe bleeding may require balanced transfusion protocol activation, with 1:1:1 (RBC to FFP to Platelet) products.

Table 3. Transfusion

Indications for transfusion
- Rapid acute hemorrhage without acute control of bleeding
- Blood loss greater than 30-40% of total blood volume with symptoms of severe blood loss
- Blood loss less than 30% but with hypovolemia despite other means of resuscitation (IV fluids)
- Comorbidities with signs or symptoms of anemia (especially chest pain or signs of ACS)

Patients with ESRD typically have chronic anemic but are also at high risk for bleeding. Uremia is associated with von Willebrand Factor disruption, abnormal vessel wall and platelet interactions, and platelet dysfunction. While the platelet number is usually normal, bleeding time increases and platelet function decreases due to uremia with defective platelet activation and adhesion.[7,11,100-102] Coagulation studies (PT, INR, aPTT/PTT) are usually normal in these patients, and stage of ESRD and uremia do not correlate with risk of bleeding.[101-104]

Sources of bleeding include the vascular access site, head, lungs, heart (effusion), abdomen, retroperitoneum, limbs, and trauma. Bleeding from the vascular access site can be life-threatening, with hemorrhage resulting from anticoagulation, aneurysm, pseudoaneurysm, site infection, and anastomosis rupture. For control, we recommend:[11,100-104]

1. Direct, focal pressure at the site. If this is insufficient, proximal and distal pressure should be applied, relative to the site of bleeding. A single stitch repairing a linear tear over the graft site can stop bleeding.
2. Topical hemostatic agents can be applied to the site, including Gelfoam, chitosan, and recombinant human thrombin. Topical TXA can be utilized as well.
3. Desmopressin results in release of vWF factor and decreases uremic effect, assisting with platelet function. Doses include 0.3mcg/kg IV, or 3mcg/kg intranasal. Other agents include protamine if the patient recently received heparin or dialysis within 1.5–2 hours (due to heparin's short half-life), as heparin is provided during HD sessions. Protamine is given in doses of 1mg for every 100 units of heparin. If the heparin dose is not known, protamine 10-20mg is sufficient.
4. Other measures include estrogen 25mg IV, cryoprecipitate 10 units over 30 minutes IV, and finally, tourniquet application proximal to the site of hemorrhage, recognizing that a tourniquet will result in thrombosis of the graft or fistula.

If bleeding was minor and responded to direct pressure, assess site patency for bruit and thrill—thrombosis at the hemodialysis site may occur after pressure.

Q#3: How should we manage someone with an infiltrate and ESRD, and how can we be fooled?

These patients have many comorbidities that can confuse the clinical picture for pneumonia, and chest x-ray is not definitive either. Many conditions can confuse the picture including CHF, PE, mass, atelectasis, or vascular emboli.[105-110]

Pneumonia classically presents with cough, purulent sputum, shortness of breath, and fever. However, these symptoms are not always present (frequency rates): cough (79%–91%), fever (75%), increased sputum production (65%), dyspnea (~ 70%), and chest pain (50%).[105-110] Elderly, immunocompromised, and debilitated patients are at greater risk for pneumonia and infection, though they may present only with altered mental status and cough, fever, or dyspnea.[105,106]

Any vital sign abnormality, especially tachypnea, warrants consideration of pneumonia in patients with ESRD.[107] Tachypnea is one of the first signs of pneumonia, but it can also be present in fluid overload. Fever is more common in patients with pneumonia as compared to pulmonary overload (odds ratio 2.01). Physical exam findings are also not reliable, including lung findings such as crackles, egophony, dullness to percussion, decreased breath sounds, and asymmetric respirations.

Unfortunately, one meta-analysis found that no combination of physical exam findings can confirm the diagnosis of pneumonia.[106] Clinical judgment is also poor, with sensitivity 74% and specificity 84% in ambulatory, febrile patients.

Chest x-ray has a sensitivity of 46–87% for pneumonia diagnosis,[105,106,111-113] with poor inter-rater reliability.[106,114] Sensitivity in patients with ESRD approaches 60% at most, and even worse, specificity is 29–50%.[106,114] Many conditions may create an infiltrate, including:

- Aspiration
- Atelectasis
- Pulmonary edema
- Effusion
- PE
- Hemorrhage
- Drug-induced lesion
- Diffuse alveolar damage
- Pneumonitis
- TB[115,116]

Our patient demonstrates left perihilar airspace disease with pulmonary edema. Is there anything else that can help? Ultrasound again provides valuable assistance, and findings for pneumonia include bronchograms, consolidations, pleural effusion, and pleural line abnormalities. Dynamic air bronchograms possess a positive LR ranging from 15.6–16.8, with negative LR 0.03–0.07.[117,118] Another option is chest CT, which should be completed if pneumonia is clinically suspected in a patient with sepsis and negative x-ray findings. Chest CT demonstrates a sensitivity that is more reliable (> 95%).[111,113]

In the patient with ESRD, the most common diseases include pneumonia and pulmonary edema. Both may have chest x-ray findings with pulmonary infiltrate or consolidation. Fever is more common with pneumonia and dyspnea without fever with pulmonary edema, but these are not definitive. Using a combination of focused history, exam, laboratory assessment, and imaging is imperative.[105-107, 109, 119]

Q#4: Which antibiotics should be given to ESRD patients with pneumonia?

Antibiotic choice in patients on ESRD is not straightforward. The classification system for pneumonia underwent recent changes to include:

1. Community-acquired pneumonia: Acute pulmonary infection in a patient who is not hospitalized or residing in a long-term care facility 14 or more days before presentation.
2. Hospital-acquired pneumonia: New pulmonary infection occurring 48 hours or more after hospital admission.
3. Ventilator-associated pneumonia: New pulmonary infection occurring more than 48–72 hours after endotracheal intubation.

There is no classification for healthcare-associated pneumonia (HCAP), which was a class designed to determine who needed broad-spectrum coverage for *Pseudomonas* and MRSA. Instead, the multidrug resistance score (MDR) can be used. Patients with any two or more of the following should receive broad-spectrum empiric coverage:

- Any antibiotics in the last 90 days.
- Hospitalization for >2 days in the last 90 days.
- Poor functional status (significant debility, incontinence, and inability to perform activities of daily living).
- Immunosuppression (absolute neutrophil count < 1000, asplenia, hematologic malignancy, congenital immunodeficiency, HIV infection, prednisone equivalent > 10mg/day for 14 days or more or any other immunosuppressive drug).[120,121]

This patient is currently intubated with concern for pneumonia. He is not on immunosuppressive medication and does not otherwise have more than 2 MDR points.[122] Table 4 details antimicrobial options based on classification of pneumonia. Patients with septic shock or intubation should be given empiric broad-spectrum antimicrobials.[17,83,120, 121, 123]

Table 4. Antibiotics for pneumonia

Pneumonia Classification		**Antimicrobial**	**ESRD Considerations**
Community-acquired	Outpatient	Levofloxacin 750 mg PO for 1 day, followed by 500 mg every 48 hours Moxifloxacin 400 mg PO for 7-14 days Amoxicillin/Clavulanate 250-500 mg PO once per day AND second agent (azithromycin 500 mg 500 mg day 1, 250 mg days 2-5 OR doxycycline 100 mg PO BID)	Levofloxacin: Dosing changed to 750 mg on day 1, with next doses 500 mg Moxifloxacin: No dose change needed Amoxicillin/Clavulanate: Decrease dose from 1g BID to 250-500 mg once per day
	Inpatient	Levofloxacin 750 mg IV/PO Moxifloxacin 400 mg IV/PO Ceftriaxone 1 g IV plus azithromycin 500 mg IV/PO once daily or doxycycline 100 mg IV/PO BID	Ceftriaxone: No dose change needed Azithromycin: No dose change needed per manufacturer, though caution recommended in GFR < 10 mL/minute Doxycycline: No dose change needed
Hospital-acquired or Ventilator-associated		Choose one from A, B, *and* C A: Cefepime 2 g IV, Ceftazidime 2 g IV, Piperacillin/tazobactam 2.25 g IV, Imipenem/cilastatin 500 mg IV, or Aztreonam 2 g IV B: Azithromycin 500 mg IV, Ciprofloxacin 400 mg IV, Levofloxacin 750 mg IV, Gentamicin 5-7 mg/kg IV C: Vancomycin 15-20 mg/kg IV or Linezolid 600 mg IV	Piperacillin/tazobactam: 2.25 g IV, rather than 4.5 g IV Ceftazidime and Cefepime: Utilize initial loading dose, but further doses require adjustment Gentamicin: Associated with worsening renal injury/failure, administer normal loading dose, then decrease to 1 mg/kg Imipenem/cilastatin: Should not be used in ESRD if HD is not available within 48 hours Aztreonam: Utilize initial loading dose, but further doses require adjustment Vancomycin: Use normal loading dose, but further doses require adjustment Linezolid: No change in dose needed

What did the actual provider do?

ATTENDING NOTE: The patient's granddaughter accompanies the medics and states that he is a full code and does want intubation if necessary. She reports that he has had gradually worsening shortness of breath over the past 2 weeks, [and significantly more] following dialysis today. At the time of medic arrival, the patient was very combative secondary to extreme hypoxia and required chemical sedation. Patient was given Versed en route, and on arrival the patient was unresponsive with minimal responsiveness to sternal rub. Patient was brought in on BiPAP and remained significantly hypoxic. Immediate preparation was made to electively intubate the patient for airway protection. The patient was also hypotensive on arrival, so sedation was selected carefully to minimize potential worsening of his hypotension.

Following ET placement, a portable chest x-ray was obtained. ET tube placement was confirmed in good position.The NG tube was in good position. Patient with consolidation of the left lower lobe questionable atelectasis versus pneumonia as well as mild pulmonary edema and cardiomegaly. Following these results, the patient was started on empiric antibiotics and was receiving gentle fluid administration for his hypotension.

The patient was placed on the ventilator, and an ABG was obtained.

The patient's laboratory values show significant anemia. Stool was sent for guaiac which was negative, and patient's power of attorney for healthcare consented for transfusion. Patient was started on 2 units packed red cells. The patient was also found to be extremely hypokalemic. Considering potassium administration in the setting of end-stage renal disease, we started with a small dose of 40 mEq and will reevaluate before any additional potassium will be infused. Patient's blood pressure has remained between 90-100 systolic. We will hold on pressors at this time.

The hospitalist has accepted the patient for admission at 2240 hrs.

Clinical Impression (22:50): Respiratory distress, Hypokalemia, Severe anemia, ESRD (end stage renal disease) on dialysis, History of CHF (congestive heart failure), History of COPD, Septic shock, CHF exacerbation, Pneumonia.

Case summary:

What could have been done to improve care at the initial encounter?

The provider appropriately managed the airway when the patient was unable to tolerate noninvasive positive pressure ventilation and was decompensating. Etomidate and rocuronium were appropriate choices permitting intubation, and dexmedetomidine was used for post-intubation sedation and analgesia. The physician was concerned for pneumonia on the x-ray, resulting in blood cultures and administration of antibiotics. Potassium replacement and RBC transfusions both occurred, all appropriate treatments in the ED.

There are several areas for potential improvement:

1. Knowing the history better would assist—the patient's dyspnea over 2 weeks, rather than acute, alters the likely causes. Ultrasound also could aid in evaluation for underlying etiologies.
2. Obtaining a full set of vital signs to include core temperature can provide valuable information and narrow the differential diagnosis.
3. Versed sedation may have added to the deterioration; another option such as ketamine would be a better choice.
4. Fluid administration was tepid—we think more fluid sooner is a better route in this patient with a baseline BP of 160–180mmHg who presented with a BP of 90–100 mmHg.

Hospital course:

(NEPHROLOGY): The patient is a 78-year-old male well known to our practice who receives dialysis at [the dialysis center of excellence] who presented to ER for shortness of breath. He has history of CHF and end-stage renal disease on hemodialysis. I saw the patient at hemodialysis yesterday where he received a full treatment and tolerated it well, walking out of the center on his own. His daughter states they talked with him on the phone for approximately an hour and he seemed fine but described some shortness of breath. EMS was called. While en route he received several doses of Versed and was placed on BiPAP/CPAP. The patient had desaturation in emergency room and became nonresponsive. Per the ER doctor, he was intubated and placed on ventilation. Chest x-ray shows possible left-sided pneumonia, and Hgb was 6.8 on admission. At the dialysis center, his Hgb was 11.4 most recently. On exam today, the patient is extubated, with daughter at bedside.

Assessment and plan:

1. Respiratory distress: Patient was extubated yesterday morning and is currently on nasal cannula and tolerating this well. Patient will be transferred out of the ICU to a telemetry bed.
2. Pneumonia: Chest x-ray showed a possible pneumonia. Vancomycin and Zosyn have been discontinued at this time. We have switched his levofloxacin to oral. We will treat his pneumonia with 500mg of levofloxacin every 48 hours.
3. ESRD (end-stage renal disease) on dialysis.
4. Hypokalemia: The patient had his potassium replaced. Current potassium is 3.8. Patient has been placed on electrolyte protocol.
5. Severe anemia: Patient initially had a hemoglobin of 6.8. Patient was transfused 2 units of blood yesterday. His repeat hemoglobin yesterday was 10.4. This morning his hemoglobin was 10.8. We will continue to monitor the patient's hemoglobin. A CT of the abdomen and pelvis was ordered yesterday and was negative for a bleed.
6. Abdominal aortic aneurysm (AAA): On the CT scan of the abdomen and pelvis the patient was found to have an abdominal aortic aneurysm measuring 3.1cm. The current recommendation is to follow up for an aneurysm this size in 3 years.
7. Elevated troponin: Patient had an elevated troponin 0.04. Troponin was repeated and was 0.04 again. Patient has chronically elevated troponin levels. When looking back in his medical record, it appears that this is baseline for him.

Chapter author note: Though an elevated troponin is often attributed to decreased renal clearance in patients with ESRD, intact troponin molecules are unlikely to be renally excreted. There are multiple etiologies for elevated troponin in this patient population, and even low-level elevations in troponin correlate with higher risk for cardiovascular complications and poor outcomes.

References:

1. United States Renal Data System (USRDS) Annual data report. Epidemiology of kidney disease in the United States. 2015. Available from: https://www.usrds.org/adr.aspx.
2. National Kidney and Urologic Diseases Information Clearinghouse (NKUDIC). Kidney disease statistics for the United States. US Department of Health and Human Services. Available at http://kidney.niddk.nih.gov/kudiseases/pubs/kustats/#7. Accessed July 4, 2017.
3. KDIGO. Chapatienter 1: Definition and classification of CKD. Kidney Int Suppl 2013; 3:19. http://www.kdigo.org/clinical_practice_guidelines/pdf/CKD/KDIGO_2012_CKD_ GL.pdf. Accessed July 4, 2017.
4. Go AS, Chertow GM, Fan D, et al. Chronic kidney disease and the risks of death, cardiovascular events, and hospitalization. N Engl J Med 2004 23;351(13):1296-305.
5. Arulkumaran N, Montero RM, Singer M. Management of the dialysis patient in general intensive care. Br J Anaesth 2012;108(2):183-92.
6. Long B, Koyfman A. Emergency medicine evaluation and management of the end stage renal disease patient. Am J Emerg Med 2017;35(12):1946-55.
7. Foley M, Mehta N, Sinert R. Chapatienter 90: End-stage renal disease. Tintinalli's Emergency Medicine: A Comprehensive Study Guide,8e. http://accessemergencymedicine.mhmedical.com/content.aspx?bookid=1658&secti onid=109433467#1121508429. Accessed 15 July 2017.
8. Bradbury BD, Fissell RB, Albert JM, et al. Predictors of early mortality among incident US hemodialysis patients in the Dialysis Outcomes and Practice Patterns Study (DOPPS). Clin J Am Soc Nephrol 2007;2:89.
9. Wolfson A. Ch. 87: Renal failure. Rosen's emergency medicine: Concepts and clinical practice, 9th ed. https://www.clinicalkey.com/#!/browse/book/3-s2.0-C20141019850.
10. Halle MP, Hertig A, Kengne AP, et al. Acute pulmonary oedema in chronic dialysis patients admitted into an intensive care unit. Nephrol Dial Transplant 2012;27(2):603-7.
11. Hodde L, Sandroni S. Emergency department evaluation and management of dialysis patient complications. J Emerg Med 1992;10:317-34.
12. Dietrich CF, Mathis G, Blaivas M, et al. Lung B-line artefacts and their use. J Thorac Dis 2016;8(6):1356-65.
13. Arntfield RT, Millington SJ. Point of care cardiac ultrasound applications in the emergency department and intensive care unit - A review. Curr Cardiol Rev 2012;8(2):98-108.
14. Hughes CG, McGrane S, Pandharipande PP. Sedation in the intensive care setting. Clin Pharmacol 2012;4: 53-63.
15. Gabardi S, Abramson S. Drug dosing in chronic kidney disease. Med Clin North Am 2005;89(3):649-87.
16. Baghdady NT, Banik S, Swartz SA, et al. Psychotropic drugs and renal failure: Translating the evidence for clinical practice. Adv Ther 2009;26(4):404-24.
17. Lexicomp. https://online.lexi.com/lco/action/home. Accessed July 2017.
18. UptoDate. https://www.upatientodate.com/contents/search. Accessed July 2017.
19. Scheppke K, Braghiroli J, Shalaby M, et al. Prehospital use of i.m. ketamine for sedation of violent and agitated patients. West J Emerg Med 2014;15(7):736-41.
20. Iwanicki JL, Barrett W, Saghafi O, et al. Prehospital ketamine for excited delirium in the setting of acute drug intoxication. Clin Toxicol 2014;52:685-6. Abstract #9.
21. Keseg D, Cortez E, Rund D, et al. The use of prehospital ketamine for control of agitation in

a metropolitan firefighter-based EMS system. Prehosp Emerg Care2015;19(1):110-5.
22. Baumgaertel MW, Kraemer M, Berlit P. Neurologic complications of acute and chronic renal disease. Handb Clin Neurol 2014;119(3):383-93.
23. Bucurescu M. Neurological manifestations of uremic encephalopathy. Medscape. Available at: http://emedicine.medscape.com/article/1135651-overview. Accessed July 4, 2017.
24. Bleck TP, Smith MC, Pierre-Louis SJ, et al. Neurologic complications of critical medical illnesses. Crit Care Med 1993;21:98.
25. Bolton, CF, Young, GB. Uremic encephalopathy. In: Bolton, CF, Young, GB, (eds), Neurological complications of renal disease, Buttersworth, Stoneham 1990. p.44.
26. Chen R, Young GB. Metabolic encephalopathies. In: Bailliere's clinical neurology, Bolton CF, Young GB (eds), London: Balliere Tindall; 1996, p.577.
27. Arieff AI. Dialysis disequilibrium syndrome: current concepts on pathogenesis and prevention. Kidney Int 1994;45(3):629-35.
28. Silver SM, Sterns RH, Halperin ML. Brain swelling after dialysis: old urea or new osmoles? Am J Kidney Dis 1996;28(1):1-13.
29. Holzmann MJ, Aastveit A, Hammar N, et al. Renal dysfunction increases the risk of ischemic and hemorrhagic stroke in the general population. Ann Med 2012;44:607-15.
30. Power A, Hamady M, Singh S, et al. High but stable incidence of subdural haematoma in haemodialysis—A single-centre study. Nephrol Dial Transplant 2010;25:2272-5.
31. Hsieh CY, Chen CH, Wu AB, et al. Comparative outcomes between hemo- and peritoneal dialysis patients with acute intracerebral hemorrhage. Am J Nephrol 2010;32:31-7.
32. Wu C-L, Tsai C-C, Kor C-T, et al. Stroke and risks of development and progression of kidney diseases and end-stage renal disease: A nationwide population-based cohort study. Burdmann EA, ed. PLoS ONE 2016;11(6):e0158533.
33. Hemphill JC 3rd, Greenberg SM, Anderson CS, et al. Guidelines for the management of spontaneous intracerebral hemorrhage: A guideline for healthcare professionals from the American Heart Association/American Stroke Association. Stroke 2015;46:2032.
34. Connolly ES Jr, Rabinstein AA, Carhuapoma JR, et al. Guidelines for the management of aneurysmal subarachnoid hemorrhage: A guideline for healthcare professionals from the American Heart Association/American Stroke Association. Stroke 2012;43:1711.
35. Jauch EC, Saver JL, Adams HP Jr, et al. Guidelines for the early management of patients with acute ischemic stroke: A guideline for healthcare professionals from the American Heart Association/American Stroke Association. Stroke 2013;44:870.
36. Demaerschalk BM, Kleindorfer DO, Adeoye OM, et al. Scientific rationale for the inclusion and exclusion criteria for intravenous alteplase in acute ischemic stroke: A statement for healthcare professionals from the American Heart Association/American Stroke Association. Stroke 2016;47:581.
37. Flythe JE, Curhan GC, Brunelli SM. Shorter length dialysis sessions are associated with increased mortality, independent of body weight. Kidney Int 2013;83(1):104-13.
38. Hajhosseiny R, Khavandi K, Goldsmith DJ. Cardiovascular disease in chronic kidney disease: Untying the Gordian knot. Int J Clin Pract 2013;67:14.
39. Kanbay M, Afsar B, Goldsmith D, et al. Sudden death in hemodialysis: An update. Blood Purif 2010;30(2):135-45.
40. Kang EW, Na HJ, Hong SM, et al. Prognostic value of elevated cardiac troponin I in ESRD patients with sepsis. Nephrol Dial Transplant 2009;24(5):1568-73.

41. Alfonzo A, Simpson K, Deighan C. Modifications to advanced life support in renal failure. Resuscitation 2007;73:12-28.
42. Maisch B, Seferovic PM, Ristic AD, et al. Guidelines on the diagnosis and management of pericardial diseases executive summary: The task force on the diagnosis and management of pericardial diseases of the European Society of Cardiology. Eur Heart J 2004;25:587-610.
43. Alpert MA, Ravenscraft MD. Pericardial involvement in end-stage renal disease. Am J Med Sci 2003;325:228-36.
44. Sterns RH, Grieff M, Bernstein PL. Treatment of hyperkalemia: Something old, something new. Kidney Int 2016;89:546-54.
45. Weisberg LS. Management of severe hyperkalemia. Crit Care Med 2008;36(12):3246-51.
46. Strayer R. Strayerisms: Why do we intubate? Emergency medicine reviews and perspectives. August 2017. Available at https://www.emrap.org/episode/challenging/strayerismswhy.
47. Hillberg RE, Johnson DC. Noninvasive ventilation. N Engl J Med 1997;337:1746.
48. Yeow ME, Santanilla JI. Noninvasive positive pressure ventilation in the emergency department. Emerg Med Clin North Am 2008;26:835.
49. Gray A, Goodacre S, Newby DE, et al. Noninvasive ventilation in acute cardiogenic pulmonary edema. N Engl J Med 2008;359:142.
50. Quon BS, Gan WQ, Sin DD. Contemporary management of acute exacerbations of COPD: A systematic review and metaanalysis. Chest 2008;133:756.
51. Lim WJ, Mohammed Akram R, Carson KV et al. Non-invasive positive pressure ventilation for treatment of respiratory failure due to severe acute exacerbations of asthma. Cochrane Database Syst Rev 2012;12:CD004360.
52. Weingart SD, Trueger NS, Wong N, et al. Delayed sequence intubation: A prospective observational study. Ann Emerg Med 2015;65(4):349-55.
53. O'Connor RE, Swor RA. Verification of endotracheal tube placement following intubation. National Association of EMS Physicians Standards and Clinical Practice Committee. Prehosp Emerg Care 1999;3:248-50.
54. Katz SH, Falk JL. Misplaced endotracheal tubes by paramedics in an urban emergency medical services system. Ann Emerg Med 2001;37:32-7.
55. Kelly JJ, Eynon CA, Kaplan JL, et al. Use of tube condensation as an indicator of endotracheal tube placement. Ann Emerg Med 1998;31:575.
56. Pollard BJ, Junius F. Accidental intubation of the oesophagus. Anaesth Intensive Care 1980;8:183.
57. Birmingham PK, Cheney FW, Ward RJ. Esophageal intubation: A review of detection techniques. Anesth Analg 1986;65:886-91.
58. Knapp S, Kofler J, Stoiser B, et al. The assessment of four different methods to verify tracheal tube placement in the critical care setting. Anesth Analg 1999;88:766-70.
59. Cummings RO, Hazinski MF. Guidelines based on the principle "first, do no harm": New guidelines on tracheal tube confirmation and prevention of dislodgment. Circulation 2000;102(8 Suppl):I380-4.
60. Williamson JA, Webb RK, Cockings J, et al. The Australian Incident Monitoring Study. The capnograph: applications and limitations: An analysis of 2000 incident reports. Anaesth Intensive Care 1993;21:551-7.
61. Jenkins WA, Verdile VP, Paris PM. The syringe aspiration technique to verify endotracheal tube position. Am J Emerg Med 1994;12:413-6.

62. Whitaker DK. Time for capnography – Everywhere. Anaesthesia 2011;66:544-9.
63. Kodali BS. Capnography outside the operating rooms. Anesthesiology 2013 Jan;118(1):192-201.
64. Manifold CA, Davids N, Villers LC, et al. Capnography for the nonintubated patient in the emergency setting. Journ Emerg Med 2013;45(4):626-32.
65. Ward KR, Yealy DM. End-tidal carbon dioxide monitoring in emergency medicine, Part 1: Basic principles. Acad Emerg Med 1998;5(6):628-36.
66. Eckstein M, Hatch L, Malleck J, et al. End-tidal CO_2 as a predictor of survival in out-of-hospital cardiac arrest. Resuscitation 2016;104:53-8.
67. Lui CT, Poon KM, Tsui KL. Abrupt rise of end tidal carbon dioxide level was a specific but non-sensitive marker of return of spontaneous circulation in patient with out-of-hospital cardiac arrest. Resuscitation 2016;104:53-8.
68. Touma O, Davies M. The prognostic value of end tidal carbon dioxide during cardiac arrest: a systematic review. Resuscitation 2013;84(11):1470-9.
69. Werner S, Smith C, Goldstein J, et al. Pilot study to evaluate the accuracy of ultrasonography in confirming endotracheal tube placement. Ann Emerg Med 2007;49(1):75-80.
70. Das S, Choupoo N, Haldar R, Lahkar A. Transtracheal ultrasound for verification of endotracheal tube placement: A systematic review and meta-analysis. Can J Anaesth 2015;62(4):413-23.
71. Tobin MJ. Principles and practice of mechanical ventilation. 3rd ed. McGraw-Hill Medical, Dallas, TX; 2013.
72. Santanilla JI, Daniel B, Yoew M-E. Mechanical ventilation. Emerg Med Clin N Am 2008;26:849-62.
73. Sutherasan, Y, Vargas, M, and Pelosi, P. Protective mechanical ventilation in the non-injured lung: Review and meta-analysis. Crit Care 2014;8:211.
74. Acute Respiratory Distress Syndrome Network, Brower RG, Matthay MA, et al. Ventilation with lower tidal volumes as compared with traditional tidal volumes for acute lung injury and the acute respiratory distress syndrome. N Engl J Med 2000;342:1301-8.
75. Reade MC, Finfer S. Sedation and delirium in the intensive care unit. N Engl J Med 2014; 370:444-54.
76. Dean M. Opioids in renal failure and dialysis patients. J Pain Symptom Manage 2004;28(5):497-04.
77. Naqvi SB, Collins AJ. Infectious complications in chronic kidney disease. Adv Chronic Kidney Dis 2006;13:199.
78. Dagher GA, Harmouche E, Jabbour E, et al. Sepsis in hemodialysis patients. BMC Emerg Med 2015;15:30.
79. Saad TF. Bacteremia associated with tunneled, cuffed hemodialysis catheters. Am J Kidney Dis 1999;34(6):1114-24.
80. Nassar GM, Ayus JC. Infectious complications of the hemodialysis access. Kidney Int 2001 Jul;60(1):1-13.
81. Allon M. Treatment guidelines for dialysis catheter–related bacteremia: An update. Am J Kidney Dis. 2009;54(1):13-7.
82. Sarnak MJ, Jaber BL. Mortality caused by sepsis in patients with end-stage renal disease compared with the general population. Kidney Int 2000;58:1758-64.

83. Rhodes A, Evans LE, Alhazzani W, et al. Surviving sepsis campaign: International guidelines for management of sepsis and septic shock: 2016. Crit Care Med 2017;45(3):486-52.
84. Rose BD, Post TW. Hypokalemia. In: Clinical Physiology of acid-base and electrolyte disorders, 5th ed, Rose BD, Post TW (eds), McGraw-Hill, New York 2001. p.836.
85. Gennari FJ. Hypokalemia. N Engl J Med 1998;339(7):451-58.
86. Knochel JP. Neuromuscular manifestations of electrolyte disorders. Am J Med 1982;72:521.
87. Knochel JP, Schlein EM. On the mechanism of rhabdomyolysis in potassium depletion. J Clin Invest 1972;51:1750.
88. Yelamanchi VP, Molnar J, Ranade V, et al. Influence of electrolyte abnormalities on interlead variability of ventricular repolarization times in 12-lead electrocardiography. Am J Ther 2001;8:117.
89. Mujais SK, Katz AL. Potassium deficiency. In: The Kidney: Physiology and pathophysiology, Seldin DW, Giebisch G (eds), Lippincott Williams & Wilkins, 2000 p.1615.
90. Cohn JN, Kowey PR, Whelton PK, et al. New guidelines for potassium replacement in clinical practice: A contemporary review by the National Council on Potassium in Clinical Practice. Arch Intern Med 2000;160:2429.
91. Huang CL, Kuo E. Mechanism of hypokalemia in magnesium deficiency. J Am Soc Nephrol 2007;18:2649.
92. Crop MJ, Hoorn EJ, Lindemans J, et al. Hypokalaemia and subsequent hyperkalaemia in hospitalized patients. Nephrol Dial Transplant 2007;22:3471.
93. Sterns RH, Cox M, Feig PU, et al. Internal potassium balance and the control of the plasma potassium concentration. Medicine (Baltimore) 1981;60:339.
94. Kim GH, Han JS. Therapeutic approach to hypokalemia. Nephron 2002;92 Suppl 1:28-32.
95. Kruse JA, Carlson RW. Rapid correction of hypokalemia using concentrated intravenous potassium chloride infusions. Arch Intern Med 1990;150(3):613-17.
96. Hamill RJ, Robinson LM, Wexler HR, et al. Efficacy and safety of potassium infusion therapy in hypokalemic critically ill patients. Crit Care Med 1991;19(5):694-99.
97. Hsu CY, McCulloch CE, Curhan GC. Epidemiology of anemia associated with chronic renal insufficiency among adults in the United States: Results from the Third National Health and Nutrition Examination Survey. J Am Soc Nephrol 2002;13(2):504-10.
98. El-Achkar TM, Ohmit SE, McCullough PA, et al. Higher prevalence of anemia with diabetes mellitus in moderate kidney insufficiency: The Kidney Early Evaluation Program. Kidney Int 2005;67(4):1483-88.
99. Astor BC, Muntner P, Levin A, et al. Association of kidney function with anemia: The Third National Health and Nutrition Examination Survey (1988-1994). Arch Intern Med 2002;162:1401.
100. Padberg F, Calligaro K, Sidawy A. Complications of arteriovenous hemodialysis access: Recognition and management. J Vasc Surg 2008;48(5 Suppl):55S-80S.
101. Linthorst GE, Avis HJ, Levi M. Uremic thrombocytopathy is not about urea. J Am Soc Nephrol 2010;21:753.
102. Galbusera M, Remuzzi G, Boccardo P. Treatment of bleeding in dialysis patients. Semin Dial 2009;22:279-86.

103. Gordz S, Mrowietz C, Pindur G, et al. Effect of desmopressin (DDAVP) on platelet membrane glycoprotein expression in patients with von Willebrand's disease. Clin Hemorheol Microcirc 2005;32(2):83-7.
104. Hedges SJ, Dehoney SB, Hooper JS, et al. Evidence-based treatment recommendations for uremic bleeding. Nat Clin Pract Nephrol 2007;3:138-53.
105. Marrie TJ. Community-acquired pneumonia. Clin Infect Dis 1994;18:501.
106. Metlay JP, Kapoor WN, Fine MJ. Does this patient have community-acquired pneumonia? Diagnosing pneumonia by history and physical examination. JAMA 1997;278:1440.
107. Wunderink RG, Waterer GW. Community-acquired pneumonia. New Engl J Med 2014;370(6):543-51.
108. Rosh AJ. Diagnosing pneumonia by medical history and physical examination. Ann Emerg Med 2005 Nov;46(5):465-7.
109. Metlay JP, Fine JM. Testing strategies in the initial management of patients with community-acquired pneumonia. Ann Intern Med 2003;138:109-18.
110. Metlay JP, Schulz R, Li YH, et al. Influence of age on symptoms at presentation in patients with community-acquired pneumonia. Arch Intern Med 1997;157(13):1453-9.
111. Self WH, Courtney DM, McNaughton DC, et al. High discordance of chest x-ray and computed tomography for detection of pulmonary opacities in ED patients: Implications for diagnosing pneumonia. Am J Emerg Med 2013;31:401-5.
112. Hash RB, Stephens JL, Laurens MB, Vogel RL. The relationship between volume status, hydration, and radiographic findings in the diagnosis of community-acquired pneumonia. J Fam Pract 2000;49:833-7.
113. Hayden GE, Wrenn KW. Chest radiograph vs. computed tomography scan in the evaluation for pneumonia. J Emerg Med 2009;36(3):266-70.
114. Judd E, Ahmed MI, Harms JC. Pneumonia in hemodialysis patients: A challenging diagnosis in the emergency room. J Nephrol 2013;26(6): 1128-35.
115. Black AD. Non-infectious mimics of community-acquired pneumonia. Pneumonia 20168:2.
116. Alves dos Santos JW, Torres A, Michel GT, et al. Non-infectious and unusual infectious mimics of community-acquired pneumonia. Respir Med 2004;98(6):488-94.
117. Hu QJ, Shen YC, Jia LQ, et al. Diagnostic performance of lung ultrasound in the diagnosis of pneumonia: a bivariate meta-analysis. Int J Clin Exp Med 2014;7(1):115-21.
118. Chavez MA, Shams N, Ellington LE, et al. Lung ultrasound for the diagnosis of pneumonia in adults: a systematic review and meta-analysis. Respir Res 2014;15:50.
119. O'Brien WT, Rohweder DA, Lattin GE, et al. Clinical indicators of radiographic findings in patients with suspected community-acquired pneumonia: Who needs a chest x-ray? J Am Coll Radiol 2006;3:703.
120. Kalil AC, Metersky ML, Klompas M, et al. Management of adults with hospital-acquired and ventilator-associated pneumonia: 2016 clinical practice guidelines by the Infectious Diseases Society of America and the American Thoracic Society. Clin Infect Dis 2016;63(5):1-51.
121. Mandell LA, Wunderink RG, Anzueto A, et al; Infectious Diseases Society of America; American Thoracic Society. Infectious Diseases Society of America/American Thoracic Society consensus guidelines on the management of community-acquired pneumonia in adults. Clin Infect Dis 2007 Mar 1;44 Suppl 2:S27-72.

122. Maruyama T, Fujisawa T, Okuno M, et al. A new strategy for healthcare-associated pneumonia: A 2-year prospective multicenter cohort study using risk factors for multidrug-resistant pathogens to select initial empiric therapy. Clin InfectDis 2013;57(10):1373-83.
123. Berman S. Infections in patients undergoing chronic dialysis. Antimicrobe Available at http://www.antimicrobe.org/e41.asp. Accessed July 2017.

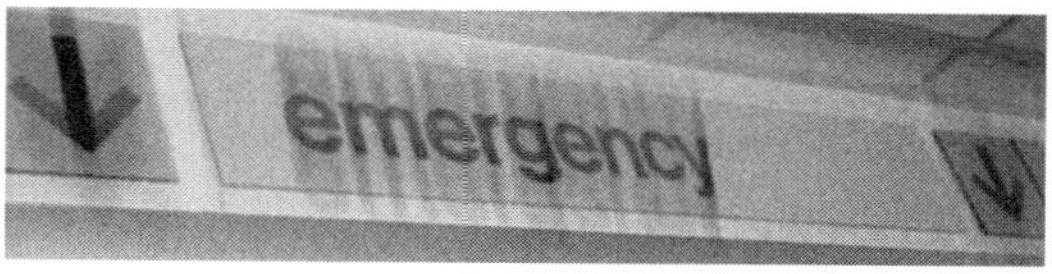

SECTION B – BREATHING/ PULMONARY

Chapter 9: A 28-year-old man with a cough

David Thompson, MD, MPH
Associate Professor
Department of Emergency Medicine
Director of Quality Improvement & Patient Safety
University of Cincinnati
Cincinnati, OH

Esther H. Chen, MD
Professor
Clinical Emergency Medicine
Department of Emergency Medicine
Director of Graduate Medical Education at ZSFG
University of California, San Francisco/
Zuckerberg San Francisco General Hospital
San Francisco, CA

Section editor:
Donald M. Yealy, MD
Chair, Department of Emergency Medicine
University of Pittsburgh/University of Pittsburgh Physicians
Vice President, Emergency and Urgent Care Services, Physician Services
UPMC Professor of Emergency Medicine, Medicine and Clinical and Translational Sciences
University of Pittsburgh School of Medicine
Pittsburgh, PA

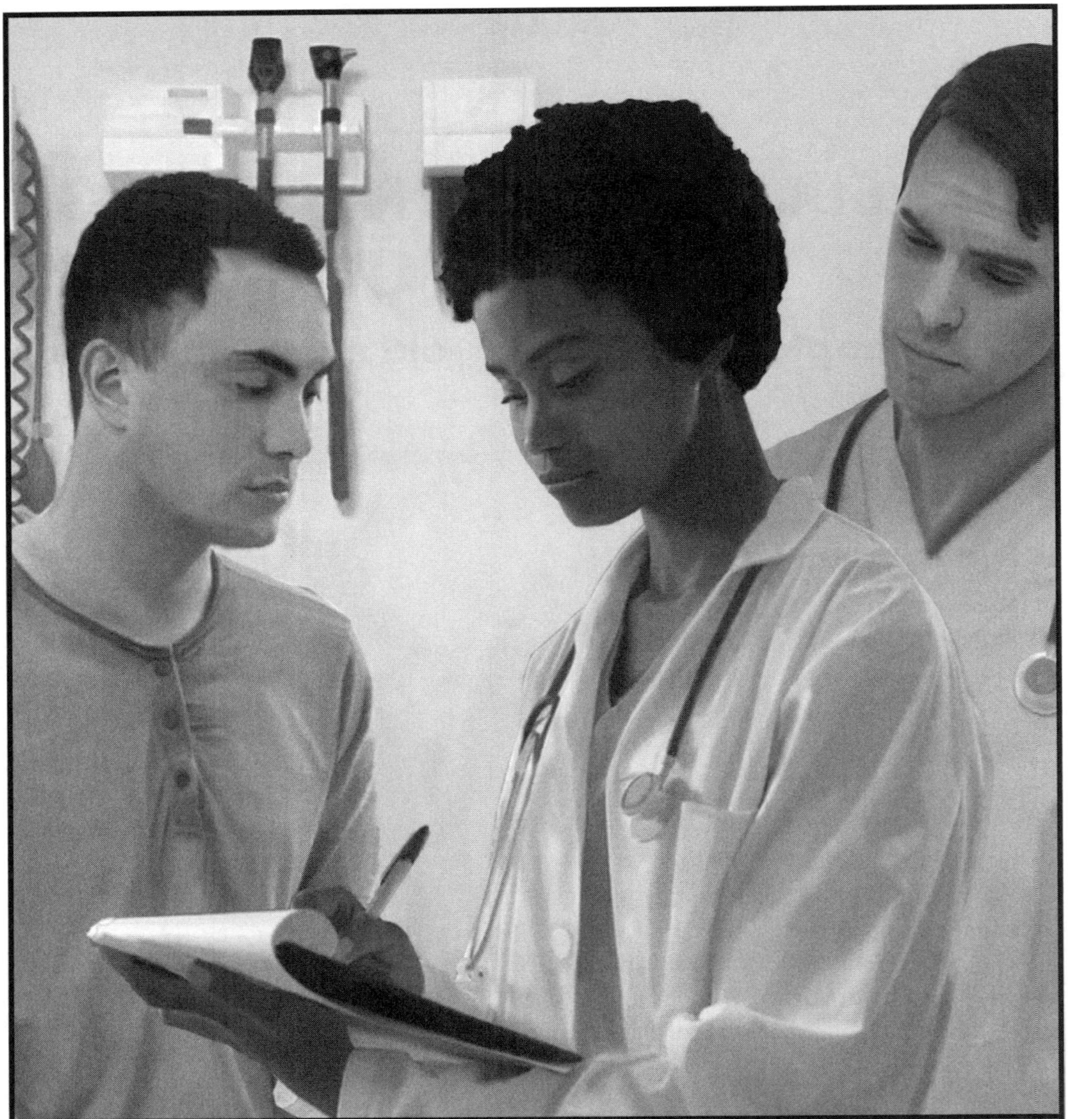

"IF YOU TAKE THESE ANTIBIOTICS FOR YOUR PNEUMONIA, YOU SHOULD BE JUST FINE."

SECTION B/CHAPTER 9

A 28-year-old man with a cough

INITIAL ED VISIT

CC (17:46):

Vitals:

Time	Temp (F)	Rt.	Pulse	Resp	Syst	Diast	Sat O2
17:46	100.5	0	102	18	108	59	97% RA

Triage: Pt. complains of productive cough and SOB since this morning.

MEDICAL HISTORY:
NKDA
PMH/PSH: Negative
Medications: None

HPI (19:48): He complains of 1 day of chest pain, shortness of breath, productive sputum. He feels a rattling sensation on the right side of the chest. He is a smoker. He denies any other significant medical or surgical history. He was seen at a local urgent care clinic today and transferred here for probable pneumonia. He denies any nausea or vomiting. He did have a temperature for 104° F at home today. Denies edema, myalgias, joint pain, headache, or rash.

EXAM (19:49)
CONSTITUTIONAL: Alert and oriented x 3, well-nourished, well appearing, in NAD
RESP: Normal chest excursion with respiration; breath sounds with rhonchi
CARDIO: Regular rhythm, without murmurs, rub or gallop
ABD: Non-distended; non-tender, soft, without rigidity, rebound or guarding
SKIN: Normal for age and race; warm and dry; no apparent lesions

RESULTS

Test	Flag	Value	Units	Ref. Range
WBC		6.1	K/uL	4.6-10.2
HGB	L	11.2	G/DL	13.5-17.5
PLT		167	K/uL	142-424

Test	Flag	Value	Units	Ref. Range
NA	L	128	MMOL/L	136-145
K	L	3.5	MMOL/L	3.6-5.1
CL	L	95	MMOL/L	98-107
CO_2		23	MMOL/L	22-32
BUN		9	MG/DL	8-20
CREAT		0.88	MG/DL	0.66-1.30

CXR: Patchy bilateral airspace opacities, consistent with acute pneumonia. Given the bilateral nature of the abnormality, this is most likely due to an atypical organism, such as Mycoplasma or PJP. Radiographic follow-up to resolution recommended. Findings communicated to Emergency Department electronically at time of dictation.

ED COURSE:
19:53 – IVF, Ceftriaxone 1g IVPB, Azithromycin 500mg IVPB
20:14 – Paged hospitalist for admission
21:57 – Phenergan 12.5mg IVP

DIAGNOSIS (20:55): Pneumonia - bacterial

DISPOSITION: Admitted. Transferred to floor at 21:38

Before we explore the return visit, let's explore a few questions:

1. With an atypical CXR appearance, we should consider other types of pneumonia—such as *Mycoplasma* or *Pneumocystis jiroveci* pneumonia (PJP), formerly known as *Pneumocystis carinii pneumonia* (PCP), as recommended by the radiologist. Did this patient have undiagnosed AIDS? What clinical features should raise our concern?
2. What other diagnoses could have the same CXR findings?

Discussion:

1. HIV infection is characterized by three phases:
   - Early phase: Occurs very quickly after exposure and includes generalized symptoms of an acute retroviral syndrome such as fever, sore throat, myalgias, headache, swollen lymph nodes, and night sweats.
   - Latent phase: The patient is asymptomatic sometimes up to 8–10 years or may have minimal symptoms such as persistent lymph node swelling.
   - Final phase: Symptoms are severe including fever, cough, night sweats, weight loss, chronic diarrhea, and rash from the underlying AIDS and presence of opportunistic infections.

Unfortunately, the clinical features of HIV infection in the early or latent phases are vague and not helpful for early diagnosis. This patient's history of recent weight loss has the highest likelihood ratio of all historical findings (LR 4.7) for HIV infection.[1] However, unless the clinician asked about possible HIV exposure by taking a thorough sexual and drug use history, he/she might not even think about ordering an HIV test. Thus, some physicians advocate using routine, universal HIV screening because it's more effective for identifying HIV disease than selective testing in high risk populations.

Once the patient has the acquired immunodeficiency syndrome (AIDS), the symptoms and signs are easier to identify.

History: In addition to weight loss, night sweats, and anorexia, ask AIDS patients about recurrent minor mucocutaneous infections which can be evidence of thrush, recurrent herpes simplex, rash, or shingles. They may also report persistent blurry vision (cytomegalovirus retinitis), cough (tuberculosis or *Pneumocystis jiroveci* pneumonia (PJP), headache (toxoplasmosis), or diarrhea (cryptosporidiosis), depending on the specific opportunistic infection.

Physical exam: Clues to late HIV infection include eye lesions (cotton wool spots from HIV retinopathy, papilledema from *Cryptococcus*, toxoplasmosis, or central nervous system lymphoma), intra-oral lesions [oral candidiasis, oral hairy leukoplakia (pathognomonic for HIV), and linear gingivitis], skin findings (dermatitis over the malar eminences, herpes zoster lesions, genital or perianal ulcers, and discrete red or purple skin patches or plaques of Kaposi sarcoma), and generalized lymphadenopathy.[2]

2. Does the CXR help or is "clinical correlation" required? The radiographic findings of bilateral airspace opacities in the clinical setting of fever and cough certainly could be atypical pneumonia from *Mycoplasma, Pneumocystis* or viral infection, as the radiologist suspected.

However, a similar pattern may also be seen in:

- non-cardiogenic pulmonary edema
- pulmonary hemorrhage
- pneumonitis
- lymphoma
- tuberculosis
- pulmonary fungal infections

Section editor comments (Yealy):

Infection with *Pneumocystis* is much less common now with improved antiviral therapies compared to the earlier years of HIV infection and AIDS; it is one malady where the clinical findings often outstrip the radiologic appearance.

Author note: The patient is appropriately admitted to the hospital and IV antibiotics are continued. A brief summary of the admission follows:

Hospital course:
CC: Fever and chest pain.

HPI: The patient is a 28-year-old white MSM male who presents with 5 days of right lower chest pain with inspiration, 3 days of fever (Tmax 104° F at home), and 1 day of nausea and vomiting.

He has nasal congestion, rhinorrhea, and a 9-pound weight loss within the last few months. No night sweats, abdominal pain, any changes in bowel or bladder habits.

Problem list:

1. Acute pneumonia. We began antibiotic therapy. We will evaluate for *Mycoplasma* vs. PJP. Will hydrate and obtain sputum culture and PPD skin test and send an HIV test.
2. DVT prophylaxis. Lovenox 40mg subcutaneous daily.
3. GI prophylaxis. Nexium 40mg p.o. daily.

Hospital course: Blood cultures are negative. He is continued on ceftriaxone and azithromycin, and his clinical condition is improved. The plan is release from the hospital with the agreement he will follow-up on an outpatient basis for his test results.

Chapter author note:
We would have ordered a CD4 count based on the suspicion of PJP on CXR, obtained sputum for acid-fast bacilli (AFB) testing to exclude tuberculosis, and assessed serum lactate dehydrogenase level (LDH). An elevated serum LDH has a high sensitivity for PJP, (100% sensitivity in a study by Quist and Hill of 42% hospitalized patients with PJP, 71% with disseminated tuberculosis (TB), 40% with pulmonary TB and 37% with bacterial pneumonia), but is not specific as it is also elevated with these other conditions.[3]

Hospitals should have processes for contacting patients when critical or actionable abnormal diagnostic tests exist, especially after discharge—in this case, the HIV test and CD4 count (if ordered) are pending. Though pneumococcal pneumonia is the most common cause of pneumonia in AIDS patients, a low CD4 count increases the probability that he may have an opportunistic infection that would not respond adequately to his prescribed discharge antibiotics. Even though he was instructed to follow up as an outpatient, we think a clear contact sequence should exist and be used to ensure the results and next steps are shared and reinforced.

Section editor comments (Yealy):

In the ED, we often use the "follow-up with your..." at discharge to cover for any new or changed information—and that often fails. Having a clear post-discharge contact which is adequately documented is best.

BOUNCEBACK ED VISIT #2

CC/quote (16:16): Pt c/o high fever and generalized weakness

HPI text (18:30): 28-year-old white male in good general health; he does not smoke cigarettes. Admitted to this hospital approximately 1 week ago for pneumonia; chest x-ray revealed atypical pneumonia, improved after several days, discharged on Zithromax feeling much better. He has done well until today when he awoke with increasing cough, right lower chest wall pain, mild shortness of breath and generalized myalgias. Shaking chills, but denies any headache or neck stiffness. His previous admission lab work reveals a CD4 count of 21, HIV is pending. No edema, n/v/d, abd pain, urinary Sx, HA, rash.

Medications: Azithromycin, Acetaminophen

Vitals:

Time	Temp (F)	Pulse	Resp	Syst	Diast	O2	Sat O2%
16:00	102.9	126	24	92	53	86%	RA

PE:
CONSTITUTIONAL: Alert and oriented X3, thin, moderate to severe respiratory distress, sitting forward on the bed. Conversational dyspnea
HEAD: Normocephalic; atraumatic.
EYES: PERRL, no scleral icterus.
NOSE: The nose is normal in appearance without rhinorrhea
RESP: Breath sounds with mild generalized crackles, there are some intercostal retractions and neck musculature is bulging out during respiration
CARDIO: Regular rhythm, without murmurs, rub or gallop
ABD: Non-distended; non-tender, soft, without rigidity, rebound or guarding
SKIN: Pt has a malar waxy rash over nose and cheeks, has some exophytic lesions on the face

Author comments (Weinstock):

We are faced with a seemingly previously healthy young man, recently discharged from the hospital, now febrile and in acute respiratory distress with tachycardia, tachypnea, hypoxemia, and hypotension. We are at the bedside in the shoes of the emergency physician. We are at decision point A:

DECISION POINT A – YOU ARE FACED WITH 4 QUESTIONS:

1. **What are the immediate airway/breathing considerations?**
2. **What are the differential diagnosis possibilities?**
3. **Should a stat chest radiograph be done or management based on clinical picture?**
4. **How should patients who return after failure of outpatient antibiotics be managed?**

Q#1: What are the immediate airway/breathing considerations?

When faced with a patient who is acutely ill and in respiratory distress, our initial management strategy is always to return to the basics: IV, O_2, and monitor. From an airway/breathing perspective, this patient is tachypneic, retracting, and hypoxemic. We would expect him to improve with supplemental oxygen. We would start with a non-rebreather face mask and call a respiratory therapist to set up for noninvasive positive pressure ventilation to decrease the patient's work of breathing and improve his oxygenation.[4,5]

Q#2: What are the differential diagnosis possibilities?

His clinical picture points to respiratory failure and septic shock, most likely from PJP or tuberculosis. He is tachypneic, tachycardic, febrile, and in acute respiratory distress. His differential diagnosis includes:

- acute respiratory distress syndrome,
- multi-focal pneumonia failing outpatient antibiotics
- pulmonary embolism, pulmonary hemorrhage
- parapneumonic effusion

While for most septic patients a venous blood gas is adequate to guide treatment, in patients with suspected PJP an arterial blood gas can be used to calculate the arterial-alveolar O_2 gradient and better assesses acid-base status, which determines the degree of illness. Other diagnostic studies include a lactate level, complete blood count with differential, comprehensive metabolic panel, LDH, 2 sets of blood cultures, portable chest radiograph, and ECG to exclude dysrhythmia as the cause of his tachycardia. From an infection control perspective, he should be placed in high respiratory isolation until tuberculosis can be excluded from after sputum AFB testing.

Consulting editor comments (Weingart):

An ABG is completely unnecessary in a patient who is already hypoxemic by pulse ox. The ABG guides nothing in PJP treatment, therefore our patient needs steroids. The acid base status is just as easily guided by VBG, if that is even important right now. This patient has type I respiratory failure, you can assess CO_2 after you fix that. Getting a lactate level is fine but does not require a blood gas.

Q#3: Should a stat chest radiograph be done or management based on clinical picture?

The management of this patient should be initiated based on his clinical picture even before imaging. In addition to considering noninvasive positive pressure ventilation, he should be treated with a 30mL/kg isotonic crystalloid bolus, IV antibiotics, and vasopressors +/- more IV fluids to maintain MAP $\geq$ 60mmHg.[6] If needed for comfort, he could be given an antipyretic agent (e.g., acetaminophen or nonsteroidal anti-inflammatory drug), even though treating the fever itself does not improve survival.[7]

Consulting editor comments (Weingart):

The mean arterial pressure (MAP) goal is 65; a 30mL/kg bolus should be given with the proviso that the patient is able to handle the volume.

Q#4: How should patients who return after failure of outpatient antibiotics be managed?

Treat empirically for hospital-acquired pneumonia with piperacillin-tazobactam or cefepime (for anti-pseudomonal and gram negative bacilli activity) along with vancomycin or linezolid (to cover methicillin-resistant *Staphylococcus aureus*).[8] Because he also has AIDS (defined by CD4 count < 200), we would also treat him for PJP with IV trimethoprim-sulfamethoxazole and IV corticosteroid therapy because of his hypoxemia (room air arterial pressure < 70mmHg or arterial-alveolar O_2 gradient > 35mmHg). Adjunctive corticosteroids may decrease the need for mechanical ventilation and decrease mortality (NNT=9).[9] Absent a drastic improvement in the ED, he would be best managed in the intensive care unit.

Section editor comments (Yealy):

In patients with sepsis or with profound infection-based organ failure, start broad therapy fast—this is not the time to ponder antibiotic stewardship and narrow choices.

What did the actual provider do?

MDM (16:18): Review of the previous record shows that the Pt. has a CD4 count of 21, with a likely initial diagnosis of AIDS. He has not improved with the antibiotics and PJP is the most likely etiology of his symptoms; so he will be started on TMP/SMZ IV and solumedrol will be ordered. He remains tachypneic but is mentating well. O26L placed on the Pt. and we will see if he improves.

Orders:
16:51 - 0.9 NS 1L bolus then 125ml/hour
17:07 – Morphine 4mg IVP
Zofran 4mg IVP
Solumedrol 40mg IVP
Bactrim IVPB
Acetaminophen 975mg PO

CXR results return: PA AND LEFT LATERAL CHEST RADIOGRAPHS, 08/20
History: Pneumonia. Comparison: 08/15
Findings (per radiology): There are ill-defined opacities noted within the upper lobes (with the right greater than left) and ill-defined opacity noted within the right lower lobe. Opacities have not significantly changed from the prior examination. Blunting of the right costophrenic angle is also stable, probably related to a pleural effusion.
IMPRESSION: Stable, multifocal opacities are most likely related to pneumonia. Recommend a follow-up chest x-ray after appropriate treatment to document clearing.

MDM (Physician): Recheck on the patient on 6L NC reveals an improvement in O2 sat to 91%, but the pt is more tachypneic with RR increased to 36. He is mentating well, but is now diaphoretic and asking for water. His partner is at the bedside.

Author comments (Weinstock):

He is "hanging in there"... but for how long? Is his care so far appropriate? Does he need to be intubated? We are at:

DECISION POINT B – YOU ARE FACED WITH 4 QUESTIONS:

1. **Should anything else have been done initially?**
2. **Our patient appears heading for respiratory failure—should we start with non-invasive ventilation or proceed directly to endotracheal intubation?**
3. **Would a CT scan be beneficial—how could this change management?**
4. **What are the considerations for initial management of pneumonia/infection with immunocompromised patients?**

Q#1: Should anything else have been done initially?

The physician narrowed the patient's treatment a little early by simply treating PJP. Patients with AIDS are also at risk for the more common causes of pneumonia—streptococcal, *Mycoplasma, Haemophilus influenzae* and others. With a critically ill patient who already failed outpatient pneumonia treatment, we suggest broad coverage: vancomycin and either cefepime, piperacillin-tazobactam, or ampicillin/sulbactam to cover PES pneumonia [***P**seudomonas aeruginosa,* ***E**nterobacteriaceae*-producing extended-spectrum beta-lactamase, and methicillin-resistant ***S**taphylococcus aureus* (MRSA)].[10] In addition, this patient has septic shock and should receive a 30mL/kg crystalloid bolus within the first 3 hours, not 125mL/hour as ordered. Steroids were appropriately given for this hypoxemic patient.[9] The typical approach would be to administer IV methylprednisolone for critically ill patients or oral prednisone for patients with milder disease.

Q#2: Our patient appears heading for respiratory failure—should we start with non-invasive ventilation or proceed directly to endotracheal intubation?

Given the patient's tachypnea and hypoxemia, we are worried about impending respiratory failure. He needs close monitoring, immediate resuscitation, and frequent reassessment to make sure that he is improving and not deteriorating. He needs to be admitted to an intensive care unit or equivalent bed. At this point, an arterial blood gas would provide a serum pH and a pCO_2, an indicator of hypercapnia.[11] While this is less important than observing the patient's overall clinical status and trajectory, a high pCO_2 and acidemia suggest that the patient may be sicker than he appears.

Despite supplemental oxygen via nasal cannula, this patient is becoming more tachypneic and likely headed for respiratory failure. Reviewing the options for preoxygenation and respiratory support available in our toolbox: high-flow nasal cannula, facemask/nonrebreather mask, continuous positive airway pressure (CPAP) support, bi-level positive airway pressure (BiPAP) support, and endotracheal intubation. All of these have their merits.

1. Oxygen delivery by nasal cannula can be low-flow (up to 15L/min) or high-flow (up to 60L/min in adults). High-flow nasal cannula (HFNC) has some important benefits. It does not cover the mouth, offers less aspiration risk to patients, and is more comfortable than strapping on a tight-fitting mask. The oxygen is usually humidified, which prevents drying of the nasal mucosa. Oxygen flow through the nasal cannula is usually high enough to generate a small amount of positive end-expiratory pressure (PEEP), providing additional ventilatory support to the lungs.[12] However, HFNC requires special equipment which may not be readily available.
2. The commonly used "nonrebreather mask" is a facemask with an oxygen reservoir. Standard facemasks deliver flow rates at 15L/min delivers about 60–70% FiO_2. However, flow rates may be turned up on most flow regulators beyond 15L/min by continuing to open the valve, which can generate a FiO_2 up to 90%.[4] Using a standard low-flow nasal cannula at 15 L/min in addition to a facemask (with the flow regulator cranked as high as possible) may offer a quick and easy way to preoxygenate patients as you prepare to escalate your airway management. The added benefit of having the nasal cannula in place is for apneic oxygenation during rapid sequence intubation.[4]

Section editor comments (Yealy):

Non-rebreather masks are notoriously difficult to use if seeking high delivered oxygen—the fit and tolerance is often poor, decreasing the impact. It is OK to try but be prepared to act more aggressively if needed.

Consulting editor comments (Weingart):

NRBs actually work fine at the flowrates the authors mention, and they are the easiest mask to use. They have reliable sealing and are leak tolerant. The problem is that this patient doesn't need high FiO_2, he needs increased Mean Airway Pressure.

3. Non-invasive positive pressure ventilation with either CPAP or BiPAP work similarly. They both offer continuously flowing oxygen into the nose and mouth.[13] Both improve lung mechanics by stenting airways open and reducing a patient's breathing effort. No-ninvasive ventilation has been used to prevent mechanical ventilation.
   - Using a CPAP machine is like breathing with your head stuck outside the window of a car or breathing into a blow dryer. There is a steady, fixed flow of oxygen blowing inward. CPAP is simpler and recommended by some experts for pre-oxygenation in patients who continue to be hypoxemic despite being on a nasal cannula and/or facemask.[1]
   - BiPAP is slightly more complex in that the machine regulates and provides different levels of inspiratory flow on the inhalation and exhalation cycles of breathing. Of the two, BiPAP is more commonly used in the ED.
4. Rapid sequence intubation is used for worsening hypoxemia or hypercapnia, declining mental status, concern for inability to protect the airway, or due to the anticipated clinical trajectory of the patient.[14] Of course, intubation is a satisfying critical procedure and we love to do it, but for the patient, spending some time on a noninvasive mask may be preferable to days spent on the ventilator!

Section editor comments (Yealy):

The "definitive airway" is the one that meets patient demands safely—endotracheal intubation is not always the best choice, but it is valuable when respiratory failure is profound or unabated after other interventions.

Q#3: Would a CT scan be beneficial—how could this change management?

In the ED, a chest CT scan is not the highest priority with this kind of critically ill patient. A chest CT is more sensitive and specific than a plain radiograph for characterizing the infiltrative pattern of PJP, so it could be used to confirm the disease if uncertain.[15] If there are other equally probable diagnostic considerations (e.g., pulmonary embolism, aortic dissection), then a chest CT may be helpful. However, the underlying important principle here is that PJP, like any other type of pneumonia, is a clinical diagnosis, not a radiographic or laboratory diagnosis. If the diagnosis is uncertain, but the patient is sick, then resuscitate the patient and delay further testing until they are more stable.

Q#4: What are the considerations for initial management of pneumonia/infection with immunocompromised patients?

For an immunocompromised patient with pneumonia, the best antimicrobial treatment is to go broad until the source of infection can be further characterized by diagnostic testing (e.g., blood cultures, sputum cultures) and clinical improvement. During hospitalization, as the patient stabilizes, the specific organism(s) can be identified, and therapy options can be narrowed.[30] In this patient, an important priority during hospitalization would be to exclude tuberculosis, as this is another common cause of pneumonia in AIDS patients. Remember to consider putting the patient in high respiratory isolation until TB is excluded.[16]

What did the actual provider do?

Physician MDM (18:13): Oxygen is increased to NRB and sat initially stabilizes at 92%, but then intermittently dips down to the high 80s. The pt remains tachypneic but mental status does not change. Labs return:

Test	Flag	Value	Units	Ref. Range
WBC	L	4.5	K/uL	4.6-10.2
HGB	L	10.6	G/DL	13.5-17.5 F
PLT		231	K/uL	142-424
NA	L	135	MMOL/L	136-145
K	L	3.5	MMOL/L	3.6-5.1
CL		102	MMOL/L	98-107
AGAP		9.0	MMOL/L	6.0-18.0
CO2		24	MMOL/L	22-32
BUN	L	6	MG/DL	8-20
CREAT		0.71	MG/DL	0.66-1.30

Urine dip – WNL
Urine antigens legionella and pneumococcus negative

Test	Flag	Value	Units	Ref. Range
ALB	L	2.1	G/DL	3.5-4.8
TP		7.3	GM/DL	6.1-7.9
BILT		0.8	MG/DL	0.3-1.2
BILD		0.1	MG/DL	0.1-0.5
BILI		0.7	MG/DL	0.0-1.0
ALT		17	U/L	14-63
ALP	H	165	U/L	32-91
AST		22	U/L	15-41
LIP	L	18	U/L	22-51

Physician MDM (19:22): The patient appears to be tiring and is placed on BiPAP.

DECISION POINT C – YOU ARE FACED WITH 4 QUESTIONS:

1. **What are the initial settings for Bilevel positive airway pressure (BiPAP) support? Does this affect bed disposition (ICU vs. other destinations)?**
2. **Is it possible to predict the CD4 count from the WBC count and the differential?**
3. **How is the diagnosis of PJP made?**
4. **Is there a disadvantage to starting Bactrim before a bronchoscopy?**

What does the literature say?

Q#1: What are the initial settings for Bilevel positive airway pressure (BiPAP) support? Does this affect bed disposition (ICU vs. other destinations)?

Most hospitals have respiratory therapists who can help with setting and titrating BiPAP settings; nevertheless, it is helpful to be familiar with the terminology and be able to suggest the initial settings. There are 3 main variables:

- FiO_2
- IPAP (inspiratory positive airway pressure)
- PEEP (positive end-expiratory pressure)

Consulting editor comments (Weingart):

If you are going to call it IPAP, then call it EPAP. Otherwise use PSV and PEEP, but don't mix the two.

Reasonable starting values would be an inspiratory pressure of 10 to 15cm H_2O (particularly if the patient has ventilation problems) and an expiratory pressure of 5cm H_2O (titrate up to 15cm H_2O as needed for oxygenation). Set the FiO_2 initially at 100% and titrate down to maintain oxygen saturation > 91%.[17] A patient being resuscitated on noninvasive ventilation is a patient who you are trying to avoid intubating, so they need admission to a closely monitored setting like an ICU or step-down unit.

Historically, pneumonia was not a condition considered appropriate for non-invasive ventilation because it is not a quickly reversible. Newer data support noninvasive ventilation (like BiPAP) in these patients, particularly when the goal is to reverse hypercapnia and avoid intubation.[18]

Consulting editor comments (Weingart):

Hypoxemia—too little oxygen in the bloodstream—is important to resolve, but hyperoxia—giving oxygen in excess of needs—also has risk. Do not target a post-treatment oxygen saturation of 100%!

Q#2: Is it possible to predict the CD4 count from the WBC count and the differential?

In developing countries, and before CD4 counts were easily obtainable in United States, the CD4 count could be estimated by multiplying the white blood cell count by the absolute lymphocyte count. This can be helpful when the CD4 count will not return in a clinically useful timeframe.[19]

Q#3: How is the diagnosis of PJP made?

PJP, caused by the fungus *Pneumocystis jiroveci*, does not respond to antifungal treatment and is one of several organisms known to cause life-threatening opportunistic infections in patients with AIDS.[20] While the definitive diagnosis occurs via bronchoscopy or sputum induction, do not delay treatment in a critically ill patient, starting promptly when the disease is strongly suspected.

Bronchoscopy does not need to occur emergently.[21] On the other hand, a well-appearing HIV patient with symptoms of acute bronchitis should not be treated with Bactrim "just in case" they have PJP. Acute bronchitis usually is not caused by bacterial organisms. If PJP is suspected, further work-up is recommended.

- The dose of TMP/SMZ DS to treat PJP is higher than the dose typically prescribed for other conditions

Q#4: Is there a disadvantage to starting Bactrim before a bronchoscopy?

In the emergency setting, the specific microorganisms causing an infection are usually unknown. Even in the AIDS patient with pneumonia, the most common causes of pneumonia are *Streptococcus pneumoniae, Haemophilus influenzae,* and *Mycoplasma,* even more than *Pneumocystis jiroveci* (PJP). If treatment for the infectious organism is delayed until bronchoscopy provides the definitive diagnosis, there is a risk that the patient may not survive to have the procedure performed. In the sick patient, initiate treatment first and focus management once a definitive diagnosis can be made.

What did the actual provider do?

MDM (19:30): I paged infectious disease [and discussed] the case.

Diagnosis:
- Pneumonia
- Fever
- Acquired immunodeficiency syndrome (AIDS)
- Hypoxemia

Hospital course:

The patient was admitted to the hospital and continued IV steroids and Bactrim. Azithromycin was added. He was seen by ID as well as pulmonary who performed a bronchoscopy which noted extensive secretions in the lungs, which were sampled and cultured. The patient was discharged home and returned a third time eight days after hospital discharge #2 and was found have an empyema. The patient had a pigtail chest tube placed, draining the empyema. *Pneumocystis jirovecii* was the causative organism of the pneumonia.

Teaching points:
- The clinical features of the early and latent phases of HIV are nonspecific. Selective testing in high risk patients or even universal HIV screening should be considered for hospitalized patients.
- Multifocal pneumonia is more likely to be caused by atypical organisms different from those commonly encountered in community-acquired pneumonia. Think of admission in these cases.
- PJP and tuberculosis are opportunistic infections that can cause concurrent illness in AIDS patients. Use respiratory isolation for hospitalized patients until TB is excluded.
- Acutely ill, hypoxemic patients with suspected PJP should be treated with both IV trimethoprim-sulfamethoxazole and IV solumedrol.
- This patient's abnormal CD4 count assessed initially, and after the first episode, the patient was not contacted about his diagnosis. Perhaps this could have averted the repeat visits and course.

- The patient history and physical exam remain the cornerstones of care. While additional testing may sometimes be necessary, pertinent clues leading to the diagnosis and guiding care are usually at the bedside, and these are not costly to obtain.

References:

1. Wood E, Kerr T, Rowell G, et al. Does this adult patient have early HIV infection?: The rational clinical examination systematic review. JAMA 2014;312(3):278-85.
2. Hare CB. Clinical Overview of HIV Disease. HIV InSite 2009: http://hivinsite.ucsf.edu/InSite?page=kb-03-01-01#S6.3X
3. Quist J, Hill AR. Serum lactate dehydrogenase (LDH) in pneumocystis carinii pneumonia, tuberculosis, and bacterial pneumonia. Chest 1995;108(2):415-18.
4. Weingart SD, Levitan RM. Preoxygenation and prevention of desaturation during emergency airway management. Ann Emerg Med 2012;59(3):165-75.
5. Torres JD, Radeos M. Noninvasive ventilation: Update on uses for the critically ill patient. EM Critical Care 2011;1(2).
6. Rhodes A, Evans LE, Alhazzani W, et al. Surviving sepsis campaign: International guidelines for management of sepsis and septic shock: 2016. Intensive Care Med 2017;43(3):304-77.
7. Young P, Saxena M, Bellomo R, et al. Acetaminophen for fever in critically ill patients with suspected infection. N Engl J Med 2015;373(23):2215-24.
8. Kalil AC, Metersky ML, Klompas M, et al. Management of adults with hospital-acquired and ventilator-associated pneumonia: 2016 clinical practice guidelines by the Infectious Diseases Society of America and the American Thoracic Society. Clin Infect Dis 2016;63(5):e61-e111.
9. Ewald H, Raatz H, Boscacci R, et al. Adjunctive corticosteroids for pneumocystis jiroveci pneumonia in patients with HIV infection. Cochrane Database Syst Rev 2015(4):CD006150.
10. Dean NC, Webb BJ. Health care-associated pneumonia is mostly dead. Long live the acronym PES? Ann Am Thorac Soc 2015;12(2):239-40.
11. Tavakol K, Ghahramanpoori B, Fararouei M. Prediction of arterial blood pH and partial pressure of carbon dioxide from venous blood samples in patients receiving mechanical ventilation. J Med Signals Sens 2013;3(3):180-4.
12. Roca O, Riera J, Torres F, et al. High-flow oxygen therapy in acute respiratory failure. Respir Care 2010;55(4):408-13.
13. Mehta S, Hill NS. Noninvasive ventilation. Am J Respir Crit Care Med 2001;163(2):540-77.
14. Orebaugh SL. Initiation of mechanical ventilation in the emergency department. Am J Emerg Med 1996;14(1):59-69.
15. Hidalgo A, Falco V, Mauleon S, et al. Accuracy of high-resolution CT in distinguishing between pneumocystis carinii pneumonia and non-pneumocystis carinii pneumonia in AIDS patients. Eur Radiol 2003;13(5):1179-84.
16. Orlovic D, Kularatne R, Ferraz V, et al. Dual pulmonary infection with mycobacterium tuberculosis and pneumocystis carinii in patients infected with human immunodeficiency virus. Clin Infect Dis 2001;32(2):289-94.
17. Meduri GU. Noninvasive positive-pressure ventilation in patients with acute respiratory failure. Clin Chest Med 1996;17(3):513-53.

18. Nicolini A, Ferraioli G, Ferrari-Bravo M, et al. Early non-invasive ventilation treatment for respiratory failure due to severe community-acquired pneumonia. Clin Respir J 2016;10(1):98-103.
19. Shapiro NI, Karras DJ, Leech SH, et al. Absolute lymphocyte count as a predictor of CD4 count. Ann Emerg Med 1998;32(3 Pt 1):323-8.
20. Stringer JR, Beard CB, Miller RF, et al. A new name (pneumocystis jiroveci) for pneumocystis from humans. Emerg Infect Dis 2002;8(9):891-6.
21. Tu JV, Biem HJ, Detsky AS. Bronchoscopy versus empirical therapy in HIV-infected patients with presumptive pneumocystis carinii pneumonia. A decision analysis. Am Rev Respir Dis 1993;148(2):370-7.

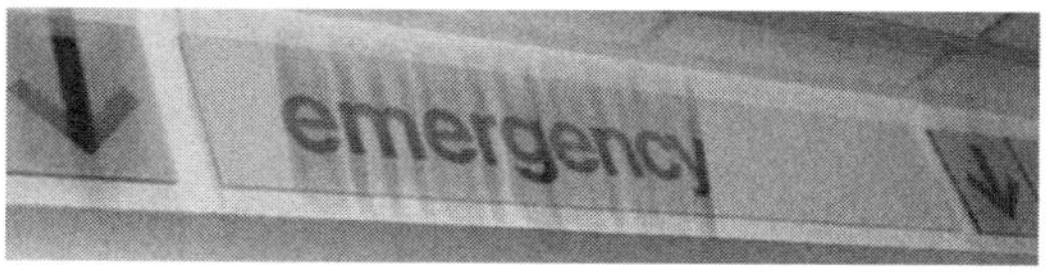

SECTION B – BREATHING/ PULMONARY

Chapter 10: A 50-year-old man with COPD and dizziness and dyspnea

Nicole Tyczynska, MD
Attending Physician
Department of Emergency Medicine
Our Lady of Lourdes Medical Center
Camden, NJ
Clinical Assistant Professor
Emergency Medicine
Thomas Jefferson University Hospital
Philadelphia, PA

Nandan Prasad, MD
Attending Physician
Department of Emergency Medicine
Tri-City Medical Center
San Diego, CA

Section editor:
Donald M. Yealy, MD
Chair, Department of Emergency Medicine
University of Pittsburgh/University of Pittsburgh Physicians
Vice President, Emergency and Urgent Care Services, Physician Services
UPMC Professor of Emergency Medicine, Medicine and Clinical and Translational Sciences
University of Pittsburgh School of Medicine
Pittsburgh, PA

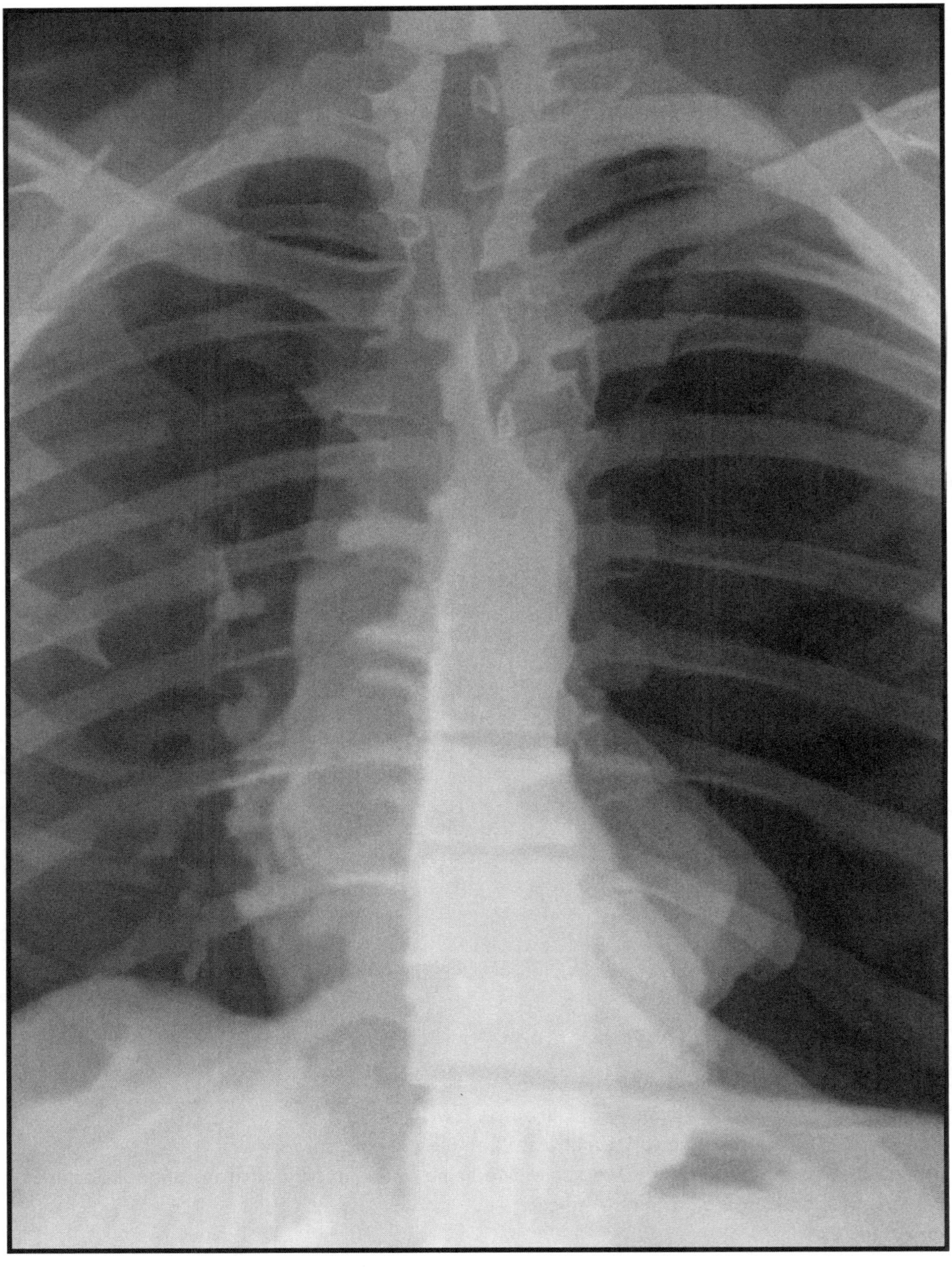

SECTION B/CHAPTER 10

A 50-year-old man with COPD and dizziness and dyspnea

Dizziness is a common symptom, with both self-limited, benign or ominous causes. Often, we order labs, CTs, x-rays, and ECGS to evaluate for potential metabolic, hematologic, orthostatic, central nervous system, or cardiopulmonary causes—fearing the worst.

How would you handle this case—could things have been done differently?

INITIAL ED VISIT

4/24/2016 19:51 EDT
Triage CC – Dizziness for 3 days.
CC (RN 19:49) – Dizziness

HPI (MD – 20:21): Patient presents per EMS with history of 4 days of intermittent lightheaded feeling. This is worse when he is walking. He does have a history of cirrhosis. He states that he drinks "… as much alcohol as I can afford." He is living with his uncle. He does not work. He denies any localized numbness or weakness of the extremities, slurred speech, facial droop or confusion, but he does have generalized weakness. He denies any pain in the head, neck, chest, abdomen or back. No vomiting or diarrhea. No blood in the urine or stool.

ROS: All other systems reviewed and are negative except as noted. Nursing triage notes were reviewed
PMH: Cirrhosis, gout, HTN
PSH: None documented
Social history: Alcohol, tobacco
Family History: No items have been selected
Allergies: None documented

PE:

Vitals:

Time	Temp (F)	Pulse	Resp	Syst	Diast	Sat
19:47	99.6	109	18	178	88	94% (RA)

GA: Alert and oriented X 3, well-nourished, well appearing, in no apparent distress
CV: Regular rhythm, without murmurs, rubs or gallops.
RESP: Normal chest excursion with respiration; breath sounds clear and equal bilaterally; no wheezes, rhonchi, or rales.
ABDOMEN: Non-distended, mild discomfort to palpation of the right upper quadrant, which he states is chronic. Elsewhere the abdomen is non-tender, soft without rigidity, rebound or guarding.
SKIN: Normal for age and race, warm and dry, no apparent lesions.

MDM (20:11): Patient does have a history of chronic cirrhosis. I have orders for IV fluids, labs, including hepatic profile, and lipase, ECG, and chest x-ray. I did review the patient's ECG showing sinus tachycardia with a rate of 103, without acute ischemic change. Labs are pending.

MDM (20:57): I did review the chest x-ray which shows a large right-sided pneumothorax, likely from a ruptured bleb, and the patient does have some element of tension.

Procedure: I did prep and drape the area in the usual sterile fashion and then used 5ml of lidocaine under the skin over the fourth rib in the midclavicular line and then placed the pigtail catheter over the rib with a good rush of air. This was hooked up to water seal. Post procedure x-ray is ordered. I did speak with the thoracic surgeon who will see the patient in consultation. Patient tolerated the procedure well.

MDM (22:20): I did review the post procedural x-ray and it does show significant expansion, but the lung is not all the way expanded.

Testing: Labs are WNL except minimal elevation of the AST and low albumin and protein. The lipase level is 69 (H).

Impression: Right-sided tension pneumothorax with placement of a Heimlich valve; history of alcoholic cirrhosis; smoker syndrome with history of COPD.

Documentation and patient safety issues:

1. Abnormal triage blood pressure, respiratory rate, and O_2 saturation are associated with increased risk of ED death, ICU admission, and in-hospital mortality.[1-3] The only normal charted vital sign in this patient is a respiratory rate of 18. However, respiratory rate values are dependent on provider technique with interobserver variability reaching as high as 35%.[4-6] If unsure, trust your evaluation or ask that vital signs be repeated.
2. The physician documents a normal physical exam, but was it simply cursory? The latter is common—we see many patients with nonspecific complaints, and on initial exam look for broader clues—but the initial exam alone may not suffice once the primary survey doesn't detect a clear cause.[7-9] Templated/macro notes may create an illusion of normalcy and detail when neither exist—be wary of using these notes if these aspects of the history and exam were not done. In a study of 200 consecutive Emergency Medicine malpractice suits, the most common physician error was a "grossly deficient examination relating to the chief complaint."[10]

3. The MDM is an opportunity to synthesize concerns. Our physician's MDM includes a plan for work-up but fails to discuss differential diagnoses related to the presenting complaint of dizziness, or the history of heavy alcohol use and potential for withdrawal.
4. The physician documented his read of the initial CXR as well as the read of the post-procedural CXR, but a repeat set of vitals post-procedure is absent. The physician documented "Patient tolerated the procedure well," but documentation of a reassessment prior to admission is needed to assure improvement.[11]

Despite these considerations, it seems like an "open and shut case." The patient presents with a pneumothorax which is decompressed using a pigtail catheter with Heimlich valve, and the patient is admitted to the hospital for monitoring until their pneumothorax resolves. What are some other considerations regarding the work-up and management of the patient's initial visit?

General discussion of COPD:
COPD patients have a high morbidity and mortality rate, often with many comorbidities and potential for drug interactions or effects.[12,13] Even absent these multipliers, COPD is a major cause of morbidity and mortality and is the 4th leading cause of death worldwide, with projections to move to the 3rd leading cause by 2020.[14-16]

Approximately 94% of COPD patients have a coexistent chronic medical condition,[17] with high rates of cardiac disease (25%), diabetes mellitus (11%), hypertension (17%), osteoporosis, and psychological disorders such as anxiety and depression.[14,18,19] Pulmonary hypertension is present in 30% of patients.[20] Over time, COPD leads to cor pulmonale, followed by right and subsequent left-sided heart failure.[21] In a study of over 45,000 patients with COPD, heart failure was the leading cause of hospitalization, followed by myocardial infarction and stroke.[22]

Other emergent medical considerations include altered mental status secondary to hypercapnic respiratory failure, severe bronchitis or pneumonia requiring intravenous (IV) antibiotics, and pneumothorax secondary to ruptured blebs. Pulmonary embolism occurs in 1.3–6.2% of patients presenting with a presumed COPD exacerbation.[23,24] Between 7 and 10% of related COPD deaths are secondary to lung cancer.[12,13]

What happened?
All is well that ends well, right? Before we detail the bounceback visit, we will review the evaluation and management of patients with alcoholism and/or pneumothorax.

Hospital course: The patient is admitted to the hospital for further management. He is seen by the thoracic surgeon, who orders a CT which confirms COPD with blebs and no air leak. The pigtail catheter is removed and the patient is discharged home. The patient's hospital course is complicated by alcohol withdrawal delirium and encephalopathy which improves after the Ativan is stopped.

Final hospital diagnosis: Right spontaneous tension pneumothorax; Alcohol dependence with withdrawal delirium.

Alcohol and the emergency evaluation:

Alcohol dependence affects 2.5% of the U.S. population and a larger percentage of ED patients. About 50% of people dependent on ETOH will experience withdrawal symptoms at some point in their lives.[26,27] This confounds care during the initial presentation with often altered vital signs and a worsening of a patient's general condition. Delirium tremens occur in 3–5% of those who are hospitalized with alcohol withdrawal.[28-30]

To diagnose alcohol withdrawal syndrome, a chronic alcohol user needs to have abruptly decreased their ethanol intake and experience two or more of the following symptoms not long after stopping: autonomic hyperactivity, increased hand tremor, insomnia, nausea or vomiting, transient visual/auditory/tactile hallucinations or illusions, psychomotor agitation, anxiety, or generalized tonic-clonic seizures.[27] Delirium tremens (DT), carry a mortality rate of 1–4%.[31-33]

The following are predictors of DT development:[34-36]

- History of previous DT
- Recent withdrawal seizures, specifically if left untreated,
- Clinical Institute Withdrawal Assessment of Alcohol Scale, revised (CIWA-Ar) ≥ 15
- History of sustained drinking
- Patients with SBP > 150mmHg, or patients with HR > 100 beats/min
- Last alcohol intake > 2 days
- Age > 30 years
- Recent misuse of other depressants such as benzodiazepines
- Concurrent medical illness such as pneumonia or active ischemia

There is no single lab value that predicts severe withdrawal or DT's; patients experience symptoms at different thresholds depending on the intensity of their consumption and the speed of ETOH metabolism. Early symptoms may begin within 6–8 hours from last drink and peak at 72 hours.[25,28] Using the Clinical Institute Withdrawal Assessment for Alcohol (CIWA) score, consider benzodiazepine therapy for a score of greater than or equal to 8, and start therapy immediately on those with a score of more than 15 or a history of withdrawal seizures.

Initiation of symptom-triggered therapy using long-acting benzodiazepines should be titrated to symptom resolution, usually spaced by an hour or two, with the option of starting a benzodiazepine IV infusion for patients in severe alcohol withdrawal.[25] In our case, the physician did not document the time of last alcohol intake; however, our patient is showing signs of autonomic instability with tachycardia, hyperthermia and hypertension. He is a prime candidate to develop DT's as an inpatient. Since he is having a painful procedure performed and will definitively be admitted to the hospital, giving 1 to 2 doses of benzodiazepines in the ED serves a dual purpose: facilitating a smooth intrathoracic catheter placement and preventing withdrawal.

Section editor comments (Yealy):

Major alcohol withdrawal is easier to prevent than to treat—anyone with a history of alcohol withdrawal or with high risk features after cessation (large and long-standing use with multiple findings of early withdrawal) should be treated with benzodiazepines early.

General discussion of pneumothorax (PTX) and blebs:
Subpleural blebs and bullae are found at the lung apices in up to 90% of cases of pneumothoraces.[37,38] Some blebs can occupy over a third of a patient's hemithorax. This condition, called idiopathic giant bullous emphysema or vanishing lung syndrome, has even been shown to mimic tension pneumothorax in its most severe form.[39, 41] Blebs can not only rupture, causing a PTX, but can also fill with fluid, become infected or even lead to bronchogenic malignancy.[12,13,42]

The treatment of pneumothoraces has been evolving, but one unified consensus as to their management remains absent. The American College of Chest Physicians (ACCP) and The British Thoracic Society (BTS) each composed their own set of practice guidelines in 2001 and 2010 respectively.[43,44] Subsequent research suggests a less invasive approach, including smaller catheters and increased outpatient treatment.

Three main decision points should be answered:
1. Is the patient stable or unstable?
2. Do I treat or not treat?
3. Can I discharge or does the patient require admission?

<u>Stable vs. Unstable:</u> Pneumothorax can be life-threatening. If tachycardia, hypoxemia or hypotension are present, immediately decompress. Our patient is stable; although the CXR shows a "large pneumothorax with initial signs of tension," this patient is still clinically well, albeit with potential for rapid deterioration.

<u>Treat vs. Not treat:</u> Both the ACCP and the BTS stratify treatment based on whether the pneumothorax is primary vs. secondary, large vs small, and symptomatic vs. asymptomatic. A primary spontaneous pneumothorax (PSP) tends to be spontaneous, unrelated to underlying lung pathology, and has milder symptoms and an easier treatment course. Secondary spontaneous pneumothorax (SSP) occurs in patients over the age of 50, often with a history of long-standing smoking or underlying lung disease. SSP tends to cause symptoms that are out of proportion to the size of the pneumothorax. Treatment of secondary pneumothoraces is driven by clinical status, as these patients typically have comorbidities that complicate the course.[45,46]

Conservative management with observation and oxygen vs. procedural intervention:
A 2014 *Cochrane* review concluded that there is a lack of quality evidence to support the current management guidelines of *primary* spontaneous pneumothoraces as current literature comparing conservative and interventional therapy is based on observational data or expert consensus.[47] Despite this, both ACCP and BTS agree that patients with small, asymptomatic *primary* pneumothoraces can be observed and that those with large, symptomatic ones should be decompressed and admitted to the hospital.

What defines a small vs. large pneumothorax?
A small pneumothorax is defined by the ACCP as < 3cm from apex to cupula (the lung dome), or < 2cm between the lung margin and the chest wall at the level of the hilum by the BTS. A 2cm radiographic pneumothorax approximates to a 50% pneumothorax by volume.[48] Four out of five pneumothoraces are estimated to be smaller than 15%, and treatment with observation alone is

less likely to lead to pneumothorax re-occurrence than in those treated with chest drains.[49] The rate of reabsorption of spontaneous pneumothoraces is 1.3–2.2% of the volume of the hemithorax every 24 hours.[45]

The ACCP recommends ED observation for 3–6 hours for small asymptomatic PSP patients, with discharge if a repeat CXR is unchanged, with follow-up in 48 hours. The BTS does not specify the exact time of ED observation and recommends follow-up within 2–4 weeks.

Management recommendations for large or symptomatic primary pneumothoraces?

The BTS recommends needle aspiration (NA) for large, symptomatic primary pneumothoraces or small, asymptomatic secondary pneumothoraces. Failure to aspirate a significant percentage of free intrathoracic air on initial attempt should trigger placement of an intrathoracic catheter and admission.[43] The ACCP does not recommend needle aspiration in any of its treatment algorithms. It recommends catheter placement and admission in both large symptomatic and asymptomatic PSPs plus *all* SSPs (regardless of size and symptoms).[44]

Back to our patient:

Our patient presents with a spontaneous, secondary pneumothorax (SSP). Except for the very small and asymptomatic PTX, all of these will have a procedural intervention. The BTS suggests needle aspiration as mentioned above, with the possibility of converting to small-bore intrathoracic device if needed, while the ACCP makes a blanket statement that all patients presenting with symptoms have a small-bore catheter placed and are admitted. Generally, SSP patients do not tolerate pneumothoraces as well as PSP patients and are more likely to have air leaks requiring intervention such as connection to water seal or suction.[51, 52] Both ACCP and BTS agree upon admitting all secondary spontaneous pneumothorax patients. All SSP patients should have an early inpatient consultation with pulmonology, and if there is persistent air leak at 48 hours, consultation with thoracic surgery for a possible video-assisted thoracoscopic surgery (VATS) procedure.[44]

Admission vs. discharge after intercostal catheter (ICC) placement:

Over the last few years, the aggressive management strategy of admitting all patients post-ICC placement has been questioned. As early as the 1970s, surgical literature documented the successful outpatient management of pneumothoraces with a 1-way Heimlich valve (HV) device.[53, 54] In 1996, the first randomized controlled trial comparing small-bore intercostal catheters (ICCs) with HV vs. larger chest tubes showed that 70% of patients with small ICCs were successfully treated as outpatients using this valve.[55]

Multiple small studies have supported the safety of outpatient management of both PSP and SSP with success rates ranging from 78–83%.[56-62]

Is it safe to send *our* patient home?

First, our patient falls into the category of the "risky" large, secondary spontaneous PTX. To date, only one observational trial by Voisin, et al. looked at outpatient management of large PSP and SSP. Success rates were not different between the two groups at 4 days (85% and 73% respectively), but the SSP arm only enrolled 22 patients.[62] Without additional research, we cannot recommend ambulatory management based on such a small data set. Secondly, despite all of the aforementioned nascent research showing good outcomes, a systematic review of 40 years of literature on the ambulatory treatment of PTX still states that the data are inconclusive.[61] A recent exploration found substantial practice variation, even though most respondents felt that outpatient management was safe if strict follow-up was arranged.[63]

Our patient arrived complaining of dizziness and a PTX, the latter incidentally discovered on routine chest-x-ray. Using the above definitions, our patient has a stable, symptomatic, large, secondary pneumothorax; he needs a procedural intervention (intrathoracic catheter) and to be admitted. This patient's initial ED visit was managed appropriately. The physician identified a life-threatening diagnosis and treated appropriately with a small-bore intrathoracic catheter and Heimlich valve, and then admitted the patient for ongoing care. The patient had an uncomplicated hospital stay and was discharged 2 days later after his pneumothorax resolved.

In a study looking at prevention of COPD-related return visits, early follow-up (within 1 month) was associated with less exacerbation-related readmissions.[64] Non-infectious lung disease is one of the three top primary discharge diagnoses which leads to death within 1 week of discharge after pneumothorax, with a frightening odds ratio of 7.1.[65] In unanticipated death among discharged patients, the following increased the likelihood of death within 7 days: atypical presentation of an unusual problem, chronic disease with decompensation, abnormal vital signs, and mental disability or psychiatric problem or substance abuse.[66] Our patient has all 4 of these concerning characteristics!

THE BOUNCEBACK (6 weeks after the initial ED visit)

6/6/16

Triage CC: Respiratory distress

HPI (01:29): Patient presents via paramedics complaining of shortness of breath for the past 3 days. I did review the previous record. The patient had a spontaneous tension pneumothorax back in April, and I did place a pigtail catheter with Heimlich valve at that time. He presents today with shortness of breath for 3 days and oxygen saturation was in the mid-60s when the paramedics arrived. He did improve with supplemental oxygen. The patient does complain of right-sided chest pain. His shortness of breath is worse with exertion. No pain or swelling to lower extremities. He does have a cough. No fevers. Social history: The patient does have a history of polysubstance abuse. I reviewed the nurses' notes.

ROS: All other systems reviewed and are negative except as noted. Nursing triage notes were reviewed
PMH: DM type 2, cirrhosis, gout, HTN
PSH: Pancreatitis
FH: No items have been selected
SH: Alcohol, tobacco
Allergies: none documented

PE:

Vitals:

Time	Temp (F)	Pulse	Resp	Syst	Diast	Sat O2
01:32	99.2	122	24	208	111	92% (NRB)

GA: Alert and oriented X3, well-nourished, ill appearing, severe respiratory distress with oxygen saturation ranging between 87 and 92% on 100% nonrebreather mask
CV: Regular rhythm, without murmurs, rubs or gallops.
RESP: Normal chest excursion with respiration; breath sounds significantly decreased on the right, clear on the left. No wheezing.
ABDOMEN: Non-distended; non-tender, soft, without rigidity, rebound or guarding.
SKIN: Normal for age and race; warm and dry; no apparent lesions.

Author comments (Weinstock):

We are at the bedside in the ED, with a patient you have seen previously, who is now in worse condition in severe respiratory distress and hypoxemic on a non-rebreather mask. We are at:

DECISION POINT A – YOU ARE FACED WITH 4 QUESTIONS:

1. **What is differential diagnosis of our patient's respiratory distress?**
2. **Should a needle decompression be done emergently, or can we wait for a portable CXR? Is a CXR showing a tension pneumothorax a "mark of shame" on the provider who ordered it?**
3. **Does the patient need a Heimlich valve/pigtail valve or chest tube?**
4. **What are some advanced tips and tricks when placing a valve or CT?**

Q#1: What is differential diagnosis of our patient's respiratory distress?

There is a 54% risk of recurrence of PSP within the first 4 years, and although our patient has an SSP, his age, smoking history and known emphysema all increase risk for a repeat episode. 67,68 Our pneumothorax patient returned, now with worsening respiratory distress. While the history and exam are highly indicative of pneumothorax recurrence, it is always critical to pause and consider other diagnoses.

Could our patient's respiratory distress be from infection? Perhaps this is a COPD exacerbation or related condition? Chronic COPD patients can suffer from a multitude of complications including hypoxemia, hypercarbia, and pulmonary hypertension and have a higher prevalence of cardiovascular diseases.[21] Surprisingly, heart failure, not reactive airway exacerbation, is the leading cause of hospitalization, followed by myocardial infarction, a diagnosis which should remain on our differential.[22] Given our patient's blood pressure in the setting of hypoxia, acute pulmonary edema is also a consideration.

How about pulmonary embolism? The data are inconclusive; the incidence of pulmonary embolism is between 1.3–6.2% of patients presenting with COPD exacerbations.[23,24] Additional conditions which can mimic a COPD exacerbation include cardiac dysrhythmia, pneumonia, drug toxicity, metabolic disorders, and cardiomyopathy.

The presenting complaint associated with the highest in-hospital mortality is dyspnea (11.5%); hypoxia and tachypnea are vital signs predictive of worse patient outcomes.[3] These all apply to our patient.

Q#2: Should a needle decompression be done emergently, or can we wait for a portable CXR? Is a CXR showing a tension pneumothorax a "mark of shame" on the provider who ordered it?

Rates of recurrence after a recent PTX can be as high as 23–37%.[69,70] In a patient who returns with another PTX, needle decompression means a likely follow-up thoracostomy, a procedure with some risk. Yet, we do not want to delay and allow progression to full tension. The decision to needle a chest is highly dependent on the pretest risk of the tension PTX, including the severity of the respiratory distress and the availability and timeliness of a portable CXR.

Are there any other, faster options? Bedside ultrasound in experienced hands is superior to chest x-ray as it allows for real time evaluation of the lungs while also helping to exclude other life threating pathologies such as tamponade or acute pulmonary edema. The sensitivity of ultrasound for clinically significant pneumothorax is 93%, and a recent study showed that a 1-view chest ultrasound is just as effective as a 4-view.[71]

Performing a needle decompression: The conventional teaching is to stick a 16 or 14 gauge standard angiocath into the 2nd intercostal space above the rib at the mid-clavicular line. A slew of studies has proven this method to be ineffective secondary to insufficient catheter length, suboptimal location, and frequent mechanical failure.

- Needle length: Decompression fails up to 65% of the time when using a standard 3.2cm catheter.[72] ATLS currently recommends using 5cm angiocatheters but in a large trauma meta-analysis in 2016, there was a 38% failure rate of anterior chest wall placement.[73] The only catheters shown to penetrate the chest wall 100% of the time were 8cm long,[74] similar in length to the 7.5cm long angiocaths found in a central line kit. Bottom line: use the longest needle you can find.
- Location: The same study analyzed chest wall thickness (CWT) at 3 common locations: the 2nd intercostal space, midclavicular line (2nd ICS-MCL), the mid-axillary line (MAL) and the anterior axillary line (AAL). Chest wall thickness was 4.3cm, 4cm, and 3.4cm respectively. In comparison to the 38% failure rate in the 2nd ICS-MCL, needle thoracostomy with a 5cm catheter failed only 13% of the time in the AAL, suggesting that the 4th/5th ICS-AAL has the lowest predicted failure rate of needle decompression.
- Source of failure: Even with use of a correct length catheter, failure occurs secondary to kinking, obstruction, or dislodgement. In a swine study, 26% of needle thoracotomies demonstrated mechanical failure within 5 minutes of placement and just under half (43%) of the remaining patent catheters failed to relieve tension physiology with an overall failure rate of 58%.[75]

Given these findings, there is growing support for finger thoracostomy (FT) as it is viewed as a safer and more definitive treatment than needle decompression.[76,77] In FT, there is a decreased risk of injury to lung parenchyma or parietal pleural. It is essentially the first steps of chest tube placement. A larger cut is made at the location of the intended chest tube, a curved hemostat is inserted, then a finger stuck into the opening. If there is a pneumothorax, insert catheter. If not, then suture the area or add a Bolin chest seal to create a one-way valve to further allow for egress of air.

For our patient, we would have used ultrasound (or chest x-ray, if immediately available), then performed a finger thoracostomy or pigtail catheter insertion.

Consulting editor comments (Weingart):

Is the x-ray of a tension pneumothorax a mark of shame? No, this is a remnant. Maybe our new learners reading this book don't know about these times, but in the old days, you would order an x-ray, and at some point, it would be shot. Then the tech would go back to the x-ray department, it might be developed 15 minutes after that, and then you would have to track down the film and read it by slapping it on a light board. So, if you have a patient with a tension pneumothorax and you're waiting that long in a crashing patient... of course you've missed the boat! But now, I have a trauma patient and I'm worried about a tension pneumo. I call x-ray, they come over in 2 minutes and then literally the second that x-ray is shot, I have it up on the screen on their actual machine; that's perfectly acceptable.

Section editor comments (Yealy):

If you supect tension pneumothorax—differing breath sounds with cardiorespiratory compromise—needle the chest using the correct length catheter. If unsure, obtain emergent imaging.

Q#3: Does the patient need a Heimlich valve/pigtail valve or chest tube?

If an immediate decompression is not performed, whether it be a needle or a finger thoracostomy, then a permanent intrathoracic catheter is needed.

Pigtail catheters are small bore intrathoracic devices (ITDs) and range from 8.5–14 Fr., which make them a tiny 2.8mm–4.7mm in internal diameter. These ITDs are thin and flexible, curling at the distal end (hence the "pigtail").

Chest tubes are less pliable and come in a wider range of sizes from 20–40 Fr. They are used to drain intrathoracic blood or other fluid and are not routinely used for uncomplicated pneumothoraces,[78] as small-bore catheters safely and effectively drain pneumothoraces with fewer complications.

In 2013, a systematic review of over four decades of PTX management with pigtails and Heimlich valves (HV) reported an overall treatment success rate of 85.8% with similar effect in draining primary and secondary pneumothoraces (83.3% vs. 88.7%). Approximately 10% of patients treated with pigtail catheters required surgical intervention, most commonly for persistent air leak.[61] Long-term pneumothorax recurrence rates averaged 15% (range 7–24) which is similar to that reported for needle aspiration (22–30%) and thoracostomy (24–27%).[79-82]

Our patient has a complicated secondary large pneumothorax and significant vital sign abnormalities. Certainly, he needs a larger chest tube to quickly drain his tension pneumothorax, right?

There is no evidence to prove that large-bore chest tubes (20–28Fr.) are any better than small-bore pigtail catheters (10–14Fr.).[83, 84] While there is only one randomized control trial and two retrospective trials comparing management with chest tubes to pigtails with HV, the available data support smaller-bore catheters.[55, 83, 84] One of the two retrospective studies reported comparable success rates when treating secondary pneumothoraces with pigtail catheters (72.5%) and large-bore catheters (72.7%).[84] Another study showed that using a small bore catheter vs. a large-bore catheter led to less complications (9.5% vs. 27.4%); faster chest tube removal (4.9 days vs. 8.3 days); and shorter hospital stays (6.9 days vs. 11.8 days).[83] Large-bore drains were associated with a greater complication rate (32% vs. 5% in smaller-bore catheters) and greater percentage of infectious complications (24% vs. 0%).[85]

Despite substantial data, there is currently no international consensus. For stable patients that are not at risk of air leak, the guidelines suggest a 16–22Fr. tube, although they support a 14Fr. or smaller if the patient has a small PTX or prefers a smaller catheter.[44]

Q#4: What are some advanced tips and tricks when placing a valve or CT?

There are 3 accepted ways of placing chest tubes/drains. We focus on blunt surgical dissection and the Seldinger technique. A trocar insertion (previously common, using a blunt, firm internal rod) method is dangerous and no longer recommended.

Size: Chest tube sizes range from 6–40Fr. (2–13.3mm in diameter) with catheters 14Fr. and below considered "small." Large chest tubes are used to drain blood and viscous fluids (> 24Fr.).[86, 87]

Location: The 5th intercostal space in the anterior axillary line is often quoted as the "ideal" location for chest tube insertion.[11, 88] The British Thoracic Society recommends placing chest tubes within the triangle of safety, found superior to the level of the nipple within the borders of the latissimus dorsi muscle laterally and pectoralis major anteriorly.[11, 99] If you find this description confusing, you are not alone, as 45–56% of junior practitioners we unable to identify these landmarks,[90, 91] with the most common error being ICC placement inferior to this "safe zone,"[92] with potential injury of the diaphragm and intra-abdominal organs. Visceral injury has been reported in 2 % of all ICC insertions and overall complication rates reach 22%.[93, 94]

Easier to remember anatomical markers include using the "mid-arm point" location (which identifies the 5th intercostal space, anterior axillary line 86% of the time)[95] or going 1 finger breadth below the inferior margin of the axillary hairline.[96]

Positioning: Have the patient semi-erect at a 45 % angle to assist with lowering the level of the diaphragm. Ask the patient to abduct their ipsilateral arm and place their hand behind their head to help spread the rib spaces (taping the hand to the stretcher helps remind the patient to stay in that position). Make sure to drape and prep a large sterile field to help keep the landmarks in view. Use towels to help prop excess adipose tissue.

The procedure: Prior to starting either blunt surgical dissection or Seldinger procedure, make sure that there is sufficient lighting, proper patient positioning, appropriate analgesia and all anticipated equipment at bedside, including eventual closed drainage system vs. Heimlich valve. You will not be able to step away once you start.

Section editor comments (Yealy):

Like virtually all emergency procedures, take time to position the patient correctly and use adequate analgesia (local and/or systemic). Unless collapse is imminent, taking the time to prepare pays dividends for all!

Blunt surgical dissection: Find your location. Anesthetize skin and subcutaneous tissue. Inject 10–20mL of 0.25% bupivacaine into the intra-pleural space for increased patient comfort.[97, 98] Make a generous incision above the rib. Use your finger to blunt dissect towards the intercostal muscle and parietal pleura just superior to the rib. Use a finer point dissection tool (such as a 16 or 18cm Kelly or Robert's forceps) to enter over the superior aspect of the rib, dissect through the intercostal muscles, and puncture the parietal pleura to enter the pleural space. Spread the forceps to increase the size of your point of entry into the pleural space. In young patients this may require significant force due to the strength of their intercostal muscles and fascia. Use 1 finger to hold open your opening in the pleural space and use the other hand to grab your ICC and enter it into the pleural space, passing it over your finger. For heavier patients, use a bougie to hold your position and guide the ICC into place. Aim your ICC superiorly and posteriorly.[77] This will prevent the tube from snaking downward or into the lung fissure. Ensure the ICC is fully in place, with the most distal drainage hole entering the pleural space. Attach the closed drainage system or Heimlich valve. Suture into place with a 1/0 silk suture using a non-slip knot.[99]

Seldinger technique: The Seldinger technique uses the same technique we use when placing central lines. Start by placing a small cut in the skin (avoid making wide incisions like in blunt dissection your cut should be only as wide as the catheter itself). We use a needle attached to a saline or bupivacaine filled syringe and aspirate back while pushing the needle forward. A rush of bubbles confirms that we are in the pleural space. We then insert the wire through the needle bevel into the hemithorax. Do not place the full length of the wire into the chest cavity as it can hit the mediastinum and deflect downwards leading to a malpositioned catheter. Approximate the desired catheter length using the patient's body and lay the patient flat prior to sliding the ICC in over the wire. This supine position prevents the pigtail from floating downward with gravity and helps it smoothly course up into the apex. As with the wire, make sure not to force the catheter all the way in as this may also result in downward positioning.

Do not suture the tube too tightly, as this may occlude the catheter. In pneumothorax patients, avoid clamping chest tubes, as this may lead to tension PTX if an undiagnosed air leak is present. Antibiotics are not recommended outside of trauma.[100]

Summary: Our patient has an unstable tension PTX and needs decompression quickly, but does not require emergent needle decompression.

DECISION POINT A – ***What did the actual provider do?***

MDM (02:44): I did prepare to place the right-sided pigtail with Heimlich valve, and at the same time, chest x-ray was done showing a large right-sided pneumothorax. I then did a timeout and prepped and draped the right side of the chest in usual sterile fashion in the mid axillary line over the third rib. I did place a pigtail with Heimlich valve with good return of air. Oxygen rapidly increased to 100% on the nonrebreather mask. A post procedure chest x-ray was done which shows the lung expanded significantly but not all the way. The tube was repositioned at this time and third x-ray was done, without change.

PE:

Vitals:

Time	Temp (F)	Pulse	Resp	Syst	Diast	Sat
02:52		116	37	190	192	93% (6L NC)

Chapter author note: The provider reacted quickly to the patient's respiratory distress. Knowing that the risk of recurrent PTX was high, they immediately prepared to place a pigtail catheter while getting a confirmatory CXR. This should have been the solution to this patient's problem, yet, post-procedural CXR shows that the lung has not completely re-expanded.

DECISION POINT B – YOU ARE FACED WITH 4 QUESTIONS:

1. **Why did the lung not re-expand?**
2. **If the water seal is not working, what is a stepwise approach to fix the problem?**
3. **Should our patient's pigtail catheter be converted to a larger-bore chest tube?**
4. **Why is the respiratory rate increased if the lung has expanded?**

Q#1: Why did the lung not re-expand?

First and foremost, check that the catheter is in the correct position, that it is not kinked or occluded, and that the most distal draining hole is in the pleural space. Check that the occlusive dressing is sealed tight and that the sutures have not pinched off the outward flow of air from the catheter.

An audit of 203 catheters placed at a large trauma center showed a 19% complication rate:[94]

- 18% (36/203) kinked
- 18% (36/203) subcutaneously placed
- 13% (27/203) not placed deep enough
- 7% (14/203) dislodged

One quick and easy initial effort to re-expand the lung is to attempt manual aspiration of the pneumothorax. Although not supported by the U.S. Consensus Guidelines, needle aspiration is safe and is recommended in the British Thoracic Societies' 2010 Guidelines. Manual needle aspiration of the lung does not lead to worse long-term outcomes and can shorten a patient's length of stay.[79, 81, 101]

This patient now has a pigtail with Heimlich valve, which is a 1-way flutter valve. Attaching the patient's pigtail to a chest tube drainage system is the next step in trying to promote lung re-expansion. A chest tube drainage system set to "water seal" is similar to a simple 1-way valve, and this will not add much in re-expanding the lung. However, checking for gentle bubbling in the suction control chamber and gentle changes in the water level with respirations (tidaling) of the seal compartment can aid in detecting a faulty pigtail set up. Aggressive bubbling in the suction control chamber can hint to an air leak while lack of tidaling in the water seal compartment can hint that your system is not patent.

Our patient has COPD with blebs, and it is possible he has ruptured a larger bleb and is failing to re-expand his lung secondary to an air leak. His water seal may need to be connected to suction at—10–20cm H_2O to remove air from the pleural cavity—a rate which exceeds the air flow into the pleural space from the hole in his visceral pleura.[44] Suction may also help by approximating the visceral and parietal pleural layers, further sealing off the defect. Use of suction is also recommended for patients with persistent air leaks (defined as greater than 48 hours), although there is otherwise no evidence for its routine use.[44,102-104] High-volume low-pressure systems such as Vernon-Thompson pumps or wall suction with low pressure adaptors are recommended.[39] Providers should be cautious when connecting patients to suction early after chest drain insertion as this can precipitate re-expansion pulmonary edema, especially with a PTX that has been present for more than a few days.[105]

Consulting editor comments (Weingart):

If pneumothorax has been there for a while, your lung may not want to expand right away. But, if you stick anything in such as a pigtail, a chest tube, a needle—you've taken care of the tension part of it, i.e. there can't be air trapped under pressure. However, we need to exercise caution with forcing the lung to expand quicker than it wants to; this is a surefire way to cause re-expansion pulmonary edema. So, if I have a patient with a spontaneous pneumothorax that's completely collapsed their lung, and it's been there for days, I don't put those patients on suction. I put in a pigtail, let it sit there, and let their lung expand when it wants to expand.

Now, there is another situation where you have a functional pigtail, or a functional small chest tube, and the lung is not an expanding lung, but you have a rambunctious air leak in the pleur-evac; this may be a bronchopleural fistula with output exceeding the capability of your pigtail or small chest tube to drain. Turn off suction for a second and if the air leak chamber is still strumming with air, this means that you have an output that is not adequately being drained. These patients need a second chest tube, and I'd probably make that second chest tube big. To summarize, if you have a continuous output from your pleur-evac, indicating that this thing's not keeping up, that is a life-threatening situation that must immediately be treated.

Q#2: If the water seal is not working, what is a stepwise approach to fix the problem?[106-109]

A chest tube drainage system or "water seal" is a 3-in-1 chamber device that functions as a 1-way valve to help facilitate the egress of air from pigtail catheters and chest tubes. When a water seal is not working, this usually means that there is an air leak either within the parenchyma, parietal pleura, or within the collection chamber or collection tubing.

Check collection tubing and chamber:

- Is the occlusive dressing sealed airtight?
- Is there crepitus in the skin surrounding the insert point?
- Is the chest tube placed beyond the first, sentinel drainage hole?
- Are all tubes patent and tightly connected to the drainage chamber?

If the tube is patent and there are no leaks within the system connections, then the air leak is likely intrathoracic.

If the air leak is persistent and the patient's lung is failing to re-expand, the drainage collection system can be attached to low wall suction. If the chest tube is already connected to suction and you are trying to troubleshoot a malfunction in the drainage system, check for the following:
Wall suction is set to at least -80mmHg

- The drainage system's suction control regulator limits the amount of suction and is preset to -20mmHg (the regulator allowance ranges from -10 to -40mmHg)
- The "suction monitor bellows" is expanded. This orange horizontal plunger is a visual indication of sufficient suction pressure and should be expanded out to the level of the small triangular "delta indicator" to indicate that the system is at the pre-set level of pressure. If the bellows is not fully expanded, increase the wall suction.

If you are trying to calculate the patient's intrathoracic pressure (ITP), remember the following:

- When the system is set to gravity seal, ITP equals the float ball water column level only
- When the system is set to suction:

ITP = suction control regulator setting + float ball water column level.

- The high negatively float valve on top of the water seal chamber:
    - o Allows patients to draw as much intrathoracic pressure as they want with every inspiration.
    - o Will automatically release pressure to protect patient against excessively elevated negative suction pressure.

Q#3: Should our patient's pigtail catheter be converted to a larger-bore chest tube?

If initial placement of a small-bore pigtail catheter with Heimlich valve does not result in lung expansion, assess a few things prior to placing a larger chest tube: pigtail catheter position, potential occlusions, and potential connection leak. Additionally, confirm that the Heimlich valve is attached in the correct direction.

In our patient with severe COPD, air may be escaping out of his ruptured bleb faster than the pigtail can drain it. A bigger catheter diameter will allow for a greater volume of air to be drained out of the pleural space within a shorter period of time (increase volumetric flow rate). Per Poiseuille's Law, there are three primary factors that dictate the flow of a fluid within a catheter: vessel diameter (or radius), vessel length, and viscosity of the fluid. Of these, the most important quantitatively and physiologically is vessel diameter as flow is related exponentially (r4) to the radius.[110]

So, bigger is better in this particular instance, which then begs the question, "If 1 larger chest tube improves drainage, then what about placing 2?"

Insertion of 1 vs. 2 chest tubes for treatment of PTX is unstudied. However, we can extrapolate data from two separate studies looking at single vs. double CT placement for fluid drainage after pulmonary lobectomy that concluded that 2 tubes were not more effective than 1.[111, 112]

For our patient, we recommend changing the pigtail catheter to a single larger-bore chest tube.

Section editor comments (Yealy):

When in doubt, carefully walk through the catheter function, and if unsure after stepwise testing, replace with a larger-bore French sized tube.

Q#4: Why is the respiratory rate still increased if the lung has expanded?

You have placed a large-bore chest tube and the lung is beginning to re-expand, but the respiratory rate is worsening.

- Is your patient in pain?
- Did you cause an unexpected injury on the way in, such as bleeding from an intercostal artery or irritation of a subcostal nerve?
- Perhaps the patient is blowing off some acidosis as oxygen starts to flush out the previously collapsed lung.

You re-auscultate your patient and now note bilateral coarse breath sounds. Could he be experiencing re-expansion pulmonary edema? In a study of 47 patients with re-expansion pulmonary edema after pneumothorax drainage, the onset occurred in less than 10 minutes in 64% of patients.[30, 113]

In one report, re-expansion pulmonary edema occurred in 14% of PTX patients treated with low continuous suction (-12mmHg).[105] However, a recent systematic review of 13 articles shows the rate to be only 0–1%, with risk factors of high negative intra-pleural pressures, larger pneumothoraxes, younger age, and greater than 7 days of pneumothorax presence prior to re-expansion.[114] Animal models suggest a correlation with duration of lung collapse and with excessive negative pleural pressures.[8, 9] The pathophysiology is thought to stem from a cytokine related increase in capillary permeability, the mechanical stress of re-expansion, and free-radical damage.[115]

The largest study on large-volume thoracentesis did not find any correlation between incidence of re-expansion pulmonary edema and measures of pleural pressure or elastance, but the study was also underpowered with only 5 of 185 patients developing re-expansion pulmonary edema. Still, looking at the collective data, the -20cm H2O cutoff is not supported by particularly strong evidence.[116]

DECISION POINT B – ***What did the actual provider do?***

MDM: I did review the blood sugar result which is only minimally elevated. I did order a chest x-ray, which did not show complete resolution of the pneumothorax, and so, I did place a second Heimlich valve, and this was done under usual sterile conditions on the right-hand side just lateral to the initial one. However, a repeat x-ray after that showed that the pneumothorax was actually increased.

(04:39): I did perform another time out and then did prep and drape the right chest in the mid-axillary line at the T4 level and I did infiltrate with 10mL of 1% lidocaine and then did incise the right chest and placed a #36 chest tube to initially 18cm and did get a final chest x-ray which did show significant expansion but not complete re-expansion of the lung. I did pull the chest tube back 2cm, and it is now at 16. It is tied in. No complications. His oxygen saturation improved; however, I did try to put him on nasal cannula at 4L he is down at 89% and so he has been placed back on a facemask.

The patient remains tachycardic and is somewhat hypoxic when he is not on the facemask. He does have increased opacity in both lungs which could be an infiltrate or could be edema. The patient may likely have had his pneumothorax for the last 3 days and may take some time to completely expand.

Chapter author comments: Einstein opined that "Insanity is doing the same the over and over again and expecting different results." Why would the physician think that a second pigtail and Heimlich valve would be a good option in this patient's case? A second small-bore catheter could have some utility; patients with COPD and multiple blebs (especially those with prior intra-thoracic procedures) have areas of scar tissue and adhesions that compartmentalize different parts of the lungs and pleura. Perhaps the initial pigtail was placed in a recess where it did not have the capability of re-expanding the larger void in the patient's hemithorax? These patients can also have multiple apical blebs that expand to take the place of prior blebs that have ruptured, causing the illusion of a persistent PTX. The one thing the physician could have tried before reaching for the larger chest tube would be to connect the patient's pigtail catheter to suction to see if suction could compete with the pleural air leak.

You can hear the physician's frustration (as well as medico-legally defensive charting) as he documents placement of a larger chest tube (he jumps right to sticking in a 36Fr). There is partial resolution of the PTX after this procedure, but the patient's O_2 sat is still sub-optimal. We are dealing with a COPD patient and long-term smoker; we are not shooting for normalcy, but rather, adequate oxygenation (at or above 91% or so).

The physician notes bilateral edema or consolidation. Could we be treating more than just a PTX? It is time to expand the differential with this new information. Let's see how this case resolves.

ED course: The nurse comes to you as the patient is saying, "I can't breathe. I feel like I am smothering. I need pain meds or something!"

DECISION POINT C – YOU ARE FACED WITH 4 QUESTIONS:

1. **The patient's condition is worsening. What is happening?**
2. **There is an infiltrate on the most recent CXR. Should we start antibiotics?**
3. **Is it time to admit or should we continue to manage in the ED?**
4. **With the persistent hypoxemia. Should he be intubated?**

Q#1: The patient's condition is worsening. What is happening?

You have now placed 3 pleural catheters, but you have not succeeded in making him feel any better.

Chest tube complications are common (19–37%), and include:

- Incorrect placement (subcutaneous, retroperitoneal).
- Damage to surrounding structures (cardiac/vascular and esophageal injuries, intercostal artery lacerations, nerve injuries).
- Complications to the heart and lungs (i.e. cardiac dysrhythmias, empyema, re-expansion pulmonary edema [REPE], re-accumulations of PTX).[94,117]

The complication rate of percutaneous chest tubes is similar to open thoracostomy, but the complications tend to be more severe as the insertion wire can migrate to undesirable locations.[78]

However, on our patient's repeat CXR, it does not seem that the patient's intracostal catheters are placed incorrectly or that there is any obvious damage to surrounding structures. The physician's chart notes edema vs. consolidations on the CXR. Could this be CHF? Re-expansion pulmonary edema? A pneumonia? Or is this still just a poorly expanding lung with a large air leak?

Q#2: There is an infiltrate on the most recent CXR. Should we start antibiotics?

COPD is more frequently associated with pneumonia when compared to other chronic diseases, and in one study that looked at community-acquired pneumonia (CAP), 19% of patients had underlying COPD. Underlying COPD antagonizes CAP as it contributes to longer hospital stays, increased intensive care admissions, and higher mortality.[118, 119]

Over a 15 year study period, Mannino, et al. found that 2.5 million patients (8.2%) had COPD listed on their death certificate.[12] A study looking at COPD-related hospitalizations reported an overall hospital mortality of 5.9%, with 43% of that mortality related to heart disease, 37% related to respiratory failure and 25% related to pneumonia.[19]

This patient is at risk for healthcare-associated pneumonia due to his recent hospitalization. He presented in respiratory distress with associated hypoxemia. With suspected infection, we recommend treating with broad-spectrum antibiotics.

Q#3: Is it time to admit or should we continue to manage in the ED?

The patient's tension PTX is alleviated and despite continued respiratory discomfort, he is stable on a non-rebreather and ready for admission. Current recommendations are to consult thoracic surgery by 2–5 days for video-assisted thoracoscopic surgery (VATS) if there is a persistent air leak or failure of the lung to re-expand.[37,51,60,113,120,121] However, there is evidence that 100% of PSP and 79% of SSP with persistent air leaks will resolve spontaneously by 14 days if treated by chest tube drainage alone.[113]

The goals of surgical intervention are to repair any persistent air leak, and to prevent re-occurrence of future pneumothoraces. This can be accomplished through resecting any visible blebs and by obliterating 7 pleural porosities under the surface of the visceral pleura.[122] The 2 opposing pleural surfaces are then brought together to cause adhesion between them.

There are 3 procedural options for pleurodesis in these patients: chemical pleurodesis, minimally invasive video-assisted thoracoscopic surgery (VATS) with pleurectomy and pleural abrasion, and finally, the full open thoracotomy with pleurectomy. Chemical pleurodesis is the least effective (9–22% re-occurrence) and should be reserved for patients that cannot tolerate surgery.[123-126]

Q#4: With the persistent hypoxemia, should he be intubated?

Use of any form of positive pressure ventilation (PPV) should be done cautiously in a patient with a pneumothorax, *especially* prior to chest tube placement. Adding PPV to a closed system will cause a simple PTX to rapidly turn into a tension PTX, risking hemodynamic collapse. Even in those with a chest tube, PPV can rapidly increase the flow rate of the pleural air leak beyond the decompressing capacity of the chest tube, resulting in tension physiology and potentially fatal consequences.

Both the BTS and ACCP recommend placement of a chest tube in a patient with a pneumothorax who is on PPV.[43,44] Traditionally, large chest tubes were placed in these patients. One study found that small chest tubes perform similarly to large chest tubes for management of spontaneous pneumothoraxes in mechanically ventilated patients. Subset analysis suggested the small chest tubes performed poorly in pneumothoraxes due to barotrauma, presumably because such air leaks are larger and require higher suctioning flow rates to treat.[127]

Our patient is having difficulty re-expanding his lung due to a large ruptured bleb with a high-flow pleural air leak. Adding PPV will force air into the pleural space at an even faster rate, increasing the flow of his air leak and worsening the pneumothorax. Beyond this, our patient is at the brink of hypoxia and likely to drop his oxygen saturation precipitously when paralyzed.

At this time, our patient should not be intubated. He is saturating adequately on the high flow Venturi mask, and even though he is tachypneic, the risk of intubation outweighs the benefits. However, should he fatigue or have worsening hypoxemia secondary to his pneumonia or re-expansion pulmonary edema, he does have 3 chest tubes in place to help blunt the insult of being intubated.

Section editor comments (Yealy):

Intubating and starting mechanical ventilation for oxygenation alone is not often needed *unless* symptoms or saturations are profoundly abnormal. Use other tools first.

What happened to the patient?

Vital Signs/Measurements:

01:58 EDT	**Pulse Rate**	**116 BPM HI**
	Respiratory Rate	**38 Br PM > HHI**
	Pulse Oximetry	100 % NML
	O_2 Device Flow	15L/min
	Device FIO_2	100 %
	Oxygen Delivery	Nonrebreather mask
	Systolic BP	171mmHg HI
	Diastolic BP	66mmHg NML

ED MDM: The patient has recently been in the hospital and has an infiltrate, and we will start Zosyn and vancomycin for possible hospital-acquired pneumonia. The patient will be admitted to the ICU. He is still in moderate respiratory distress and hypoxemic.

Diagnosis: Right-sided pneumothorax with pigtail and Heimlich valve placement ×2 and chest tube placement ×1

Hospital course: Patient was admitted to the ICU for hypoxemia. He received oxygen via Venturi Mask to maintain 95% O_2 saturation and antibiotics for healthcare-associated pneumonia (vancomycin and Piperacillin/Tazobactam), with added albuterol and ipratropium for concomitant chronic COPD. CIWA protocol was begun for prevention of alcohol withdrawal.

Cardiothoracic surgery consultants detected a large right-sided air leak and did video-assisted thoracic surgery (VATS). The patient had a wedge resection of the right upper lobe to remove a "giant bleb" at the right apex. The remainder of hospital course was unremarkable, and the chest tube removed by the thoracic surgeon prior to discharge home.

Chapter take home points:

- There is a high probability of pneumothorax recurrence (up to 37% of patients).
- Needle decompress or use rapid, finger-assisted thoracostomy for all with suspected tension pneumothorax.
- 1-view ultrasound detects most hemodynamically significant PTX.
- Use the longest angiocatheter available for needle decompression. The central line kit angiocath is 3 inches (7.5cm) long. Inserting at the 4th/5th ICS-AAL has the highest predicted success rate.
- Small-bore catheters are as safe and efficient at draining PTX as large-bore catheters and have lower complication rates.
- In pneumothoraces that fail to expand after initial pigtail or chest tube placement, consider adding or increasing suction flow, followed by placing a second pigtail or chest tube if necessary.
- Avoid intubation or BiPAP in a patient with a PTX unless they have a chest tube/pigtail in place. PPV will increase the pneumothorax, leading to tension physiology and hemodynamic collapse.

References:

1. LaMantia MA, Stewart PW, Platts-Mills TF, et al. Predictive value of initial triage vital signs for critically ill older adults. West J Emerg Med 2013;14(5):453-60.
2. Hong W, Earnest A, Sultana P, et al. How accurate are vital signs in predicting clinical outcomes in critically ill emergency department patients. Eur J Emerg Med 2013;20(1)27-32.
3. Barfod C, Lauritzen MM, Danker JK, et al. Abnormal vital signs are strong predictors for intensive care unit admission and in-hospital mortality in adults triaged in the emergency department - a prospective cohort study. Scand J Trauma Resusc Emerg Med 2013;(20)28.
4. Hewson P, Humphries S, Roberton D, et al. Markers of serious illness in infants under 6 months old presenting to a children fs hospital. Arch Dis Child 1990;65(7):750-6.
5. Hooker EA, O fBrien DJ, Danzl DF, et al. Respiratory rates in emergency department patients. J Emerg Med 1989;7(2):129-32.
6. Simoes EA, Roark R, Berman S, et al. Respiratory rate: measurement of variability over time and accuracy at different counting periods. Arch Dis Child 1991;66(10):1199-1203.
7. Mangione S, Nieman LZ. Pulmonary auscultatory skills during training in internal medicine and family practice. Am J Respir Crit Care Med 1999;159(4 Pt 1):1119-24.
8. Peterson MC, Holbrook JH, Von Hales D, et al. Contributions of the history, physical examination, and laboratory investigation in making medical diagnoses. West J Med 1992;156(2):163-5.
9. Leuppia JD, Dieterlec T, Kocha G, et al. Diagnostic value of lung auscultation in an emergency

room setting. Swiss Med Wkly 2005;135(35/36):520-4.
10. Traulhein JJ, Lambert RL, Miller J. Malpractice in the emergency department \A review of 200 cases. Ann Emerg Med 1984; 13(9 Pt 1) 709-11.
11. Yu KT, Green RA. Critical aspects of emergency department documentation and communication. Emerg Med Clin North Am 2009;27(4):641-54.
12. Mannino DM, Brown C, Giovino GA. Obstructive lung disease deaths in the United States from 1979 through 1993. An analysis using multiple-cause mortality data. Am J Respir Crit Care Med 1997;156(3 Pt 1):814-8.
13. Hansell AL, Walk JA, Soriano JB. What do chronic obstructive pulmonary disease patients die from? A multiple cause coding analysis. Eur Respir J 2003;22(5):809-4.
14. Global initiative for chronic obstructive lung disease. Pocket guide to COPD diagnosis, management, and prevention. A guide for health care professionals. 2017 ed. Available at: https://goldcopd.org/wp-content/uploads/2016/12/wms-GOLD-2017-Pocket-Guide.pdf
15. Lozano R, Naghavi M, Foreman K, et al. Global and regional mortality from 235 causes of death for 20 age groups in 1990 and 2010: a systematic analysis for the Global Burden of Disease Study 2010. Lancet 2012;380(9859): 2095-128.
16. Mathers CD, Loncar D. Projections of global mortality and burden of disease from 2002 to 2030. PLoS Med 2006;3(11):e442.
17. van Manen JG, Bindels PJ, IJzermans CJ, et al. Prevalence of comorbidity in patients with a chronic airway obstruction and controls over the age of 40. J Clin Epidemiol 2001;54(3):287-93.
18. Chatila WM, Thomashow BM, Minai OA, et al. Comorbidities in chronic obstructive pulmonary disease. Proc Am Thorac Soc 2008;5(4)549-55.
19. 19. Holguin F, Folch E, Redd SC, et al. Comorbidity and mortality in COPD-related hospitalizations in the United States, 1979 to 2001.Chest 2005;128(4):2005-11.
20. Grimminger J, Ghofrani HA, Weissmann N, et al. COPD-associated pulmonary hypertension: clinical implications and current methods for treatment. Expert Rev Respir Med 216;10(7):755-66.
21. Curkendall SM, DeLuise C, Jones JK, et al. Cardiovascular disease in patients with chronic obstructive pulmonary disease, Saskatchewan Canada cardiovascular disease in COPD patients. Ann Epidemiol 2006;16(1):63-70.
22. Sidney S, Sorel M, Quesenberry CP Jr, et al. COPD and incident cardiovascular disease hospitalizations and mortality: Kaiser Permanente Medical Care Program. Chest 2005;128(4):2068-75.
23. Rutschmann OT, Cornuz J, Poletti PA, et al. Should pulmonary embolism be suspected in exacerbation of chronic obstructive pulmonary disease? Thorax 2007;62(2):121-5.
24. Tillie-Leblond I, Marquette CH, Perez T, et al. Pulmonary embolism in patients with unexplained exacerbation of chronic obstructive pulmonary disease: prevalence and risk factors. Ann Intern Med 2006;144(6):390-396.
25. Kosten TR, O'Connor PG. Management of drug and alcohol withdrawal N Engl J Med 2003;348(18):1786-95.
26. Schuckit MA. Alcohol-use disorders. Lancet 2009;373(9662):492-501.
27. American Psychiatric Association. Diagnostic and statistical manual of mental disorders. 5th ed., Washington DC: American Psychiatric Publishing, 2013.
28. Mainerova B, Prasko J, Latalova K, et al. Alcohol withdrawal delirium - diagnosis, course and treatment. Biomed Pap Med Fac Univ Palacky Olomouc Czech Repub 2015;159(1):44-52.

29. Eyer F, Schuster T, Felgenhauer N, et al. Risk assessment of moderate to severe alcohol withdrawal - predictors for seizures and delirium tremens in the course of withdrawal. Alcohol Alcohol 2011;46(4):427-33.
30. Berggren U, Fahlke C, Berglund KJ, et al. Thrombocytopenia in early alcohol withdrawal is associated with development of delirium tremens or seizures. Alcohol Alcohol 2009;44(4):382-6.
31. Schmidt KJ, Doshi MR, Holzhausen JM, et al. Treatment of severe alcohol withdrawal. Ann Pharmacother 2016;50(5):389-401.
32. Mayo-Smith MF, Beecher LH, Fischer TL, et al. Management of alcohol withdrawal delirium. An evidence-based practice guideline. Arch Intern Med 2004;164(13):1405-12.
33. Hjermo I, Anderson JE, Fink-Jensen A, et al. Phenobarbital versus diazepam for delirium tremens - a retrospective study. Dan Med Bull 2010;57(8):A4169.
34. Ferguson JA, Suelzer CJ, Eckert GJ, et al. Risk factors for delirium tremens development. J Gen Intern Med 1996;11(7):410-4..
35. Cushman Jr P. Delirium tremens. Update on an old disorder. Postgrad Med 1987; 82(5):117-22.
36. Schuckit MA, Tipp JE, Reich T, et al. The histories of withdrawal convulsions and delirium tremens in 1648 alcohol dependent subjects. Addiction 1995;90(10):1335-47.
37. Donahue DM, Wright CD, Viale G, et al. Resection of pulmonary blebs and pleurodesis for spontaneous pneumothorax. Chest 1993;104(6):1767-9.
38. Lesur O, Delorme N, Frogamet JM, et al. Computed tomography in the etiologic assessment of idiopathic spontaneous pneumothorax. Chest 1990;98(2):341-7.
39. Sharma N, Justaniah AM, Kanne JP, et al. Vanishing lung syndrome (giant bullous emphysema): CT findings in 7 patients and a literature review. J Thorac Imaging 2009;24(3):227-30.
40. 40. Stern EJ, Webb WR, Weinacker A, Muller NL. Idiopathic giant bullous emphysema (vanishing lung syndrome): imaging findings in nine patients. AJR Am J Roentgenol 1994; 162(2):279-82.
41. Chen CK, Cheng HK, Chang WH, et al. Giant emphysematous bulla mimicking tension pneumothorax. Am J Med Sci 2009;337(3):205.
42. Chandra D, Rose SR, Carter RB, et al. Fluid-containing emphysematous bullae: a spectrum of illness. Eur Respir J 2008;32(2):303-6.
43. MacDuff A, Arnold A, Harvey J, et al. Management of spontaneous pneumothorax: British Thoracic Society pleural disease guideline 2010. Thorax 2010;65 Suppl 2:ii18-31.
44. Baumann MH, Strange C, Heffner, et al. Management of spontaneous pneumothorax: an American College of Chest Physicians Delphi consensus statement. Chest 2001;119(2):590-02.
45. Wait MA, Estrera A. Changing clinical spectrum of spontaneous pneumothorax. Am J Surg 1992;164(5):528-31.
46. Tanaka F, Itoh M, Esaki H, et al. Secondary spontaneous pneumothorax. Ann Thorac Surg 1993;55(2):372-6.
47. Ashby M, Haug G, Mulcahy P, et al. Conservative versus interventional management for primary spontaneous pneumothorax in adults. Cochrane Database Syst Rev 2014;(12):CD010565.
48. Engdahl O, Toft T, Boe J. Chest radiograph--a poor method for determining the size of a pneumothorax. Chest 1993;103(1):26-9.
49. O'Rourke JP, Yee ES. Civilian spontaneous pneumothorax. Treatment options and long-term results. Chest 1989;96(6):1302-6.
50. Kelly AM, Loy J, Tsang AY, et al. Estimating the rate of re-expansion of spontaneous

pneumothorax by a formula derived from computed tomography volumetry studies. Emerg Med J 2006;23(10):780-2.
51. Schoenenberger RA, Haefeli WE, Weiss P, et al. Timing of invasive procedures in therapy for primary and secondary spontaneous pneumothorax. Arch Surg 1991;126(6):764-6.
52. Heimlich HJ. Valve drainage of the pleural cavity. Dis Chest 1968;53(3):282-7.
53. Mercier C, Page A, Verdant A, et al. Outpatient management of intercostal tube drainage in spontaneous pneumothorax. Ann Thorac Surg 1976;22(2):163-5.
54. Cannon WB, Mark JB, Jamplis RW. Pneumothorax: a therapeutic update. Am J Surg 1981;142(1):26-9.
55. Roggla M, Wagner A, Brunner C, et al. The management of pneumothorax with the thoracic vent versus conventional intercostal tube drainage. Wien Klin Wochenschr 1996;108(11):330-3.
56. Campisi P, Voitk AJ. Outpatient treatment of spontaneous pneumothorax in a community hospital using a Heimlich flutter valve: a case series. J Emerg Med 1997;15(1):115-19.
57. Hassani B, Foote J, Borgundvaag B. Outpatient management of primary spontaneous pneumothorax in the emergency department of a community hospital using a small-bore catheter and a Heimlich valve. Acad Emerg Med 2009;16(6):513-518.
58. Ho KK, Ong ME, Koh MS, et al. A randomized controlled trial comparing minichest tube and needle aspiration in outpatient management of primary spontaneous pneumothorax. Am J Emerg Med 2011;29(9):1152-1157.
59. Massongo M, Leroy S, Scherpereel A, et al. Outpatient management of primary spontaneous pneumothorax: a prospective study. Eur Respir J 2014;43(2):582-90.
60. Marquette CH, Marx A, Leroy S, et al. Simplified stepwise management of primary spontaneous pneumothorax: a pilot study. Eur Respir J 2006;27(3):470-6.
61. Brims FJ, Maskell NA. Ambulatory treatment in the management of pneumothorax: a systematic review of the literature. Thorax 2013;68(7):664-9.
62. Voisin F, Sohier L, Rochas Y, et al. Ambulatory management of large spontaneous pneumothorax with pigtail catheters. Ann Emerg Med 2014;64(3): 222-8.
63. Trueger NS, Murray H, Kobner S, et al. Global Emergency Medicine Journal Club: A social media discussion about the outpatient management of patients with spontaneous pneumothorax by using pigtail catheters. Ann Emerg Med 2015;66(4):409-16.
64. Gavish R, Levy A, Dekel OK, et al. The association between hospital readmission and pulmonologist follow-up visits in patients with COPD. Chest 2015;148(2):375-81.
65. Gabayan GZ, Derose SF, Asch SM, et al. Patterns and predictors of short-term death after emergency department discharge. Ann Emerg Med 2011;558(6):551-8.e2.
66. Sklar DP, Crandall CS, Loeliger E, et al. Unanticipated death after discharge home from the emergency department. Ann Emerg Med 2007;49(6):735-45.
67. Lippert HL, Lund O, Blegrad S, et al. Independent risk factors for cumulative recurrence rate after first spontaneous pneumothorax. Eur Respir J 1991;4(3):324-31.
68. Videm V, Pillgram-Larsen J, Ellingsen O, et al. Spontaneous pneumothorax in chronic obstructive pulmonary disease: complications, treatment and recurrences. Eur J Respir Dis 1987;71(5):365-71.
69. Schramel FM, Postmus PE, Vanderschueren RG. Current aspects of spontaneous pneumothorax. Eur Respir J 1997;10(6):1372-9.
70. Chambers A, Scarci M. In patients with first-episode primary spontaneous pneumothorax is video-assisted thoracoscopic surgery superior to tube thoracostomy alone in terms of time to

resolution of pneumothorax and incidence of recurrence? Interact Cardiovasc Thorac Surg 2009;9(6):1003-8.
71. Helland G, Gaspari R, Licciardo S, et al. Comparison of four views to single-view ultrasound protocols to identify clinically significant pneumothorax. Acad Emerg Med. 2016;23(10):1170-5.
72. Ball CG, Wyrzykowski AD, Kirkpatrick AW, et al. Thoracic needle decompression for tension pneumothorax: clinical correlation with catheter length. Can J Surg. 2010;53(3):184-8.
73. Laan DV, Vu TD, Thiels CA et al. Chest wall thickness and decompression failure: A systematic review and meta-analysis comparing anatomic locations in needle thoracostomy. Injury 2016;47(4):797-04.
74. Aho JM, Thiels CA, El Khatib MM, et al. Needle thoracostomy: clinical effectiveness is improved using a longer angiocatheter. J Trauma Acute Care Surg 2016;80(2):272-7.
75. Martin M, Satterly S, Inaba K, et al. Does needle thoracostomy provide adequate and effective decompression of tension pneumothorax? J Trauma Acute Care Surg 2012;73(6):1412-7.
76. Weingart S. Podcast 62 . Needle vs. Knife II: Needle Thoracostomy? EMCrit Blog 2011. Available at: https://emcrit.org/emcrit/needle-finger-thoracostomy/
77. Fitzgerald M, Mackenzie CF, Marasco S, et al. Pleural decompression and drainage during trauma reception and resuscitation. Injury 2008;39(1):9-20.
78. Inaba K, Lustenberger T, Recinos G, et al. Does size matter? A prospective analysis of 28-32 versus 36-40 French chest tube size in trauma. J Trauma Acute Care Surg 2012;72(2):422-7.
79. Noppen M, Alexander P, Driesen P, et al. Manual aspiration versus chest tube drainage in first episodes of primary spontaneous pneumothorax: a multicenter, prospective, randomized pilot study. Am J Respir Crit Care Med 2002;165(9):1240-4.
80. Harvey J, Prescott RJ. Simple aspiration versus intercostal tube drainage for spontaneous pneumothorax in patients with normal lungs. British Thoracic Society Research Committee. BMJ 1994;309(6965):1338-9.
81. Ayed AK, Chandrasekaran C, Sukumar M. Aspiration versus tube drainage in primary spontaneous pneumothorax: a randomised study. Eur Respir J 2006;27(3):477-82.
82. Andrivet P, Djedaini K, Teboul JL, et al. Spontaneous pneumothorax. Comparison of thoracic drainage vs immediate or delayed needle aspiration. Chest 1995;108(2):335-9.
83. Iepsen UW, Ringbak T. Small-bore chest tubes seem to perform better than larger tubes in treatment of spontaneous pneumothorax. Dan Med J 2013;60(6):A4644
84. Tsai WK, Chen W, Lee JC, et al. Pigtail catheters vs. large-bore chest tubes for management of secondary spontaneous pneumothoraces in adults. Am J Emerg Med 2006;24(7):795-800.
85. Benton IJ, Benfield GF. Comparison of a large and small-calibre tube drain for managing spontaneous pneumothoraces. Resp Med 2009;103(10):1436-40.
86. Fysh ETH, Smith NA, Lee YCG. Optimal chest drain size: the rise of the small-bore pleural catheter. Semin Respir Crit Care Med 2010;31(6):760-68.
87. Cooke DT, David EA. Large-bore and small-bore chest tubes. Thorac Surg Clin 2013;23(1):17-24.
88. Bowness J, Kilgour P, Whiten S, et al. Guidelines for chest drain insertion may not prevent damage to abdominal viscera. Emerg Med J 2014;32(8):620-5.
89. Laws D, Neville E, Duffy J, et al. BTS guidelines for the insertion of a chest drain. Thorax 2003;58 Suppl 2:ii53-9.

90. Griffiths JR, Roberts N. Do junior doctors know where to insert chest drains safely? Postgrad Med J 2005;81(957):456-8.
91. Elsayed H, Roberts R, Emadi M, et al. Chest drain insertion is not a harmless procedure . are we doing it safely? Interact Cardiovasc Thorac Surg 2010;11(6):745-8.
92. Carter P, Conroy S, Blakeney J, et al. Identifying the site for intercostal catheter insertion in the emergency department: is clinical examination reliable? Emerg Med Australas 2014;26(5):450-5.
93. Kong VY, Clarke DL. The spectrum of visceral injuries secondary to misplaced intercostal chest drains: Experience from a high volume trauma service in South Africa. Injury 2014;45(9):1435-9.
94. Kong VY, Oosthuizen G, Sartorius B, et al. An audit of the complications of intercostal chest drain insertion in a high volume trauma service in South Africa. Ann R Coll Surg Engl 2014;96(8):609-13.
95. Bing F, Fitzgerald M, Olaussen A, et al. Identifying a safe site for intercostal catheter insertion using the mid-arm point (MAP), J Emerg Med Trauma Acute Care 2017;2017(1).
96. Butson B., Kwa P. Intercostal Catheter Insertion. Emerg Med Australas 2015;27(1)66-8.
97. Knottenbelt JD, James MF, Bloomfield M. Intrapleural bupivacaine analgesia in chest trauma: a randomised double blinded controlled trial. Injury 1991;22(2):114-6.
98. Engdahl O, Boe J, Sandstedt S. Interpleural bupivacaine for analgesia during chest drainage treatment for pneumothorax. A randomised double blind study. Acta Anaesthesiol Scand 1993;37(2):149-53.
99. Kirsch TD. Tube thoracostomy. In: Roberts JR, Hedges JR, eds. Clinical Procedures in Emergency Medicine. 5th ed. Philadelphia PA: Elsevier, 2010:175-96.
100. Havelock T, Teoh R, Laws D, et al. Pleural procedures and thoracic ultrasound: British Thoracic Society Pleural Disease Guideline 2010. Thorax. 2010;65(Suppl 2):ii61-ii76.
101. Devanand A, Koh MS, Ong TH, et al. Simple aspiration versus chest-tube insertion in the management of primary spontaneous pneumothorax: a systematic review. Respir Med 2004;98(7):579-90.
102. So SY, Yu DY. Catheter drainage of spontaneous pneumothorax: suction or no suction, early or late removal? Thorax1982;37(1):46-8.
103. Sharma TN, Agrihotri SP, Jain NK, et al. Intercostal tube thoracostomy in pneumothorax: factors influencing re-expansion of lung. Ind J Chest Dis All Sci 1988;30(1):32-5.
104. Reed MF, Lyons JM, Luchette FA, et al. Preliminary report of a prospective, randomized trial of underwater seal for spontaneous and iatrogenic pneumothorax. J Am Coll Surg 2007;204(1):84-90.
105. Matsuura Y, Nomimura T, Nurikami H, et al. Clinical evidence of reexpansion pulmonary edema. Chest 1991;100(6):1562-6.
106. Atrium's Ocean Chest Drain Setup and Operation. 2018. Available at: www.youtube.com/watch?v=bLf5WexvsEk
107. Atrium's Ocean Chest Drain Setup and Operation Part 2. 2013. Available at: https://www.youtube.com/watch?v=3co3MxdbWwk
108. Atrium's Ocean Chest Drain Setup and Operation Part 3. 2013. Available at: https://www.youtube.com/watch?v=tXKpOWzK-ZQ
109. Oasis Training - Atrium. 2011. Available at: www.youtube.com/watch?v=pH4XMTJXQY8&t=
110. Sutera SP, Skalak R. The history of Poiseuille's Law. Annu Rev Fluid Mech 1993;25:1-19.

111. Okur E, Baysungur V, Tezel C, et al. Comparison of the single or double chest tube applications after pulmonary lobectomies. Eur J Cardiothorac Surg 2009;35(1):32-5.
112. Alex J, Ansari J, Bahalkar P, et al. Comparison of the immediate postoperative outcome of using the conventional two drains versus a single drain after lobectomy. Ann Thorac Surg 2003; 76(4):1046-9.
113. Chee CB, Abisheganaden J, Yeo JK, et al. Persistent air-leak in spontaneous pneumothorax. clinical course and outcome. Respir Med 1998;92(5):757-61.
114. Echevarria C, Twomey D, Dunning J, et al. Does re-expansion pulmonary oedema exist? Interact Cardiovasc Thorac Surg. 2008;7(3):485-9.
115. Ritchie M, Brown C, Bowling M. Chest tubes: Indications, sizing, placement, and management. Clin Pulm Med 2017;24(1):37-53.
116. Feller-Kopman D, Berkowitz D, Boiselle P, et al. Large-volume thoracentesis and the risk of reexpansion pulmonary edema. Ann Thorac Surg 2007,84(5):1656-61.
117. Sethuraman KN, Duong D, Mehta S, et al. Complications of tube thoracostomy placement in the emergency department. J Emerg Med 2011;40(1):14-20.
118. Pifarre R, Falguera M, Vicente-de-Vera C, et al. Characteristics of community-acquired pneumonia in patients with chronic obstructive pulmonary disease. Respir Med 2007;101(10):2139-44.
119. Lieberman D, Lieberman D, Gelfer Y, et al. Pneumonic vs nonpneumonic acute exacerbations of COPD. Chest 2002;122(4):1264-70.
120. Granke K, Fischer CR, Gago O, et al. The efficacy and timing of operative intervention for spontaneous pneumothorax. Ann Thorac Surg 1986;42(5):540-2.
121. Shah SS, Cohen AS, Magee PG, et al. Surgery remains a late and under-utilised option in the management of spontaneous pneumothorax: should the British Thoracic Society guidelines be revisited? Thorax 1998;53.
122. Schramel F, Meyer CJ, Postmus P. Inflammation as a cause of spontaneous pneumothorax (SP) and emphysematous like changes (ELC)? Results of bronchoalveolar lavage (BAL). Eur Respir J 1995;8(Suppl 19):397.
123. Light RW, O'Hara VS, Moritz TE, et al. Intrapleural tetracycline for the prevention of recurrent spontaneous pneumothorax. Results of a Department of Veterans Affairs Co-operative Study. JAMA 1990;264(17):2224-30.
124. Almind M, Lange P, Viskum K. Spontaneous pneumothorax: comparison of simple drainage, talc pleurodesis and tetracycline pleurodesis. Thorax 1989;44(8):627-30.
125. Olsen PS, Anderson HO. Long-term results after tetracycline pleurodesis in spontaneous pneumothorax. Ann Thorac Surg1992;53(6):1015-17.
126. Massard G, Thomas P, Wihlm JM. Minimally invasive management for first and recurrent pneumothorax. Ann Thorac Surg1998;66(2):592-9.
127. Lin YC, Tu CY, Liang SJ, et al. Pigtail catheter for the management of pneumothorax in mechanically ventilated patients. Am J Emerg Med 2010;28(4):466-71.

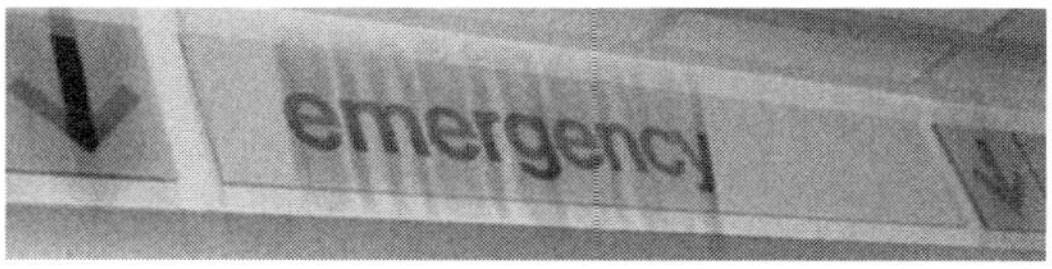

SECTION C – CARDIAC/ VASCULAR

Chapter 11: A 63-year-old man with shortness of breath after a fall

Sarah A. Stahmer, MD
Clinical Associate Professor
Emergency Medicine
Director of Emergency Ultrasound
University of North Carolina
Chapel Hill, NC

Robert Stenberg, MD
Attending Emergency Physician
Ultrasound Fellow
VCU Health
Richmond, VA

Section editor:
John C. Greenwood, MD
Assistant Professor
Department of Emergency Medicine
Department of Anesthesiology and Critical Care
Perelman School of Medicine
University of Pennsylvania
Philadelphia, PA

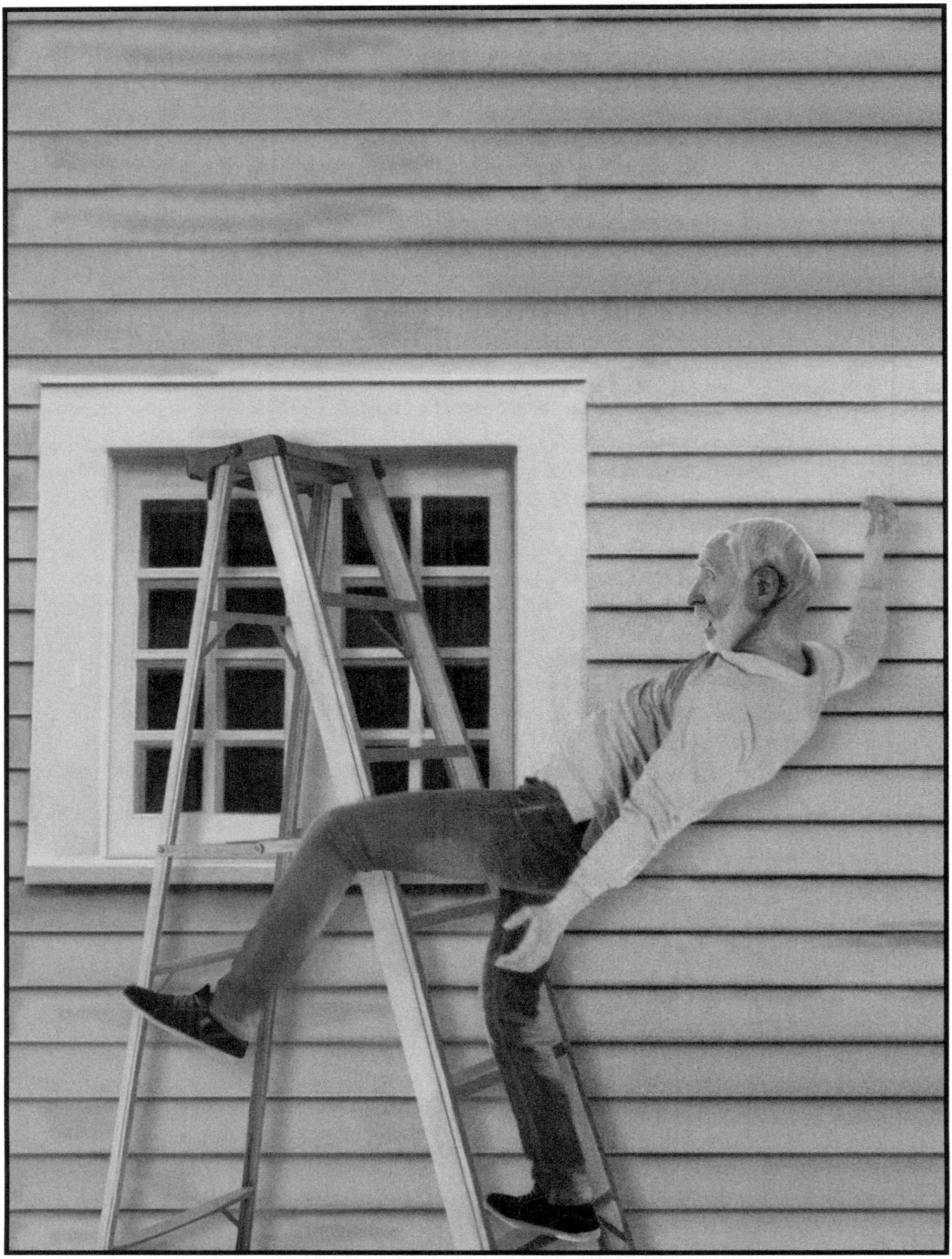

SECTION C/CHAPTER 11

A 63-year-old man with shortness of breath after a fall

The patient's story:
Ben Russ is a 63-year-old attorney. He has been successful in his career but has been unlucky with his genetics; despite maintaining his weight, exercising regularly, and stopping smoking in his mid-40s, he suffered his first deep vein thrombosis (DVT) at the age of 52 and was found to have factor V Leiden.

On a warm fall day, while standing on a ladder to clean his gutters, he falls onto his left side. His wife rushes outside, finding him still laying on the ground. She helps him to a sitting position, but after 30 minutes of significant pain with breathing, they decide he needs medical attention, so he is helped into the car, and his wife drives to the local emergency department. He is found to have 3 fractured ribs and is admitted for pain control, but during the night develops CO_2 retention, becomes confused and is intubated by the hospitalist physician.

He improves, is extubated, and is eventually discharged home, but only days later he is again short of breath. Waking from sleep with significant respiratory distress, his wife calls 911 and he is taken to a larger, regional hospital where he is diagnosed with pneumonia and a congestive heart failure (CHF) exacerbation. He undergoes a heart catheterization and is found to have 95% occlusion of the right coronary artery (RCA) which is stented. He is discharged in "good" condition, but six days later he is again experiencing chest pain and shortness of breath. EMS is activated.

ED VISIT #3

CC: Chest pain/shortness of breath

HPI (PA-C) (19:41): Patient is a 64-year-old male with history of hypertension, diabetes, DVT, COPD, atrial fibrillation, CHF and factor V Leiden. His recent history is notable for a fall resulting in multiple rib fractures requiring intubation for hypoventilation. He was then hospitalized 2 days later for shortness of breath and found to have pneumonia and pleural effusions for which was started on Levaquin. He also underwent cardiac catheterization and underwent PTCA of his RCA. He did require Foley placement for urinary retention. The patient was discharged from this hospital 6 days ago after being admitted for roughly 5 days. He is on Coumadin. Had an INR checked earlier this week and it was over 5. He was told to hold his Coumadin and reduce the dosage. He was discharged to home 6 days ago.

He returns today with chest pain/shortness of breath which worsened today. He states he feels dizzy and lightheaded. Has been nauseated but no vomiting. Family believes he is still on Levaquin for pneumonia. He denies any abdominal pain. States his blood sugars were in the 400s today. Normally poorly controlled but usually in the 200s. No fever, blood in urine/stool bruising, rash, extremity pain, paresthesias. He has not had his INR rechecked.

PMH:
Atrial fibrillation
CHF (congestive heart failure)
COPD (chronic obstructive pulmonary disease)
DM (diabetes mellitus)
DVT (deep venous thrombosis)
Factor 5 Leiden mutation, heterozygous
HTN (hypertension)
Macular degeneration
Recent rib fractures

PSH:
Stent in branch of right coronary artery
Gunther Tulip Vena Cava Filter
Ankle
Knee

Medications: Atorvastatin, budesonide-formoterol inh, metoprolol, montelukast, tamsulosin, tiotropium inh, colace, Januvia, klor-con, Lantus insulin, nitrostat 0.4mg PRN, Plavix, aspirin 81mg, ferrous sulfate, warfarin 4mg QD
SH: No smoking or alcohol

PE (PA):

Vitals:

Time	Temp (F)	Pulse	Resp	Syst	Diast	Sat
19:39	95.7	121	18	78	58	97% (3L NC)

CONSTITUTIONAL: Alert and aware, chronic ill-appearing appearance, holding an emesis bag which is empty.
RESP: Normal chest excursion with respiration; breath sounds clear and equal bilaterally; no wheezes, rhonchi, or rales.
CARDIO: Regular rhythm, without murmurs, rub or gallop, distant heart sounds.
ABD: Non-distended; non-tender, soft, without rigidity, rebound or guarding.
SKIN: Normal for age and race; warm and dry; no apparent lesions
EXT: Chronic venous stasis changes.

MDM (MD @ 20:16): I discussed the case with [the PA who] saw the patient, spoke with him and examined him. Lungs are clear with equal breath sounds. Heart tones are distant. Abdomen is soft. No pulsatile abdominal mass but does have bilateral lower extremity edema which appears chronic. The patient had chest pain and shortness of breath during the day today. EKG shows low voltage QRS.

Author comments (Weinstock):

The ECG below is a reproduction but is not the actual patient's ECG. Note our patient's heart rate is 121 bpm but the ECG below shows a slower rate.

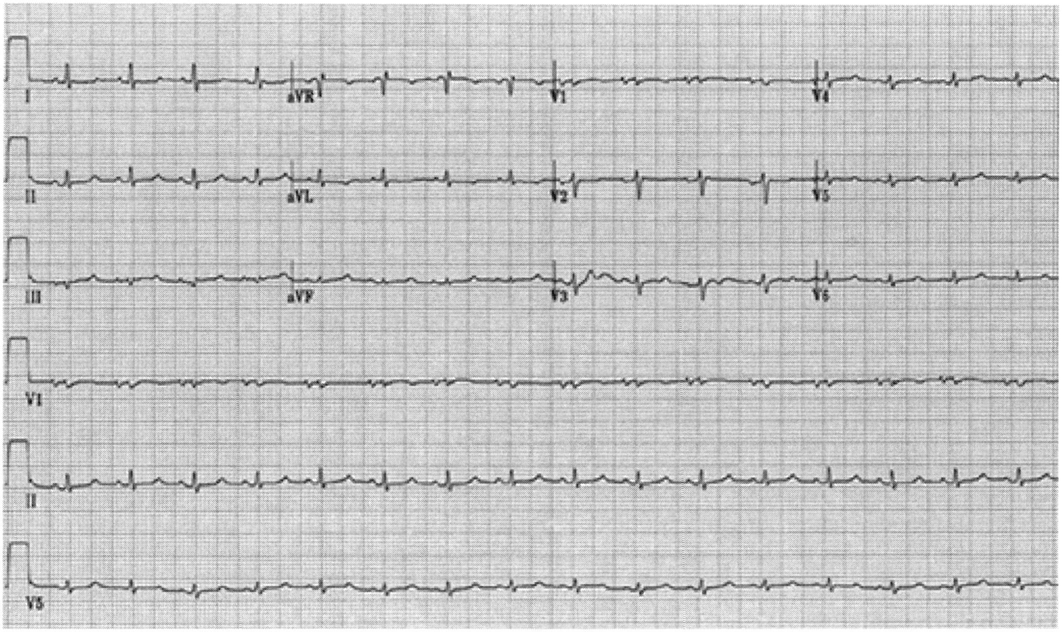

Author comments (Weinstock):

We are at the bedside of a hypotensive, tachycardic, anticoagulated patient with a concerning ECG who has just arrived per EMS. We are at:

DECISION POINT A – YOU ARE FACED WITH 4 QUESTIONS:

1. **What is the differential diagnosis?**
2. **Which tests should be done to start the work-up?**
3. **How should the hypotension be managed initially? How does the history of CHF change the indication for IV fluids?**
4. **How does the history of an elevated INR play into the differential diagnosis?**

Q#1: What is the differential diagnosis?

This patient is critically ill based on his presenting vital signs; HR 121 and BP 78/58. The differential diagnosis is broad given his history of chest trauma, heart catheterization and two recent hospitalizations during which he was immobilized and intubated. I recommend starting by organizing a differential based on his recent history.

Trauma:

The remote history of thoracic trauma and rib fractures puts him at risk for bleeding, which could be delayed given his recent history of elevated INR. Possible sites of bleeding are pleural (hemothorax), pericardial and intraperitoneal, particularly if this is a delayed presentation of splenic injury. Intubation in the setting of torso trauma and rib fractures also places him at risk for pneumothorax, which causes RV dysfunction and shock when tension pathophysiology is present.

Cardiac cath/Possible recent MI:

He had a recent cardiac catheterization with PTCA of his RCA, which places him at risk for reocclusion and myocardial ischemia. In-stent thrombosis causing RV infarct/hypotension usually occurs in the first 30 days. It is not clear from the history as to whether he sustained an MI during his most recent hospitalization, but if he had, he is also at risk for myocardial rupture, and pericardial effusion (Dressler's syndrome, hemorrhagic). Causes of hypotension in both scenarios include:

- Systolic dysfunction if ischemic etiology, diastolic dysfunction if effusion present
- Isolated RV dysfunction
- Pericardial tamponade
- Papillary muscle dysfunction—should be considered as the RCA is the sole coronary artery supplying the posteromedial papillary muscle. With dysfunction or rupture, the patient will have resultant acute mitral regurgitation, pulmonary edema, and cardiogenic shock.

Hospitalizations:

He has been hospitalized twice in recent weeks. Commonly encountered complications arising from hospitalization are infectious and thrombotic. Potential sources of infection in this patient are urine and lung. He reportedly had a pneumonia, pleural effusions and was recently intubated; he could have an empyema, parapneumonic effusion, abscess, or failed outpatient antibiotics. Hypotension in the setting of infection would be due to distributive shock.

Pulmonary embolism in a recently hospitalized hypotensive/tachycardic patient cannot be ruled out by his supratherapeutic anticoagulation; however, the suspicion is lower given that the patient has a secondary protection from an IVC filter.

Medications:

An elevated INR would not be surprising considering that he recently started levofloxacin,[1] placing him at risk for bleeding in all listed above locations plus other mucosal sites (e.g., GI tract). Other considerations of medication related conditions include uremic pericarditis from nephrotoxic medications such as levofloxacin, aspirin, contrast dye, or loop diuretics.

Summary:

Included in the differential are also mechanical causes of shock, specifically pericardial tamponade and tension pneumothorax, both of which require urgent needle decompression.

These varied scenarios create a "shock" differential that includes the following:

Cardiogenic, distributive and obstructive. The initial interventions are drastically different... Volume, inotropes or pressors? Each of these therapies holds certain risk if treating the wrong condition, such as erroneously giving a large fluid bolus when the patient actually has CHF. Delays in appropriate interventions are high-risk, particularly when considering hemorrhagic tamponade in a patient with a coagulopathy!

In the "old days" before the use of bedside sonography, pericardiocentesis was often considered only when the patient was in PEA arrest, and the chances of meaningful recovery at this point in the disease course were slim to none. This is the true value of point-of-care ultrasound (POCUS); early identification of life threatening conditions while there is still time to intervene.

Section editor comments (Greenwood):

Patients with low stroke volume as a result of external compression or reduced systolic function are fully dependent on an elevated heart rate to maintain their cardiac output. The patient is presenting with tachycardia and a particularly narrow pulse pressure, which is an important sign pointing towards hypovolemic, cardiogenic, or obstructive shock over a wide pulse pressure that's often present in septic shock as a result of severe vasoplegia.

Q#2: Which tests should be done to start the work-up?

There is a growing body of data showing that early use of ultrasound is effective in reducing diagnostic uncertainty and narrowing the differential diagnosis. Additional benefits of early POCUS include an increase in the absolute proportion of patients with a definitive diagnosis, appropriate changes in the use of IV fluids, vasoactive agents, or blood products in addition to significant changes in major diagnostic imaging, consultation and emergency department disposition.[2–4]

This is a critically ill patient and he should be placed in an acute care resuscitation bed. Once IV access is established, blood should be sent for CBC to check for anemia, serum chemistries to measure electrolytes and serum glucose, renal function and anion gap and a VBG and lactate to assess tissue perfusion and hypoxia. Clearly his INR should be checked in addition to a type and screen, in the case that he will need blood. A troponin should also be sent and if positive, a CK-MB may also be helpful to determine timing of myonecrosis if he did have an MI within the past 14 days. The patient should be on telemetry and his BP frequently checked. A portable CXR should be performed to look for pulmonary infiltrate/consolidation, status of his known pleural effusions and to assess his cardiac contour. Importantly, the ECG is notable for a sinus tachycardia, low voltage and electrical alternans, so pericardial tamponade should be high on the differential.

This patient needs a diagnosis, now! The ultrasound machine should be brought to the bedside specifically looking for findings that would sufficiently narrow this broad differential diagnosis.

A number of US protocols have been proposed to organize the sonographic approach to the critically ill patient.[5-8] What they have in common is an organ-based approach to the patient with undifferentiated hypotension, assessing the heart, IVC, lung, and abdomen to identify causes of hypotension.

	CARDIOGENIC	RV DYSFUNCTION	TAMPONADE	HYPOVOLEMIC DISTRIBUTIVE	PNEUMOTHORAX
HEART	Poor systolic function, hypokinetic	Septal bowing, Enlarged RV	Effusion with RV end-diastolic collapse	Underfilled hyperdynamic	Likely underfilled and hyperdynamic
IVC	Plethoric	Plethoric	Plethoric	Collapsibility with respirations	Plethoric
LUNG	Diffuse B lines	(-)	(-)	(-)	No lung sliding, Barcode/stratosphere sign, A lines
AORTA Abdomen for free fluid	(-)	(-)	(-)	AAA Free IP fluid	(-)

1. **Cardiogenic shock:** LV systolic dysfunction, lung B lines, plethoric IVC with minimal respiratory variation.
2. **RV dysfunction (PE, Inferior MI):** RV free wall hypokinesis, McConnell's sign, RV dilatation, paradoxical RV septal systolic motion, dilated IVC with lack of respiratory collapse.
3. **Pericardial tamponade:** Pericardial effusion, RA systolic collapse, RV diastolic collapse.
4. **Hypovolemic shock (bleeding):** Hyperdynamic heart and flat IVC with exaggerated respiratory variation. AAA and/or free intraperitoneal fluid.
5. **Distributive shock (sepsis):** Note that unless the sepsis picture has affected the cardiac function, distributive and hypovolemic shock will appear similar on the RUSH ultrasound.
6. **Pneumothorax:** Absence of lung sliding, barcode/stratosphere sign on M-Mode, lung point.

Q#3: How should the hypotension be managed initially? How does the history of CHF change the indication for IV fluids?

POCUS is exceptionally useful when assessing volume responsiveness, particularly when the IVC is flat with exaggerated respiratory variation.[9] In this case, fluids are clearly of benefit. In patients with pulmonary or cardiac disease resulting in high RA/RV pressures, the respiratory collapsibility of IVC, while not perfect, may help predict fluid responsiveness. If there is any respiratory variation in the IVC, then a small bolus of fluids (500cc) may be helpful. The risk of a 500mL fluid bolus with history of CHF becomes a risk/benefit ratio, and the risk is lower when using a trial with a smaller volume.

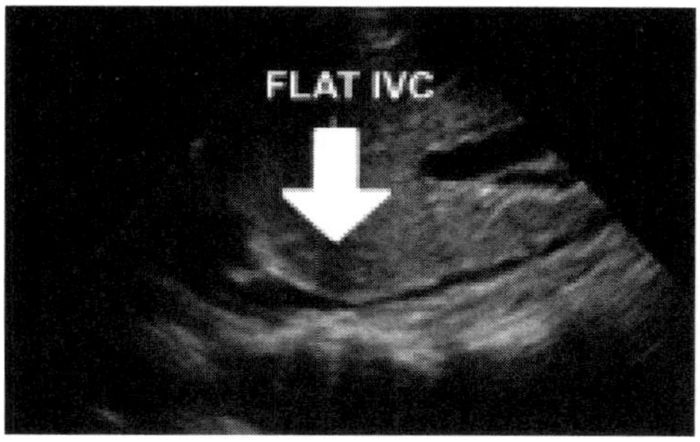

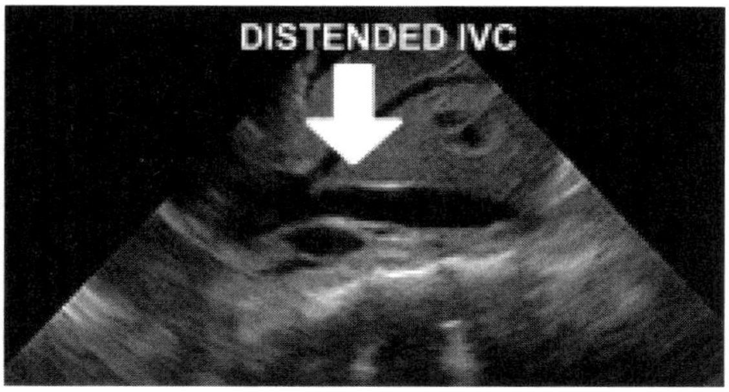

In the patient who is not in florid pulmonary edema, tripoding and gasping for air, a fluid bolus trial is usually a safe and effective intervention. Fluid resuscitation is an appropriate and effective intervention in both hypovolemic and distributive shock.

POCUS has been shown to aid in assessing fluid responsiveness by assessing the IVC for diameter and respiratory variation with the patient supine and with straight raising.[9]

Section editor comments (Greenwood):

In general, IV fluids are an effective strategy in temporizing the shocked patient with pericardial tamponade. Fluids will increase intracardiac filling pressure relative to the intrapericardial pressure while arranging for pericardiocentesis.

Consulting editor comments (Weingart):

At our facility, we routinely temporize tamponade with volume loading.

Q#4: How does the history of an elevated INR play into the differential diagnosis?

Atraumatic bleeding in patients with an elevated INR can occur anywhere but most commonly in the GI tract, lung, and brain. In the setting of thoracic trauma, as in this patient, we have additional concerns regarding bleeding in the pleural, pericardial, and intraperitoneal cavities. Hypotension caused by bleeding within the pericardial space is most often due to myocardial contusion, wall rupture, or laceration of an epicardial vessel. These often cause hemodynamic instability with small volumes because of the speed of accumulation within the pericardial space. Slowly accumulating effusions can become quite large before becoming symptomatic. These tend to be due to malignancies that have involved the pericardium, uremia, rheumatologic diseases that cause inflammation of the serosal surfaces, (e.g., SLE, familial Mediterranean fever and indolent infections such as tuberculosis). Pericardial effusion due to any one of these conditions can also be hemorrhagic, particularly in the setting of an elevated INR.[10,11]

We know that the patient had a supratherapeutic INR and that his warfarin dose was reduced. We would have to assume that INR is still elevated, increasing the chance that bleeding may be contributing to his hypotension, either into his pericardium, pleural spaces and/or GI tract.

DECISION POINT A – ***What did the provider actually do?***

MDM (20:31): One consideration is pericardial tamponade and for that reason I will ask for a stat echocardiogram. Patient may have congestive heart failure and a saline well will be started. Additional labs are pending. Chest x-ray ordered. I did speak with the echocardiogram technician who asked that I call [the cardiologist]. I spoke with him and he agrees with an echocardiogram and he will call the echocardiogram technician to ask her to come in from home to do a stat echocardiogram. His lungs are clear, and he still could have congestive heart failure as etiology of his symptoms; however, the concern would be for fluid around the heart.

The ED physician was correct in being concerned about a pericardial effusion. It is not clear if he/she had access to a bedside ultrasound and/or training to screen for a pericardial effusion. ED physicians are now expected to have the ability to screen for a pericardial effusion, since this is one component of the FAST exam![12,13] If there was a machine then why wasn't it used? The 30 seconds it would take to look for a pericardial effusion would provide a diagnosis and shorten time to definitive care.

The diagnosis and treatment of a hemodynamically significant pericardial effusion is nearly impossible to treat without US at the bedside. Although it is something you might suspect, you are not going to blindly stick a needle in, unless the patient is actually in arrest. Any ED treating sick patients should have a US capable of performing the RUSH exam in any patient who presents hypotensive or in shock.

If there was no machine, then the ED physician needed to appreciate the severity of this patient's condition. The patient is hypotensive and tachycardic, and if the cause is a pericardial effusion, then it is causing tamponade physiology. While the potential causes of pericardial effusions are numerous, those conditions that present as tamponade are usually due to trauma or malignancy; we can be fairly certain that in addition to all his other problems, he is not likely to have developed cancer in the interim! He did suffered a significant blow to his torso breaking ribs, is anticoagulated and recently underwent a cardiac procedure. One must be concerned that he has a hemopericardium that is already of sufficient size to create hemodynamic instability to the point that it is imminently life threatening.

Section editor comments (Greenwood):

Rapid bedside echocardiography could also provide time sensitive information to get the correct consultant team assembled. In the setting of a recent AMI (approximately 3–7 days post-MI), one must be concerned about free wall rupture. Visualization of simple/clear fluid could not only represent a serious or inflammatory effusion but also fresh blood. A complex fluid collection, concerning for pericardial clot, may lead the EP to consider early surgical evaluation as well.

ED course:

The nurse approaches the physician, "I rechecked the blood pressure and it is now 72. Has the cardiologist called back?"

You respond, "Yeah. I just spoke with him and we are calling in the ECHO tech to see if there is pericardial tamponade."

"Do you want me to give a fluid bolus," asks the nurse. "We only have a saline well right now."

"How does the patient look?" you ask, hoping for a positive response.

"Sleeping…" responds the nurse.

DECISION POINT B – YOU ARE FACED WITH 4 QUESTIONS:

1. **What is the sensitivity and specificity of physical exam and ECG findings for pericardial effusion/tamponade?**
2. **Which POCUS findings support tamponade vs. effusion?**
3. **Should the EP perform a pericardiocentesis or wait for the cardiologist?**
4. **What is the best option for the EP to emergently drain the effusion/tamponade?**

Q#1: What is the sensitivity and specificity of physical exam and ECG findings for pericardial effusion/tamponade?

In medical school we learned that the "classic" findings for pericardial tamponade are Beck's Triad (Muffled heart + JVD + hypotension) and pulses paradoxus; measuring Korotkoff sounds when first heard compared to when they are heard throughout the respiratory cycle. When the difference is > 10mmHg, there is a 98% sensitivity and 70% specificity with + LR of 3.3.

A 2007 JAMA review described the presence of physical findings in pericardial tamponade as reported in 8 studies.[14] Five features were found in most patients with tamponade:

- dyspnea (sensitivity range, 87%–89%).
- tachycardia (pooled sensitivity, 77%; 95% confidence interval [CI], 69%–85%).
- pulsus paradoxus (pooled sensitivity, 82%; 95% CI, 72%–92%).
- elevated jugular venous pressure (pooled sensitivity, 76%; 95% CI, 62%–90%).
- cardiomegaly on chest radiograph (pooled sensitivity, 89%; 95% CI, 73%–100%).

The most common ECG finding is tachycardia (sensitivity 77%)! The three other findings associated with pericardial effusion are low voltage QRS, electrical alternans, and PR depression. These findings have good specificity but poor sensitivity for pericardial effusion/tamponade.[15]

The bottom line is that physical findings associated with tamponade are nonspecific and present in a variety of conditions that include congestive heart failure, pulmonary embolus and COPD exacerbation. Pulsus paradoxus is the only exam finding unique to the diagnosis of tamponade.

Q#2: Which POCUS findings support tamponade vs. effusion?

Early signs of tamponade reflect the fact that pressure within the pericardial sac has reached a point at which ventricular filling is restricted by the surrounding fluid/blood. During diastole, LV filling begins slightly before the RV. As the muscular LV fills, the less robust RV is essentially compressed and cannot completely fill. The rate of accumulation is more significant in cardiac tamponade than the absolute size or composition of the pericardial fluid. Rapidly developing pericardial effusions can abruptly increase the intrapericardial pressure and produce cardiac tamponade with as little as 100–200mL of pericardial fluid. But slowly accumulating effusions, as seen in malignancy or connective tissue diseases, can allow pericardial distention with tamponade not seen until the accumulation of 1–2L of pericardial fluid.

Transudative effusions as seen in rheumatic disease, hypothyroidism and uremia will be echo free, but those effusion related to trauma, infection or inflammatory conditions may contain echogenic debris (blood, pus, fibrin).[16]

The size of the effusion roughly correlates with the pericardial fluid volume as follows:
- Trace effusion: < 0.5cm
- Small effusion: < 1cm (roughly corresponds to < 100cc)
- Moderate effusion: 1–2cm (roughly corresponds to 100–500cc)
- Large effusion: > 2cm (roughly corresponds to > 500cc)

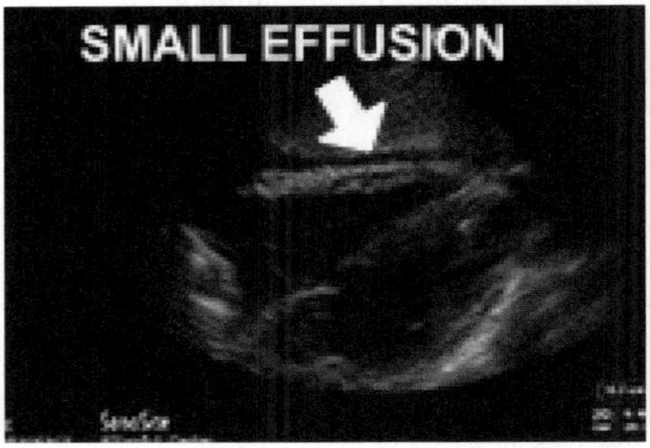

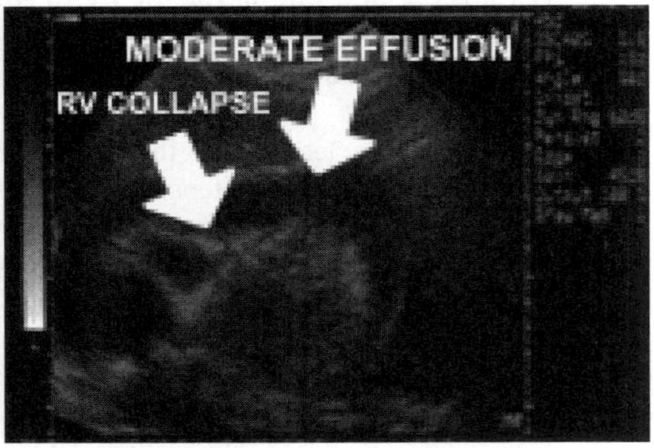

Major sonographic signs of tamponade are:
- Large pericardial effusion with swinging heart.
- Systolic collapse of RA.
- Diastolic collapse of RV.
- Inferior vena cava (IVC) plethora (dilatation > 20mm and < 50% reduction in the diameter of IVC with respiratory phases).
- Variations in E velocities during respiration across the mitral valve, tricuspid valve, and pulmonary outflow that are greater than 25, 50, and 30%.

Figure 1. Subxiphoid view of the heart showing a small pericardial effusion due to chest wall trauma that is already hemodynamically compromising as seen by RA collapse.

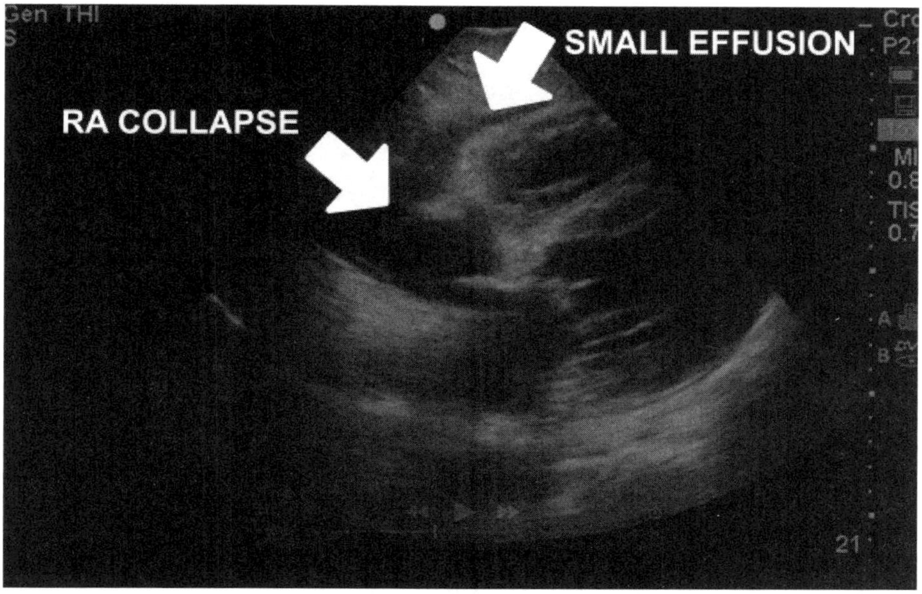

Figure 2. Large pericardial effusion in a patient with lung cancer that is now hemodynamically significant as seen by end-diastolic RV collapse.

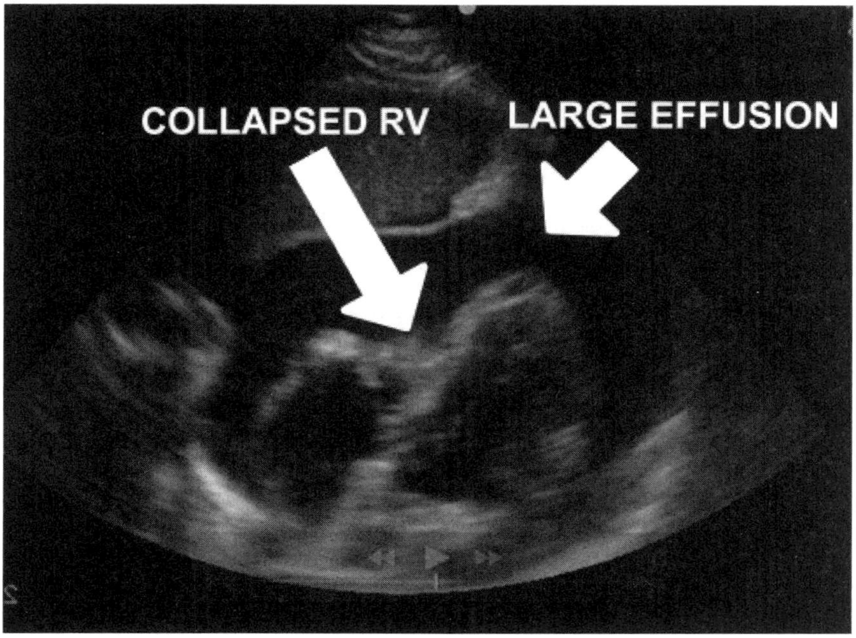

Figure 3. This is a patient with recent minor thoracic trauma, on warfarin, who presented with syncope. There is blood within the pericardial space that has partially clotted. Clot has the same echogenicity as the adjacent myocardium, which can lead to underdiagnosis of the effusion or size estimates.

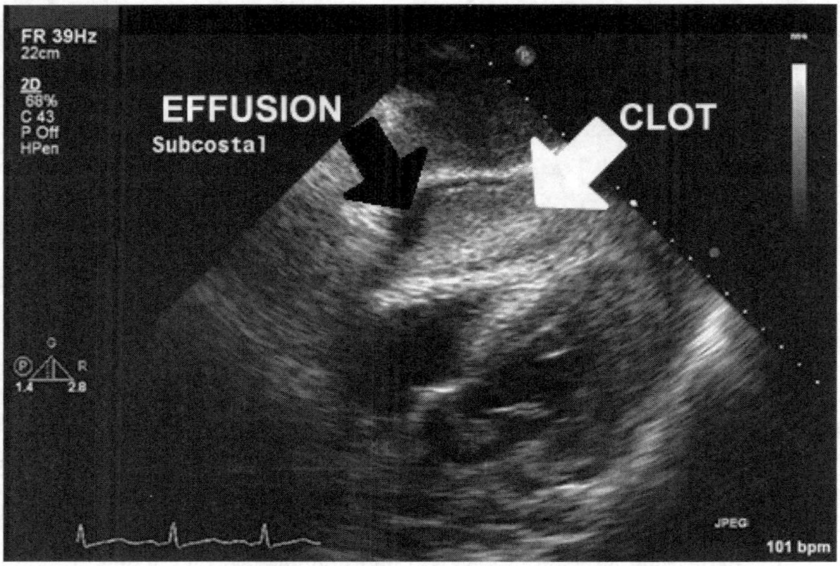

Q#3: Should the EP perform a pericardiocentesis or wait for the cardiologist?

This is a tough call, because it is a procedure that is rarely performed and usually only under stressful conditions! I would venture to say that even a consultant cardiologist would have limited experience in performing emergent pericardiocentesis. Yet the performance of procedures in the setting of life-threatening conditions is what emergency physicians do, even if done infrequently. Pericardiocentesis falls in the same category as cricothyrotomy, an uncommon procedure that is essential and time-dependent when needed. As with emergent "crics," all ED physicians should take advantage of educational opportunities to maintain skills learned in residency through simulation and a wide variety of online instructional materials.

Consulting editor comments (Weingart):

This is a critical time to assess the confidence of the emergency physician to successfully perform US guided pericardiocentesis; if you can see a big pocket that you can reach with no intervening structures, the barrier to pull the trigger should be much smaller. If there is only the ability to perform a Hail-Mary/blind pericardiocentesis, I would wait until the last moment if a consultant is coming in, and they can do this under fluoroscopic guidance or US at the bedside.

Consulting editor comments (Weingart):

Note: Blind placement of a needle into a suspected pericardial effusion is very likely to just drain the ventricle and not the effusion. There should be no blind pericardiocentesis short of cardiac arrest—this is potentially deadly.

Q#4: What is the best option for the EP to emergently drain the effusion/tamponade?
Breathe, use POCUS and believe that you are the best person to save this person's life!

Pericardiocentesis procedural pearls:

1. Prep: Clean skin, elevate the head of bed to angle 30–45 degrees if possible to draw the heart more anteriorly. Use an 18Ga spinal needle, 20mL syringe. Methods for ongoing drainage include using a 3-way stopcock with tubing and also placing a catheter (8fr.pigtail/catheter).
2. Approach to pericardiocentesis when using sonographic guidance:
   a. The optimal approach is at the level of the 5th intercostal space, lateral to where you imagine the internal mammary artery.
   b. Apical, 1 interspace below and 1cm lateral to PMI toward right shoulder.
   c. Blind pericardiocentesis (PEA arrest): The subxiphoid approach is 45 degrees along subxiphoid and left costal margin aiming towards left shoulder.
3. Procedure: Enter skin, aspirate continuously. Upon blood return, can use 3-way stopcock to drain.
4. After procedure: Use ultrasound if available to evaluate for improvement in effusion. Get chest x-ray to evaluate for pneumothorax and hemothorax.

Figure 4. This is a phantom view of needle aspiration of a pericardial effusion that closely represents the images seen in "real-life."

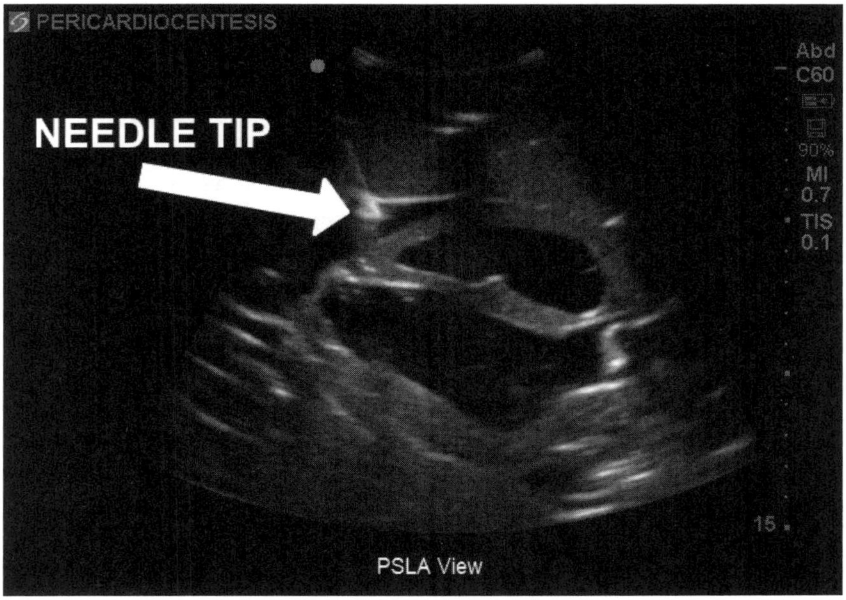

http://www.bluephantom.com/product/Transthoracic-Echocardiography-and-Pericardiocentesis-Ultrasound-Training-Model.aspx?cid=411. Image provided courtesy of CAE Healthcare.

The key question here is whether the EP should "wait." A consensus committee by the European Society of Cardiology in 2015 developed a scoring system to guide the timing of the intervention.[11]

Our patient has a score of 7 without ECHO! Consideration of his physical findings, CXR and ECG, mandates urgent pericardiocentesis.

- Dyspnea (1)
- Hypotension (0.5)
- Progressive tachycardia (1)
- Rapid worsening of sx (2)
- Cardiomegaly on CXR (1)
- Electrical Alternans (0.5)
- Microvoltage on ECG (1.5)

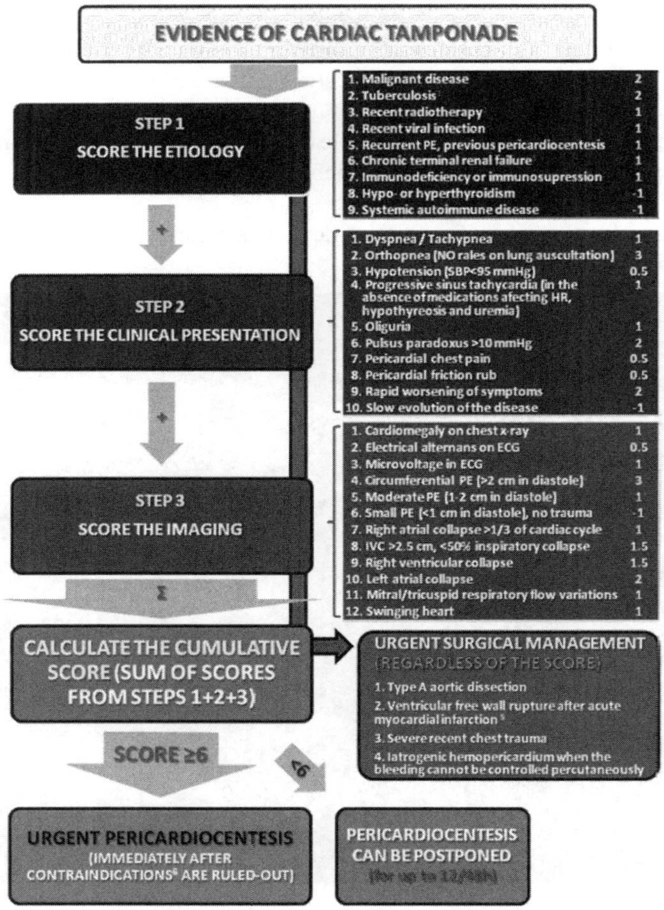

Ristić AD, Imazio M, Adler Y, et al. Triage strategy for urgent management of cardiac tamponade: a position statement of the European Society of Cardiology Working Group on Myocardial and Pericardial Diseases. Eur Heart J. 2014 Sep 7;35(34):2279-84. Copyright © 2014, Oxford University Press. Used with permission.

DECISION POINT B – ***What did the actual provider do?***

MDM 20:38: I did review the chest x-ray from today. This was done as a stat portable chest x-ray. Does show an enlarged heart which sometimes can be present with the portable chest x-rays. I did compare to previous. Today's film does show a large heart as has been seen in the past; however, the patient's lungs do appear mostly clear and do appear improved compared to previous x-ray. The blood pressure did now decrease to 72 systolic. Will give a 500mL normal saline bolus. I will go back and see the patient. He has been moved to the trauma room. Labs have returned:

Results review:

WBC Count	**13.7thou/mcL**	**HI**
Hemoglobin	**9.9gm/dL**	**LOW**
Platelet Count	284thou/mcL	
Sodium Level	**123mmol/L**	**LOW**
Potassium Level	**6.1mmol/L**	**CRIT**
Chloride Level	**91mmol/L**	**LOW**
Carbon Dioxide Level	**16mmol/L**	**LOW**
Anion Gap	16.0mMol/L	
Glucose Level	**438mg/dL**	**HI**
BUN	**171mg/dL**	**HI**
Creatinine	**5.61mg/dL**	**HI**
Lactic Acid Level	**2.6 mmol/L**	**HI**
B Type Natriuretic Peptide	**131Picogram/ml**	**HI**
Prothrombin Time (PT)	**96.9Sec**	**HI**
INR	**8.43**	**CRIT**
Troponin I POCT	0.01ng/mL	

MDM (continued): I did review the patient's labs. Lactate elevated 2.6. INR is elevated at 8.4. I did speak with [the cardiologist] as the echocardiogram is being done at this time. The patient does have a large pericardial effusion. He is coming in to perform emergent pericardiocentesis.

Expert commentary: Was the action of the EP appropriate? What could have been done better?
As written, this physician's actions do not suggest an appropriate urgency in managing this very sick patient! Even if unable to perform a bedside ECHO, they should be at the bedside and watching the technician. On seeing the effusion, it should have been clear that this was the cause of the patient's hypotension (no surprise) and the physician should be concerned that it may be hemorrhagic because of the markedly elevated INR. They should have been on the phone with the blood bank to order PCC, type and cross-matched blood, and then called the cardiologist to inform them of the findings and to drive to the hospital faster! At the same time a needle and syringe with alligator clamps should be clamped to the leads on the ECG in readiness to perform an emergent

pericardiocentesis if the patient were to lose pulses (PEA arrest). In the majority of mechanical causes of PEA arrest (tamponade, tension pneumothorax, pulmonary embolism), RV filling is compromised. Chest compressions directly over the RV may further limit RV filling and hence LV filling! I would suggest that they have a 500mcg dose of phenylephrine at hand for pressor support until the pericardium is drained.

DECISION POINT C – YOU ARE FACED W ITH 2 QUESTIONS:

1. **Should the patient undergo emergent pericardiocentesis or be sent to surgery for a pericardial window?**
2. **What is the quickest way to reverse the anticoagulation?**

Q#1: Should the patient undergo emergent pericardiocentesis or be sent to surgery for a pericardial window?

The patient is in obstructive shock and is decompensating while in the ED. They have a problem which can be temporized by a procedure within the scope of practice of the EP. In the setting of his coagulopathy, it would be advised to leave a drain in place (i.e., 8 fr. catheter or catheter from pericardiocentesis kit) in case it was to reaccumulate.

Echocardiography or fluoroscopy-guided pericardiocentesis is the usual method of choice for drainage of pericardial effusions, with surgery is reserved for the following 4 scenarios:

1. Type-A aortic dissection.
2. Free wall rupture after a myocardial infarction.
3. Recent and severe chest trauma.
4. Iatrogenic hemopericardium when bleeding cannot be controlled through percutaneous access.[17-19]

This patient has had both trauma and a catheterization in the recent past and is anticoagulated. He is at great risk for hemopericardium, so that a catheter (rather than needle aspiration) should be placed within the pericardium to allow for continued drainage and CT surgery notified as back-up.

Section editor comments (Greenwood):

In the setting of hemopericardium from type-A dissection or free wall rupture, one additional consideration of the EP would be to perform a controlled pericardial drainage as a bridge to the OR instead of a complete pericardial drainage. The goal is to improve the patient's hemodynamics enough to maintain systemic perfusion but not to excessively increase the patient's blood pressure to encourage re-bleeding. An interval drainage of 5–10 mLs of pericardial fluid to achieve a systolic blood pressure goal between 80–90mmHg, should be sufficient to improve the patient's clinical status and prevent further deterioration.[20]

Consulting editor comments (Weingart):

I agree!! I took 3mLs off of a dying type A dissection recently and the patient was rock solid stable through 60-minute transfer after the procedure.

Q#2: What is the quickest way to reverse the anticoagulation?

Patient is having tamponade which is likely hemorrhagic and an INR > 8. The INR needs to be urgently corrected prior to performance of pericardiocentesis. Once a drain/window has been established, there will be the ongoing concern for continued bleeding. He should receive vitamin K 10mg IV and 4-factor prothrombin complex concentrate (PCC) which is dosed based on INR and body weight. For this patient with an INR of 8.0, he should receive 50U/kg; max dose 5,000U capped at 100 kg body weight for VKA reversal. Per unit volume, 4F-PCCs contain approximately 25 times the concentration of vitamin K–dependent factors as compared with plasma (1U/mL). Therefore, PCC can be given in a much smaller volume at a much faster infusion rate (8×) compared with plasma.[21]

DECISION POINT C – ***What did the actual provider do?***

MDM (21:08): I did speak with the pharmacist and we will do a prothrombin complex concentrate and they will send that down emergently. His blood pressure is now 60/palp and he is lethargic and diaphoretic. I asked for 250mcg of phenylephrine to be administered and a spinal needle to perform an emergent pericardiocentesis. I was able to withdraw 50cc of bloody fluid with improvement the patient's BP to 110 systolic. He had a brief run of VT and is now more alert.

Expert commentary: This is where the EP physician got lucky. A blind pericardiocentesis was performed and the observed VT was likely due to minor myocardial injury. There was improvement in the patient's BP which is a good thing and may have been due to the phenylephrine as well as the small volume drained.

MDM (22:23): [The cardiologist] did arrive and placed a catheter in the pericardial space and at this point has removed 300mL of dark red hemorrhagic fluid. The patient is receiving prothrombin complex concentrate (PCC) and IV vitamin K. The patient did receive Versed 2mg and morphine 2mg prior to the procedure. I have reviewed the labs. For the hyperkalemia he did receive dextrose, insulin and sodium bicarbonate. Patient does have significant hyperkalemia and significantly worsened renal failure.

Critical care time: 98 minutes

Final diagnosis:

Pericardial tamponade secondary to hemorrhage secondary to over coagulation from Coumadin, tachycardia, hypotension, acute on chronic renal failure, anemia, severe hyponatremia, hyperkalemia.

The patient is admitted to the intensive care unit with a consult to the intensivist and the cardiologist.

Final discussion/chapter author expert opinion:

This is a patient who presented in triage at 19:39 with vital signs showing a HR of 121 and BP 78/58. Patient presumptively was seen by a PA where H&P was obtained. Forty minutes later the hypotensive patient is first seen by MD at 20:16. This seem to be an excessively long delay in MD notification when seeing a patient with unstable vital signs at triage. MD notes that heart tones are distant, and the ECG shows low voltage QRS with a rate of 104. An ECHO is then ordered "stat" at 20:31. The CXR is reviewed and shows an enlarged heart. Labs are reviewed at 20:40 and show that he is hyperglycemic, acidotic, coagulopathic and uremic. The patient then becomes more hypotensive, and a fluid bolus is given. Over the next 2 hours the patient was treated with fluids, PCC, and Vitamin K awaiting the arrival of the echocardiographer and cardiologist. Fortunately, the patient survived despite what can be interpreted as delays in care owing to the failure to perform a bedside echo on the patient's arrival.

Timeline (a look back at this case): Arrival 19:39 > Pericardiocentesis @ 22:23 = 2 hours and 44 minutes

An alternative scenario including the use of echocardiography would be the following:

19:39 - Pt arrives with unstable VS.

20:00 Physician made aware and obtains history of trauma, recent instrumentation and medications. Requests immediate assistance from staff to start IV fluids and send off INR, lactate, VBG, Type and Screen. ECG obtained showing sinus tachycardia and low voltage.

20:15 Bedside ECHO performed by physician that identifies pericardial effusion with tamponade physiology.

20:30 Physician reviews labs and sees elevated INR. Orders PCC.

21:00 PCC given. Equipment assembled to perform pericardiocentesis (Betadine, Lidocaine and 18-gauge needle). Aspiration of hemorrhagic fluid until aspiration is dry and/or BP improves.

Timeline (optimal/improved): Arrival 19:39 > Pericardiocentesis @ 21:00 = 1 hour 21 minutes

Inpatient course:

Cardiology consultation: Patient with recent hospitalization for CP/PNA with an echo showing a trivial pericardial effusion presented with elevated INR/distant heart tones/low voltage ECG per ED. Stat echo was ordered showing a large pericardial effusion. Bedside pericardiocentesis was performed in the setting of coagulopathy due to hypotension and tamponade. Improved hemodynamics after procedure. Effusion likely a combination of uremia and coagulopathy. Resume warfarin when effusion and renal function stabilized. Will follow.

References:

1. Jones CB, Fugate SE. Levofloxacin and Warfarin interaction. Ann Pharmacother 2002;36(10):1554-7.
2. Jones AE, Tayal VS, Sullivan DM, et al. Randomized, controlled trial of immediate versus delayed goal-directed ultrasound to identify the cause of nontraumatic hypotension in emergency department patients. Crit Care Med 2004;32(8):1703-8.

3. Volpicelli G, Lamorte A, Tullio M, et al. Point-of-care multiorgan ultrasonography for the evaluation of undifferentiated hypotension in the emergency department. Intensive Care Med 2013;39:1290.
4. Shokoohi H, Boniface KS, Pourmand A, et al. Bedside ultrasound reduces diagnostic uncertainty and guides resuscitation in patients with undifferentiated hypotension. Crit Care Med 2015;43:2562–9.
5. Perera P, Mailhot T, Riley, et al. The RUSH Exam 2012: Rapid ultrasound in shock in the evaluation of the critically ill patient. Ultrasound Clin 2012;7(2):255-7.
6. Atkinson P, Bowra J, Milne J, et al. International Federation for Emergency Medicine Consensus Statement: Sonography in hypotension and cardiac arrest (SHoC): An international consensus on the use of point of care ultrasound for undifferentiated hypotension and during cardiac arrest. CJEM 2016;21:1-12.
7. Milne J, Atkinson P, Lewis D, et al. Sonography in hypotension and cardiac arrest (SHoC): Rate of abnormal findings in undifferentiated hypotension and during cardiac arrest as a basis for consensus on a hierarchical point of care ultrasound protocol. Cureus 2016;8(4):e564.
8. Atkinson PRT, McAuley DJ, Kendall RJ, et al. Abdominal and cardiac evaluation with sonography in shock (ACES): An approach by emergency physicians for the use of ultrasound in patients with undifferentiated hypotension. Emerg Med J 2009;26:87-91.
9. Monnet X, Marik P, Teboul JL. Passive leg raising for predicting fluid responsiveness: A systematic review and meta-analysis. Intensive Care Med 2016;42(12):1935-47.
10. Spodick DS. Acute Cardiac Tamponade. N Engl J Med 2003;349:684-90A.
11. Adler Y, Charron P, Imazio M, et al. 2015 ESC Guidelines for the diagnosis and management of pericardial diseases: The Task Force for the Diagnosis and Management of Pericardial Diseases of the European Society of Cardiology (ESC). Eur Heart J 2015;36(42):2921-64.
12. Labovitz AJ, Noble VE, Bierig M. Focused cardiac ultrasound in the emergent setting: A consensus statement of the American Society of Echocardiography and American College of Emergency Physicians. J Am Soc Echocardiogr 2010;23(12):1225-30.
13. Akhtar S, Theodoro D, Gaspari R, et al. Resident training in emergency ultrasound: Consensus recommendations from the 2008 Council of Emergency Medicine Residency Directors Conference. Acad Emerg Med 2009;16:S32–6.
14. Roy CL, Minor MA, Brookhart MA, et al. Does this patient with a pericardial effusion have cardiac tamponade? JAMA 2007;297(16):1810–8.
15. Eisenberg MJ, de Romeral LM, Heidenreich PA. The diagnosis of pericardial effusion and cardiac tamponade by 12-lead ECG. A technology assessment. Chest 1996;110(2):318-24.
16. Imazio M, Adler Y. Management of pericardial effusion. Eur Heart J 2013;34(16):1186-97.
17. Tsung T, Enriquez-Sarano M, Freeman WK, et al. Consecutive 1127 therapeutic echocardiographically guided pericardiocenteses: Clinical profile, practice patterns, and outcomes spanning 21 years. Mayo Clin Proc 2002;77:429-36.
18. Callahan JA, Seward JB, Nishimura RA, et al. Two-dimensional echocardiographically guided pericardiocentesis: Experience in 117 consecutive patients. Am J Cardiol 1985;55:476–9.
19. Silvestry FE, Kerber RE, Brook MM, et al. Echocardiography-guided interventions. J Am Soc Echocardiogr 2009;22:213-31.

20. Hayashi T, Tsukube T, Yamashita T, et al. Impact of controlled pericardial drainage on critical cardiac tamponade with acute type A aortic dissection. Circulation 2012;126(11 Suppl 1):S97-S101.
21. Tomaselli GF, Mahaffey KW, Cuker A, et al. 2017 ACC expert consensus decision pathway on management of bleeding in patients on oral anticoagulants. J Am Coll Cardiol 2017;70(24):3042-67.

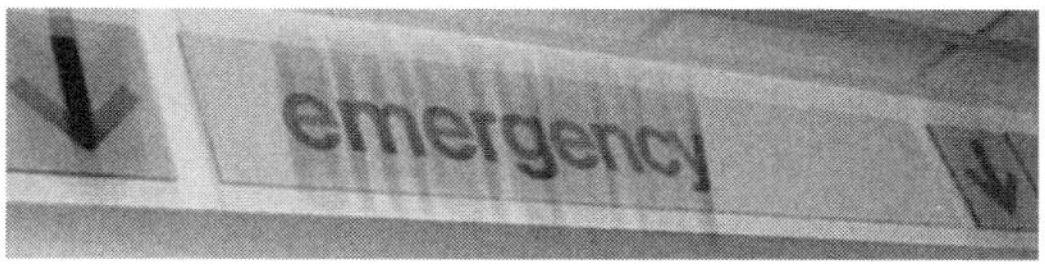

SECTION C – CARDIAC/ VASCULAR

Chapter 12: A 59-year-old methamphetamine user with nontraumatic back pain

Rene Ramirez, MD
Assistant Clinical Professor
Emergency Medicine
Community Regional Medical Center Department of Emergency Medicine
UCSF Fresno, Fresno CA

Miranda Lewis, MD
Department of Emergency Medicine, PGY4 UCSF Fresno
Fresno, CA

Eileen Shu, MD
Assistant Clinical Professor
Community Regional Medical Center Department of Emergency Medicine
UCSF Fresno, Fresno, CA
Assistant Clinical Professor, Antelope Valley Hospital Department of Emergency Medicine
UCLA, Lancaster, CA

Jessica Mason, MD
Assistant Clinical Professor
Emergency Medicine
Department of Emergency Medicine
UCSF Fresno, Fresno, CA

Section editor:
John C. Greenwood, MD
Assistant Professor
Department of Emergency Medicine, Department of Anesthesiology and Critical Care
Perelman School of Medicine
University of Pennsylvania, Philadelphia, PA

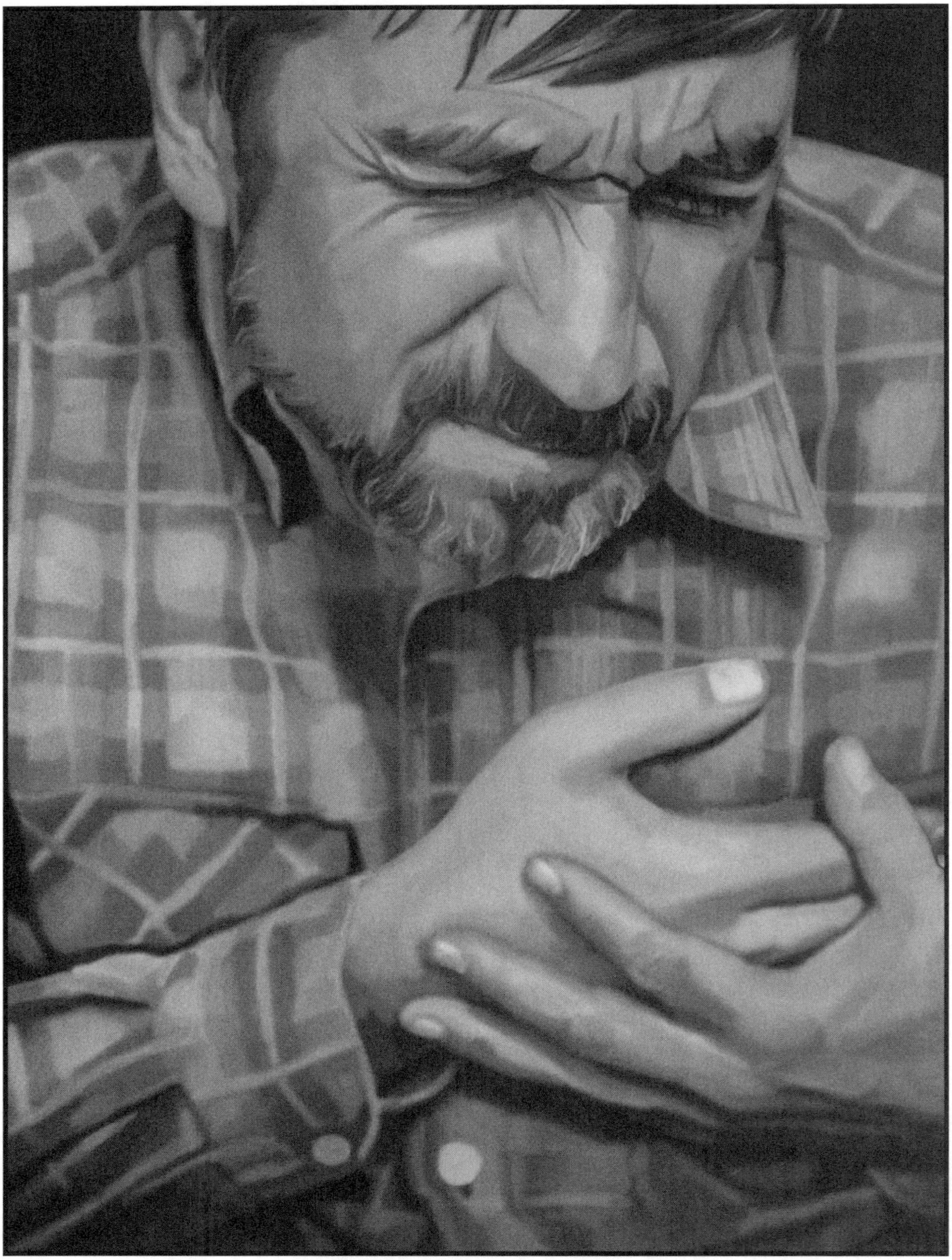

SECTION C/CHAPTER 12

A 59-year-old methamphetamine user with nontraumatic back pain

Nontraumatic back pain is a common complaint in the emergency department (ED), accounting for 2–3% of all ED visits[1]. Usually, the etiology is benign and self-limited; however, there is a small percentage of patients who have dangerous pathology. This patient was seen in the ED on three separate occasions, the first two with the complaint of back pain—it was not until his final visit that the accurate diagnosis was made.

INITIAL ED VISIT

HPI (19:19): 59 y.o. male presents for medical clearance after being tased. Patient complaining of severe back pain, writhing in pain and states he has difficulty speaking or taking a deep breath due to pain. Denies medical problems, felt fine prior to taser application. Nursing note and vitals reviewed

PMH/PSH: denies
SH: in custody
Medications and allergies have been reviewed

ROS:
CONSTITUTIONAL: Negative for fever.
RESP: Positive for shortness of breath. Negative for cough.
CARDIO: Negative for palpitations.
NEURO: Negative for syncope, weakness and numbness.

PE:
BP: 168/112 mmHg | Heart Rate: 78 | Temp: 37° C (98.6° F) | Temp src: Oral
Resp: 18 | SpO_2: 97 % | O_2 Device: None (Room air)

CONSTITUTIONAL: He is oriented to person, place, and time. He appears well-developed and well-nourished. He appears distressed (writhing).
HEAD: Normocephalic and atraumatic.
EYES: Pupils are equal, round, and reactive to light.
NECK: Neck supple.
CARDIO: Normal rate, regular rhythm and normal heart sounds.

PULM/CHEST: Effort normal and breath sounds normal. No respiratory distress. He has no wheezes. He has no rales. Clear, equal, good volumes. Two small wounds from taser application, no hematoma.
ABDOMINAL: Soft. He exhibits no distension. There is no tenderness.
MUSCULOSKELETAL: He exhibits no edema.
NEURO: He is alert and oriented to person, place, and time.
SKIN: Skin is warm and dry. He is not diaphoretic.

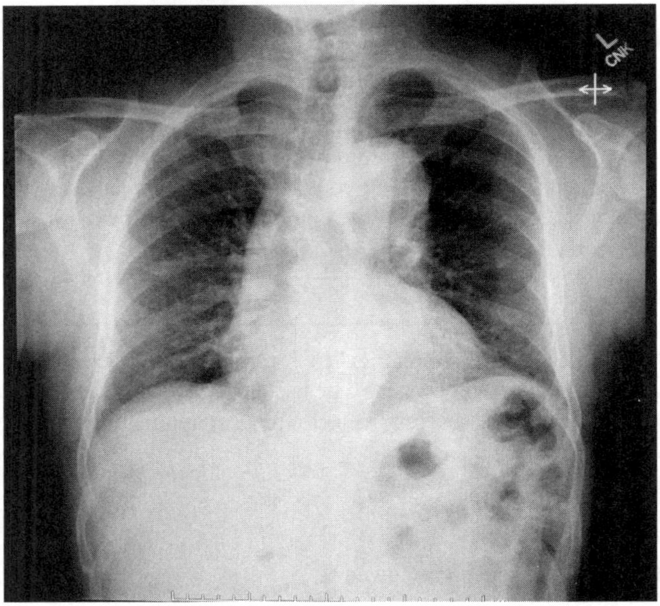

ED Course (22:20): patient sleeping comfortably, no distress, vitals improved. Feels well.
MDM: 59 y.o. male with pain and subjective shortness of breath after taser application, satting well on room air, chest x-ray normal, lung exam normal. Improved during stay. Medically clear for jail.
Clinical Impression: Medical clearance for incarceration

Documentation issues at visit #1:

The initial visit note is very brief, which is typical. This appears to be a cursory visit, likely required by jail policy. The exam is thorough, including documentation that there are no taser probes embedded in the back. The chest x-ray (CXR), likely ordered because of the pleuritic pain and concern for pneumothorax or rib fractures, is read as negative by the emergency provider. The patient is reassessed, and he is no longer distressed, looks and feels well, and is discharged to jail.

Note: The overread of the CXR after the patient has left states: "Possible ascending thoracic aortic aneurysm." There is no follow-up on this interpretation.

Differential of a widened mediastinum:

A widened mediastinum, > 8cm measured near the aortic knob, can be seen on a CXR view due to:

- Magnification of the heart and mediastinal structures
- An unfolded aortic arch
- Mediastinal lymphadenopathy
- Retrosternal thyroid
- Thymoma
- Paravertebral mass
- Dilation of the esophagus
- Ruptured aorta[2]
- Sternal fracture with retrosternal mediastinal hematoma[3]
- Mediastinal lipomatosis[4]
- Tortuous atherosclerotic vessels[5]
- Cardiac tamponade[6]
- Thoracic aortic aneurysm (TAD)
- Rare causes (reported as single case studies alone) include:
    - Pulmonary artery aneurysm
    - Pulmonary artery dissection[7]
    - Loculated pleural effusion[8]

Patients may have widened mediastinum, depending on how the image is taken, given that the mediastinal width is directly related to type of film (PA vs. AP) as well as degree of inspiration. Several studies have found that upright chest films with full inspiration are the most sensitive for actual pathology; some studies recommend only this type of image be used.[9,10]

Section editor comments (Greenwood):

The overread of this chest x-ray places the emergency physician (EP) at significant risk of litigation if not promptly followed up. Reading standard radiography is well within the skill set of emergency physicians. However, there needs to be a mechanism to address discrepancies after the specialist read. The clinician's documentation provides no medical decision-making narrative of EP CXR interpretation, making it difficult to know if an aortic dissection was considered.

ED VISIT #2 (9 months later at 03:33)

ED provider note: Rapid Medical Evaluation

HPI: Patient is complaining of left sided para thoracic muscle pain after laying down x 3 days.

PMH: Negative

Social history: Negative

ROS:
CONSTITUTIONAL: Negative for fever.
RESP: Negative for cough and shortness of breath.

CARDIO: Negative for chest pain.
GASTRO: Negative for abdominal pain.
GENITOURINARY: Negative for dysuria and flank pain.
MUSCULOSKELETAL: Positive for back pain. Negative for neck pain.
SKIN: Negative for rash.
NEURO: Negative for dizziness and headaches.
PSYCHIATRIC/BEHAVIORAL: The patient is not nervous/anxious.

PE:
BP: 143/108 mmHg | Heart Rate: 84 | Heart Rate Source: Monitor | Temp: 36.6° C (97.9° F)
Temp src: Oral | Resp: 18 | SpO2: 98 % | O2 Device: None (Room air)
CONSTITUTIONAL: He is oriented to person, place, and time and well-developed, well-nourished, and in no distress.
EYES: Conjunctivae are normal.
CARDIO: Normal rate, regular rhythm and normal heart sounds.
PULM/CHEST: Breath sounds normal.
ABDOMINAL: Soft. There is no tenderness.
MUSCULOSKELETAL: Tender to right parathoracic muscle area
NEURO: He is alert and oriented to person, place, and time.
SKIN: Skin is warm and dry.

IMPRESSION: Muscle strain
MDM and Plan: I will discharge with ibuprofen for pain. Discharge instructions for muscle strain.

Hmmm, this work-up seems very basic for the patient's complaint, and the documentation leaves a lot of unanswered questions.

Documentation issues visit #2:
HPI: The HPI is short without descriptors of pain (severity, radiation, exacerbating/alleviating factors, associated symptoms). Luckily, we do have a review of systems with pertinent negatives including no chest pain or dyspnea. Classic "red flags" were only addressed on a cursory basis; the patient denied fever, but it is not clear if he was asked about neurological symptoms such as numbness/tingling of limbs, gait problems, bowel or bladder incontinence. Social history is documented as "negative," but it is unclear if intravenous drug use (IVDU) was specifically addressed.
PE: The patient is hypertensive with a diastolic blood pressure of 108 during this visit without prior history of hypertension; this is not addressed by the provider. Left-sided parathoracic pain is documented in the history of present illness, but right-sided parathoracic muscle tenderness is documented in the exam. Could this represent radiation of pain or was it just a laterality error in documentation? The neurological exam is inadequate.
MDM: There is no documentation of the provider's thought process; we are left to guess if serious diagnoses were considered. It is unlikely that the provider reviewed past imaging documenting a widened mediastinum.

Follow-up: There is no follow-up plan, return precautions, or counseling of the patient documented. If there is diagnostic uncertainty, the patient needs to know when to return and why.

Medical and risk management/patient safety issues visit #2:
How reliable is reproducible pain at ruling out dangerous causes of chest/back pain?
Although we palpate the chest wall in patients with chest pain, tender pectoral muscles or ribs do not prove a musculoskeletal etiology11 and do not rule out serious causes, such as acute coronary syndrome (ACS)[12,13] or acute MI.[12-15] In fact, no single descriptor in the chest pain history can be used alone to rule out dangerous causes of chest pain.[14] How about PE? Le Gal and colleagues found that there was no association between chest wall tenderness and lower prevalence of pulmonary embolism.[16] Lastly, how about reproducible pain and dissection? This is even less studied; we only identified one case study, in which a 73-year-old man with a thoracic aortic dissection (TAD) presented with only left-sided pleuritic chest pain and minor tenderness to palpation of the left lower chest wall.[17] We are left with inadequate data to make a conclusive recommendation.

So how do we balance patient safety with over testing and over admitting? Much depends on our pre-test suspicion as well as a mechanism of injury. For example, a 22-year-old who has a sudden onset of chest pain while lifting a couch and has point tenderness at the left lower sternal border does not likely require admission, whereas a 60-year-old with a history of coronary artery bypass surgery and a gradual onset of exertional pain with diaphoresis and generalized chest pain reproducible with palpation might be managed differently. The key is that reproducible pain can occur with serious causes of chest pain and does not definitively rule them out.

1. How sensitive and specific is back pain in the diagnosis of TAD?
In their 2015 publication, Pape, et al.,[18] reviewed 17 years of data among 4,428 patients with aortic dissection and found that only 43% of those with type A (ascending) dissection had back pain compared to 70% of patients with a type B (descending) dissection. In contrast, the rates for chest pain were 85% and 67% for type A and B dissections, respectively.[18] China created a Registry of Aortic Dissection in 2011 (Sino-RAD), which covers 15 different Chinese centers; of the 1,003 patients in their cohort, 77% of all patients (71.9% of type A dissection and 80.8% of type B dissection) had back pain.[19] Though percentages were higher in the Chinese cohort overall, the data from the two groups are consistent in that more type B dissections present with back pain than type A dissections.

In summary, back pain is often but not always present in aortic dissection, no matter the type of dissection (A or B), but the finding is not sensitive enough to forgo additional testing in a high-risk patient without back pain.

2. How sensitive and specific is a widened mediastinum on CXR?
A 2002 JAMA review looking at 21 studies between 1966 and 2000 found that the pooled sensitivity of widened mediastinum for dissection was 64% (95% CI: 44–80%).[20] Of note, there may be other abnormalities:

CXR findings concerning for TAD (see Table 1).

Table 1. Chest x-ray Findings in Thoracic Aortic Dissection

1. Widened mediastinum
2. Aortic knob blurring or widening
3. Difference in diameter of ascending and descending aorta
4. Blurring of aortic margin
5. Unilateral or bilateral effusion
6. Calcium sign (>5mm separation of intimal calcification to outmost border of the aortic knob)

They report a pooled sensitivity of 90% (95% CI: 87–92%) for any abnormal chest radiograph findings, and with a normal mediastinum and aortic contour on CXR, the negative likelihood ratio was 0.3, 95% CI 0.2–0.3.[20] This study reported that no particular single radiographic abnormality was dependably present in all cases of aortic dissection.

In 2004, von Kodolitsch and his colleagues specifically addressed the diagnostic accuracy of routine CXR for diagnosing aortic syndromes (dissection, aneurysm, ulcer, and intramural hematoma), and found CXR to be 64% sensitive and 86% specific in those with suspected aortic disease. For dissection, sensitivity was 67% and specificity 70%.[21]

The International Registry of Acute Aortic Dissection (IRAD) is an international consortium of 30 large referral centers in 11 countries that have been collecting data on aortic dissections since 1996. They reviewed data of CXRs of 464 patients with TAD and found mediastinal widening in only 62.6% of patients, with a completely normal CXR in 12.4%.[22]

In summary, CXR is not sensitive nor specific enough to exclude aortic disease.

3. What do the guidelines say?

Several groups have developed "rules" to rule out low risk patients by identifying variables that are independent predictors of acute aortic dissection, but they missed an unacceptably large subset of patients with active aortic disease.[20,23,24] This is in part because aortic dissection has such a variable presentation and is not exclusively an acute onset of tearing or ripping pain, mediastinal widening on CXR, or systolic pulse differential between extremities. In fact, one study found that the probability of having a dissection was still 7% absent all of these classic findings.[24] In 2015 an American College of Emergency Physicians (ACEP) committee addressed this question in a clinical policy, with level C recommendations that those with very low risk for acute nontraumatic thoracic aortic dissection cannot be identified with existing clinical decision rules alone.[25]

So how can we decide who needs further imaging to rule out aortic pathology? The key to making the diagnosis is to have a high level of suspicion, obtain a thorough history and be alert for history and exam findings that suggest the diagnosis such as: sudden and severe onset of pain, radiation to the back, chest pain plus neurologic complaints, symptoms above and below the diaphragm, unexplained tachycardia, widened mediastinum, pulse/blood pressure differential, or when there is no alternative explanation for the patient's symptoms. While there is no decision rule to rule out the diagnosis, the above findings should raise suspicion for TAD and prompt further work-up.

4. When is it appropriate to discharge a patient with only a rapid medical evaluation?
Rapid medical evaluation (RME) units in emergency departments are becoming more common to decrease length of stay and to decrease those leaving before being seen. They are typically staffed by physician assistants, nurse practitioners, and physicians. Though there are papers that commend RME units[26] and many departments are shifting toward this model, there is an inherent risk to missing serious but rare diseases. The Chartier paper called their RME unit "a new pathway of care for patients with lower acuity presentations," prompting the question: who determines if a patient is low risk/acuity? Low acuity is often defined by a low Emergency Severity Index (ESI), which can under-triage as many as 27% of patients.[27] How much does triage cueing, ascertainment bias, diagnostic momentum, and anchoring bias play a role?

5. Radiology call backs:
The quality control process for radiology overreads needs to be tight, with institutional procedures in place so patients are alerted on reads where there is a discrepancy. Not only is there a moral and ethical duty to disclose errors such as a missed CXR interpretation,[28] but data suggests that there may be decreased litigation and increased physician trust if the error is disclosed by the physician.[29,30] Even removing the question of physician risk, we have a professional obligation.

THE BOUNCEBACK (approximately 11 months after initial visit)

Patient arrives at 06:34

Advanced Practice Provider (APP) Note (09:48):
CC: Patient presents with Pain Abdomen mid epigastric, + Meth and ETOH use tonight.

HPI: 60-year-old male here with acute onset mid upper epigastric abdominal pain last night. Non radiating. Pain has been constant since onset. Began at 8pm + n/v. No hematemesis. No diarrhea. Endorses some body aches and chills. No similar illness in others
Despite cc above and triage provider note, patient is adamant that he has not drank since August 2014. He also denies meth use since 2011.
Some chest pain when vomiting. Not well described. Spanish speaking.

Past medical and/or surgical history: Denies pertinent medical or surgical history
SOC: Former ETOH; denies meth and alcohol use
Medications: none

ROS:
CONSTITUTIONAL: Negative for fever and chills.
RESP: Negative for cough and shortness of breath.
CARDIO: Negative for chest pain.
GASTRO: Positive for nausea, vomiting and abdominal pain. Negative for diarrhea, constipation and rectal pain.
GENITOURINARY: Negative for dysuria, hematuria and flank pain.
MUSCULOSKELETAL: Positive for myalgias.

NEURO: Negative for dizziness, weakness and headaches
HEMATOLOGICAL: Negative for adenopathy
All other systems reviewed and are negative

PE:
Initial Vitals:
BP: 105/77mmHg | Heart Rate: 70 | Temp: 37.1° C (98.8° F) | Temp src: Oral | Resp: 22
SpO2: 96 % | O2 Device: None (Room air)
CONSTITUTIONAL: He is oriented to person, place, and time. He appears well-developed. He appears distressed.
CARDIO: Normal rate and normal heart sounds.
No murmur heard.
PULM/CHEST: Effort normal and breath sounds normal. He has no wheezes. He has no rales.
ABDOMINAL: Soft. Bowel sounds are normal. He exhibits no distension. There is tenderness in the epigastric area and left lower quadrant. There is no rebound, no guarding, no tenderness at McBurney's point and negative Murphy's sign.
NEURO: He is alert and oriented to person, place, and time. No cranial nerve deficit.
SKIN: Skin is warm. No rash noted.
MDM (10:00): Uncomfortable appearing 60-year-old male here with acute onset upper epigastric abdominal pain, vomiting. On exam, exquisitely tender upper abdomen and LLQ. Ddx includes acute gastroenteritis, appy, cholecystitis, diverticulitis. Doubt acute coronary syndrome, AAA

Author comments (Weinstock):

The patient has a concerning differential diagnosis but only mildly abnormal vitals at this time. You are now in the footsteps of the provider. How should the work-up be started? Is the systolic blood pressure of 105mmHg concerning?

DECISION POINT A – YOU ARE FACED WITH 3 QUESTIONS:

1. **What is the differential diagnosis?**
2. **How should the work-up be initiated?**
3. **Which management options (IV, medications) should be started at this time?**

Q#1: What is the differential diagnosis?

Abdominal pain is one of the most common reasons that adults present to the emergency department.[31] The differential diagnosis for epigastric pain includes:

- Gastritis
- Peptic ulcer disease
- Gastric outlet obstruction
- Foreign body impaction
- Esophagitis
- Boerhaave syndrome
- Cholecystitis, cholelithiasis, choledocholithiasis, cholangitis

- Perforated viscous
- Acute coronary syndrome
- Abdominal aortic dissection
- Thoracic aortic dissection

Q#2: How should the work-up be initiated?

Most patients presenting with epigastric pain will receive a similar battery of tests including a (CBC) to evaluate for possible blood loss and infection, metabolic panel, LFTs, and lipase to evaluate for hepatobiliary pathology/pancreatitis, and based on age and presentation, an ECG and troponin to evaluate for ACS. This is a reasonable place to start. When advanced imaging is considered, we are more selective based on clinical assessment. In our patient with undifferentiated sudden onset severe epigastric pain, nausea, and emesis, it is reasonable to start with a bedside ultrasound (US) to evaluate for biliary pathology. Computed tomography (CT) can be helpful in identifying visceral and vascular pathology. The clinical appearance and relative hypotension compared with prior visits are concerning placing sepsis and hypovolemia on the differential. Given our patient's age, the "exquisitely tender" abdomen, acute onset pain, distress, and lack of similar prior presentation, many providers may order the above labs and a CT abdomen immediately upon arrival, but there is a risk to just "shotgunning" tests before an adequate H&P.

Q#3: Which management options (IV, medications) should be started at this time?

Based on the patient's initial clinical appearance (distress, severe abdominal pain and tenderness, borderline hypotension), these authors recommend obtaining 2 large-bore IVs, 1 to 2L IVF bolus (given no cardiac or fluid overload history), antiemetics, and pain control (as blood pressure tolerates) as a starting point while waiting for labs and imaging. That is, until the patient starts to decompensate.

DECISION POINT A – ***What did the actual provider do?***

Time (10:02): 12-lead ECG: Sinus tachycardia, rate 117; no ischemic ECG changes. Left axis deviation (no previous for comparison). A 1 liter normal saline bolus, 4mg IV ondansetron, and 6mg IV morphine were ordered.

MDM: Limited bedside ultrasound showed some pericholecystic fluid and GB wall thickening. This is worrisome for acute cholecystitis. Will order formal abdominal ultrasound.

ED course:
Labs show WBC 11.8, normal Hgb, CO_2 20, T bili 1.4, glucose 296

MDM (11:30): Review of the previous records shows a prior chest x-ray that was read as "widened mediastinum."

MDM (12:05): Notified by ultrasound tech that the patient has a 2cm pericardial effusion.

Section editor comments (Greenwood):

At 11:30, the ED provider (an APP) documents a records review that includes language on the previous radiology read that would raise concern for acute aortic pathology, yet there is no follow-up diagnostic test or intervention to investigate these findings further. If they are documenting a concern for possible acute aortic syndrome, a STAT CT angiogram to rule out acute aortic syndrome should be ordered. In addition to the CBC, metabolic panel, liver function tests, and cardiac enzymes, a critical test is a serum or point-of-care lactate. This test could lead the EP to be more aggressive in their decision to immediately obtain a CT angiogram to look for acute mesenteric ischemia, even if the patient is still in the radiology department finishing the ultrasound. The pericholecystic fluid is tricky. Certainly, it could be the cause for the patient's symptoms but could potentially be a sign of a dissection-related malperfusion, leading to visceral edema.

DECISION POINT B – YOU ARE FACED WITH 6 QUESTIONS:

1. **How sensitive and specific is point of care ultrasound (POCUS) for cholecystitis?**
2. **How does the widened mediastinum on CXR factor into the clinical decision-making?**
3. **Which historical and lab factors, such as D-dimer, help with the diagnosis?**
4. **What are ECG differences between acute coronary syndrome (ACS) and thoracic aortic dissection (TAD)?**
5. **What is on the differential diagnosis for nontraumatic pericardial effusion?**
6. **Who needs advanced imaging?**

Q#1: How sensitive and specific is point of care ultrasound (POCUS) for cholecystitis?

Emergency physicians can accurately detect acute cholecystitis by ultrasound,[32,33] but the findings should be taken in the context of the patient's presentation. Gallbladder wall thickening is not specific for acute cholecystitis and is seen in heart failure, renal failure, cirrhosis, malignancy, and even with physiologic contraction.[34]

Gallstones are one of the major criteria for ultrasound diagnosis of acute cholecystitis, present in most cases.[35] Gallstones and a sonographic Murphy's sign (neither of which were observed in our patient), have a positive predictive value of 92% for acute cholecystitis.[36] The isolated findings of gallbladder wall thickening and pericholecystic fluid, however, are not specific enough to make the diagnosis of acute cholecystitis. Some of our patient's symptoms may be consistent with acute cholecystitis. However, there are other concerning causes of epigastric pain, including the documented left lower quadrant pain which requires more investigating.

Q#2: How does the widened mediastinum on CXR factor into the clinical decision-making?

Although a widened mediastinum alone is not sensitive nor specific for the diagnosis of aortic dissection, our patient is now presenting with sudden onset severe pain and a BP of 105, significantly increasing the possibility of TAD. This should alert the ED provider to immediately order definitive diagnostic testing.

Q#3: Which historical and lab factors, such as D-dimer, help with the diagnosis?

The pain associated with aortic dissection is highly variable and depends on the location of the dissection. Most patients complain of chest pain, with back pain and abdominal pain also common,[37,18] but 5–6% of patients will not have any pain.[22,38] The most common pain characteristics in aortic dissection is sudden onset and "worst ever" pain, present in over 90% of cases.[37,18] Our patient is described as "uncomfortable appearing" and "distressed," which arguably meets this criterion. Visceral symptoms, such as the nausea and vomiting seen in our patient, are also common in dissection.[39]

D-dimer has been proposed as a screening test to exclude the diagnosis of aortic dissection in low risk patients with multiple studies suggesting that D-dimer has a high sensitivity.[40,25] Suzuki, et al., has presented prospective data suggesting risk stratification within the first 24 hours after symptom onset. They suggest a D-dimer of < 100ng/mL has an NPV 100% and a value of < 500ng/mL has an NPV 95%, with a negative likelihood ratio of 0.07 in the first 24 hours. In patients with a high pre-test probability they suggest a D-dimer of > 1600ng/mL within the first 6 hours may also help to support the diagnosis of an aortic dissection.[41] This takes into account time of onset of symptoms, but some patients present without any pain and may have a normal CXR.[42,22,38] While these studies show some promise, the use of D-dimer has not been validated in any large clinical trials and is not widely accepted as a screening lab. ACEP does not recommend using a D-dimer to assess for TAD.[25]

Q#4: What are ECG differences between acute coronary syndrome (ACS) and thoracic aortic dissection (TAD)?

ECG characteristics in aortic dissection are quite variable. Patients may have a normal ECG or have nonspecific changes, as was the case for our patient; 15–27% of patients with aortic dissection have some ECG evidence of ischemia.[22,43]

Aortic dissection is commonly misdiagnosed as ACS,[44-46] which is not surprising given type A TADs may dissect into the coronary arteries and cause a STEMI appearing ECG! Accordingly, many patients misdiagnosed as ACS receive antiplatelet or antithrombotic agents,[45-46] the last thing we want to do with TAD. In summary, ischemic ECG changes increase our suspicion for ACS but do not eliminate the possibility of TAD.

Section editor comments (Greenwood):

While rare (< 2%) there are no current recommendations from the *Journal of the American College of Cardiology* (JACC) or other leading bodies on how to risk stratify aortic dissection versus STEMI. In our patient, a CXR with a wide mediastinum or a history confirming back pain or chest pain radiating to the back might push the EP to get a CT angiogram (CTA) before activating the cath lab.

Q#5: What is on the differential diagnosis for nontraumatic pericardial effusion?

The most common causes of nontraumatic pericardial effusion are pericarditis, malignancy, infection, uremia, collagen vascular disease, and idiopathic effusions.[47-49] Pericardial effusion is commonly seen in type A aortic dissection, occurring in up to one-half of cases.[50] The abrupt onset of severe pain described by this patient combined with a pericardial effusion should prompt consideration for aortic dissection.

Q#6: Who needs advanced imaging?

Aortic dissection is a particularly difficult diagnosis to make. It is rare, affecting only around 2.9 to 4.7 in 100,000 people,[51-53] is variable in its presentation, and is deadly. It is a "ZERO MISS" diagnosis, but it would be cost-prohibitive and inefficient to use CT with every patient with aortic dissection on the differential diagnosis. We cannot rely on decision rules but need to consider the entire clinical picture to determine which patients warrant further investigation.

Transthoracic echocardiogram is best for visualizing the proximal aorta and pericardial effusion, but it has a poor negative predictive value and can't be used to rule out the diagnosis.[54,55] If there are findings suggestive of aortic dissection seen on bedside transthoracic echocardiogram (TTE), a cardiothoracic surgeon should be consulted emergently, even if definitive imaging is pending.[25] CT is the most commonly used test to diagnose aortic dissection and is quick and easy,[22] but the type of imaging selected should be based on what is most readily available[56] as MRI, transesophageal echocardiogram (TEE), and CT are all very accurate for diagnosis of dissection.[57,58] Given the history and differential in this case, these authors absolutely recommend CT. As a side note, even in patients with chronic kidney disease or pregnancy, an emergent CTA should be done without waiting for labs as morbidity and mortality increased with delay in diagnosis.[59]

DECISION POINT B – ***What did the actual provider actually do?***

MDM (12:05): CT chest abdomen pelvis ordered for evaluation of LLQ pain, not likely explained by acute cholecystitis. The 12-lead is not suggestive of ACS. Will obtain troponin for further differentiation. Chest x-ray pending and will add CT chest for further differentiation. Patient moved to red zone for further monitoring. I have also asked for cardiology consultation of pericardial effusion and ordered a formal echocardiogram.

Section editor comments (Greenwood):

At this point, we have correctly identified the acuity of this patient and transitioned them to an appropriate clinical area. The findings of a pericardial effusion, in the setting of a lower blood pressure, should raise the suspicion of the ED Provider for early tamponade. If the clinician had an ultrasound available to them, evaluating for tamponade should be a priority, as it may take time to obtain a CT angiogram.

ED course:

Radiology read at 13:20:

1. Stanford type-A aneurysm dissection likely involving the origin of the right coronary artery with aortic rupture and hemopericardium. There is mass effect upon the right ventricular free wall concerning for pericardial tamponade. The abdominal extension of the dissection involves the celiac axis trunk. There is marked gallbladder wall thickening. This may be on the basis of hepatic venous congestion from pericardial tamponade or gallbladder ischemia on the basis of impaired arterial inflow. Additionally, the dissection extends up to and involves the origin of the left renal artery with impaired arterial inflow to the left kidney.

2. Incidental bilateral inguinal direct hernia defects, the right hernia containing a short-segment knuckle of small bowel which appears unincarcerated and unobstructed.

Repeat vitals (13:22): HR 122, BP 158/113, RR 26, SpO_2 99%

Author comments (Weinstock):

The patient's heart rate has increased from 70 to 122bpm, but he is *hypertensive*. We have confirmation of a TAD. We are back at the bedside. We are at:

DECISION POINT C – You are faced with 2 questions:

1. **What is the emergent medical management of aortic dissection in a crashing patient?**
2. **What is the goal blood pressure and pulse?**

Q#1: What is the emergent medical management of aortic dissection in a crashing patient?

Initial management of aortic dissection involves:

- pain control
- heart rate control
- blood pressure management

Pain management is critical not only because it is humane, but also because of its effect on blood pressure.

Consulting editor comments (Weingart):

Use fentanyl. Longer acting pain meds only come into effect for post-op or type B dissections.

Q#2: What is the goal blood pressure and pulse?

A heart rate of 60–70 and systolic blood pressure < 120mmHg should be targeted. Aggressive rate control can minimize additional aortic injury by reducing the frequency of left ventricular ejection and sheer force on the dissection flap.[56,60] Esmolol is a cardioselective, beta-1 antagonist which has a quick onset of about 60 seconds and duration of action about 10–20 minutes, making it the "ideal" beta-adrenergic blocker for use in critically ill patients. The dose of Esmolol is 50–100mcg/kg bolus, followed by an infusion at 50mcg/kg/min increasing to 300mcg/kg/min as necessary.[61] In patients with contraindications to beta-blockers, calcium channel blockers can be used.[56,57]

Essential hypertension is a known risk factor for aortic dissection, present acutely in 75% of cases.[62] Higher blood pressure on presentation is associated with a higher mortality.[63]

In patients who still have systolic pressure > 120mmHg, a vasodilator such as nicardipine should be initiated. Nicardipine is a dihydropyridine calcium channel blocker that offers pure blood pressure control via alpha-blockade. Nitroprusside is no longer recommended unless other medications are not available. Antihypertensive effects can be unpredictable, can cause coronary steal, excessive reflex tachycardia, and cyanide toxicity in patients with liver dysfunction.[61] Vasodilators should not be given prior to beta-blockers due to the risk of reflex tachycardia which may worsen the dissection.[56,57,64] These hemodynamic goals, while not validated, are accepted based on the principle that lower heart rate and blood pressure means less shear stress on the aortic wall and less risk of propagation and rupture. If there is adequate perfusion to the brain, heart, and kidneys, then lower is better.

Clevidipine is a fourth generation dihydropyridine L-type calcium channel blocker; it has an ultra-short half-life of 1 minute and faster onset of action compared with nicardipine. It decreases blood pressure by direct arterial vasodilation without any preload reduction, unlike sodium nitroprusside or nitroglycerin. Initial IV infusion is at 0.4mcg/kg/min or 1–2mg/hr. The dose is doubled every 90 seconds up to 3.2mcg/kg/min. Above that dose, increments are by 1.5mcg/kg/min depending on patient's response with a maximum of 8mcg/kg/min.[64]

Note that there may be involvement of the innominate or left subclavian artery with the dissection flap so measuring blood pressure in an affected limb may show an inaccurately low blood pressure.[56] The CT scan should help identify any evidence of malperfusion to limbs or organs. If there is a limb blood pressure discrepancy, and an arterial line should be placed for invasive blood pressure monitoring. The limb with the higher blood pressure should be used, to avoid undertreating the patient's hypertension.

Consulting editor comments (Weingart):

Labetalol is not an alternative for acute TAD. It has its primary effects on inotropy but not chronotropy. If you have a type B dissection and need to transition, they will need metoprolol for heart rate control and then labetalol for blood pressure. Labetalol is inappropriate for acute aortic emergencies.

DECISION POINT C – ***What did the actual provider do?***

MDM (13:23): Esmolol and nitroprusside drips ordered. Goal BP 90–100 SBP. Patient is neurologically intact with normal grip strength BUE and intact dorsi and plantar flexion bilaterally. Pericardiocentesis and intubation equipment at bedside.

MDM (13:40): CT surgery consulted for evaluation. I have also spoken with Dr. ICU resident. Further care and disposition per ICU team and Dr. CT surgeon.

Section editor comments (Greenwood):

We need to be prepared for other potential complications when initiating medical management for an acute Type A dissection. First, a Type A dissection or any type B dissection with an associated malperfusion syndrome is a *surgical emergency that requires emergent, definitive repair.* In our patient, there is a known pericardial effusion which means the dissection flap has extended to the aortic root and opened into the pericardial space. Documentation (with a time stamp) should include the discussion of the communication with the cardiac surgeon and that the diagnosis of Type A dissection has been discussed, as well as the presence of an effusion and consideration of immediate operative repair.

While awaiting the surgical evaluation, the ED provider has correctly initiated treatment to provide both heart rate and blood pressure control. Blood pressure management in our patient is challenging since he not only has an acute aortic dissection but is also intoxicated with methamphetamines. Did the clinician use nitroprusside due to the patient's recent methamphetamine use?

A trial of benzodiazepines may have also helped in managing the hypertension. For non-intoxicated patients, nitroprusside is not my first-line antihypertensive as it is a potent arterial and venodilator, which can have very unpredictable effects on the patient's blood pressure, particularly with a pericardial effusion. Nicardipine (a pure alpha-antagonist) tends to be a more reliable blood pressure lowering agent. The one adverse reaction to nicardipine is "shunting," where patients with underlying lung disease or pulmonary edema lose their physiologic, hypoxic pulmonary vasoconstriction leading to hypoxemia.

In some cases, patients will remain tachycardic despite aggressive titration of negative chronotropic agents, such as esmolol or labetalol. This is often an ominous sign that the patient's type A dissection may involve the aortic valve causing acute aortic insufficiency. Aggressive heart rate control in these patients can lead to a significant reduction in cardiac output secondary to aortic regurgitation and or subsequent pulmonary edema. If the patient has a wide pulse pressure (indicating aortic regurgitation) or develops respiratory symptoms after aggressive heart rate control, it may be necessary to tolerate a higher heart rate while awaiting transportation to the OR.

Consulting editor comments (Weingart):

With cocaine intoxication, diltiazem plus nicardipine may be the best combination.

DECISION POINT D – You are faced with 2 questions:

1. **Should we perform pericardiocentesis in the ED?**
2. **Should the patient be intubated now? If so, what drugs should be used?**

Q#1: Should we perform pericardiocentesis in the ED?

Cardiac tamponade is present in 14–19% of cases of aortic dissection[65,66] and while tamponade occurs in a minority of patients, it is the leading cause of death in type A aortic dissection.[22] However, pericardiocentesis in patients with aortic dissection and tamponade leads to worse outcomes.[67,68] This is based on the theory that the cardiac tamponade itself reduces the bleeding into the pericardial sac by compressing the aortic leak and that the increase in blood pressure precipitated by relief of the tamponade may lead to propagation of the dissection.[68] Pericardiocentesis is listed as a Class III management strategy and is not recommended by the European Society of Cardiology.[60]

Newer guidelines from the American Heart Association (AHA) state that in patients who are unlikely to survive until surgery, limited pericardiocentesis with removal of just enough fluid to restore perfusion is an acceptable temporizing measure.[56] Several studies have confirmed that controlled, small volume, pericardiocentesis with incremental removal of fluid (approximately 10 cc at a time) is safe for patients who are tenuous and need a bridge to surgery.[69,70]

Q#2: Should the patient be intubated now? If so, what drugs should be used?

This patient is at high risk for peri-intubation cardiac arrest given his already tenuous hemodynamic status and the catecholamine surge associated with laryngoscopy, and intubation may just be enough to tip the balance. If intubation becomes absolutely necessary, we need to maintain our treatment goals of control of heart rate and blood pressure, with rapid sequence intubation (RSI) medications that support these goals. Pretreatment with fentanyl can be used to attenuate the catecholamine release associated with laryngoscopy.[71] Etomidate is a good because of its relatively neutral hemodynamic effects.[72] Propofol has both calcium channel and beta-receptor antagonist properties, so is a reasonable choice in the hypertensive and tachycardic patient.[71] For neuromuscular blockade, succinylcholine or rocuronium are both acceptable. Ketamine is not a good choice for the patient with aortic dissection because it stimulates catecholamine receptors and increases heart rate, and in some cases, blood pressure.

Section editor comments (Greenwood):

The author correctly advocates for the ED provider to generally avoid the urge to intubate the hemodynamically unstable patient with a pericardial effusion. In the setting of early tamponade, cardiac filling and output are often dependent on the negative transpleural pressure changes that occur with spontaneous respiration.[73] Introducing positive pressure ventilation, analgesia, and sedation can reduce venous return and rapidly cause cardiovascular collapse in the setting of a worsening pericardial effusion.[74] At some point, intubation may be unavoidable, but in this case the concept of resuscitation prior to intubation should include aggressive volume resuscitation to improve intracardiac filling pressures and a controlled pericardiocentesis prior to intubation.

What was the patient outcome?

The ED provider did not perform pericardiocentesis. The patient was taken emergently to the operating room. He underwent induction of anesthesia, but 6 minutes later he went into PEA arrest. Efforts at resuscitation were unsuccessful.

Final hospital impression: Aortic Dissection, PEA arrest.

Chapter summary:

Although first described over 200 years ago, the diagnosis of aortic dissection can be a challenging feat even today. Annual incidence of acute aortic dissection is about 3–5 cases per 100,000 people per year, and about 10% of patients are without classic symptoms of tearing chest pain and a pulse deficit. Common risk factors include hypertension, advanced age, atherosclerosis, congenital connective tissue disorders, aortic aneurysm, penetrating atheromatous ulcers, and previous cardiovascular or aortic surgeries.[37]

CT angiography, MRI, and transesophageal echocardiography each have >95% sensitivity and specificity for diagnosis. CT is better at excluding aortic dissection in patients with low pre-test probability, whereas MRI is better diagnostically in patients with a high pre-test probability and should considered for those unable to have an iodinated contrast study,[37] with the only absolute contraindication being those with a true anaphylactic reaction to contrast. As mentioned, given the high mortality of dissection, we recommend CT angiography even in those with acute or chronic renal failure unless another imaging modality (MRA, TEE) can be completed faster. D-dimer does not have validated cutoffs and is not recommended by ACEP to rule out TAD.

Many people with aortic dissections die before reaching the emergency department. Type A dissections are surgical emergencies given their mortality rate of 1–2% per hour at onset of symptoms vs. Type B dissections which are usually treated medically.[59] With intubation, there is a high-risk for peri-intubation cardiac arrest. RSI medications should be aligned with heart rate and blood pressure goals. Pericardial tamponade has been correlated with worse outcomes, but a controlled pericardiocentesis as a bridge to surgery can be performed.

Our goals include early diagnosis, prompt blood pressure control, and emergent surgical evaluation and repair.

References:

1. Edlow JA. Managing acute nontraumatic back pain. Ann Emerg Med 2015;66(2):148-53.
2. Lai V, Tsang WK, Chan WC, et al. Diagnostic accuracy of mediastinal width measurement on posteroanterior and anteroposterior chest radiographs in the depiction of acute nontraumatic thoracic aortic dissection. Emerg Radiol 2012;19(4):309-15.
3. Pozek I, Hurt CJ, Stern EJ. The wide mediastinum: Don't forget about sternal fractures. Curr Probl Diagn Radiol 2012;41(4):124-5.
4. Mohapatra PR, Janmeja AK. Images in clinical medicine. Asymptomatic mediastinal lipomatosis. N Engl J Med 2010;363(13):1265.
5. Geusens E, Pans S, Prinsloo J, et al. The widened mediastinum in trauma patients. Eur J Emerg Med 2005;21(4):179-84.
6. Chandra S, Laor YG. Lung scan and wide mediastinum. J Nucl Med 1974;16(4):324-5.
7. Pillow MT, Kaul B. A rare cause of widened mediastinum. J Emerg Med2012;43(2):346-7.
8. Mohapatra PR, Garg K, Prashanth C, et al. Pleural effusion presenting as mediastinal widening. Lung India 2013;30(4):354-6.
9. Lee FT Jr, Katzberg RW, Gutierrez OH, et al. Reevaluation of plain radiograph findings in the diagnosis of aortic rupture: The role of inspiration and positioning on mediastinal width. J Emerg Med 1993;11(3):289-96.
10. Schwab CW, Lawson RB, Lind JF, et al. Aortic injury: Comparison of supine and upright portable chest films to evaluate the widened mediastinum. Ann Emerg Med 1984;13(10):896-9.
11. Bickley LS, Szilagyi PG. The thorax and lungs. In: Bickley LS, Szilagyi PG. Bates' Guide to Physical Examination and History Taking. 10th ed. Philadelphia: Lippincott Williams & Wilkins, 2009.
12. Goodacre S, Locker T, Morris S et al. How useful are clinical features in the diagnosis of acute, undifferentiated chest pain? Acad Emerg Med 2002;9(3):203-8.
13. Woo KC, Schneider JI. High-risk chief complaints I: Chest pain—the big three. Emerg Med Clin N Am 2009;27(4):685-712.
14. Swap CJ, Nagurney JT. Value and limitations of chest pain history in the evaluation of patients with suspected acute coronary syndrome. JAMA 2005;294(20):2623-9.
15. Fanaroff AC, Rymer JA, Goldstein SA, et al. Does this patient with chest pain have acute coronary syndrome? The rational clinical examination systematic review. JAMA 2015;314(18):1955-65.
16. Le Gal G, Testuz A, Righini M, et al. Reproduction of chest pain by palpation: Diagnostic accuracy in suspected pulmonary embolism. BMJ 2005;330(7489):452-3.
17. Hado HSH, Scarpello JHB, Barton T, et al. A case of thoracic aortic dissection presenting as lateral pleuritic chest pain. Emerg Med J 2005;22(3):229-30.
18. Pape LA, Awais M, Woznicki EM, et al. Presentation, diagnosis, and outcomes of acute aortic dissection: 17-year trends from the international registry of acute aortic dissection. J Am Coll Cardiol 2015;66(4):350-8.
19. Wang W, Duan W, Xue Y, et al. Clinical features of acute aortic dissection from the Registry

of Aortic Dissection in China. J Thorac Cardiovasc Surg 2014;148(6):2995-3000.
20. Klompas M. Does this patient have an acute thoracic aortic dissection? JAMA 2002;287(17):2262-72.
21. von Kodolitsch Y, Nienaber CA, Dieckmann C, et al. Chest radiography for the diagnosis of acute aortic syndrome. Am J Med 2004;116(2):73-7.
22. Hagan PG, Nienaber CA, Isselbacher EM, et al. The International Registry of Acute Aortic Dissection (IRAD): New insights into an old disease. JAMA 2000;283(7):897-903.
23. Rogers AM, Hermann LK, Booher AM, et al. Sensitivity of the aortic dissection detection risk score, a novel guideline-based tool for identification of acute aortic dissection at initial presentation: Results from the international registry of acute aortic dissection. Circulation 2011;123(20):2213-8.
24. von Kodolitsch Y, Schwartz AG, and Nienaber CA. Clinical prediction of acute aortic dissection. Arch Intern Med 2000;160(19):2977-82.
25. Diercks DB, Promes SB, Schuur JD, et al. Clinical policy: Critical issues in the evaluation and management of adult patients with suspected acute nontraumatic thoracic aortic dissection. Ann Emerg Med 2015;65(1):32-42.e12
26. Chartier L, Josephson T, Bates K, et al. Improving emergency department flow through Rapid Medical Evaluation unit. BMJ Qual Improv Rep 2015;4(1).
27. Jordi K, Grossmann F, Gaddis GM, et al. Nurses' accuracy and self- perceived ability using the Emergency Severity Index triage tool: A cross-sectional study in four Swiss hospitals. Scand J Trauma Resusc Emerg Med 2015;23:62.
28. Rosner F, Berger JT, Kark P, et al. Disclosure and prevention of medical errors. Committee on Bioethical Issues of the Medical Society of the State of New York. Arch Intern Med 2000;160(14):2089-92.
29. Banja JD. Does medical error disclosure violate the medical malpractice insurance cooperation clause? In: Henriksen K, Battles JB, Marks ES, et al., eds. Advances in Patient Safety: From Research to Implementation (Volume 3: Implementation Issues). Rockville, MD: Agency for healthcare research and quality. US 2005.
30. Wolf ZR, Hughes RG. Error reporting and disclosure. In: Hughes RG, ed. Patient Safety and Quality: An Evidence-Based Handbook for Nurses. Rockville, MD: Agency for Healthcare Research and Quality; US 2008.
31. Niska R, Bhuiya F, Xu J. National Hospital Ambulatory Medical Care Survey: 2007 emergency department summary. Natl Health Stat Report 2010;(26):1-31.
32. Seyedhosseini J, Nasrelari A, Mohammadrezaei N, et al. Inter-rater agreement between trained emergency medicine residents and radiologists in the examination of gall bladder and common bile duct by ultrasonography. Emerg Radiol 2017;24(2):171-6.
33. Kendall JL, Shimp RJ. Performance and interpretation of focused right upper quadrant ultrasound by emergency physicians. J Emerg Med 2001;21(1):7-13.
34. Blanco P, Volpicelli G. Common pitfalls in point-of-care ultrasound: A practical guide for emergency and critical care physicians. Crit Ultrasound J 2016;8(1):15.
35. Villar J, Summers SM, Menchine MD, et al. The absence of gallstones on point-of-care ultrasound rules out acute cholecystitis. J Emerg Med 2015;49(4):475-80.
36. Ralls PW, Colletti PM, Lapin SA, et al. Real-time sonography in suspected acute cholecystitis: Prospective evaluation of primary and secondary signs. Radiology 1985;155(3):767-71.

37. Golledge J, Eagle KA. Acute aortic dissection. Lancet 2008;372(9632):55-66.
38. Park SW, Hutchison S, Mehta RH, et al. Association of painless acute aortic dissection with increased mortality. Mayo Clin Proc 2004;79(10):1252-7.
39. Upadhye S, Schiff K. Acute aortic dissection in the emergency department: Diagnostic challenges and evidence-based management. Emerg Med Clin North Am 2012;30(2):307-27.
40. Asha SE, Miers JW. A systematic review and meta-analysis of D-dimer as a rule-out test for suspected acute aortic dissection. Ann Emerg Med 2015;66(4):368-78.
41. Suzuki T, Isselbacher EM, Nienaber CA, et al. Type-selective benefits of medications in treatment of acute aortic dissection (from the International Registry of Acute Aortic Dissection [IRAD]). Am J Cardiol 2012;109(1):122-7.
42. Spittell PC, Spittell JA Jr, Joyce JW, et al. Clinical features and differential diagnosis of aortic dissection: Experience with 236 cases (1980 through 1990). Mayo Clinic Proc 1993;68(7):642-51.
43. Biagini E, Lofiego C, Ferlito M, et al. Frequency, determinants, and clinical relevance of acute coronary syndrome-like electrocardiographic findings in patients with acute aortic syndrome. Am J Cardiol 2007;100(6):1013-9.
44. Zhan S, Hong S, Shan-Shan L, et al. Misdiagnosis of aortic dissection: Experience of 361 patients. J Clin Hypertens 2012;14(4):256-60.
45. Pourafkari L, Tajlil A, Ghaffari S, et al. The frequency of initial misdiagnosis of aortic dissection in the emergency department and its impact on outcome. Intern Emerg Med 2017;12(8):1185-95.
46. Kurabayashi M, Miwa N, Ueshima D, et al. Factors leading to failure to diagnose acute aortic dissection in the emergency room. J Cardiol 2011;58(3):287-93.
47. Sagrista-Sauleda J, Merce J, Permanyer-Miralda G, et al. Clinical clues to the causes of large pericardial effusions. Am J Med 2000;109(2):95-101.
48. Corey GR, Campbell PT, Van Trigt P, et al. Etiology of large pericardial effusions. Am J Med 1993;95(2):209-13.
49. Imazio M, Mayosi BM, Brucato A, et al. Triage and management of pericardial effusion. J Cardiovasc Med 2010;11(12):928-35.
50. Sato F, Kitamura T, Kongo M, et al. Newly diagnosed acute aortic dissection: Characteristics, treatment modifications, and outcomes. Int Heart J 2005;46(6):1083-98.
51. Meszaros I, Morocz J, Szlavi J, et al. Epidemiology and clinicopathology of aortic dissection. Chest 2000;117(5):1271-8.
52. Pacini D, Di Marco L, Fortuna D, et al. Acute aortic dissection: Epidemiology and outcomes. Int J Cardiol 2013;167(6):2806-12.
53. Clouse WD, Hallet JW Jr, Schaff HV, et al. Acute aortic dissection: Population-based incidence compared with degenerative aortic aneurysm rupture. Mayo Clin Proc 2004;79(2):176-80.
54. Nazerian P, Vanni S, Castelli M, et al. Diagnostic performance of emergency transthoracic focus cardiac ultrasound in suspected acute type A aortic dissection. Intern Emerg Med 2014;9(6):665-70.
55. Evangelista A, Carro A, Moral S, et al. Imaging modalities for the early diagnosis of acute aortic syndrome. Nat Rev Cardiol 2013;10(8):477-86.
56. Hiratzka LF, Bakris GL, Beckman JA, et al. 2010

ACCF/AHA/AATS/ACR/ASA/SCA/SCAI/SIR/STS/SVM Guidelines for the diagnosis and management of patients with thoracic aortic disease. Circulation 2010;121(13):e266-369.
57. Tsai TT, Nienaber CA, Eagle KA. Acute aortic syndromes. Circulation 2005;112(24):3802-13.
58. Shiga T, Wajima Z, Apfel CC, et al. Diagnostic accuracy of transesophageal echocardiography, helical computed tomography, and magnetic resonance imaging for suspected thoracic aortic dissection: Systematic review and meta-analysis. Arch Intern Med 2006;166(13):1350-6.
59. Salameh MJ, Ratchford EV. Aortic dissection. Vasc Med 2016;21(3):276-80.
60. Erbel R, Alfonso F, Boileau C, et al. Diagnosis and management of aortic dissection: Recommendations of the Task Force on Aortic Dissection, European Society of Cardiology. Eur Heart J 2001;22:1642-81.
61. Varon, J. Treatment of acute severe hypertension: Current and newer agents. Drugs 68(3):283-97.
62. Neinaber CA, Clough RE. Management of acute aortic dissection. Lancet 2015;385(9970):800-11.
63. Howard DP, Banerjee A, Fairhead JF, et al. Population-based study of incidence and outcome of acute aortic dissection and premorbid risk factor control: 10-year results from the Oxford Vascular Study. Circulation 2013;127(20):2031-7.
64. Gupta PK, Gupta H, Khoynezhad A. Hypertensive emergency in aortic dissection and thoracic aortic aneurysm—A review of management. Pharmaceuticals 2009;2(3):66-76.
65. Sato F, Kitamura T, Kongo M, et al. Newly diagnosed acute aortic dissection: Characteristics, treatment modifications, and outcomes. Int Heart J 2005;46(6):1083-98.
66. Gilon D, Mehta RH, Oh JK, et al. Characteristics and in-hospital outcomes of patients with cardiac tamponade complicating type A acute aortic dissection. Am J Cardiol 2009;103(7):1029-31.
67. Norman PH, Mycyk T. Dissection of ascending thoracic aorta complicated by cardiac tamponade. Can J Anaesth 1989;36(4):470-2.
68. Isselbacher EM, Cigarroa JE, Eagle KA. Cardiac tamponade complicating proximal aortic dissection: Is pericardiocentesis harmful? Circulation 1994;90(5):2375-8.
69. Cruz I, Stuart B, Caldeira D, et al. Controlled pericardiocentesis in patients with cardiac tamponade complicating aortic dissection: Experience of a centre without cardiothoracic surgery. Eur Heart J Acute Cardiovasc Care 2015;4(2):124-8.
70. Hayashi T, Tsukube T, Yamashita T, et al. Impact of controlled pericardial drainage on critical cardiac tamponade with acute type A aortic dissection. Circulation 2012;126(11 Suppl 1):S97-S101.
71. Stollings JL, Diedrich DA, Oyen LJ, et al. Rapid-sequence intubation: A review of the process and considerations when choosing medications. Ann Pharmacother 2014; 48(1):62-76.
72. Zed PJ, Abu-Laban RB, Harrison DW. Intubating conditions and hemodynamic effects of etomidate for rapid sequence intubation in the emergency department: An observational cohort study. Acad Emerg Med 2006;13(4):378-83.
73. Faehnrich JA, Noone RB, White WD, et al. Effects of positive-pressure ventilation, pericardial effusion, and cardiac tamponade on respiratory variation in transmitral flow velocities. J Cardiothorac Vasc Anesth 2003;17(1):45-50.
74. Ho AM, Graham CA, Ng CS, et al. Timing of tracheal intubation in traumatic cardiac tamponade: A word of caution. Resuscitation 2009;80(2):272-4.

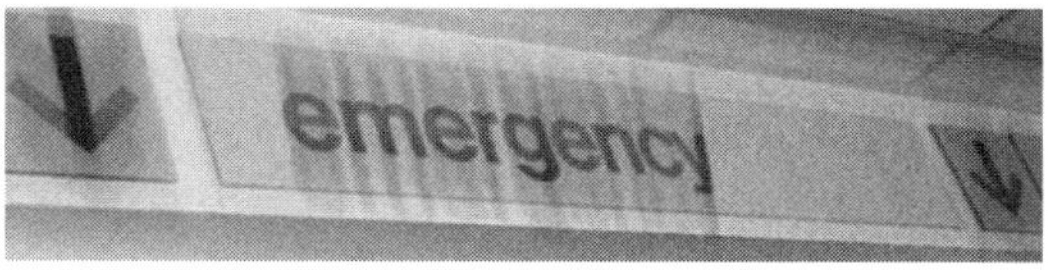

SECTION C – CARDIAC/ VASCULAR

Chapter 13: A 33-year-old man with abdominal pain who leaves AMA

Brad S. Goldman, MD, FACEP, FAAEM

Core faculty
Adena Emergency Medicine Residency
EMS Rotation Director
SIM lab Co-Director
Adena Heath Systems
Chillicothe, OH

Jesse Nichols, DO

Emergency Medicine Attending
Langley Air Force Base, Hampton, VA

Legal Commentary:

Gregory L. Henry, MD

Former President of The American College of Emergency Physicians (ACEP)
Former Professor of Emergency Medicine at the University of Michigan
Former CEO of Medical Practice Risk Assessment, Ann Arbor, MI

Section editor:

John C. Greenwood, MD

Assistant Professor
Department of Emergency Medicine
Department of Anesthesiology and Critical Care
Perelman School of Medicine
University of Pennsylvania, Philadelphia, PA

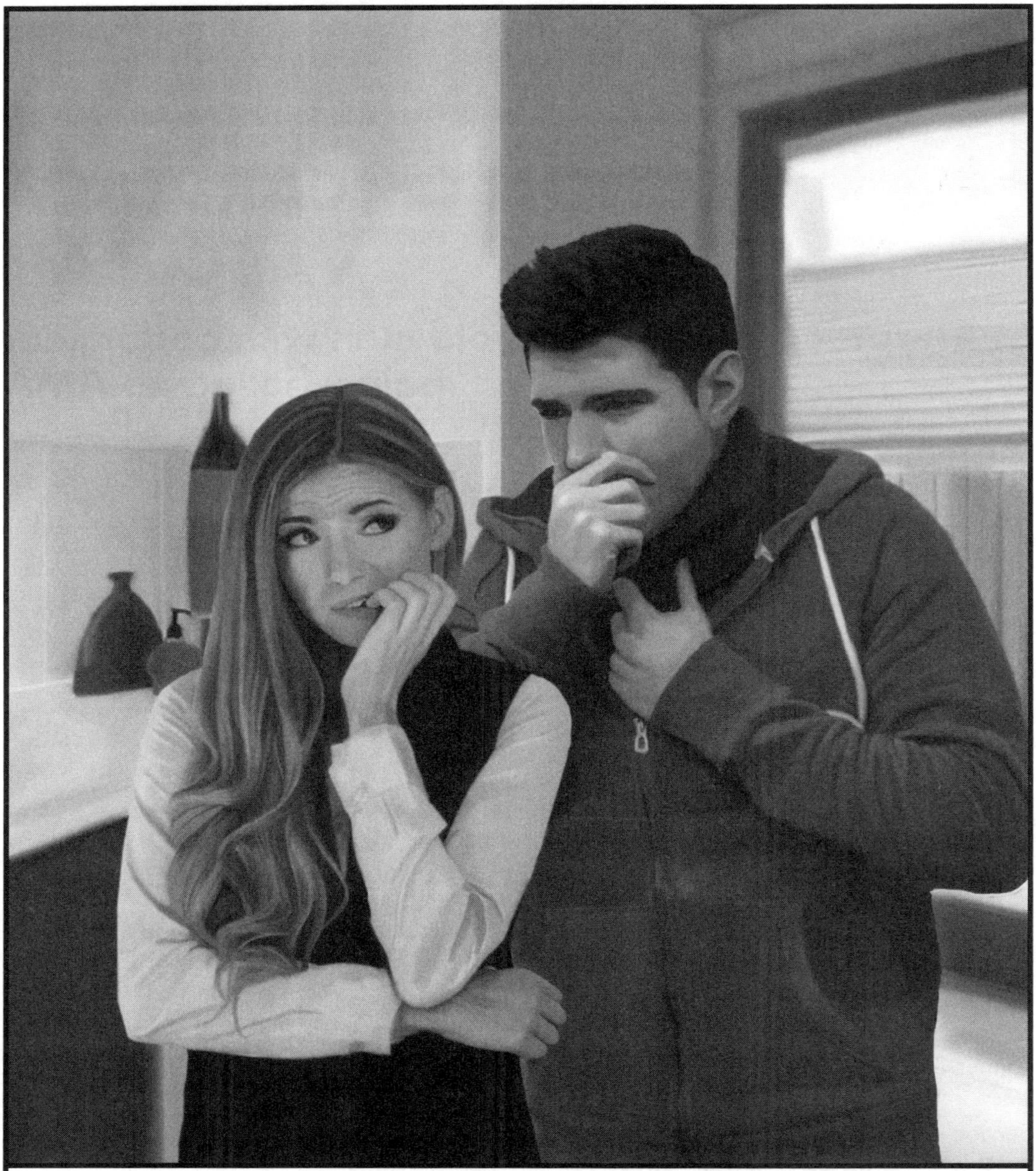

"I REALLY HAVE TO LEAVE, ARE YOU COMING WITH ME OR NOT?"

SECTION C/CHAPTER 13

A 33-year-old man with abdominal pain who leaves AMA

INITIAL ED VISIT

CC (23:29): Abdominal pain

Vitals:

Time	Temp (F)	Pulse	Resp	Syst	Diast	Pos.	O2	(SatO2%)
23:34	96.5	107	18	67	36	S	96	RA

PH:
Allergies: X-ray dye and shellfish
Medications: Quetiapine, hydrocodone, esomeprazole, celecoxib, furosemide, tizanidine
PMH: Ehlers-Danlos syndrome, depression, anxiety, sickle cell anemia, bipolar disorder, enlarged heart, post-traumatic stress disorder, substance-abuse, heart murmur
PSH: Left foot surgery, bilateral toe surgery, splenectomy
SH: Tobacco, occasional alcohol, marijuana and crack cocaine
Family History: Hypertension, diabetes

HPI (00:25): Pt. is a 33-year-old male with "horrible" abdominal pain which is a pressure sensation and started at 6:20 this evening. He did have two episodes of vomiting. He did use crack cocaine this evening. Felt fine until his symptoms started at 6:20. He has never had pain like this in the past. He has not had a normal bowel movement the last couple days and is on chronic Vicodin. He has not been taking the recommended stool softeners. He does have a history of Ehlers-Danlos syndrome with multiple digestive problems and vascular issues and has had blood clotting problems and a splenectomy in the past. He denies any respiratory complaints, chest pain, coughing, shortness of breath, recent travel, or sick contacts.
ROS: Extensive review of 10 systems is negative.

EXAM (00:27):
CONSTITUTIONAL: Thin male appearing older than stated age and marked discomfort but no other acute distress
HEAD: Normocephalic, atraumatic.
EYES: Pupils are round and react to light
NOSE: Nose appears normal. No rhinorrhea.
NECK: Supple, full range of motion, no tenderness, no lymphadenopathy or JVD
RESP: Normal chest excursion with respiration, no stridor.

CARDIO: Regular rate and rhythm with a holosystolic murmur loudest at the left lower sternal border, no rubs or gallops
GASTRO: There is a well-healed surgical scar. Firm, diffusely tender, moderate guarding but no rebound.
NEURO: Patient is awake, alert, cooperative, no focal motor or sensory deficits
ORDERS: Dicyclomine, famotidine, metoclopramide, IV fluids. (Benadryl and hydrocortisone premedication for CT scan)

RESULTS:

Test	**Flag**	**Value**	**Units**	**Ref. Range**
WBC	H	18.0	K/uL	4.6-10.2
HGB	L	8.7	G/DL	12.0-16.0
PLT		160	K/uL	142-424

Test	**Flag**	**Value**	**Units**	**Ref. Range**
BUN		18	MG/DL	8-20
CREAT		1.7	MG/DL	0.6-1.3

Lytes, LFT, lipase – WNL
Sed rate = 2
Glucose 276
Lactate 4.6
Urine – Protein 40, glucose 150, other normal

Acute abdominal series: Negative without signs of obstruction or free air

PROGRESS NOTE: The patient's significant other was irritated and wanted the patient to sign out against medical advice because she needed to get to work. I did go back and reevaluate the patient. He had drank one dose of contrast was able to drink another cup and at that point said he would be willing to stay.

When the CT tech arrived to transport him to the scanner his significant other refused to let him go to the CT scan and said she needed to get to work and wanted him discharged. Repeat blood pressure was 103/54, heart rate 136, respirations 18, and oxygen saturation 99% on room air. I did go back and speak with the patient and family members again; at this point he was sleeping comfortably. The family member was markedly irritated and agitated and was refusing to wait any longer stating that we should discharge him at this time.

We did discuss the incomplete workup and marked lab abnormalities and the patient did sign the AMA forms and leave in spite of having continued abdominal pain. I've had extensive discussion with the patient and family members. We attempted to complete the workup but ultimately, they decided to leave.

DIAGNOSIS: Abdominal pain of uncertain etiology, cocaine abuse, leukocytosis, anemia, elevated lactic acid, renal insufficiency, hyperglycemia

Initial visit discussion:

1. What are the etiologies of abdominal pain in patients with a history of drug abuse?

Though we often end up with "abdominal pain of unknown etiology," the patient demographic, history, physical exam, as well as the clinician's differential diagnosis, often determines the need for further diagnostic testing; discharge may be appropriate for low-risk pediatric patients, imaging and consultation in the post-surgical patient, and an expanded differential for the elderly, but how about the drug user?

Unique issues to the drug abusing patient with abdominal pain include a likely lower economic status, decreased access to medical care and overall poorer health, not to mention an often difficult and perhaps inaccurate history in an altered patient who may delay seeking medical care.

Our patient's symptoms appeared *suddenly*, approximately 6 hours prior to arrival. The character of the pain is a non-localized "pressure sensation," which may increase concern for visceral etiology. But even more worrisome is the past medical history, social history, and surgical history including collagen vascular disease (Ehlers-Danlos syndrome), sickle cell anemia, a "blood clotting disorder," depression and anxiety, enlarged heart, and a heart murmur combined with a history of splenectomy and use of marijuana and crack cocaine. The differential is quite extensive including:

- Small bowel obstruction
- Sickle cell crisis
- Thoracic/Abdominal aortic dissection
- Mesenteric ischemia
- Endocarditis with septic emboli
- Bacteremia and sepsis

Now combine the patient's symptoms with the testing we have been able to obtain (he left before a CT scan was done) including hypotension, leukocytosis, acute renal failure and an elevated lactate level. Imagine observing him physically leaving the ED; did he ambulate or was he pushed in a wheelchair? Would involvement of a social worker, a warm meal, or fuzzy slippers have encouraged him to stay?

Section editor comments (Greenwood):

This patient has multiple risk factors for acute aortic dissection with a clinical concern for multiple sites of malperfusion (bowel ischemia indicated by the lactate of > 4 that could be secondary to acute thrombosis, vasospasm, or intimal flap, as well as renal malperfusion indicted by the elevated creatinine). It is unclear what type of CT scan was ordered; however, if the patient was asked to drink oral contrast it was unlikely the CT angiogram would be needed to evaluate vascular competency and patency. This type of study may have shown late findings of bowel ischemia such as transmural edema, hyperemia, pneumatosis, and free fluid, but would have significantly impaired the radiologist's (and vascular surgeon's) ability to identify vascular pathology. In addition, the requirement of oral contrast also likely delayed this patient's throughput, which may have also factored into his decision to leave.

2. What should the EP do in a high-risk patient who wants to leave against medical advice (AMA)?

Whereas the provider did have some uncertainty about the specific *diagnosis*, there was certainly no uncertainty about the *disposition*; this patient was sick and needed further evaluation and management!

The quandary for the EP is palpable; we can hear the agitated words of disagreement and frustration clashing with our medical knowledge and experience. On one side resides the patient whose wishes appear clear in the documentation. Their demands appear to be primarily represented by the "significant other" who is adamant about leaving.

On the other side is the provider who applied reason and knowledge to evaluate the etiology of the pain; with the patient's history of collagen vascular disease, multiple digestive and vascular problems, and clotting issues and who admits to crack cocaine use, we can only imagine the "black box" of pathology that will eventually be discovered in the patient's abdomen. Though the provider obviously cared and spent a lot of time trying to talk the patient into changing his mind, did the documentation address the seminal issue?

We establish decision-making capacity in every patient encounter; it is usually clear that the patient has the ability to reason and think logically. On the other hand, when the patient is severely intoxicated or altered, they may lack ability to make informed decisions.

The Against Medical Advice (AMA) form represents a cornerstone of a larger ethical decision which occurs in 1–2% of ED encounters,[1] generating our ethical gymnastics; balancing the patient's right of autonomy with the provider's beneficence and need to act in the patient's best interest.

It was 1914 when Justice Benjamin Cardozo wrote a decision that set a standard regarding informed consent and the patient's right to refuse treatment. The patient was Mary Scholendorff. The hospital was the New York Hospital.

Justice Benjamin Cardozo (1870-1938):

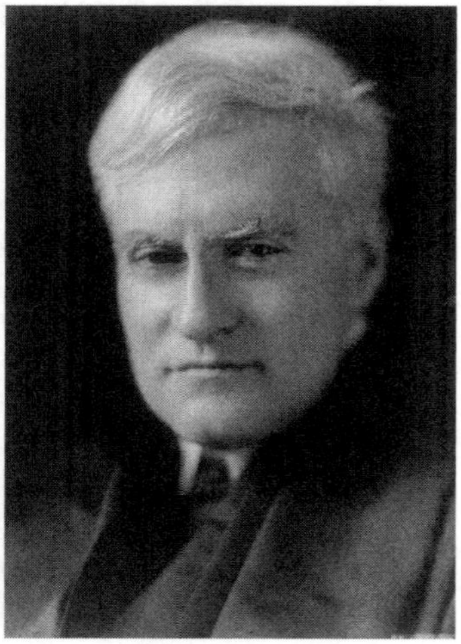

Mary Schloendorff presented to New York Hospital with abdominal symptoms and was diagnosed with a fibroid tumor. The patient consented to examination under general anesthesia with ether, but there was no consent for surgery. The surgeon upon finding the fibroid performed surgery, but there were unfortunately infectious complications that ultimately lead to gangrene of the fingers with eventual amputation and chronic pain.

She filed suit against New York Hospital claiming that she consented to examination under anesthesia but explicitly excluded surgical intervention from her consent. The surgeon who performed the examination and removal of the malignant tumor was excluded from the litigation. Schloendorff's claim was based on trespass or medical battery, which the hospital permitted, as the proximate cause to her injuries.

In her case, *Schloendorff v. Society of New York Hospital*, the court found in favor of the defendant citing that the hospital was not responsible for the actions of the physicians. Schloendorff appealed the case to the New York Court of Appeals.

It was the New York Court of Appeals (1914) that established principles of informed consent and respondeat superior in United States law.

"Every human being of adult years and sound mind has a right to determine what shall be done with his own body; and a surgeon who performs an operation without his patient's consent commits an assault for which he is liable in damages. This is true except in cases of emergency where the patient is unconscious and where it is necessary to operate before consent can be obtained."
- Justice Benjamin Cardozo

Five components to establish and document when the patient is being discharged AMA:
1. Patient is adult or emancipated minor
2. Patient has medical decisional capacity
3. Patient has been informed of potential consequences of non-treatment & alternatives offered
4. Involve family, friends, or patient's physician
5. Signature on AMA form of patient (consider adding family members, physician and discharging nurse)

3. Was the documentation adequate?
The ED physician certainly realized the risk of leaving with an incomplete work-up and documented the recognition of marked abnormalities in the work-up, but there was only a cursory exploration of the patient's capacity to decide; the refusal to complete the work-up was initiated and encouraged by the "significant other." She did not have power of attorney.

Without documentation explicitly noting normal capacity, a clear mental status exam (even establishing date, month, and year), or documentation of a "repeat back" of risks, would make a stronger case for allowing the patient to leave. We have many reasons to suspect the patient may have had decreased capacity including cocaine/drug intoxication, malperfusion, and the underlying medical process.

It is the opinion of these authors, that despite the MDM note and obvious concern, we do not feel that the provider established the patient's capacity or met the requirements for adequate documentation of AMA. As we will soon see, this is the critical point where appropriate intervention may have altered his outcome.

Section editor comments (Greenwood):

There are a number of clinical documentation concerns, as well as the obvious medicolegal issues of a high-risk patient wanting to leave prior to receiving a thorough evaluation. The progress note really does not discuss the clinician's risk assessment for an emergent differential diagnosis in a patient with documented hypotension (67/36 at triage), an elevated lactic acid, and likely acute kidney injury. The documented abdominal exam is concerning for a surgical abdomen. Given these concerns, the EP appropriately ordered an emergent CT scan, but unfortunately, it would likely not have shown the most emergent cause of this patient's abdominal pain. An emergent surgical consult prior to the abdominal CT would have been reasonable quickly after leaving the room.

Risk management issues with initial chart:

It was not documented if patient had the medical decisional capacity to decide to leave AMA.

- No documentation if he or significant other understood implications/risks of leaving.
- No documentation of offer to return or alternative treatments/arrangements.

Despite the decision to leave, providing an acceptable/alternative approach to management is advisable and encouraged. For example, antibiotics for a sick pneumonia patient or aspirin for a patient with a TIA. In the end, as physicians we are here to give advice, and it is the patient's right to accept or reject the advice.

Author comments (Weinstock):

Before presentation of the bounceback visit, we will insert potential legal considerations. Of note, unlike the previous two cases which did proceed to legal action, this case did not, but that does not diminish the importance of appropriate documentation, especially with such a high-risk patient. I agree with the chapter authors that more should have been done to establish and document capacity; Greg Henry, has a different viewpoint.

Gregory L. Henry, MD
Former President of The American College of Emergency Physicians (ACEP)
Former Professor of Emergency Medicine at the University of Michigan
Former CEO of Medical Practice Risk Assessment, Ann Arbor, MI

Schloenforff vs. Society of New York Hospitals

I am glad to see that the *Schloenforff vs. Society of New York Hospitals* was referenced by the authors. Interestingly, just after this ruling, Benjamin Cardoza moved from the NY Appellate Bench to the U.S. Supreme Court; he unfortunately died way too early in his judicial career. Justice Cardozo's doctrine which has guided medicine for the last 104 years, is simple and direct. It is Cardozo who defines the fact that it is the patient who is in charge of their care. Because a patient does not agree with the physicians does not mean they are incompetent to make their own health care decisions, and his dictum of patients of adult years and sound mind is revisited almost daily in the ED.

Against medical advice:

The elements of against medical advice are relatively straightforward. A ten-year-old, whether parents are present or absent, is not allowed to make a decision on withholding care; the reasonable person doctrine would perceive to cover a physician who acted in the best interest of the child until the parents were in attendance. Equally straightforward is that "sound mind," though not absolute, is still recognized as the primary indicator to proceed in adults. A patient who comes to the ED in a stupor or coma or clear psychosis has essentially, by arriving at the department, given consent for examination and treatment. But just because a patient has an impressive list of diseases does not mean they cannot think. An adult patient has the right to control their own destiny.

Documentation:
There is no evidence in this chart that the patient did not have decision-making capacity. There is not a nursing note that says the patient is confused or cannot follow direction. There is no family input that the patient is unable to think or perform normal daily functions. Although it has been commented upon, the mental status is not extensively documented. Clearly there is nothing on the opposite side of the table. If a claim of incapacitation is made by the plaintiff, they're going to need someone or something to back up this up. Multiple people saw this patient. Where is the documentation that they considered the patient to be non-compos mentis? If this case proceeded to legal action, the plaintiff would have a long way to go to show that the physician did not act in his best interest.

But there are a few areas where a plaintiff's councel could attack the chart. The comment that the patient had "marked discomfort, but no acute distress" is a little contradictory. But there is no evidence that the discomfort in any way changed the thought-making process. In fact, most people would argue that the presence of pain would make patients more attentive to the physician's recommendation to stay. There is no inability to follow orders, to respond or cooperate with the examination, outbursts of anger, or anything else that might show that the patient was not functioning in a reasonable capacity.

Defense expert strategy:
Serving as the defense witness would be relatively easy; multiple people saw the patient, and no one had trouble interacting or explaining medical activities to this gentleman. The exact nature of the discussions will never be completely known but it would be expected that the physician would testify that if he had thought there was a decrease in mental status, he would have recorded such and proceeded to act for the patient's best interest. The defense posture here has been reiterated by multiple courts since the time of Cardozo.

Within the past few years, multiple medical legal actions have been dismissed because the patient could not be shown to have decreased intellectual capacity. The very same appellate court which wrote the *Schloendorff* decision 104 years ago has since reiterated that decision and said that if an emergency physician had held a patient down or prevented them from leaving, they would be guilty of assault and battery. This is good news for emergency physicians. There is no question that independence of the individual is a paramount tenet of American jurisprudence.

Approach to the AMA patient + would a jury find against this physician?
It is always wise for the emergency physician to get family members involved; there is nothing as useful as having a patient's family be able to testify to the degree in which the physician has informed the patient, and the degree to which the patient was able to interact in the decision-

making process. I believe that family involvement tends to handle the vast majority of AMA cases. Documenting these discussions is also useful. It is my opinion that an insurance company would be very hesitant to settle the against medical advice-based case for this patient. Juries are humans. They understand the difficulties involved with cocaine-addicted patients. This is a hospital. It is not a prison. Nor is it a place where physicians can casually suspend civil liberties. It is unlikely that the average juror would hold the doctor responsible when a patient seems to be awake and alert and able to cooperate with medical decision-making.

The authors comment that one to two percent of patients are signing out against medical advice; my thought is that if an individual physician has a rate at this level, they need to be rethinking their practice. The vast majority of patients want help and the intelligent and crafty physician can almost always find common ground. A physician who has an unusual number of against medical advice forms signed may constitute a risk management problem for the hospital.

Though input can come from all members of the health care team, it is the physician's responsibility to incorporate the data available and to recommend that the patient stay for further evaluation. Suggesting that "we are caring for the patient in the same way as with our own family member" is a powerful argument.

It is the overall gestalt of the patient's ability to cooperate which dictates if he has reasonable decision-making capacity. On the other hand, if the patient lacks capacity, it is the job of the physician to act in their best interest. If the physician has in good faith determined that the decision-making capacity is significantly diminished, it is extremely difficult for a plaintiff to prevail. Of course, it is important that the staff reassess to ensure that they are still incapacitated. But in general, acting in defense of the patient is never a mistake.

Author comments (Weinstock):

And finally... to the bounceback.

ED RETURN VISIT (7 hours later–presents to a different ED – within minutes of arrival begins to seize)

CC(09:04): Abdominal pain

RN: Nurse received report from the EMS medics. The patient was moaning in the room upon arrival. After report the nurse went into the room to assess patient. Patient was lying on his left-hand side. The nurse asked the patient what we were seeing him for today. The patient responded, "I need to pee." The nurse then began to explain to the patient it was important to hook him up to the monitor and check him out and then he would be allowed to urinate. The patient suddenly began to seize. The RN placed the patient on the pulse ox and cardiac monitor and given O_2. The physician was called immediately to the room.

HPI text/documented later (09:56): This is a 33-year-old male who has a history of Ehler Danlos syndrome and questionable hemophilia. He arrives here by ambulance from home when his son initially called for possible constipation and abdominal pain. The patient did also call an ambulance last night and was transported to [an outlying hospital] for chest and abdominal pain. He was observed for several hours and was discharged home. His wife states that he has recently started smoking cocaine and was at a friend's house last night. Upon immediately transferring him from the ambulance stretcher to the bed, the patient had a possible seizure and then became apneic, and went into cardiac arrest.

PE/documented later (9:41):
CONSTITUTIONAL: cardiac arrest within 1 minute of arrival, asystole on the monitor
HEAD: Normocephalic; atraumatic.
EYES: pupils and dilated
NOSE: The nose is normal in appearance
RESP: B BS with bagging
CARDIO: No rhythm
ABD: firm
SKIN: warm, no peripheral pulses

We start at decision point A:

DECISION POINT A – YOU ARE FACED WITH 5 QUESTIONS:

1. **What are the first steps in the evaluation of an actively seizing patient?**
2. **What is the differential diagnosis in a patient who is speaking and then begins to seize?**
3. **What are the first steps in the management of an actively seizing patient?**
4. **The patient has no IV access—how long should we wait before placing an IO?**
5. **Should we intubate now or wait to see if the medications are effective?**

What does the literature say?

Q#1: What are the first steps in the evaluation of an actively seizing patient?

Our patient does not give us much time to think, beginning to seize within minutes of ED arrival. Ensuring IV access, placement of a cardiac monitor/pulse-ox, and bedside point-of-care glucose are the first steps that should be done in concert while obtaining history from EMS, bystanders and family, while at the same time observing the patient, palpating the femoral artery and firing up the ultrasound machine. With time, determining PMH, reviewing prior medical records and determining medications should be completed. The physical exam begins with vitals and a bedside glucose. With an actively seizing patient, the provider should include focusing on any localizing signs of the seizure activity, skin color, deviation of the patient's eyes, posturing, as well as signs of trauma, or lateral tongue biting.[2]

Ideally treatment focuses on the etiology; however, the exact cause of the seizure may be unknown, therefore, the evaluation should be contemporaneous with the treatment.

Q#2: What is the differential diagnosis in a patient who is speaking and then begins to seize?

Seizure was described by Hippocrates, in 400 B.C., as "the sacred disease."[3] Status Epilepticus can be defined as epileptic seizures which follow one another without interval recovery of consciousness. While the etiologies of seizure are extensive, first differentiate seizure from mimics including syncope, migraines, movement disorders, and psychogenic non-epileptic seizures.

Findings that suggest a seizure:

- History of seizures
- Lateral tongue biting
- Postictal period
- Age < 45
- Preceding aura
- Observed seizure activity-not just myoclonic activity. Brief myoclonic activity may also be observed with syncope

The mortality of status epilepticus ranges from 10–40% and is related to the underlying etiology.[3]

Section editor comments (Greenwood):

In the adult without a previous seizure history, attention should be made to nonprimary neurologic causes of seizure. These may include eclampsia in the young female, cerebral malperfusion due to a cardiac dysrhythmia or aortic dissection into carotid arteries, acute ischemic or hemorrhagic stroke, toxidromes (including sympathomimetics, isoniazid overdose, etc.), acute intracranial hypertension, or CNS infectious causes such as encephalitis.

Q#3: What are the first steps in the management of an actively seizing patient?

A clinical diagnosis of status epilepticus is defined as 5+ minutes of continuous seizure activity or recurrent seizure activity not returning to baseline.[4] Early termination of seizure is priority and allows for prompt diagnostic evaluation. Neurologic damage may occur within 30 minutes despite adequate oxygenation and respiratory status.[5] The goal of therapy is to prevent neuron damage from prolonged seizure activity.

Seven recommended actions for status epilepticus are listed below.[4] We correlate how these are relevant to our patient:

1. **Airway protection and support gas exchange:**
    - The airway assessment should begin with non-invasive airway protection and head position to allow for adequate gas exchange.
2. **Intubation:**
    - If the airway appears compromised or increased intracranial pressure is suspected, rapid sequence intubation should be performed with an induction agent and short-acting paralytic. A post-sedation agent for our patient is unlikely necessary if he has already received multiple doses of benzodiazepines. A long-acting paralytic is contraindicated unless capabilities of continuous EEG monitoring are available, as prolonged paralysis can mask the persistent electrical activity of the brain.
3. **Vital signs:**
    - Establish a baseline and use them to direct therapies.

4. **Support circulation with IV fluids and/or vasopressor support:**
   - o Maintain cerebral perfusion pressure by ensuring SBP > 90 (or MAP > 65).
5. **Bedside glucose:**
   - o Diagnose hypoglycemia. It's embarrassing/possibly fatal to miss an easily treatable cause of seizures.
6. **Peripheral IV access:**
   - o At this point our patient has no IV access as they have just arrived, and will be a nursing priority to check point of care lab values and administer IV benzodiazepines as a first line treatment for seizure.
7. **Abortive therapies:**
   - o There are multiple abortive therapies available (below). Once IV access is obtained, we recommend starting with lorazepam 2mg IV push with reassessment 3–5 minutes. If seizure persists, then increasing to 4mg IV push. The potential to stop seizures with initial abortive medications decreases the longer the seizure occurs.
   - o First line medications: Use benzodiazepines aggressively and early.[4]
     - i. Lorazepam: 0.1mg/kg IV up to 4mg IV per dose, may be repeated in 5–10 minutes
     - ii. Diazepam: 0.15mg/kg IV up to 10mg per dose, may be repeated in 5 minutes
     - iii. Midazolam 0.2mg/kg up to 10mg (route: intramuscular)
   - o Second line medications:
     - i. Fosphenytoin (20–30mg/kg at 150mg/min) IV or
     - ii. Valproic Acid (20–40mg/kg at 5mg/kg/min) IV or
     - iii. Levetiracetam (60mg/kg with max 4500mg/dose) IV or
     - iv. Phenobarbital (20mg/kg at 50–75mg/min) IV
   - o Refractory medications- prepare to intubate:
     - i. Propofol (2–5mg/kg, 2–10mg/kg/hr) IV or
     - ii. Midazolam (0.2mg/kg, 0.05–2mg/kg/hr) IV or
     - iii. Ketamine[6] (0.5–3mg/kg, 0.3–4mg/kg/hr) IV

Section editor comments (Greenwood):

Initial benzodiazepine dosing is often *too low*. Current guidelines recommend a 0.1mg/kg dose of lorazepam up to a MAX dose of 4mg, that can be repeated every 5–10 minutes.

Q#4: The patient has no IV access—how long should we wait before placing an IO?

Multiple attempts to establish IV access have failed and the patient continues to seize. What is the next course of action?

Concurrently with attempts at access, the first line abortive therapies can be administered via intramuscular, rectal, nasal, or buccal routes. With no peripheral IV access, Midazolam is the preferred therapy.[6]

Midazolam and lorazepam given IM have good absorptive profiles, but diazepam IM is not recommended due to the unpredictable absorption. When IV access is established, the preferred agent is lorazepam given the extended duration of effect. In pre-hospitalized patients, IM midazolam was found to be as effective as IV lorazepam.[7] Diazepam is formulated for rectal administration, but is not always practical with a seizing patient. The anticonvulsant effects of benzodiazepines are most effective when administered early.

IO access has been demonstrated to have fewer complications than placing central lines and is faster than obtaining a peripheral IV.[8-10] While there are no specific guidelines about when to place an IO, it is reasonable to allow for 2 attempts over a time span of 60 seconds in a critical, crashing patient, and if unsuccessful, then an IO should be placed. It's quick, easy and safe.

Q#5: Should we intubate now or wait to see if the medications are effective?

As emergency medicine providers, anticipating and recognizing the need for a definitive airway intervention is priority, but deciding when to intubate the seizure patient is less well-defined. The indications for endotracheal intubation are:

- to support oxygenation and ventilation
- to protect the patency of the airway
- anticipated decline in clinical course

Status epilepticus is a neurological emergency with respiratory failure as one of the serious complications,[4] stemming from a combination of the seizure or the side-effects of medications used to abort the seizure. Most patients who are poorly responsive after a seizure will recover without any airway support or intervention.

The rates of endotracheal intubation in patients with status epilepticus vary. The Rapid Anticonvulsant Medication Prior to Arrival Trial (RAMPART) found that 21% of the patients with status epilepticus were intubated, with the majority occurring in the hospital setting vs. the pre-hospital. Of those intubated, 42% were for a duration of less than 24 hours with the primary indications being respiratory depression, decreased mental status, and recurrent convulsions following the initial interventions.[11] The postictal period is a harmonizing balance between the potentially quick resolution of the postictal depressed mental status versus the risk for airway compromise and complications of aspiration.

Once the decision is made to proceed with endotracheal intubation, the patient should be adequately resuscitated and pre-oxygenated. The use of apneic oxygenation during rapid sequence intubation (RSI) is associated with increased first pass success without resulting hypoxemia.[12]

For our patient, we recommend immediate abortive therapy with parenteral benzodiazepines. If the patient remains in status epilepticus despite the first and second-line therapy as defined above, a definitive airway with RSI should have been obtained.

DECISION POINT A – *What did the actual provider do?*

1. The provider did not meet the EMS at the door and had no information when entering the room. The nurse explained this history while care was being initiated.
2. Fingerstick blood sugar was not documented. There were no signs of head trauma. It was unknown if patient had a seizure history or any ingestions.
3. A code was called to mobilize resources. There were 2 peripheral IV lines quickly and easily placed.
4. The physician started to examine the patient while the nurse was opening an Ambu bag and monitor lines were placed at the same time. The monitor shows sinus tachycardia, but when the physician palpates for a femoral pulse, none is found.

ED course:

RN documentation: The seizure lasted for approximately 1–2 minutes. The patient then became apneic and pulseless post seizure-like activity and CPR was initiated.

Code sheet:

- 09:10 – Pt. becomes apneic and pulseless – code called
- 09:11 – Connected to monitor = PEA
- 09:11 – CPR initiated. Pt. is bagged. Code cart to bedside
- 09:13 – Epi 1mg
- 09:14 – Respiratory therapy arrives. Pharmacy arrives
- 09:17 – Pt. intubated per ED MD
    - o MD procedure note: Orotracheal intubation: The patient was intubated orotracheally, with an 8.0mm endotracheal tube using A curved Macintosh blade with direct visualization and advanced. Tube position is 24cm at the lips. Breath sounds were auscultated bilaterally.
    - o Respiratory note: Tube secured at 22 at the lips. Breath sounds ausc bilaterally. Good color change with CO_2 detector. Pt bagged with 100% O_2.
- 09:17 – CPR continues
- 09:20 – Epi 1mg, bicarb 1 amp

Time CPR Started: 0910
Ventilation: ☒ Ambu ☐ Mouth to Mask
Fi 02 100% ☒
Intubation: Time 0912 ☒ Oral ☐ Nasal
Tube Size 8 cm 22
Tube Placement Verified By: ☐ CXR ☐ AUSC ☐ End Tidal CO2

Precipitating Symptoms
☐ Resp. Distress
☐ Resp. Arrest
☒ Cardiopulmonary Arrest
☐ Sudden Unconsciousness
☐ Other

IV ACCESS:
Peripheral:
1. 20 LAC .9NS
2.
3.
4.
5.
CVC: Site
Time
Placed By

Family Notified of Code:
☒ Yes Relationship Wife
☐ No Unable to Reach
Outcome:
☐ Successful
☒ Unsuccessful
Termination Time: 0936

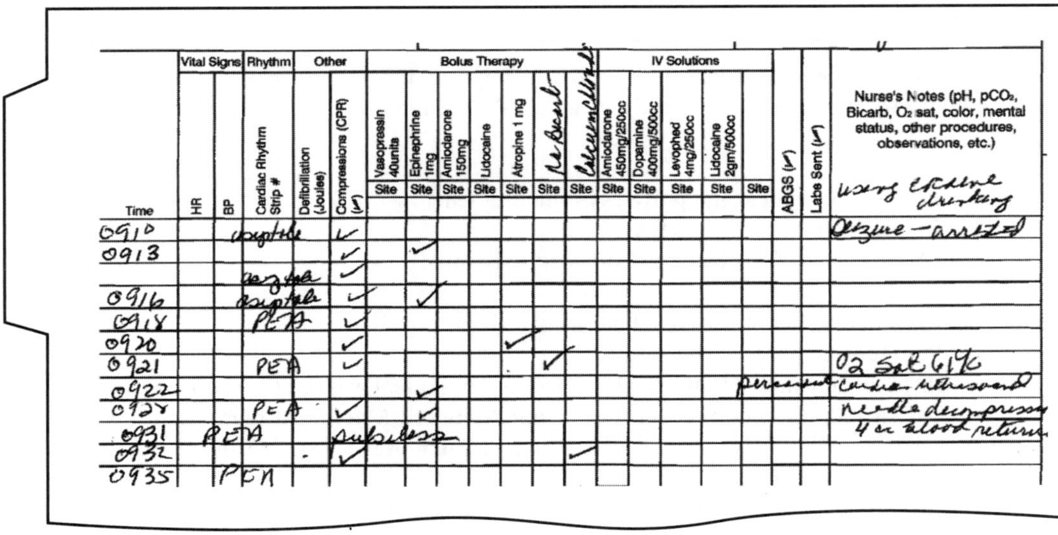

Time	HR	BP	Cardiac Rhythm Strip #	Defibrillation (Joules)	Compressions (CPR) (✓)	Vasopressin 40units Site	Epinephrine 1mg Site	Amiodarone 150mg Site	Lidocaine Site	Atropine 1 mg Site	Na Bicarb Site	Calcium chloride Site	Amiodarone 450mg/250cc Site	Dopamine 400mg/500cc Site	Levophed 4mg/250cc Site	Lidocaine 2gm/500cc Site	Site	ABGS (✓)	Labs Sent (✓)	Nurse's Notes (pH, pCO₂, Bicarb, O₂ sat, color, mental status, other procedures, observations, etc.) using cocaine drinking
0910			asystole		✓															Seizure – arrested
0913					✓		✓													
			asystole		✓															
0916			asystole		✓		✓													
0918			PEA		✓															
0920					✓					✓										
0921			PEA		✓						✓									O2 Sat 61%
0922							✓											pericardial		cardiac ultrasound
0928			PEA		✓		✓													needle decompress
0931	PEA				pulseless															4 cc blood return
0932					✓							✓								
0935		PEA																		

DECISION POINT B – YOU ARE FACED WITH 4 QUESTIONS:

1. **What are the initial steps in resuscitating a patient who arrives talking and then arrests?**
2. **What are steps post-intubation to confirm tube placement and adequate ventilation?**
3. **The patient had a history of Ehlers-Danlos syndrome—should blood be given empirically with consideration of aortic dissection or rupture?**
4. **What is the role of US and how might it change management?**

What does the literature say?

Q#1: What are the initial steps in resuscitating a patient who arrives talking and then arrests?

As team leader, the ED physician assigns roles with direct dialogue to all ancillary staff and conducts the primary survey with assessment of the airway, breathing, and circulation.

- **Airway:** Air exchange may be improved with repositioning with head tilt-chin lift or head tilt-jaw thrust. A decrease in survival to hospital discharge has been associated with early attempts at intubation during in-hospital cardiac arrest,[13] possibly due to a focus on the airway that distracts from high-quality CPR and defibrillation. If mechanical ventilation is needed, an LMA may be easier to place in certain clinical circumstances, and has been shown to be associated with similar outcomes compared to endotracheal intubation.[14]
- **Breathing:** Assisted breathing with bag-valve-mask should be initiated while preparing for intubation. Once an advanced airway such as an endotracheal tube or laryngeal mask airway (LMA) is secured, start with a ventilation rate of 10 breaths/minute.
- **Circulation:** Target is 100–120 compressions/minute with a depth of 1/3 of the anterior-posterior diameter or a depth of 5–6cm in adults. High-quality CPR includes adequate rate, adequate depth, full chest recoil, minimized interruptions, and appropriate ventilations. With a focus on circulation, the concept of cardiocerebral resuscitation and continuous chest compressions developed. This strategy was conducted initially with animal studies,[15-18] which suggested improved survival at 24hrs and improved survival neurologic outcomes at 24hrs when compared to standard CPR. When that same concept was applied to human studies and

lay rescuers the results varied, and it was found that there were no differences in survival.[19-23] The 2015 AHA guidelines recommend that all rescuers should provide chest compressions to cardiac arrest victims. Untrained lay rescuers should provide compression-only CPR to adult victims at a minimum. If a trained lay rescuer is able to provide rescue breaths should that should be at a ratio of 30 compression to 2 rescue breaths.[24] The high-quality CPR and defibrillation helps establish an organized rhythm to allow for coronary perfusion and subsequent cerebral perfusion of oxygen starved tissues of the heart and brain.

Electromechanical dissociation (EMD) as referred to as pulseless electrical activity (PEA) is present in 32–37% of in-hospital cardiac arrest,[25,26] prompting consideration of reversible causes. Traditional teaching centers on the "H's and T's" that include:

- Hypovolemia
- Hypoxia
- Hydrogen ion (acidosis)
- Hyper/hypokalemia
- Hypothermia
- Hypoglycemia
- Toxins
- Tamponade
- Tension pneumothorax
- Thrombosis (coronary and pulmonary)
- Trauma

Section editor comments (Greenwood):

More recently, an alternative strategy has been proposed to help the clinician more effectively treat PEA arrest.[27]

The evaluation of a patient in PEA should include a bedside echocardiogram and a rhythm strip to determine if the QRS is narrow or wide (normal 0.12s–0.2s).[27] This alternative strategy may be used in conjunction with the patient's clinical presentation and only mentioned here to help diagnosis possible etiologies of the cardiac arrest and guide therapies and should not be used to definitively evaluate PEA.

- If the QRS is narrow, the etiology is likely mechanical in nature and is caused by inflow or outflow obstruction of the right ventricle.The initial treatment options include fluid resuscitation plus therapies that focus on frequent causes including cardiac tamponade, tension pneumothorax, mechanical hyperinflation, and pulmonary embolism. The clinical history combined with bedside ultrasound are key.
- If the QRS is wide, the etiology is likely metabolic with severe hyperkalemia or sodium channel blocker toxicity. The initial therapies should focus on correction of the metabolic abnormalities such as IV calcium and IV sodium bicarbonate. The clinical exam, ancillary studies such as labs, and bedside ultrasound will help confirm the diagnosis.

Patients with epilepsy have an increased mortality compared to the general population.[28,29] Sudden unexpected death in epilepsy (SUDEP) is witnessed or unwitnessed, nontraumatic and non-drowning death which excludes status epilepticus.[30] One of the proposed pathophysiologic mechanisms includes autonomic dysfunction with increased parasympathetic tone causing bradycardia and asystole following a seizure.[30] Stecker, et al. found that the majority of patients with epilepsy did not have witnessed seizure activity prior to the cardiac arrest.[31]

Seizure preceding arrest may be from cerebral hypoperfusion secondary to the underlying process. Our patient did not have a history of seizures, making this possibility much more likely.

Q#2: What are steps post-intubation to confirm tube placement and adequate ventilation?

The most reliable means of confirmation is visualization of the tube progressing through the cords. Other means that help confirm placement are capnography or colorimetric end-tidal CO_2 ($EtCO_2$) after a couple cycles of ventilation.[32] The condensation of the tube, symmetric chest movement and listening for bilateral and equal breath sounds over the lung fields with absence of sounds over the stomach are adjuncts but are not confirmatory. A post-intubation CXR will confirm the depth of the ET tube above the carina but does not rule out esophageal intubation.[32]

In emergent endotracheal intubation, $EtCO_2$ can be used in conjunction with other modalities. There is a false-negative failure rate of 7% and a false positive rate of 3% with colorimetric CO_2 devices which may occur due to air or gas in the stomach, excessive secretions, or during cardiac arrest due to decreased circulation.[33] Point-of-care ultrasound may also be used (as discussed in greater detail below).[34,35]

Section editor comments (Greenwood):

Newer continuous capnography and capnometry is very sensitive/specific (100%)!

With our patient, the endotracheal tube was confirmed in the appropriate position and the patient is able to be ventilated. Use of a continuous $EtCO_2$ monitor can provide a numeric and graphical waveform representation of the concentration of CO_2 at the end of exhalation. $EtCO_2$ monitoring can provide effective feedback regarding CPR quality. With no spontaneous circulation and poor CPR quality, the $EtCO_2$ is generally less than 10mmHg. Effective CPR that achieves an $EtCO_2$ of at least 20mmHg is desirable, and an abrupt rise may indicate ROSC. [36]

Q#3: The patient had a history of Ehlers-Danlos syndrome—should blood be given empirically with consideration of aortic dissection or rupture?

Ehlers-Danlos Syndrome is a collection of inherited disorders that involve a defect in the collagen and connective tissues, increasing the risk of dissection and rupture, the most common cause of death is Ehlers-Danlos Syndrome.[37]

Given this risk, a type and screen along with obtaining large-bore peripheral intravenous access should have been obtained. If the bedside US is consistent with dissection or shows signs of hemorrhage, then emergent transfusion should be initiated.

Q#4: What is the role of US and how might it change management?

When time is of the essence in this critical patient, bedside ultrasound is a useful adjunct to assist with airway confirmation, evaluating lung sliding, and assess circulatory function with cardiac echo/ vascular studies in hopes of diagnosing the cause of the arrest. Like all streamline time-sensitive processes, a well-defined algorithm with POCUS in cardiac arrest has been proposed. Cardiac Arrest Sonographic Assessment (CASA) is a 3-step process that utilizes the <10 seconds during the rhythm check.[38] Each assessment should be completed every 2 minutes in coordinating with the ACLS algorithm.

Step 1: Cardiac tamponade?

The initial phase of pericardial tamponade causes an impaired filling of the right ventricle. As the fluid accumulates, the pericardial pressure becomes greater than the right ventricular (RV) filling pressure. A decline in cardiac output occurs when pericardial pressure is equal to the left ventricular (LV) filling pressure.[39] When evaluating the RV on ultrasound, if it is collapsed in diastole (when the AV valves are open) the diagnosis of tamponade is suggested. If there is a question to whether the fluid seen on ultrasound is pericardial or pleural, use the long axis parasternal view; fluid anterior to the descending aorta is consistent with pericardial fluid. Ultrasound allows for real-time guidance as the pericardium is evacuated. Once a return of fluid is noted, a small amount of agitated saline may be injected; presence of bubbles in the pericardial space confirms the needle is in correct position.

Step 2: Right heart strain?

Pulmonary embolism – With the apical 4-chamber view, findings include a dilated right ventricle that is grossly the same size or larger than the left ventricle or right ventricle septal flattening (consistent with elevated right ventricle pressures). The McConnell sign, used to help diagnose PE, is a pattern of akinesia of mid free wall and normal apex motion.

Step 3: Cardiac activity?

Finally evaluating the overall global activity of the heart can provide prognostic and diagnostic information. Organized hypodynamic activity in PEA is profound shock and initiating an epinephrine or norepinephrine drip titrating to hemodynamic response is recommended. Alternatively, absence of cardiac activity in PEA is a poor prognostic sign and can assist with when to call "time of death."

- Aorta – Evaluation of the aorta in an actively coding patient is difficult, but especially relevant in this patient with Ehlers-Danlos Syndrome and cocaine use. Ensure adequate compression of the probe to allow for displacement of bowel gas. Any focal dilation in an artery with greater than 50% increase in size is classified as an aneurysm. If the abdominal aorta is > 3cm or an increase in aortic diameter to 1.5 times the normal expected diameter, it is considered an aneurysm. If free fluid is noted in the abdomen, one can speculate rupture. Ultimately, for the critical patient with a suspected thoracic aortic dissection and concerning vital signs, a bedside TEE while waiting for the cardiothoracic surgeon may provide the diagnosis.

Returning to our patient, with compressions ongoing, it is time for a rhythm check; the goal is to not interrupt chest compressions for more than 10 seconds. Though the information learned from POCUS is valuable, ultrasound during CPR is associated with delays in chest compressions.[40] Minimize pauses by having the probe in appropriate position, loop record the images, and if the image cannot be obtained, then resume chest compressions. An international consensus expert panel for cardiac arrested patients recommends core views that include cardiac subxiphoid and parasternal long axis with supplementary views of lung and IVC.[41] The core views should only be attempted during rhythm checks without interruption of chest compressions. Evaluating for pericardial fluid, ventricular form including right heart strain, and overall function of organized cardiac activity is the purpose of the cardiac views. Perhaps evaluating each of these during separately rhythm checks ensures less than 10-second interruption of CPR.

After countless minutes of resuscitation, several cycles of chest compressions, multiple dosages of IV medications, we are faced with the decision; when should we call the code?

DECISION POINT B – *What did the actual provider do?*

1. CPR was initiated, and provider helps with bagging until respiratory therapy arrives. Patient is intubated 7 minutes into the cardiac arrest
2. Blood sugar is not documented
3. Blood was not ordered
4. POCUS was performed showing pericardial effusion (see below)
5. The code was continued

ED course:

A bedside ultrasound is performed and shows a large amount of pericardial fluid

- 09:22 – Bedside US > pericardial tamponade > pericardiocentesis with 10mL blood aspirated, no systemic response to pericardiocentesis
    - MD procedure note: Pericardiocentesis: A pericardiocentesis was performed using the paraxiphoid approach with an 18-gauge needle, (spinal needle) 10mL blood was aspirated. Patient's condition did not improve
- 09:22 – Compressions continued
- 09:28 – Epi 1mg
- 09:32 – CaChloride

DECISION POINT C – YOU ARE FACED WITH 3 QUESTIONS:

1. **What US findings support pericardial tamponade?**
2. **With the additional information about cocaine toxicity, does this change management?**
3. **When should a code be called?**

Q#1: What US findings support pericardial tamponade?

Decompensation from tamponade occurs not only due to a quantity of fluid, but the rate of accumulation, initially impairing relaxation and filling of the ventricles and eventually causing decreased cardiac output, occurring with as little as 150mL of fluid.[39,42]

Cardiac tamponade is a clinical diagnosis. Early symptoms and signs include dyspnea, tachycardia, jugular venous distension, hypotension and pulsus paradoxus. ECG findings may include electrical alternans (alternation of the axis of the QRS complexes on ECG).

Ultrasound diagnosis starts with the phase array or curvilinear probe. The sub-xiphoid and apical 4-chamber reveals the presence of pericardial fluid with right atrial collapse on systole with eventual right ventricle collapse during diastole.[43] Other findings include "swinging of the heart" within the fluid collection.

The provider did find tamponade and a pericardiocentesis was performed without improvement in the patient's condition. The technique that was once described in the 1840's, percutaneous pericardiocentesis, has been modified over the decades with the advent of echocardiography. The ultrasound helps to identify the most optimal site for fluid collection seen by a para-apical approach.[44] Materials include a No.11 blade scalpel and an 18ga spinal needle connected to a 20-mL or 60-mL syringe. With continuous negative pressure on the plunger, the needle is advanced with blood aspirated. With our patient, 10mL of blood was withdrawn, but the patient remained pulseless.

Q#2: With the additional information about cocaine toxicity, does this change management?

The substance abuse history adds to the complexity of the case. Cocaine acts primarily by inhibiting reuptake of serotonin, norepinephrine, and dopamine, and has an effect on nearly every organ system.[45] With the extensive release of catecholamines, and sodium channels, the myocardium has more potential for irritability,[46,47] creating the perfect storm for circulatory failure and cardiac arrest—an increase in myocardial infarction rate of 24-fold in the first hour following administration.[48] The enhanced sympathetic activity predominates at lower levels and the sodium channel blockade is more evident at higher doses.[49] When these pathways are activated, the patient is at risk of cardiovascular dysfunction, dysrhythmias, and ultimately cardiac arrest.

The reasons for cardiac arrest in a cocaine user include acute ischemia and myocardial infarctions predisposing to arrhythmias. In one study, 81% of the time there was no post-mortem cause of death found, with the etiology presumed to be a fatal arrhythmia.[50] Sustained ventricular tachycardia has been found to occur in cocaine abusing patients in the absence of ischemia.[51,52]

In our patient with a history of an underlying connective tissue disorder, cocaine use, and who is in cardiac arrest with a pericardial tamponade—a type A aortic dissection rises to the top of the differential. The International Registry for Aortic Dissection sites approximately 0.5% of 921 cases to have cocaine reported aortic dissection.[53] A retrospective study in an urban center reported numbers as high as 37%.[54]

The cornerstone of treatment of cocaine toxicity is supportive care with benzodiazepines. But our patient is pulseless in cardiac arrest—should we really just "cookbook" the ACLS algorithm and give epinephrine, which may potentiate the sympathomimetic effects? The evidence from the American Heart Association (AHA) and American College of Cardiology Foundation (ACCF) offer some recommendations that are primarily based on class C evidence.

The AHA specific recommendation is as follows:[55]

"There are no data to support the use of cocaine-specific interventions in the setting of cardiac arrest due to cocaine overdose. Resuscitation from cardiac arrest should follow standard BLS and ACLS algorithms, with specific antidotes used in the post-resuscitation phase if severe cardiotoxicity or neurotoxicity is encountered. A single case series demonstrated excellent overall and neurologically intact survival (55%) in patients with cardiac arrest associated with cocaine overdose who were treated with standard therapy."[52]

Vasopressin offers a potential pathophysiologic advantage in the setting of cocaine arrest with augmentation of coronary blood flow.[56,57] Vasopressin also appears to exhibit inotropic effects, even with the acidosis which is common in cocaine toxicity.[58] In cases of refractory ventricular tachycardia or ventricular fibrillation, it is advised to consider withholding subsequent dosages of epinephrine due to potential concerns of excessive catecholamines.

Section editor comments (Greenwood):

As mentioned, acute cocaine toxicity can lead to a number of devastating hemodynamic consequences including severe hypothermia, rhabdomyolysis, acidosis, coronary vasospasm, QT prolongation, and ventricular tachycardia. Early sodium bicarbonate therapy may benefit these patients to reverse cocaine's sodium-blocking effect and correcting severe metabolic acidosis. In patients with refractory ventricular tachycardia, therapy should attempt to reduce adrenergic stimulation and the reduction of circulating cocaine and its metabolites. Nonselective beta-blockers are likely a useful treatment, despite historical dogma that beta-blockade is contraindicated. Intravenous lidocaine should also be considered. Intravenous lipid emulsion (ILE) therapy can be used to compartmentalize the highly lipophilic circulating cocaine and reduce any further cardiovascular toxicity.[59,60]

Author comments (Weinstock):

Scott has a slightly different take, but keep in mind that once the patient is in refractory V-fib, this is a "Hail Mary"...

Consulting editor comments (Weingart):

The coding cocaine user is handled the same as other patients with the only difference—and probably not even worth commenting on—using esmolol due to refractory V-fib. "Is it going to cause undifferentiated constriction of their heart vasculature?" If I knew they were doing copious amounts of cocaine, I would probably not use esmolol, but other than that, I probably wouldn't do anything differently.

Q#3: When should a code be called?

A resuscitation should be stopped when (1) the patient has an advanced directive, (2) the patient's condition is futile, (3) all appropriate interventions have been unsuccessful. Factors that need to be considered include:

- Witnessed or unwitnessed arrest?
- Initial rhythm?
- Onset of CPR?
- Time to defibrillation? (if applicable)
- Reversible causes have been addressed?

As our patient had a witnessed arrest and there are still some reversible causes to exclude, we agree with continued resuscitation at this time. When the patient enters the hospital with chest compression in progress, the overall chance of survival is primarily dependent on time to defibrillation and

ROSC. When the initial rhythm on arrival is asystole, the prospect of survival is minimal. A rhythm of asystole for 20 minutes is generally considered non-viable. Our patient is different; he arrested right in front of us, changing some of the approaches as well as the potential outcome.

One study found a ROSC rate of > 50% if cardiac activity was detected on POCUS with an overall survival rate to hospital discharge of 3.8% in patients with cardiac activity, but when no cardiac activity was present on initial ultrasound, only 0.6% survived to hospital discharge.[61]

Section editor comments (Greenwood):

Other things to consider, such as CPR > 20 min with $EtCO_2$ < 10 show a poor chance of survival and that it may be reasonable to discontinue ACLS in these cases.

In the AHA 2015 guidelines[62] for out-of-hospital cardiac arrest (OHCA), termination of resuscitation should be considered when all of the following criteria are present:

- Arrest was not witnessed by emergency medical personnel.
- No ROSC prior to transport.
- No AED shock was delivered.

The National Association of EMS Physicians for non-traumatic OHCA supports cessation of resuscitation in the following situations:[63]

- Sudden cardiac death likely to be medical.
- Unwitnessed arrest with a delay in CPR of 6 minutes and/or delay in defibrillation beyond 8 minutes.
- In absence of advanced directives, full resuscitative effort with definitive airway, appropriate medications, defibrillation as necessary, with at least 20 minutes of ACLS guidelines.
- Persistent ventricular fibrillation or ventricular tachycardia rhythm should have continued efforts where asystole and PEA OHCA should be ceased.
- Other factors such as family wishes and the safety of crew.
- Online medical direction with a consensus decision between on-scene paramedic and directed physician.
- Providers and family access to resources that include clergy, social workers.
- Quality review to define an appropriate termination protocol and to ensure all resources involved.

When considering the termination of resuscitation, one should investigate the potential for advanced techniques such as extracorporeal membrane oxygenation CPR (ECPR) as a bridge until definitive therapy with suspected reversible etiology. In 2015 the International Liaison Committee on Resuscitation (ILCOR) conducted a systematic review that compared manual or mechanical CPR with the use of ECPR. The study was a prospective, observation cohort of 162 OHCA patients who did not achieve ROSC with more than 20 minutes of standard CPR. The post hoc analysis showed that at 3-month follow-up ECPR was associated with higher rate of neurologically intact survival compared with standard CPR.[64]

The 2015 AHA summarizes and states "insufficient evidence to recommend routine use of ECPR for patients with cardiac arrest. In settings where it can be rapidly implemented, ECPR may be considered for select cardiac arrest patients for whom the suspected etiology of the arrest is potentially reversible during a limited period of mechanical cardiorespiratory support."[62]

Summary: If there is not ROSC, viable cardiac rhythm, or reversible causes identified after 20 minutes of high-quality CPR, the probability of neurologic intact survival is diminished. The provider's experience, judgment of futility, family wishes, resources available, and patient comorbidities are all considered in the decision. In our patient, considering the interventions which we have unsuccessfully employed and lack of response to pericardiocentesis, we feel that this is an appropriate time to call the code.

Consulting editor comments (Weingart):

If we had known that this patient had mesenteric ischemia/infarction, this is probably not going to be a successful code. By the time you code for mesenteric ischemia, there's not too much that can be done. Even if you got the patient back and operated, there's a lot of dead gut. Which is not to say don't try, but just don't feel so bad when you can't get them back.

DECISION POINT C – ***What did the actual provider do?***

ED course:

- **09:36:** Code called and Pt. pronounced dead (26 minutes of ACLS)

Physician post-code note (MDM at 10:08): Upon arrival here, the patient stated he needed to urinate and then immediately became unresponsive with possible seizure activity. We immediately started bagging and followed CPR protocol with chest compressions and intubation. His initial rhythm appeared to show PEA. He received numerous rounds of epinephrine and received atropine. I did do a quick bedside ultrasound and he appeared to have a significant pericardial effusion as well as free fluid in the abdomen. I attempted pericardiocentesis but obtained less than 10 cc of blood. We continued resuscitation for a half hour but never regained a pulse and he remained in PEA. I wonder if he had an aortic catastrophe given his underlying connective tissue disease and cocaine abuse. I should also note that one piece of info in the [initial] HPI was inaccurate—the outlying hospital states he did sign out AMA.

Post-code (chaplain at 10:58): Chaplaincy consult required for intervention with family. Note: The following family/significant other support was given: I have been with the [wife]. She found out when she got here that her husband had died. I did grief work with her and death paperwork. She went home to tell her son. The Pt. is going to the Coroner.

ED Diagnosis:

1. Cardiac arrest
2. Cocaine abuse

15:56: The body was taken to the morgue

Autopsy (next day):

1. Cocaine positive toxicology
2. Mesenteric ischemia

Teaching points:

Identifying medical decision capacity in patients with illicit drug use leaving AMA.

- Ultimately, the patient must demonstrate the following abilities:[65,66]
    1. To understand the decisions.
    2. To appreciate the information presented.
    3. To reason with the treatment options.
    4. To express a choice.
- Speaking patient who subsequently seizes with refractory management.
    - o Seizure management involves initial management with benzodiazepines in concert with formation of a differential diagnosis. Did an underlying process cause the seizure or did the seizure cause the arrest?
- In patients with underlying connective tissue disease, consider aortic dissection and potential for cardiac tamponade early in their care.

Chapter author "debrief:"

The emergency department diagnosis was (1) cardiac arrest and (2) cocaine abuse. The autopsy revealed (1) cocaine positive toxicology and (2) mesenteric ischemia; this has been described in the literature.[67] In retrospect, the patient's limited history and physical exam support the post-mortem diagnosis. The patient's chief complaint was abdominal pain on the initial visit and acute mesenteric ischemia is on the differential of generalized abdominal pain with exam findings of pain out of proportion.[68] The "ischemia" is also evident given the elevated lactate during the evaluation. Perhaps if the patient would not have left AMA, the treating clinician would have eventually arrived at the diagnosis. Cocaine has been attributed to causing myocardial ischemia with the pathophysiology attributed to its vasoactive properties. By extension, the vasoactive properties may affect the visceral vascular beds and is likely compounded in this case by the collagen vascular disease. Chronic cocaine use has been attributed to accelerated atherosclerotic disease and thrombosis.[69]

Author comments (Weinstock):

Our patient had a serious process occurring; it is unknown if his decision to leave was clouded by his metabolic encephalopathy secondary to ischemic bowel and it is unknown if his outcome would have been different if he had not left AMA, but he may have had a chance...

References:

1. Glasgow JM, Vaughn-Sarrazin M, Kaboli PJ. Leaving against medical advice (AMA): risk of 30-day mortality and hospital readmission. J Gen Intern Med 2010;25(9):926-9.
2. Benbadis S, Wolgamuth BR, Goren H, et al. Value of tongue biting in the diagnosis of seizures. Arch Intern Med 1995;155(21):2346-9.
3. Shearer P, Park D, Bowman A, et al. Seizures and status epilepticus: Diagnosis and management in the emergency department. Emerg Med Pract 2006;8(8):1-32.
4. Brophy, GM, Bell R, Claassen J, et al. Guidelines for the evaluation and management of status epilepticus. Neurocrit Care 2012;17(1): 3-23.
5. Meldrum BS, Horton RW. Physiology of status epilepticus in primates. Arch Neurol 1973;28(1):1-9.
6. Glauser T, Shinnar S, Gloss D, et al. Evidence-based guideline: Treatment of convulsive status

epilepticus in children and adults: report of the guideline committee on the American Epilepsy Society. Epilepsy Curr 2016;16(1):48-61.
7. Silbergleit R, Durkalski V, Lowenstein D, et al. Intramuscular versus intravenous therapy for prehospital status epilepticus. N Engl J Med 2012;366(7)591-600.
8. Leidel BA, Kirchhoff C, Bogner V, et al. Is the intraosseous access route fast and efficacious compared to conventional central venous catheterization in adult patients under resuscitation in the emergency department? A prospective observational pilot study. Patient Saf Surg 2009;3(1):24.
9. Neuhaus D, Weiss M, Engelhardt T, et al. Semi-elective intraosseous infusion after failed intravenous access in pediatric anesthesia. Paediatr Anaesth 2010;20(2):168-71.
10. Lamhaut L, Dagron C, Apriotesei R, et al. Comparison of intravenous and intraosseous access by pre-hospital medical emergency personnel with and without CBRN protective equipment. Resuscitation 2010;81(1):65-8.
11. Vohra TT, Miller JB, Nicholas KS, et al. Endotracheal intubation in patients treated for prehospital status epilepticus. Neurocrit Care 2015;23(1):33-43.
12. Sackles JC. Mosier JM. Patanwala AE, et al. First pass success without hypoxemia is increased with use of apneic oxygenation during rapid sequence intubation in the emergency department. Acad Emerg Med 2016;23(6):703-10.
13. Anderson LW, Granfeldt A, Callaway CW, et al. Association between tracheal intubation during adult in-hospital cardiac arrest and survival. JAMA 2017;317(5): 494-506.
14. Benger JR, Kirby K, Black S, et al. Effect of a strategy of a supraglottic airway device vs tracheal intubation during out-of-hospital cardiac arrest on functional outcome: The AIRWAYS-2 Randomized Clinical Trial. JAMA. 2018;320(8):779-91.
15. Kern KB, Hilwig RW, Berg RA, et al. Importance of continuous chest compressions during cardiopulmonary resuscitation: improved outcome during a simulated single lay-rescuer scenario. Circulation 2002;105(5):645-9.
16. Sanders AB, Kern KB, Berg RA, et al. survival and neurologic outcome after cardiopulmonary resuscitation with four different chest compression-ventilation ratios. Ann Emerg Med 2002;40(6):553-62.
17. Wang S, Li C, Ji X, et al. Effect of continuous compressions and 30:2 cardiopulmonary resuscitation on global ventilation/perfusion values during resuscitation in a porcine model. Crit Care Med 2010;38(10):2024-30.
18. Mader TJ,Kellog AR, Walterscheid JK, et al. A randomized comparison of cardiocerebral and cardiopulmonary resuscitation using a swine model of prolonged ventricular fibrillation. Resuscitation 2010;81(5):596-02.
19. Svensson L, Bohm K, Castren M, et al. Compression-only CPR or standard CPR in out-of-hospital cardiac arrest. N Engl J Med 2010;363(5):434-42.
20. Iwami T, Kawamura T, Hiraide A, et al. Effectiveness of bystander-initiated cardiac-only resuscitation for patients with out-of-hospital cardiac arrest. Circulation 2007;116(25):2900-7.
21. Kitamura T, Iwami T, Kawamura T, et al. Time-dependent effectiveness of chest compression-only and conventional cardiopulmonary resuscitation for out-of-hospital cardiac arrest of cardiac origin. Resuscitation 2011;82(1):3-9.
22. SOS-KANTO Study Group. Cardiopulmonary resuscitation by bystanders with chest compression only (SOS-KANTO): an observational study. Lancet 2007;369(9565):920-6.
23. Bobrow BJ, Spaite DW, Berg RA, et al. Chest compression-only CPR by lay rescuers and

survival from out-of-hospital cardiac arrest. JAMA 2010;304(13):1447-54.
24. Neumar RW, Shuster M, Callaway, et al. Part 1: Executive Summary: 2015 American Heart Association Guidelines Update for Cardiopulmonary Resuscitation and Emergency Cardiovascular Care. Circulation 2015;132(18 Suppl 2):S315-67.
25. Nadkarni VM, Larkin GL, Peberdy MA, et al. First documented rhythm and clinical outcome from in-hospital cardiac arrest among children and adults. JAMA 2006;295(1):50-7.
26. Meaney PA, Nadkarni VM, Kern KB, et al. Rhythms and outcomes of adult in-hospital cardiac arrest. Crit Care Med 2010;38(1):101-8.
27. Littmann L, Bustin, DJ, Haley, MW. A simplified and structured teaching tool for the evaluation and management of pulseless electrical activity. Med Princ Pract 2014;23(1):1-6.
28. Duncan JS, Sander JW, Sisodiya SM, et al. Adult epilepsy. Lancet 2006;367(9516):1087-1100.
29. Devinsky O. Sudden, unexpected death in epilepsy. N Engl J Med 2011;365(19):1801-1811. doi: 10.1056/NEJMra1010481
30. Mehvari J, Fadaie F, Omidi S, et al. Cardiac arrest associated with epileptic seizures: A case report with simultaneous EEG and ECG. Epilepsy Behav Case Rep 2014;2:145-151.
31. Stecker EC, Reinier K, Uy-Evanado A, et al. Relationship between seizure episode and sudden cardiac arrest in patients with epilepsy: A community-based study. Circ Arrhythm Electrophysiol 2013;6(5):912-6. after 26 on page 305:
32. Grmec S. Comparison of three different methods to confirm tracheal tube placement in emergency intubation. Intensive Care Med 2002;28(6):701-4.
33. Li J. Capnography alone is imperfect for endotracheal tube placement confirmation during emergency intubation. J Emerg Med 2001;20(3):223-9.
34. Das SK, Choupoo NS, Haldar R, et al. Transtracheal ultrasound for verification of endotracheal tube placement: a systematic review and meta-analysis. Can J Anaesth 2015;62(4):413-23.
35. Chou HC, Chong KM, Sim SS, et al. Real-time ultrasonography for confirmation of endotracheal tube placement during cardiopulmonary resuscitation. Resuscitation 2013;84(12):1708-12.
36. Einav S, Bromiker R, Weiniger CF, et al. Mathematical modeling for prediction of survival from resuscitation based on computerized continuous capnography: Proof of concept. Acad Emerg Med 2011;18(5):468-75.
37. Pepin M, Schwarze U, Superti-Furga A, et al. Clinical and genetic features of Ehlers-Danlos syndrome type IV, the vascular type. N Engl J Med 2000;342(10):673-80.
38. Gardner KF, Clattenburg EJ, Wroe P, et al. The Cardiac Arrest Sonographic Assessment (CASA) Exam - A standardized approach to the use of ultrasound in PEA. Am J Emerg Med 2018;36(4):729-31.
39. Reddy PS, Curtiss EI, Uretsky BF. Spectrum of hemodynamic changes in cardiac tamponade. Am J Cardiol 1990;66(20):1487-91.
40. Huis in 't Veld, Allison MG, Bostick DS, et al. Ultrasound use during cardiopulmonary resuscitation is associated with delays in chest compressions. Resuscitation 2017;119:95-8.
41. Atkinson P, Bowra J, Milne J, et al. International Federation for Emergency Medicine Consensus Statement: Sonography in hypotension and cardiac arrest (SHoC): An international consensus on the use of point of care ultrasound for undifferentiated hypotension and during cardiac arrest. CJEM 2017;19(6):459-70.
42. Saito Y, Donohue A, Attai S, et al. The syndrome of cardiac tamponade with "small" pericardial effusion. Echocardiography 2008;25(3):321-7.
43. Budhram G, Reardon R, Plummer D. Critical Care. In: Ma OJ, Mateer J, Reardon R, et al.

Ma & Mateer's Emergency Ultrasound. 3rd ed. New York, NY: McGraw-Hill, 2014:191-224.
44. Tsang TS, Enriquez-Sarano M, Freeman WK, et al. Consecutive 1127 therapeutic echocardiographically guided pericardiocenteses: clinical profile, practice patterns, and outcomes spanning 21 years. Mayo Clin Proc 2002;77(5):429-436.
45. Pomara C; Cassano T, D'Errico S, et al. Data available on the extent of cocaine use and dependence: biochemistry, pharmacologic effects and global burden of disease of cocaine abusers. Curr Med Chem 2012;19(33):5647-57.
46. Kanani PM, Guse PA, Smith WM, et al. Acute deleterious effects of cocaine on cardiac conduction, hemodynamics, and ventricular fibrillation threshold: effects of interaction with a selective dopamine D1 antagonist SCH 39166. J Cardovasc Pharmacol 1998;32(1):42-8.
47. O'Leary ME, Hancox JC. Role of voltage-gated sodium, potassium and calcium channels in the development of cocaine-associated cardiac arrhythmias. Br J Clin Pharmacol 2010;69(5):427-42.
48. Mittleman MA, Mintzer D, Maclure M, et al. Triggering of myocardial infarction by cocaine. Circulation 1999;99(21):2737-41.
49. Egashira K, Morgan KG, Morgan JP. Effects of cocaine on excitation-contraction coupling of aortic smooth muscle from the ferret. J Clin Invest 1991;87(4):1322-8.
50. Bauman JL, Grawe JJ, Winecoff AP, et al. Cocaine-related sudden cardiac death: a hypothesis correlating basic science and clinical observations. J Clin
51. Hollander JE, Hoffman RS, Burstein JL, et al. Cocaine-associated myocardial infarction. Mortality and complications. Cocaine-Associated Myocardial Infarction Study Group. Arch Intern Med 1995;155(10):1081-6.
52. Hsue PY, McManus D, Selby V, et al. Cardiac arrest in patients who smoke crack cocaine. Am J Cardiol 2007;99(6):822-4.
53. Eagle KA, Isselbacher EM, DeSanctis RW, et al. Cocaine-related aortic dissection in perspective. Circulation 2002;105(13):1529-30.
54. Hsue PY, Salinas CL, Bolger AF, et al. Acute aortic dissection related to crack cocaine. Circulation 2002;105(13):1592-5.
55. Lavonas EJ, Drennan IR, Gabrielli A, Part 10: Special circumstances of resuscitation. 2015 American Heart Association guidelines update for cardiopulmonary resuscitation and emergency cardiovascular care. Section 3: cardiac or respiratory arrest associated with opioid overdose. Circulation 2015; 132(18 Suppl 2):S501-18.
56. Field JM. Toxicology in emergency cardiovascular care. In: Advanced Cardiovascular Life Support Experienced Providers. Dallas, TX: American Heart Association, 2008:259-87. Available at: https://cpr.heart.org/en/courses/advanced-cardiovascular-life-support-for-experienced-providers.
57. McIntyre KM. Vasopressin in asystolic cardiac arrest. N Engl J Med 2004;350(2):179-81.
58. Wenzel V. Krismer AC. Arntz HR, et al. A comparison of vasopressin and epinephrine for out-of-hospital cardiopulmonary resuscitation. N Engl J Med 2004;350(2):105-13.
59. Richards JR, Garber D, Laurin EG, et al. Treatment of cocaine cardiovascular toxicity: a systematic review. Clin Toxicol (Phila) 2016;54(5):345-64.
60. Havakuk O, Rezkalla SH, Kloner RA. The cardiovascular effects of cocaine. J Am Coll Cardiol 2017;70(1):101-13.
61. Gaspari R, Weekes A, Adhikari S, et al. Emergency department point-of-care ultrasound in out-of-hospital and in-ed cardiac arrest. Resuscitation 2016;109:33-9.

62. American Heart Association. Part 3: Ethical Issues. Web-based Integrated 2010 & 2015 American Heart Association guidelines for cardiopulmonary resuscitation and emergency cardiovascular care. Available at https://eccguidelines.heart.org/index.php/circulation/cprecc-guidelines-2/part-3-ethical-issues/?strue=1&id=4-1-6
63. Bailey ED, Wydro GD, Crone DC. Termination of resuscitation in the prehospital setting for adult patients suffering nontraumatic cardiac arrest. National Association of EMS Physicians Standard and Clinical Practice Committee. Prehosp Emerg Care 2000;4(2):190-5.
64. Maekawa K, Tanno K, Hase M, et al. Extracorporeal cardiopulmonary resuscitation for patients with out-of-hospital cardiac arrest of cardiac origin: A propensity-matched study and predictor analysis. Crit Care Med 2013;41(5):1186-96.
65. Appelbaum P. Clinical practice. Assessment of patients' competence to consent to treatment. N Engl J Med 2007;357(18):1834-40.
66. Dunn LB, Nowrangi MA, Palmer BW, et al. Assessing decisional capacity for clinical research or treatment: a review of instrument. Am J Psychiatry 2006; 163(8):1323-34.
67. Schulz J, Sumpio BE, Gusberg RJ. Cocaine-associated myocardial and mesenteric ischemia: A case report and review of the literature. Int J Angiol 1998;7(1):1-5.
68. Byard RW. Acute mesenteric ischaemia and unexpected death. J Forensic Leg Med 2012;19(4):185-90.
69. Thomas VK, Paul C, Rajeev PC, et al. Reliability of ultrasonography in confirming endotracheal tube placement in an emergency setting. Indian J Crit Care Med 2017;21(5):257-61.

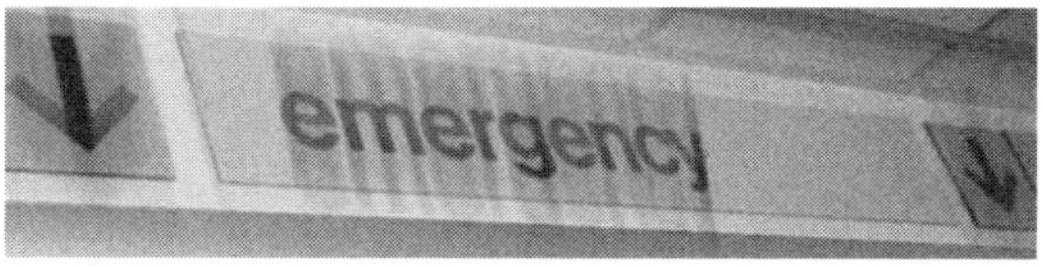

SECTION C – CARDIAC/ VASCULAR

Chapter 14: A 70-year-old woman with STEMI and hypotension

Nathan M. Finnerty, MD, FACEP
Assistant Professor, Adjunct
Emergency Medicine
Department of Emergency Medicine
The Ohio State University Wexner Medical Center
Columbus, OH

Section editor:
John C. Greenwood, MD
Assistant Professor
Department of Emergency Medicine
Department of Anesthesiology and Critical Care
Perelman School of Medicine
University of Pennsylvania
Philadelphia, PA

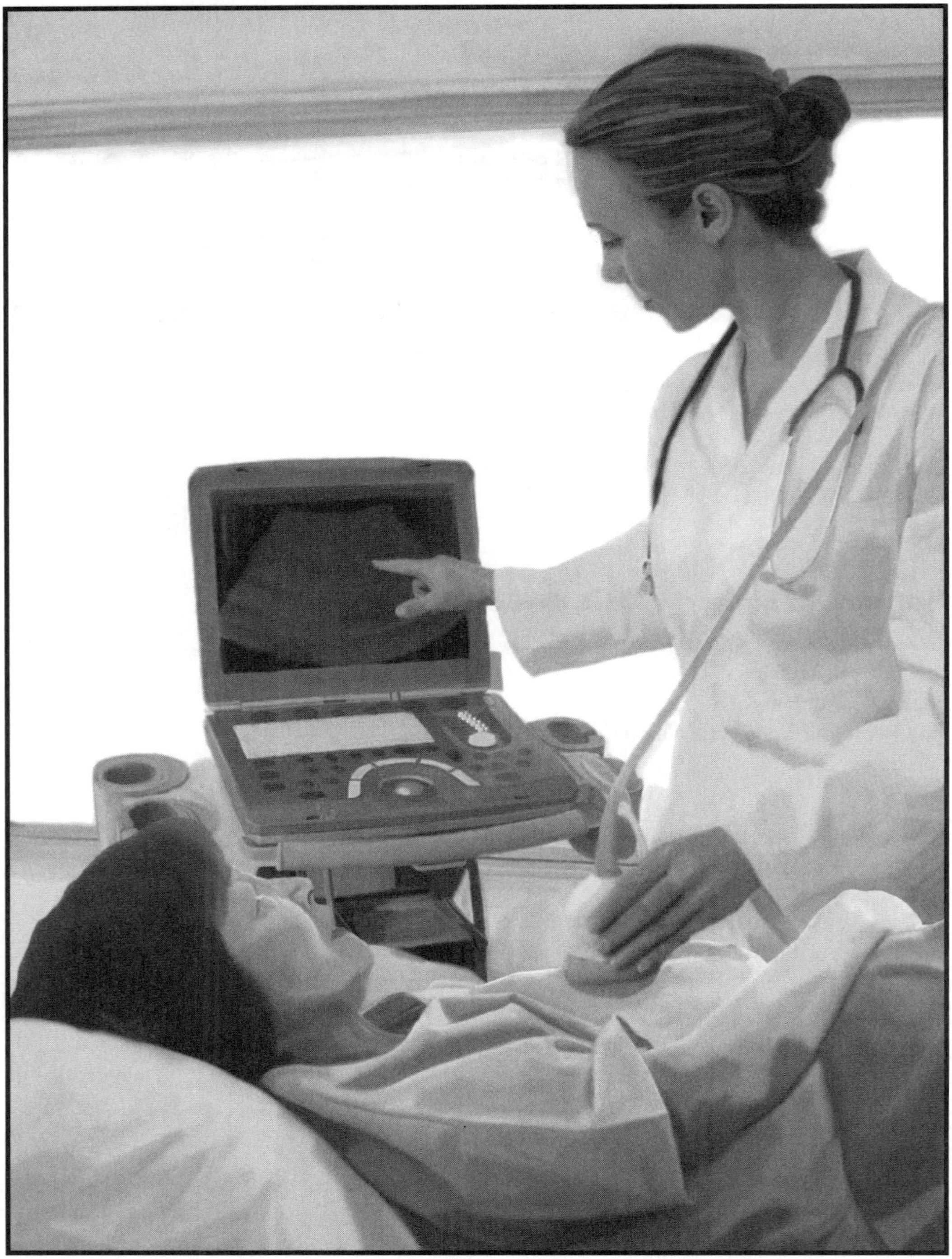

SECTION C/CHAPTER 14

A 70-year-old woman with STEMI and hypotension

The patient's story:
Suzanne is a 72-year-old woman, healthy and full of life. She is happily married to Joseph, who is 9 years her senior. She has recently sold her restaurant, a small building in an old firehouse, which has been in her family for the last three generations, with plans to spend more time with her two daughters and five grandchildren, both who still live in the same town. Though she is a smoker, she is otherwise well, attributing her energy to a good diet and a 1 mile walk each day.

On a cool spring morning, early in May, she develops chest pain. It is initially minimal, but when it worsens, she asks her husband to drive her to the ED, where she undergoes testing including labs, a chest XR, and a troponin, all of which return negative. An ECHO and a stress test are done in the observation unit, and when they return negative, she is discharged home and is asked to follow up with a cardiologist. When she calls the next day for a time, she is told the next appointment is June.

Suzanne is an early riser, but a week later, she finds it hard to even get out of bed, finally making it to the bathroom, brushing her teeth, and deliberately making it downstairs where she lays down on the couch. When her husband comes down for breakfast, he finds her there, pale and sweaty. He dials 911.

When EMS arrive, they perform an ECG showing ST elevation in leads II, III, and AVF with reciprocal changes. She is taken to the ED.

ED VISIT #2

CC (10:32): Chest pain

HPI (07:18): She presents with shortness of breath, sweatiness and weakness. She was admitted to [an outside] hospital a couple weeks ago. She had an echo and a stress test at that time and she was told everything was okay. She was discharged home and seemed to be doing well until several days ago when she started getting nauseated. Today, she developed shortness of breath. She has felt weak the last several days. She called EMS who saw the patient and found that she had an inferior STEMI. She was brought here after being given aspirin. She was hypotensive so they started some IVs and gave her fluids.

The patient denies chest pain on arrival here but it did develop it later in the visit. Substernal achiness that seems to radiate and move around. She has had nausea but no vomiting. No fevers, cough or cold symptoms that are new that she chronically has a smoker's cough that is unchanged. No swelling.

No fever, rhinorrhea, abd pain, n/v/d, blood in the stool or urine, rash, syncope, HA, vision changes, numbness.

NKDA
Medications: ASA just prior to arrive by EMS
PMH: Negative
PSH: Wrist surgery
FH: Negative
SH: Smoker, no alcohol or drugs

Vitals:

Time	Temp	Pulse	Resp	Syst	Diast	Sat
07:12	N/A	62	22	51	40	96% (NRB)

PE:
CONSTITUTIONAL: A&O, well-nourished. Pale and dyspneic. Anxious. Appears very ill. diaphoretic.
MOUTH: Mucous membranes are moderately dry, no erythema or exudates.
NECK: trachea is midline. voice is normal.
RESP: Normal chest excursion with respiration; breath sounds slightly diminished but essentially clear and equal bilaterally; no wheezes, rhonchi, or rales. Mild to moderate diffuse tenderness anteriorly
CARDIO: Normal S1, S2. Regular rate and rhythm, without murmurs
ABD: Non-distended; non-tender (though later developed abdominal tenderness while in CT scan); abdomen is soft, without rigidity, rebound or guarding. Normal BS. No masses or organomegaly
BACK: No CVA, midline or paraspinal muscle tenderness.
EXTREM: well perfused w/o cyanosis or edema. MOE x 4 easily. 1+ radial and faintly palp DP pulses equal bilaterally.

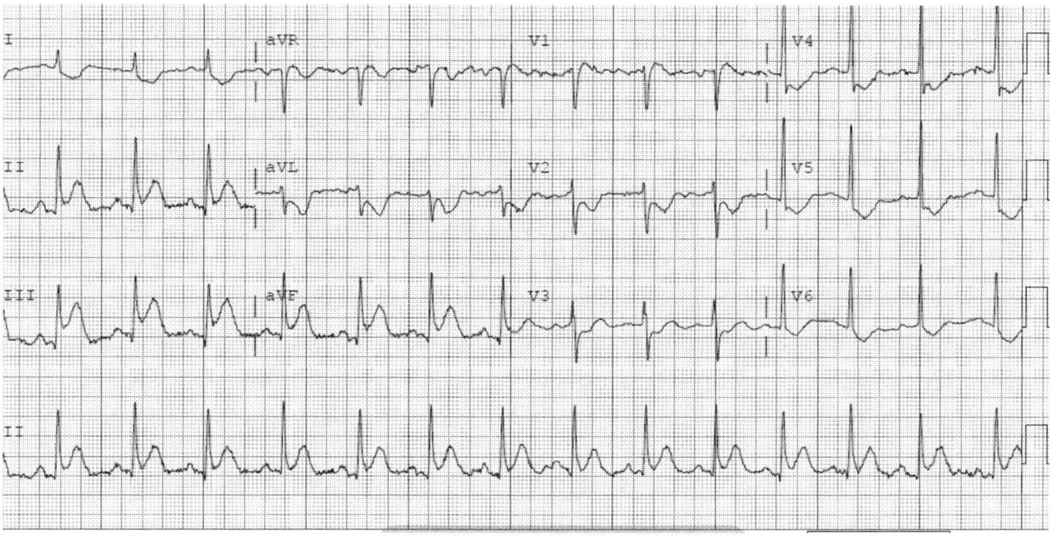

Electrocardiogram showing normal sinus rhythm with ST elevations in II, III, aVF and V1. Courtesy of V. Namana et al.[1] *Note: This is an example ECG, not the actual ECG in the case.*

Author comments (Weinstock):

Seems like the easiest case of the day; an inferior STEMI requiring cath lab activation... next patient. But a closer look reveals an SBP of 51 unresponsive to IV fluids. Could this be an RV infarct? Which immediate interventions should be done on our patient? We are at:

DECISION POINT A – YOU ARE FACED WITH 4 QUESTIONS:

1. **Which immediate interventions are helpful for this patient?**
2. **Why is our patient hypotensive and what should we do about it?**
3. **If there is a delay in interventional cardiac catheterization, is systemic thrombolytic therapy helpful?**
4. **How can point-of-care ultrasonography (POCUS) help with our patient?**

Q#1: Which immediate interventions are helpful for this patient?

There is no doubt that the patient is critically ill. Our initial approach focuses on airway, breathing and circulation. From the documentation, her airway is intact and breath sounds are clear and unlabored, so we can quickly shift our focus to the hypotension and hypoperfusion with cardiogenic shock (CS) being the most likely cause;[2] the evaluation does not suggest neurogenic or anaphylactic shock or a toxidrome such as beta-blocker or calcium channel overdose.[3,4]

Cath-lab activation or transfer to an appropriate care center should be initiated immediately, as early invasive strategy with appropriate revascularization is the reference standard of care for patients with suspected acute coronary syndrome (ACS)-associated CS.[4] In one study, early revascularization resulted in a 13.2% absolute risk reduction (ARR) in 6-year survival compared with initial medical stabilization, giving a number needed to treat (NNT) of 7.6.[5] In the setting of CS in a patient with resulted in a 13.2% absolute risk reduction (ARR) in 6-year survival compared with initial medical stabilization, giving a number needed to treat (NNT) of 7.6.[5] In the setting of CS in a patient with clear lungs, an initial volume challenge is recommended while awaiting definitive care, though over-aggressive volume replacement may do more harm than good.[6] The right ventricle (RV) is a pre-load dependent chamber and volume resuscitation remains the cornerstone of management for right ventricular infarction (RVI) to maintain adequate cardiac output.[4,6] In the setting of pulmonary edema, volume loading may be detrimental and precipitate respiratory failure and should be avoided or administered judiciously. Agents that reduce ventricular preload such as diuretics, nitrates, beta-blockers, and opioids should be avoided.[4,6,7] In most cases of CS, hypoperfusion will be refractory to volume resuscitation alone, and the addition of vasopressor support will be required.

In the setting of severe bradycardia, atropine can be given, though such patients will likely require temporary pacing.[6] Where available, temporary mechanical circulatory support (MCS) may be initiated in cases of refractory CS or cardiac arrest.[4] Though they may temporarily increase cardiac indices and mean arterial pressure, neither intra-aortic balloon pumps or percutaneous MCS have been shown to improve mortality.[4] Veno-arterial extracorporeal membrane oxygenation (ECMO) has shown promising results for temporizing CS.[4]

What about her underlying ACS? Traditional teaching for the management of ACS has been morphine, oxygen, nitroglycerine, and aspirin (MONA). But MONA for the management of ACS is not without controversy.

Morphine:
Morphine use in STEMI is associated with enhanced platelet reactivity, reduced spontaneous myocardial reperfusion, and larger infarct size for those treated with dual-antiplatelet therapy (DAPT) and primary percutaneous coronary intervention (PCI).[8] The use of morphine alone or in combination with nitroglycerin for patients presenting with non-ST-segment elevation ACS has been associated with increased mortality.[9] For ED patients diagnosed with acute heart failure, the use of IV morphine may be associated with increased 30-day mortality.[10] Though fentanyl has been shown to delay antiplatelet effects as well, its shorter time to peak effect, shorter duration of action, and reduced histamine release with subsequent hypotension may make it a superior choice for refractory pain in the setting of ACS with CS.[11]

Oxygen:
Despite its theoretical benefits, the routine use of supplemental oxygen in patients with suspected myocardial infarction without hypoxemia was not found to reduce 1-year all-cause mortality. Supplemental oxygen may increase early myocardial injury and lead to larger infarct size in patients with STEMI but without hypoxia.[12,13] Routine oxygen is not recommended in patients with $SaO_2 > 90\%$.[2]

Nitroglycerin:
Though nitrates have been shown to reduce mortality at 2 days when administered within 24 hours of symptom onset of acute myocardial infarction (AMI),[14] the suspected benefits of sublingual administration is primarily extrapolated from data on IV or long-acting nitrate use and their utility for STEMI is less clear.[2,14] In the setting of RVI and CS, administration of nitroglycerine may

significantly reduce preload and precipitate or worsen hypotension.[6,15] For patients presenting with inferior AMI or known acute RVI, nitrates should be avoided.[2,4,15]

Aspirin:

In the largest and most cited study on the topic, aspirin was found to reduce re-infarction (ARR=1.5%; NNT=67), cardiac arrest (ARR=1.2%; NNT=83), vascular deaths (ARR=2.4; NNT=42), and stroke (ARR=0.4%; NNT=250) with no significant difference in major bleeding.[16] It's hard to argue with those numbers.

So, the old habits die hard… we started with "MONA" and ended with an "A." Can we call it progress?

Q#2: Why is our patient hypotensive and what should we do about it?

Cardiogenic shock (CS):

CS results from ineffective cardiac output resulting in both clinical and biochemical manifestations of inadequate tissue perfusion.[4] AMI with left ventricular dysfunction is the most frequent cause of CS.[4,17] The resultant depression in myocardial contractility leads to reduced cardiac output and systemic hypoperfusion, which worsens coronary ischemia and precipitates further reductions in myocardial contractility.[4,17] As this death spiral continues, compensatory mechanisms are activated including sympathetic stimulation to increase heart rate and contractility and renal fluid retention to increase preload.[17] However, these compensatory mechanisms ultimately increase myocardial oxygen demand, reduce coronary perfusion, further inhibit cardiac output, worsen systemic hypoperfusion and may lead to pulmonary edema and respiratory failure.[17]

Right ventricular infarction (RVI):

Another cause of hypotension is RVI, usually the extension of an inferior left ventricular (LV) infarction with septal involvement.[18] Isolated RVI is uncommon; however, roughly one-third of patients suffering an acute inferoposterior STEMI will present with concomitant RVI with resultant higher in-hospital morbidity and mortality.[4,6,19] Proximal right coronary artery (RCA) occlusion is most commonly the culprit lesion resulting in RV ischemic dysfunction; however, RV performance can be maintained via collateral flow or spontaneous reperfusion.[19] The infarcted RV becomes stiff and dilated resulting in decreased RV compliance, reduced filling and decreased RV stroke volume.[6] This leads to decreased LV filling and a drop in cardiac output even in the setting of normal LV contractility.[6,17]

ECG changes with (RVI):

RVI is suspected when there is ST-segment elevation in lead V_1 along with inferoposterior ST-segment elevation (Leads II, III, AVF).[6] ST-segment elevations in precordial leads V_1 to V_5 may result from acute RVI, mimicking anterior ST-elevation MI.[6,20] In such cases, the distribution of ST-segment elevation in the anterior leads is greater in leads V_1–V_2 and decreased toward V_5–V_6 in RVI compared with anterior wall MI.[6,21]

Obtaining an ECG with right-sided precordial leads is essential in confirming RVI and should be performed early in the work-up as ST-segment changes in this distribution are transient and may be absent in up to 50% of patients > 12 hours after symptom onset.[6] ST-segment elevation in-hospital mortality.[6,23] To add insult to injury, RVI secondary to proximal RCA occlusion may also lead to right atrial (RA) and sinoatrial node (SAN) ischemia.[6,24] The symptoms of RVI may be more pronounced with associated right atrial infarction as RA dysfunction decreases RV filling leading to further reductions in LV preload and subsequent cardiac output; another problem is that SAN involvement predisposes to significant arrhythmias.[6]

Consulting editor comments (Weingart):

Oh yeah, so there's so much inherent in this! It's a weird dichotomy between a right ventricular involved MI—they have an inferior wall STEMI with right ventricular involvement—vs. your prototypical right-sided heart failure (your acute pulmonary embolism or pulmonary hypertension patient), in which fluids are the worst thing you can do for those patients in most circumstances. You have to be really sure of yourself to give fluids to those patients and yet you're like, "Oh no, the treatment for STEMI with right ventricular involvement is just give them a lot of fluid; give them a liter of fluid and that will fill that right side and passively send blood over to the left." And all of this is based on a really sketchy foundation. So, I would say if you want to try it, a liter is the top amount of fluid you could give those patients. For me it's 500 cc's, and then I'm going to start treating them like I would right-sided failure in the setting of a PE or a pulmonary hypertension, which means things like ionotropic support with dobutamine, or a low-dose epinephrine, as a way to bolster their output, as opposed to giving them more than 500 or 1,000 cc's of fluid. So that would be my transition point.

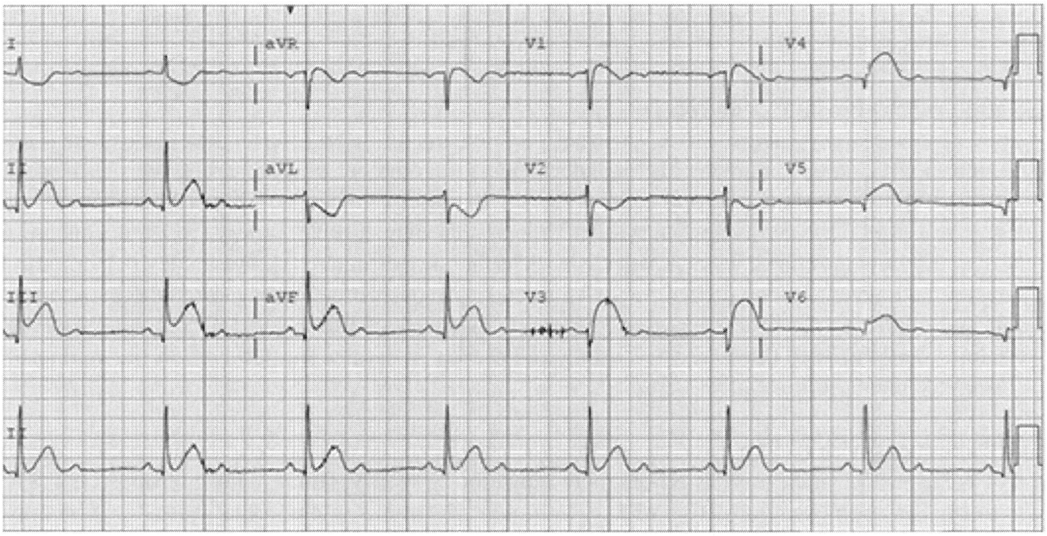

Right-sided precordial lead electrocardiogram showing 2:1 atrioventricular block and ST elevations in leads V3R–V6R. Courtesy of V. Namana et al.1

Note: This is an example ECG demonstrating Right-sided precordial leads, but not the actual ECG in the case.

Q#3: If there is a delay in interventional cardiac catheterization, is systemic thrombolytic therapy helpful?

Patients with CS are typically excluded from clinical trials of thrombolytic agents and, as a result, data is limited.[25] In one trial, CS developed significantly less frequently in patients receiving recombinant tissue-type plasminogen activator (rt-PA) though there were fewer deaths in patients who presented with CS and were treated with streptokinase plus heparin.[26] However, only angioplasty was associated with a significantly lower mortality rate.[26] When compared to placebo, streptokinase has not been shown to improve survival.[4,25] Thrombolysis may be more effective if increased aortic pressure is achieved, following the administration of an inotropic agent, for example, but the data is very limited.[27] Current guidelines suggest that when an early invasive approach cannot be completed in a timely fashion, fibrinolysis can be considered for STEMI with associated CS.[4] Given the lack of benefits currently reported, the risks of systemic thrombolysis may out-weigh the benefits and an early invasive strategy with appropriate revascularization remains the reference standard of care—it should not be delayed for STEMI with associated CS.[2,4]

Q#4: How can point-of-care ultrasonography (POCUS) help with our patient?

There are multiple potential applications for point-of-care ultrasonography (POCUS) in the ED and ICU.[28] As in our patient, early POCUS has been shown to reduce diagnostic uncertainty and increase diagnostic accuracy for patients with hypotension.[29-31] Though it may change management in selected cases, there is little data addressing patient centered outcomes, such as mortality.[29-33] The utility of POCUS is dependent on the clinical setting as well as the training of the provider performing and interpreting the exam. For example, POCUS has been found to be sensitive for the diagnosis of heart failure, whereas standard ED evaluation performed better in the diagnosis of COPD, asthma, and pulmonary embolism.[34] In other settings, POCUS may interfere with patient care and even cause harm, for example during cardiac arrest there is an association with significantly increased duration of pulse checks, nearly doubling the duration recommended in current guidelines.[35] Additionally, given the variation in POCUS training among ED providers, the sensitivity/specificity of a given exam may vary widely.[36] In the right setting and in the hand of the right provider, POCUS can guide resuscitative interventions and be lifesaving. However, the indiscriminate use of POCUS could lead to unnecessary testing and interventions in the case of false positive findings, or inadequate work-up and management for false negative findings.[32] Ultimately, providers should be aware of their limitations and maintain regular training.[36] In our patient we can make the argument that POCUS was warranted; but was it helpful or harmful?

DECISION POINT A – ***What did the actual provider do?***

MDM:
5/21/2017 07:25 – Pacer pads placed on Pt. during initial resuscitation due to risk of heart block. Spoke w [the interventional cardiologist], who is en route.

Portable CXR: no acute findings per ED interpretation

RESULTS (07:38):

WBC Count	5.8thou/mcL
Hemoglobin	**4.9gm/dL (L)**
Platelet Count	**71thou/mcL (L)**
Sodium Level	**145mmol/L (L)**
Potassium Level	**1.6mmol/L (L)**
Chloride Level	**129mmol/L (H)**
Bicarbonate	**8mmol/L (L)**
Anion Gap	8mmol/L
Glucose Level	**144mg/dL (H)**
BUN	16mg/dL
Creatinine	0.6mg/dL
Prothrombin Time (PT)	19 Sec

INR 1.7

Type and Cross match

Author comments (Weinstock):

So now things get interesting... our patient has drastically unexpected lab findings with severe anemia, hypokalemia, and acidosis, not to mention the abnormal POCUS findings below. There are some important bedside decisions to be made which may change the trajectory of the outcome.

PROCEDURE: 5/21/2017 07:32

EP bedside ECHO – re: hypotension and dyspnea-transthoracic echo shows pericardial effusion and possible depressed RV function; no evidence of tamponade; heterogeneous material in effusion noted though not clear what it is.

Impression: Pericardial effusion without tamponade. Decision to defer transfer to cath lab made based on this pending more comprehensive echo done by cardiac echo sonographer who is en route.

FAST – re: hypotension of unclear origin; 3 quadrants of abd evaluated including echo done previously; negative for intraperitoneal free fluid though pericardial effusion noted;
Impression: no evidence of intra-abd free fluid though pericardial effusion noted.

Aorta – re: hypotension of unclear origin; aorta evaluated without evidence of enlargement.
Impression: negative for aneurysm.

- **5/21/2017 07:55** – working with the interventional cardiologist at bedside. spoke with lab about blood products needed.
- **5/21/2017 07:59** – paging cardiothoracic surgery
- **5/21/2017 08:04** – spoke with physician covering – cardiothoracic surgery is in the OR

Vitals:

Time	Temp	Pulse	Resp	Syst	Diast	Sat
08:18	N/A	96	26	48	palp	95% (NRB)

- **5/21/2017 08:24** – Pt. has become more hypotensive. Serial echo—stable pericardial effusion with depressed RV function. FAST exam—no free fluid in the abd. Aorta—not enlarged and no obvious dissection. Spoke with cardiothoracic surgery about Pt. and continued discussions with the interventional cardiologist.

DECISION POINT B – YOU ARE FACED WITH 4 QUESTIONS:

1. **The patient remains hypotensive after IV fluids. Uncross matched blood has been started. Which vasoactive agent should be started?**
2. **What are the potential complications of AMI/STEMI?**
3. **How do we reconcile the severe anemia and hypokalemia?**
4. **Does knowledge of the patient's first encounter help or hinder the work-up at the second encounter?**

Q#1: The patient remains hypotensive after IV fluids. Uncross matched blood has been started Which vasoactive agent should be started?

There is little available data on clinical outcomes to guide the initial selection of vasoactive therapies in patients with CS.[4] In general, norepinephrine is associated with a lower incidence of arrhythmia and may be the vasopressor of choice for CS; however, dobutamine or dopamine (despite dopamine's increased risk for arrhythmia) may be considered in CS related to RVI.[4,6]

Section editor comments (Greenwood):

Initiating vasopressor therapy prior to inodilator therapy is critical to prevent worsening hypotension that is associated with dobutamine and milrinone therapy.

Q#2: What are the potential complications of AMI/STEMI?

In addition to arrhythmia, the major mechanical complications include rupture of the left ventricular free wall, papillary muscle rupture, and ventricular septal rupture. Each is extremely uncommon with an incidence of 0.52%, 0.26%, and 0.17%, respectively.[37,38]

Rupture of left ventricular free wall:

Rupture of the left ventricular free wall carries a high mortality.[2,37] Risk factors include older age, female gender, first MI, poor coronary artery collateralization, lack of reperfusion, or late fibrinolysis.[2,38] There are no presenting symptoms specific to free wall rupture. Patients may present with sudden onset of pain and/or cardiovascular collapse, though subacute presentations are not uncommon.[2,38] Non-specific symptoms such as repetitive emesis, restlessness, and agitation have been reported to be more common in those with AMI and rupture compared to AMI alone.[39] Finally, rupture may be preceded by one or more episodes of abrupt, transient hypotension and bradycardia.[39]

The diagnosis is confirmed by echocardiography with color-flow Doppler and definite treatment is surgical repair of the defect, though revascularization is recommended to reduce further ischemia and necrosis.[2,38]

Pericardiocentesis is controversial. In early rupture, partial sealing of the ruptured site by thrombus formation and the pericardium may permit time to perform a pericardiocentesis for hemodynamic stabilization in preparation for emergent surgery; however, it can cause a dangerous increase in blood pressure with increased tension on the damaged myocardium and the potential for extension to a full rupture.[2,38] Though ventricular wall rupture does not typically present immediately following an MI, *our* patient initially presented a week prior, increasing her risk for complications related to myocardial infarction. Pericardial blood on US is concerning for ventricular wall rupture.

Papillary muscle rupture:
Acute papillary muscle rupture is usually diagnosed between 2 to 7 days after AMI, though the median time to rupture is 13 hours.[2,38] Papillary muscle dysfunction due to partial or complete rupture most commonly follows an inferior or posterior AMI, given the single blood supply to the posteromedial papillary muscle from the posterior descending coronary artery.[38,41] Severe dysfunction or rupture of the papillary muscle leads to acute mitral regurgitation, pulmonary edema, and cardiogenic shock.[38] Clinically, a new pansystolic murmur heard loudest at the cardiac apex with radiation to the axilla is characteristic and chest x-ray demonstrates pulmonary edema.[38] Echocardiography with color-flow Doppler is the standard for diagnosis, and definitive treatment is via emergent surgery, though cardiac catheterization is recommended as concomitant revascularization during mitral valve surgery is associated with improved outcomes.[42-44] With medical therapy alone, in-hospital mortality is 70% and 80%.[45]

Section editor comments (Greenwood):

I'd also consider early mechanic support with an intra-aortic balloon pump (IABP) in this patient. Acute, ischemic mitral regurgitation has sound physiologic rationale and reasonable mortality data to support early IABP therapy to reduce regurgitant and VSD shunt fraction in patients with shock. [Kenner, et al. Am J Cardio – below]

Ventricular septal rupture:
Since the introduction of early reperfusion therapy, the incidence of ventricular septal rupture (VSR) has decreased from 1–2% to 0.17% and is usually diagnosed within the first 24 hours of AMI.[26,38] VSR may occur following posteroinferior, posterolateral or anteroseptal AMI.[2,38,46] Ischemia and necrosis of the interventricular septum leads to a septal defect and shunting of blood from the LV to the RV, leading to volume overload and RV dysfunction.[38] Ultimately, the combination of AMI and VSR may lead to LV and RV failure and CS.

Clinical presentation is similar to left ventricular free wall rupture; VSR may precede free wall rupture, emphasizing the need for revascularization and early surgical repair.[47] A harsh pansystolic murmur heard loudest at the left sternal edge is present in up to 90% of patients, with an associated parasternal thrill palpable in 50% of patients.[38,48] This may differentiate VSR from MR due to papillary muscle rupture.

Echocardiography with color-flow Doppler is the reference standard for diagnosis.[49] Surgical repair with concomitant revascularization is recommended as medical management alone is almost universally fatal at 30 days.[2,50,51]

Q#3: How do we reconcile the severe anemia and hypokalemia?

Acute anemia should alter the care for this patient… if it is real. Consider this, of the various forms of statistical analysis reported in clinical studies, the P-value is often used to assess significance. Generally, a P-value less than 0.05 is considered significant and indicates that the results of an experiment are due to more than just chance.[52] With a traditional cutoff of 0.05, we accept that for every 20 variables analyzed, one may be "abnormal" by random chance alone. With that in mind, in the ED evaluation of chest pain, we generally measure over 20 variables, meaning that we will have at least 1 abnormal test by chance alone! Though we often joke about the radiologist's mantra—"clinical correlation required"—we need to repeat these "sage" words at times also: if the results do not fit the clinical picture, we should question the results and perform confirmatory testing. In this context, we have not only found anemia, but also hypokalemia. Does this fit into our clinical picture? Answer: No.

If we were truly dealing with acute pancytopenia, there could very easily be a component of cell lysis leading to *hyper,* and not *hypo*kalemia which is almost always the result of potassium loss with prescribed medications being the most common cause.[53] In the absence of an inciting medication, hypokalemia can result from inadequate intake or abnormal loss through the kidney due to metabolic alkalosis or through the gastrointestinal tract secondary to diarrhea.[53] None of these etiologies for hypokalemia fit our patient's clinical picture. So, the single unifying diagnosis could be dilution. If available, POC testing can be utilized, as there is excellent agreement with central laboratory testing.[54,55] This would be an effective means to avoid unnecessary and potentially life-threatening deviations from essential interventions. If POC testing affirms our suspicion of dilution, then arrangements should be made for angiography and revascularization.

Q#4: Does knowledge of the patient's first encounter help or hinder the work-up at the second encounter?

At the index visit, the patient presented with chest pain. As the differential diagnosis for chest pain is broad, the focus of the ED provider is often on risk stratification, not necessarily on diagnosis. Of the available risk stratification tools, the HEART score has come to the forefront of emergency medicine practice. It was designed to assess patients presenting to the ED with possible acute coronary syndrome and identify those at low, moderate, or high risk for adverse events.[56]

The HEART score utilizes a composite outcome of a major adverse cardiac event (MACE), which includes AMI, PCI, coronary artery bypass graft surgery (CABG), and all-cause death measured at 6 weeks.[56] We don't have all the information needed to accurately risk stratify this patient, but given that she was placed in observation for urgent stress testing, we will assume she was deemed to be moderate; with a risk of MACE at 6 weeks from 17–20%.[56,57]

There is no definitive data to suggest that ED observation reduces the risk of short-term MACE,[58,59] and cardiovascular testing has not been shown to reduce admissions for AMI.[60,61] Given the specificity of STEMI for AMI, emergent coronary angiography and revascularization are the reference standard of care followed by additional diagnostic testing after ruling out obstructive coronary artery disease.[2] What happened with our patient? Unfortunately, knowledge of the patient's recent observation stay and subsequent stress testing may have led the provider to search for an alternative source of her hypotension and STEMI. Had she presented initially with STEMI, likely her care would have differed considerably.

DECISION POINT B – ***What did the actual provider do?***

- **5/21/2017 08:28** – KCl ordered and blood infusion started (uncross matched initially). Dopamine started.
- **5/21/2017 08:54** – Spoke with the intensivist. Pt.'s pressure improving. Pt. may have had progressive anemia. No s/sx of blood loss at this time.
- **5/21/2017 08:59** – Rectal: intact tone. Dark brown stool that is guaiac negative.
- **5/21/2017 09:00** – Records arrived from outside hospital. D/c 5/4/2017. Hgb there was 14. Consider accidental dilutional effects as well—will recheck CBC and BMP.
- Stat bedside formal echo in progress. Floating substance around heart not causing evidence of tamponade. RV maybe slightly less function.
- **5/21/2017 09:27** – Spoke with hospitalist—admit. Spoke with staff about holding potassium pending chemistries. I am concerned of dilutional effect causing initial results.
- **5/21/2017 10:01** – Pt. is more SOB. Lung sounds distant. Notes soreness in chest with coughing when asked to cough purposely; limited ability to do so. Chest wall is tender. Pt. still cyanotic in neck and face. Will try neb and recheck ECG and CXR.

RESULTS (09:04):

WBC Count	14.8thou/mcL
Hemoglobin	14.2gm/dL
Platelet Count	**133thou/mcL (L)**
Sodium Level	**136mmol/L (L)**
Potassium Level	3.8mMol/L
Chloride Level	**109mmol/L (L)**
Bicarbonate	**15mmol/L (L)**
Anion Gap	12mMol/L
Glucose Level	**292mg/dL (H)**
BUN	13mg/dL
Creatinine	**1.4mg/dL (H)**
ALT	**349U/L (H)**
AST	**495U/L (H)**
Total Bilirubin	0.9mg/dL

MDM note: The patient was due to undergo PFTs for COPD in a couple of weeks. She may indeed have COPD but I suspect her symptoms today are from her inferolateral (RCA) STEMI. She has evidence of RCA occlusion on her CT angiogram when we reviewed this with the radiologist. However, given her pericardial effusion and the risk of worsening this with intervention, the decision was made not to do cardiac catheterization because of the need for anticoagulants. If she does have RV rupture, it currently is contained and not causing tamponade.

Her initial lab work was extremely concerning but then as we started evaluating her more, we opted to reconsider. I ordered new blood work to be done which showed different information. We did spend a fair amount of time looking for blood loss sources and thankfully did not find any. Her second round of bloodwork was more consistent with her clinical picture. She did get several units of blood before the second hemoglobin returned. However, we were able to limit how much potassium she got and ended up giving her half of the originally intended amount.

We continue to keep the family updated as well as the patient. In the end, I suspect the patient's primary issue is her STEMI though we continued to consider several other potential causes such as pericarditis and other causes of the pericardial effusion like RV rupture, aortic dissection, G.I. bleeding, infectious causes/sepsis, etc. We opted to place her in the ICU for further evaluation and treatment. The patient and her family were agreeable to the plan of care with no further questions.

DECISION POINT C– YOU ARE FACED WITH 2 QUESTIONS:

1. **With the return of the "normal" labs, should an emergent cardiac catheterization be done *now*?**
2. **How do we reconcile a difference of management between the emergency physician (EP) and specialist?**

Q#1: With the return of the "normal" labs, should an emergent cardiac catheterization be done *now*?

As expected, repeat serum studies confirm our suspicion that the abnormalities first noted were due to dilution. The confounding factor is the fact that the patient received an unspecified amount of uncross matched packed red blood cells (PRBCs) and potassium. On average, 1 unit of packed red blood cells transfused increases hematocrit by about 2–3% and hemoglobin by about 1g/dL.[62,63] It is unlikely that the patient received 10 units of PRBCs to account for the difference in initial serum results and follow-up testing! Additionally, her repeat serum studies are consistent with previous labs obtained from her recent ED visit. In general it is expected that for every 10mEq of potassium given the serum potassium would be expected to rise by about by 0.1mEq/L.[64] At a rate of 20mEq/hr, the repeat potassium level is clearly not from repletion.[53] On a side note, supplemental potassium administration is also the most common cause of severe hyperkalemia in hospitalized patients and can reach life threatening levels.[53] Finally, if the anemia were the primary source of the patient's hypotension with associated demand ischemia in the form of STEMI, then we would expect to see significant improvement in her clinical status and even resolution of her ECG findings with resolution of her anemia. This wasn't the case. Overall, PRBCs and potassium could have been withheld and confirmatory testing performed to prevent iatrogenic harm, but both interventions should be discontinued at this point.

Chapter author expert opinion: As the initially erroneous lab results would not expect to account for the patient's symptoms, this chapter author recommends a reconsideration of emergent cardiac catheterization.

Q#2:How do we reconcile a difference of management between the emergency physician (EP) and specialist?

Communication breakdowns are among the most frequent contributors to adverse events in medicine, with the majority involving verbal communication between two providers.[65] Emergency operations are at increased risk for information loss,[65] in other words, ED consultations are at high risk for miscommunication and subsequent medical errors. There is limited data addressing consultation practices and methods in the ED;[66] however, a standardized means of communication in these high risk situations may reduce the risk of communication errors.[67] Situation, Background, Assessment, Recommendations (SBAR) is thought to create conditions for accurate information exchange and is recommended by the World Health Organization to increase patient safety.[68] In one study, the proportion of incident reports due to communication errors decreased from 31% to 11% after the implementation of SBAR (ARR=20%; NNT=5).[68]

Regardless of how communication with a consultant is approached, the primary goal should be to reduce ambiguity about roles and responsibilities.[65] It is the ED provider's responsibility to give a concise and clear case presentation, the limitations of continued ED care, and the role and responsibility of the consultant. In this case, the only intervention that may make a difference for our patient is PCI; it is the responsibility of the ED provider to communicate this to the consultant. Clearly explaining the lab error that led to the perception of anemia and the role of angiography even in the setting of pericardial effusion may have reduced case ambiguity and focused the conversation on the need for cardiovascular intervention. In the end, a strong knowledge base of current evidence and practice guidelines, an effective means of communication, and a firm commitment to do what is right for the patient may subvert a difficult consultant.

Author comments (Weinstock):

The discussion should be documented in a clear and truthful fashion. An example for our case, with the initial interaction, could be, "I spoke with Dr. ____, the interventional cardiologist at ____ and we discussed the patient's history, presentation, vital signs including severe hypotension and her ECG. [They] said that I should wait to activate the cath lab and that they would be into the ED within 20 minutes."

Final diagnosis:
1. Acute inferolateral STEMI with pericardial effusion, hypotension and dyspnea
2. Acute pericardial effusion and pericarditis, etiology unclear—infectious vs. hemorrhagic vs. inflammatory vs. other
3. Acute hypokalemia
4. Acute acidosis
5. Acute thrombocytopenia
6. ARI and abnormal LFTs

Inpatient course:

Cardiology consult: Patient was seen in the ED earlier today. Records from outside hospital reviewed. Echo from 1 week ago without pericardial effusion. Current echo findings consistent with a large inferoposterior infarct and probable contained myocardial rupture with blood in the pericardial space. Initial CBC was erroneous-Hb now 14g. Regardless, the patient is not a candidate for any procedure requiring anticoagulation or antiplatelet tx. Discussed option for surgery with [cardiothoracic]. Due to late presentation and current medical issues, he felt she is not a surgical candidate for revascularization at this time. Despite ongoing CP and ECG changes, there is nothing we can offer this patient without risking further clinical deterioration from cardiac tamponade. Repeat echo with less effusion and surprisingly improved LV function. Will manage medically close surveillance.

ICU Note (next day): Patient was initially admitted in for acute inferolateral wall MI and started on medical management only. Her symptoms had started to improve with nitrates. Last night, her BP started to fall. This AM she became bradycardic and unresponsive. CPR was initiated after the patient was found to be in PEA. ACLS protocol was initiated at 0549 hours. The patient received multiple rounds of epinephrine and was intubated successfully. Throughout the entire course of the code the patient remained in PEA. During several pulse checks, bedside cardiac ultrasonography was used to perform direct visualization of cardiac activity. Although a small pericardial effusion could be seen, there was complete cessation of all cardiac activity.
She could not be revived with the advanced cardiac resuscitation efforts.
She was pronounced at 6:14 a.m.
Cause of death: Cardiac arrest 2/2 Inferior wall STEMI

Final discussion/chapter author expert opinion/debrief:
There are two seminal facts pertinent to this case:
- CS is the leading cause of in-hospital mortality complicating STEMI.[2,4,69]
- Revascularization is the only treatment proven to decrease mortality rates.[2,4]

There were several complicating factors that altered the clinical course:
1. **Associated pericardial effusion deterred early revascularization.** This may have been incidental but was also possibly secondary to early free wall rupture. Risk of bleeding is the most commonly cited contraindication to PCI and has been shown to contribute to in-hospital mortality; however, it is not listed as an absolute contraindication for angiography and revascularization.[69-71] Instead, bleeding risk reduction strategies are suggested.[2,69] In the

setting of free wall rupture, revascularization is recommended to reduce further ischemia and necrosis followed by surgical repair.[2,38] In one case report, a 62-year-old woman presenting with inferior AMI and evidence of free wall rupture successfully underwent RCA PCI without the subsequent need for surgery.[72] As serial echos demonstrated reduced pericardial effusion, the patient should have been reconsidered for revascularization. Though PCI is not recommended in patients with STEMI in whom the risks of revascularization are likely to outweigh the benefits, that was not necessarily the case here.[69]

2. **Anemia and hypokalemia.** These two findings did not fit the clinical picture and further delayed care and deterred revascularization efforts. Early recognition of erroneous results and rapid confirmation could prevent deviations from definitive care as well as iatrogenic harm from unnecessary repletion and interventions. It is the ED provider's responsibility to recognize these inconsistencies, redirect care, and emphasize the need for revascularization.
3. **Previous ED visit.** Understanding the limitations of observation care and non-invasive testing in the setting of acute chest pain is critical. The patient's previous ED visit and subsequent testing did not significantly reduce her likelihood for MACE. STEMI on ECG is infarction until proven otherwise. Mimics, such as aortic dissection presenting with STEMI are rare (< 1%).[73] Though CT angiography may delay definitive care, it may be unavoidable in some cases and we can't fault the ED provider in this case. However, there are case reports in which aortic dissection has been diagnosed during emergency coronary angiography followed by successful surgical repair.[73] Either way, once dissection has been ruled out, revascularization should have been revisited.
4. **ICU care included the use of nitrates.** In the setting of RVI and CS, nitrates are contraindicated. This may have contributed to her progressive hypotension and ultimate PEA arrest, though it may also have occurred due to persistent infraction without revascularization.

Given the high mortality associated with CS due to STEMI and the possibility of an underlying ventricle free wall rupture, there is no guarantee that a change in clinical management would have improved this patient's outcome. However, there were opportunities for improvement.

Section editor comments (Greenwood):

Agreed, would have probably also ordered a CTAngio—to rule out aortic dissection with RCA/pericardial extension once it was determined the patient was not eligible for the cath lab.

Author comments (Weinstock):

This is a tragic case; the patient presented with a STEMI and we were not able to save her. In the end we can advocate for our patients, as was done by this EP, but we cannot do the cardiac cath ourselves... still, I wonder if it had been done, would we still be reading about this case now?

References:

1. Namana V, Balasubramanian R. Images in clinical medicine. Right ventricular infarction. N Engl J Med 2016;374(9):872.
2. Ibanez B, James S, Agewall S, et al. 2017 ESC Guidelines for the management of acute

myocardial infarction in patients presenting with ST-segment elevation: The Task Force for the management of acute myocardial infarction in patients presenting with ST-segment elevation of the European Society of Cardiology (ESC). Eur Heart J 2018;39(2):119-77.
3. St-Onge M, Anseeuw K, Cantrell FL, et al. Experts consensus recommendations for the management of calcium channel blocker poisoning in adults. Crit Care Med 2017;45(3):e306-15.
4. van Diepen S, Katz JN, Albert NM, et al. Contemporary management of cardiogenic shock: A scientific statement from the American Heart Association. Circulation 2017;136(16):e232-68.
5. Hochman JS, Sleeper LA, Webb JG, et al. Early revascularization and long-term survival in cardiogenic shock complicating acute myocardial infarction. JAMA 2006;295(21):2511-5.
6. Namana V, Gupta SS, Abbasi AA, et al. Right ventricular infarction. Cardiovasc Revasc Med 2018;19(1 Pt A):43-50.
7. Caplin JL. Acute right ventricular infarction. BMJ 1989;299(6697):515-6.
8. Farag M, Spinthakis N, Srinivasan M, et al. Morphine analgesia pre-PPCI is associated with prothrombotic state, reduced spontaneous reperfusion and greater infarct size. Thromb Haemost 2018; 118(3):601-12.
9. Meine TJ, Roe MT, Chen AY, et al. Association of intravenous morphine use and outcomes in acute coronary syndromes: Results from the CRUSADE Quality Improvement Initiative. Am Heart J 2005;149(6):1043-9.
10. Miro O, Gil V, Martin-Sanchez FJ, et al. Morphine use in the ED and outcomes of patients with acute heart failure: A propensity score-matching analysis based on the EAHFE registry. Chest 2017;152(4):821-32.
11. McEvoy JW, Ibrahim K, Kickler TS, et al. Effect of intravenous fentanyl on ticagrelor absorption and platelet inhibition among patients undergoing percutaneous coronary intervention: The PACIFY randomized clinical trial (platelet aggregation with ticagrelor inhibition and fentanyl). Circulation 2018;137(3):307-9.
12. Hofmann R, James SK, Jernberg T, et al. Oxygen therapy in suspected acute myocardial infarction. N Engl J Med 2017;377(13):1240-9.
13. Stub D, Smith K, Bernard S, et al. Air versus oxygen in ST-segment-elevation myocardial infarction. Circulation 2015;131(24):2143-50.
14. Perez MI, Musini VM, Wright JM. Effect of early treatment with anti-hypertensive drugs on short and long-term mortality in patients with an acute cardiovascular event. Cochrane Database Syst Rev 2009;(4):CD006743.
15. Ferguson JJ, Diver DJ, Boldt M, et al. Significance of nitroglycerin-induced hypotension with inferior wall acute myocardial infarction. Am J Cardiol1989;64(5):311-4.
16. Randomised trial of intravenous streptokinase, oral aspirin, both, or neither among 17,187 cases of suspected acute myocardial infarction: ISIS-2. ISIS-2 (Second International Study of Infarct Survival) Collaborative Group. Lancet 1988;2(8607):349-60.
17. Hollenberg SM, Kavinsky CJ, Parrillo JE. Cardiogenic shock. Ann Intern Med.1999;131(1):47-59.
18. Lopez-Sendon J, Coma-Canella I, Alcasena S, et al. Electrocardiographic findings in acute right ventricular infarction: Sensitivity and specificity of electrocardiographic alterations in right precordial leads V4R, V3R, V1, V2, and V3. J Am Coll Cardiol 1985;6(6):1273-9.
19. Bowers TR, O'Neill WW, Pica M, et al. Patterns of coronary compromise resulting in acute right ventricular ischemic dysfunction. Circulation 2002;106(9):1104-9.

20. Geft IL, Shah PK, Rodriguez L, et al. ST elevations in leads V1 to V5 may be caused by right coronary artery occlusion and acute right ventricular infarction. Am J Cardiol 1984;53(8):991-6.
21. Mavric Z, Zaputovic L, Matana A, et al. Prognostic significance of complete atrioventricular block in patients with acute inferior myocardial infarction with and without right ventricular involvement. Am H J 1990;119(4):823-8.
22. van der Bolt CL, Vermeersch PH, Plokker HW. Isolated acute occlusion of a large right ventricular branch of the right coronary artery following coronary balloon angioplasty. The only true 'model' to study ECG changes in acute, isolated right ventricular infarction. Eur Heart J 1996;17(2):247-50.
23. Zehender M, Kasper W, Kauder E, et al. Right ventricular infarction as an independent predictor of prognosis after acute inferior myocardial infarction. N Engl J Med 1993;328(14):981-8.
24. Vikse J, Henry BM, Roy J, et al. Anatomical variations in the sinoatrial nodal artery: A meta-analysis and clinical considerations. PLoS One 2016;11(2):e0148331.
25. Col NF, Gurwitz JH, Alpert JS, et al. Frequency of inclusion of patients with cardiogenic shock in trials of thrombolytic therapy. Am J Cardiol 1994;73(2):149-57.
26. Holmes DR, Jr., Bates ER, Kleiman NS, et al. Contemporary reperfusion therapy for cardiogenic shock: The GUSTO-I trial experience. The GUSTO-I investigators. Global utilization of streptokinase and tissue plasminogen activator for occluded coronary arteries. J Am Coll Cardiol 1995;26(3):668-74.
27. Garber PJ, Mathieson AL, Ducas J, et al. Thrombolytic therapy in cardiogenic shock: Effect of increased aortic pressure and rapid tPA administration. Can J Cardiol 1995;11(1):30-6.
28. Emergency ultrasound imaging criteria compendium. American College of Emergency Physicians. Ann Emerg Med 2006;48(4):487-510.
29. Ahn JH, Jeon J, Toh HC, et al. SEARCH 8Es: A novel point of care ultrasound protocol for patients with chest pain, dyspnea or symptomatic hypotension in the emergency department. PLoS One 2017;12(3):e0174581.
30. Jones AE, Tayal VS, Sullivan DM, et al. Randomized, controlled trial of immediate versus delayed goal-directed ultrasound to identify the cause of nontraumatic hypotension in emergency department patients. Crit Care Med 2004;32(8):1703-8.
31. Shokoohi H, Boniface KS, Pourmand A, et al. Bedside ultrasound reduces diagnostic uncertainty and guides resuscitation in patients with undifferentiated hypotension. Crit Care Med 2015;43(12):2562-9.
32. Moore CL, Copel JA. Point-of-care ultrasonography. N Engl J Med 2011;364(8):749-57.
33. Rose JS. Ultrasonography and outcomes research: one small step for mankind or another drop in the bucket? Ann Emerg Med 2006;48(3):237-9.
34. Zanobetti M, Scorpiniti, M, Gigli C, et al. Point-of-care ultrasonography for evaluation of acute dyspnea in the ED. Chest 2017;151(6):1295-01.
35. Huis in't Veld MA, Allison MG, Bostick DS, et al. Ultrasound use during cardiopulmonary resuscitation is associated with delays in chest compressions. Resuscitation 2017;119:95-8.
36. Pedraza GJ, Valle AJ, Ceballos GP, et al. Comparison of the accuracy of emergency department performed point-of-care-ultrasound (POCUS) in the diagnosis of lower-extremity deep vein thrombosis. J Emerg Med 2018; 54(5):656-64.
37. French JK, Hellkamp AS, Armstrong PW, et al. Mechanical complications after percutaneous coronary intervention in ST-elevation myocardial infarction (from APEX-AMI). Am J Cardiol 2010;105(1):59-63.

38. Kutty RS, Jones N, Moorjani N. Mechanical complications of acute myocardial infarction. Cardiol Clin 2013;31(4):519-531, vii-viii.
39. Oliva PB, Hammill SC, Edwards WD. Cardiac rupture, a clinically predictable complication of acute myocardial infarction: Report of 70 cases with clinicopathologic correlations. J Am Coll Cardiol 1993;22(3):720-6.
40. Nozoe M, Sakamoto T, Taguchi E, et al. Clinical manifestation of early phase left ventricular rupture complicating acute myocardial infarction in the primary PCI era. J Cardiol 2014;63(1):14-8.
41. Voci P, Bilotta F, Caretta Q, et al. Papillary muscle perfusion pattern. A hypothesis for ischemic papillary muscle dysfunction. Circulation 1995;91(6):1714-18.
42. Chevalier P, Burri H, Fahrat F, et al. Perioperative outcome and long-term survival of surgery for acute post-infarction mitral regurgitation. Eur J Cardiothorac Surg 2004;26(2):330-5.
43. Lorusso R, Gelsomino S, De Cicco G, et al. Mitral valve surgery in emergency for severe acute regurgitation: Analysis of postoperative results from a multicentre study. Eur J Cardiothorac Surg 2008;33(4):573-82.
44. Russo A, Suri RM, Grigioni F, et al. Clinical outcome after surgical correction of mitral regurgitation due to papillary muscle rupture. Circulation 2008;118(15):1528-34.
45. Kishon Y, Oh JK, Schaff HV, et al. Mitral valve operation in postinfarction rupture of a papillary muscle: Immediate results and long-term follow-up of 22 patients. Mayo Clin Proc 1992;67(11):1023-30.
46. Vlodaver Z, Edwards JE. Rupture of ventricular septum or papillary muscle complicating myocardial infarction. Circulation 1977;55(5):815-22.
47. Figueras J, Cortadellas J, Soler-Soler J. Comparison of ventricular septal and left ventricular free wall rupture in acute myocardial infarction. Am J Cardiol 1998;81(4):495-7.
48. Lemery R, Smith HC, Giuliani ER, et al. Prognosis in rupture of the ventricular septum after acute myocardial infarction and role of early surgical intervention. Am J Cardiol 1992;70(2):147-51.
49. Fortin DF, Sheikh KH, Kisslo J. The utility of echocardiography in the diagnostic strategy of postinfarction ventricular septal rupture: A comparison of two-dimensional echocardiography versus doppler color flow imaging. Amer Heart J 1991;121(1 Pt 1):25-32.
50. Poulsen SH, Praestholm M, Munk K, et al. Ventricular septal rupture complicating acute myocardial infarction: Clinical characteristics and contemporary outcome. Ann Thorac Surg 2008;85(5):1591-6.
51. Perrotta S, Lentini S. In patients undergoing surgical repair of post-infarction ventricular septal defect, does concomitant revascularization improve prognosis? Interact Cardiovasc Thorac Surg 2009;9(5):879-87.
52. Farrell MB. Statistics refresher for molecular imaging technologists, Part 2: Accuracy of interpretation, significance, and variance. J Nucl Med Technol 2018;46(2):76-80.
53. Gennari FJ. Hypokalemia. N Eng J Med 1998;339(7):451-8.
54. Dashevsky M, Bernstein SL, Barsky CL, et al. Agreement between serum assays performed in ED point-of-care and hospital central laboratories. West J Emerg Med 2017;18(3):403-9.
55. McIntosh BW, Vasek J, Taylor M, et al. Accuracy of bedside point of care testing in critical emergency department patients. Am J Emerg Med 2018; 36(4):567-70.
56. Six AJ, Backus BE, Kelder JC. Chest pain in the emergency room: Value of the HEART score. Neth Heart J 2008; 16(6):191-6.

57. Backus BE, Six AJ, Kelder JC, et al. A prospective validation of the HEART score for chest pain patients at the emergency department. Int J Cardiol 2013;168(3):2153-8.
58. Holly J, Hamilton D, Bledsoe J, et al. Prospective evaluation of the treatment of intermediate-risk chest pain patients in an emergency department observation unit. Crit Pathw Cardiol 2012;11(1):10-3.
59. Wang H, Watson K, Robinson RD, et al. Chest pain risk scores can reduce emergent cardiac imaging test needs with low major adverse cardiac events occurrence in an emergency department observation unit. Crit Pathw Cardiol 2016;15(4):145-51.
60. Sandhu AT, Heidenreich PA, Bhattacharya J, et al. Cardiovascular testing and clinical outcomes in emergency department patients with chest pain. JAMA Intern Med 2017;177(8):1175-82.
61. Foy AJ, Dhruva SS, Peterson B, et al. Coronary computed tomography angiography vs functional stress testing for patients with suspected coronary artery disease: A systematic review and meta-analysis. JAMA Intern Med 2017;177(11):1623-31.
62. Elzik ME, Dirschl DR, Dahners LE. Correlation of transfusion volume to change in hematocrit. Am J Hematol 2006;81(2):145-6.
63. Armas-Loughran B, Kalra R, Carson JL. Evaluation and management of anemia and bleeding disorders in surgical patients. Med Clin North Am 2003;87(1):229-42.
64. DeCarolis DD, Kim GM, Rector TS, et al. Comparative dose response using the intravenous versus enteral route of administration for potassium replenishment. Intensive Crit Care Nurs 2016;36:17-23.
65. Greenberg CC, Regenbogen SE, Studdert DM, et al. Patterns of communication breakdowns resulting in injury to surgical patients. J Am Coll Surg 2007;204(4):533-40.
66. Lee RS, Woods R, Bullard M, et al. Consultations in the emergency department: a systematic review of the literature. Emerg Med J 2008;25(1):4-9.
67. Flemming D, Hubner U. How to improve change of shift handovers and collaborative grounding and what role does the electronic patient record system play? Results of a systematic literature review. Int J Med Inform 2013;82(7):580-92.
68. Randmaa M, Martensson G, Leo Swenne C, et al. SBAR improves communication and safety climate and decreases incident reports due to communication errors in an anaesthetic clinic: A prospective intervention study. BMJ Open 2014;4(1):e004268.
69. Levine GN, Bates ER, Blankenship JC, et al. 2011 ACCF/AHA/SCAI guideline for percutaneous coronary intervention: A report of the American College of Cardiology Foundation/American Heart Association Task Force on practice guidelines and the society for cardiovascular angiography and interventions. Circulation 2011;124(23):e574-651.
70. Jaski BE, Grigoriadis CE, Dai X, et al. Factors associated with ineligibility for PCI differ between inpatient and outpatient ST-elevation myocardial infarction. J Interv Cardiol 2016;29(4):363-9.
71. Chhatriwalla AK, Amin AP, Kennedy KF, et al. Association between bleeding events and in-hospital mortality after percutaneous coronary intervention. JAMA 2013;309(10):1022-9.
72. Vervaeke H, Becaus N, Penicka M, et al. Self-limiting left ventricular wall rupture following myocardial infarction: A case report and literature review. Acta Cardiol 2014;69(2):209-12.
73. Zhu QY, Tai S, Tang L, et al. STEMI could be the primary presentation of acute aortic dissection. Am J Emerg Med 2017;35(11):1713-17.

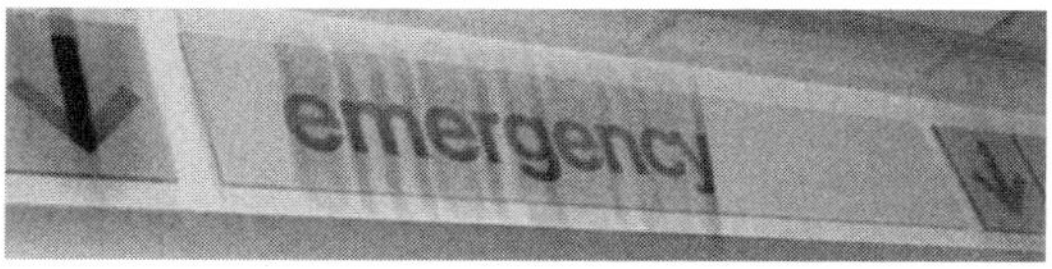

SECTION C – CARDIAC/ VASCULAR

Chapter 15: An 81-year-old man with shortness of breath 5 days after TURP surgery

Alan Janssen, DO, FACOEP-D
Medical/Program Director
Ascension Genesys
Assistant Clinical Professor
Michigan State University College of Osteopathic Medicine
East Lansing, MI

Emily Hammer, DO
Assistant Clinical Professor
Michigan State University College of Osteopathic Medicine
East Lansing, MI

Section editor:
John C. Greenwood, MD
Assistant Professor
Department of Emergency Medicine
Department of Anesthesiology and Critical Care
Perelman School of Medicine
University of Pennsylvania
Philadelphia, PA

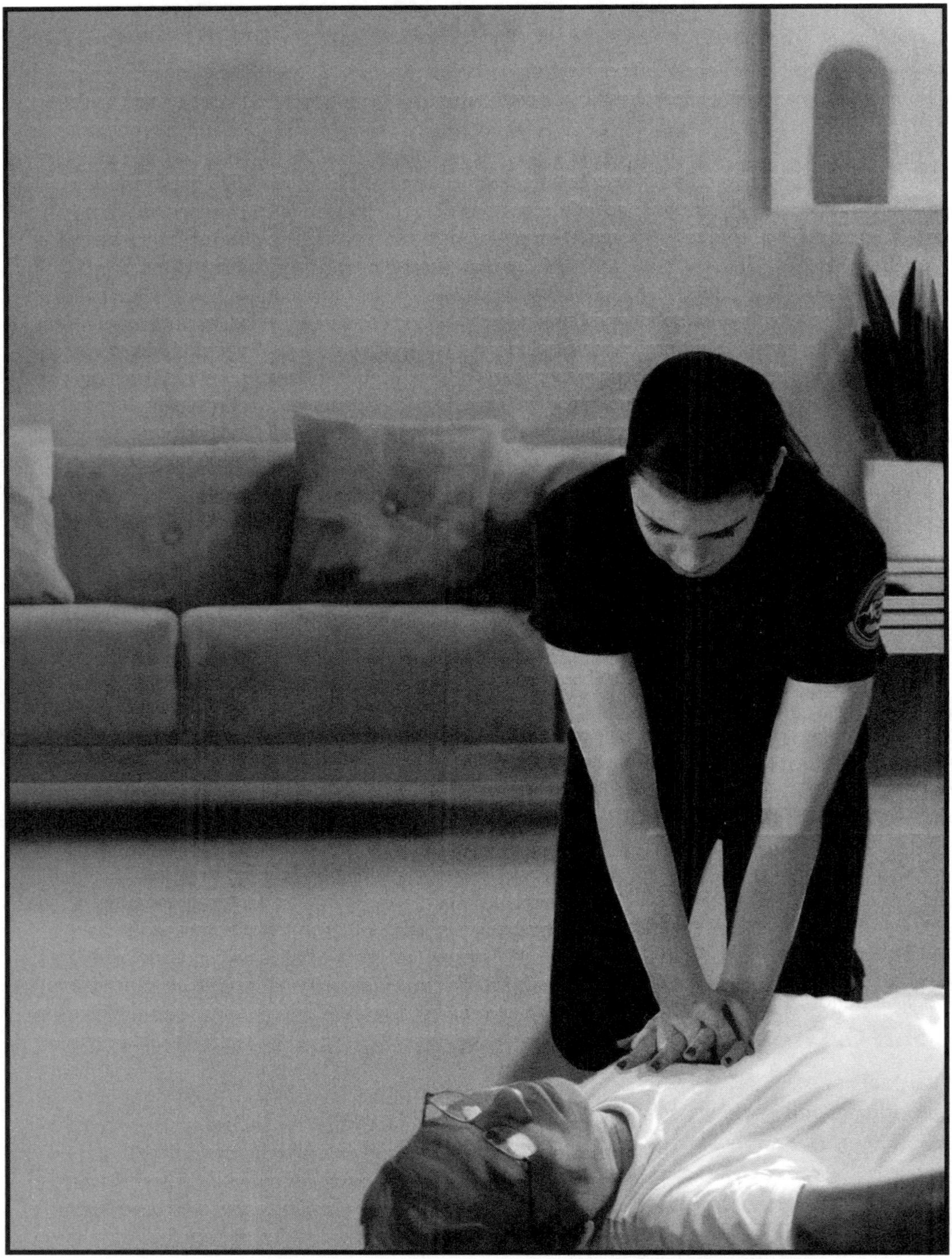

SECTION C/CHAPTER 15

An 81-year-old man with shortness of breath 5 days after TURP surgery

The patient's story:
Thomas Wynam is an 81-year-old man with BPH who has failed medical therapy. On June 17th, he has an outpatient TURP, which is uneventful. The Foley catheter is left in but is removed in the office 2 days later and he is discharged for routine outpatient follow-up.

Home life begins to return to normal, but on post-op day five, he awakens, not feeling "quite right." Tom gets dressed and comes down for breakfast, but is not hungry, and sits in front of the plate prepared by his wife, not eating, eventually retiring to the family room to watch TV.

At 10:07, his wife realizes that she has not heard from him in a while and upon entering the room, finds her husband still on the couch, conscious, but confused and gray in appearance. She tries to get him to the car but is unable. She feels panicky and calls 911.

ED VISIT

CC (10:32): Cardiac arrest

HPI (documented later): I did see the patient upon arrival and also spoke with the paramedics. The story is that they were called because the patient was short of breath when they arrived the patient was in full cardiac arrest and asystole. The patient did have prostate surgery 5 days ago. They did give epinephrine ×3, bicarbonate times one and intubated the patient. He did regain a pulse when they were leaving the house, but did lose the pulse en-route so compressions were resumed with a LUCAS device.

The patient is unresponsive and not able to give a history secondary to his medical condition. Family has not yet arrived. I reviewed the nurse's notes.
ROS: Unable to obtain secondary to alt LOC

NKDA
Medications (from previous):
Actoplus Met XR, Avodart 0.5mg, amLODIPine 5mg, aspirin 325mg oral tablet: 1 Tab, PO, Daily, 30 Tab, 0 Refill(s), atenolol 25mg, furosemide 20mg, glipiZIDE 10 mg, oxybutynin 5mg, sertraline 50mg, simvastatin 10mg, tamsulosin 0.4mg, traMADol 50mg

PMH Problem List

1. BPH (benign prostatic hyperplasia)
2. Diabetes
3. HTN (hypertension)

Surgical history: No active procedure history items have been selected or recorded.
Family history: No family history items have been selected or recorded.
Social history: No qualifying data available.

Vitals:

Time	Temp (C) Rt.	Pulse	Resp	Syst	Diast	Sat
10:38	34.8	90	20 (bagged)	0	0	0

PE:
CONSTITUTIONAL: Unresponsive, pupils are normal size and fixed
HEAD: Normocephalic; atraumatic.
EYES: PER
NOSE: The nose is normal in appearance without rhinorrhea
RESP: Good and equal breath sounds with bagging. No air over the stomach
CARDIO: The LUCAS device was turned off and auscultation revealed a regular rhythm, without murmurs, rub or gallop
ABD: Non-distended
SKIN: Normal for age and race; warm and dry; no apparent lesions
EXT: Femoral pulse present with compressions and remains present after compressions stopped

Author comments (Weinstock):

We are in the footsteps of the EP with an 81-year-old man post-arrest. He has a pulse and is intubated with good bilateral breath sounds. He is 5 days post-surgical, narrowing the differential. Should he be empirically treated for a pulmonary embolism (PE) or should he leave the department for a CT scan first? Should therapeutic hypothermia be initiated now or after imaging? Is this anemia or an electrolyte abnormality? The staff is busy obtaining the ECG, monitor, ventilctor, IV lines, pulse oximetry and BP; they will soon look for direction. We are at:

DECISION POINT A – YOU ARE FACED WITH 5 QUESTIONS:

1. **What immediate initial actions should be taken in a post-arrest patient?**
2. **Was the use of a prehospital device for mechanical chest compressions useful?**
3. **How should the EMS tube placement be confirmed; are a colorimetric CO_2 detector and physical exam enough?**
4. **What is the differential diagnosis at this point and how should the initial work-up proceed?**
5. **Should the patient go for immediate cardiac catheterization?**

What does the literature say?

Q#1: What immediate initial actions should be taken in a post-arrest patient?

Out of hospital cardiac arrest survival rate is dismal with some studies estimating a survival rate to be between 8–10%.[1] The most important initial actions to maximize a successful outcome are early access to high quality CPR and defibrillation. Some studies suggest that an advanced airway should not be completed in the field but reserved for arrival at the hospital.[2] Management of the patient who has return of spontaneous circulation (ROSC) is fast-paced and multifactorial with a focus on:

- Confirmation of airway placement by:
  - Direct visualization
  - Auscultation
  - Capnography
  - Use of a colorimetric device
  - Pulse oximetry and chest x-ray (not reliable)
  - Esophageal detector devices (not reliable)
  - Ultrasonography(experienced users)

Utilization of multiple methods are often beneficial to maximize safety in confirming placement.

- Optimal airway support should be confirmed with a goal of maintaining an oxygen saturation of 94%–99%. Animal studies have shown hyperoxia may exacerbate brain injury post-cardiac arrest.[3]
- Establishing appropriate IV access with 2 peripheral IV lines. If peripheral IV access is not immediately attainable then interosseous access should be initiated. While central venous access may be required later; it is not necessary for this to be instituted on an urgent basis. This is true regardless of the need for administration of vasopressors early in their treatment.
  - Loubani OM, et al. conducted a systematic review based on 85 articles and 270 patients, reviewing extravasation and local tissue injury from administration of vasopressors through peripheral intravenous catheters and central venous catheters. The mean duration of infusion was 55 hours and over 85% of line placements were distal to the antecubital vein. They concluded, "short term administration (< 2 hours) of vasopressor infusions via proximal, well-placed peripheral intravenous lines are unlikely to cause local tissue injury."[4]
  - Cardenas-Garcia, et al. conducted a single arm, consecutive patient study in which vasoactive medications were administered through a peripheral intravenous line. This study was comprised of 783 medication administration events with a duration of 49 +/- 22 hours and found that 19 patients (2%) had extravasation of medication, but with no tissue injury noted after local treatment with phentolamine.[5]
  - Recommendation: Given the appropriate clinical condition, these investigations support the safe administration of vasoactive medications to avoid hypotension with the intent of maintaining a systolic blood pressure of > 90mmHg or a MAP of 65,[6,7] even without administration through a central venous access.
- Post-arrest lab studies should be done to evaluate for reversible causes.
- An ECG is recommended to evaluate for STEMI or rhythm abnormalities.
- If the patient is unresponsive, consider therapeutic hypothermia with a goal of 32–36° C.

One way to remember post-cardiac arrest tasks would be BLEACHO:

- **B**lood pressure, systolic > 90mmHg
- **L**abs – Obtain post-arrest cardiac labs
- **E**CG
- **A**irway, definitive airway
- **C**O_2, end tidal, to maintain CO_2 35–45mmHg
- **H**ypothermia protocol
- **O**$_2$ sats 94–99%

Section editor comments (Greenwood):

And hypoglycemia! Early finger stick blood sugar (FSG) is a must, particularly with the prolonged arrest and use of secretagogue (glipizide). One other point is location of the peripheral IV's being used for vasopressors. It is briefly mentioned in the Loubani article summary; it is imperative that peripheral vasopressors be administered through a proximal, well-running peripheral IV, preferably > 20 gauge. Also, an evidence-based review would suggest that norepinephrine, phenylephrine, epinephrine, and dopamine are likely safe to be administered peripherally, at lower doses. Vasopressin should be avoided, as there is no treatment for vasopressin extravasation, as there is for catecholamines.

Author comments (Weinstock):

Scott's comments on targeted temperature management (from Chapter 1) are reproduced and expanded here:

Consulting editor comments (Weingart):

Some people think that a patient immediately post-op (a little different than our patient who is 5 days out) cannot be cooled, as it might affect their bleeding. Now, there *are* some platelet effects at 32–34° F, and maybe at this temperature we are even at the very beginning of affecting coagulation cascade, but cooling to 36° F (a level which a lot of us have moved to), has no effect whatsoever on platelets or the anticoagulation cascade; it's 100% safe. If we stop at 36° F, it's too easy for them to slide up into temps I don't want, so I like a little buffer. The goal temp with brain injury patients, post-arrest and post-surgical patients is 35° F, knowing it's not going to affect their bleeding but still allow the lion's share of any benefits.

Q#2: Was the use of a prehospital device for mechanical chest compressions useful?

Our patient received CPR in the field and chest compressions were instituted using a mechanical device.While this makes the duties of EMS easier and frees up rescuers for other tasks; is it the best method for compressions? Li, et al. completed a systematic review and meta-analysis comparing mechanical vs manual chest compressions for cardiac arrest. They looked at 12 trials including 9 out-of-hospital and 3 in-hospital studies comprising 11,162 participants. The results found no differences in the Cerebral Performance Category scores, survival to hospital admission and survival to discharge between manual cardiopulmonary resuscitation, and mechanical CPR for out-of-hospital cardiac arrest patients. Out-of-hospital cardiac arrest patients receiving manual resuscitation were more likely to attain ROSC compared with a load-distributing band chest compression device. They concluded the use of mechanical compression device could not be a recommended replacement for manual CPR. A 2014 *Cochrane* review had similar findings; there is insufficient evidence to conclude that mechanical chest compressions during CPR for cardiac arrest are associated with benefit or harm and cannot support mechanical devices.[8,9]

Section editor comments (Greenwood):

We cannot support *routine* use of mechanical devices, as poor quality mechanical compressions (improper location/placement) are just as ineffective as with the human hand. But note that these studies should not be interpreted as showing that mechanical devices should never be used or that they cause harm.

Q#3: How should the EMS tube placement be confirmed; are a colorimetric CO_2 detector and physical exam enough?

Verifying tube placement can be a challenge, especially in the field. Numerous methods exist for verifying endotracheal tube placement, with the simplest being direct visualization and physical auscultation of breath sounds, but is this enough? Physical exam can be misleading or difficult in the field, and calorimetric end tidal carbon dioxide can be used, but in low flow states such as cardiac arrest, it may yield a false result. Fogging of the tube can be used but is not a reliable enough practice to use for verification. Trans-tracheal ultrasound has also been shown to be an effective method but is not an accessible intervention in an out-of-hospital setting.[10] The gold standard is waveform capnography, though it may still be unreliable in low flow states. Silvestri, et al. was able to demonstrate 100% sensitivity and specificity with sustained 4-phase capnographic waveforms in intubated cadaveric models,[11] supporting capnography as the optimal method for verifying tube placement.

Q#4: What is the differential diagnosis at this point and how should the initial work-up proceed?

With the history of recent surgery, our patient is clearly at high risk for pulmonary embolism. Additionally, based on his medication list and past medical history, he is also at high risk for STEMI. Other considerations include cardiac arrhythmia from ischemia, heart failure (HF), or an electrolyte disturbance. The initial suggestion of dyspnea is also concerning for an aortic catastrophe such as dissection, aneurysmal rupture, or a central event such as an intracranial hemorrhage or massive stroke. Finally, post-surgery, an infectious etiology including pneumonia, urosepsis, or another source of sepsis needs to be considered.

For unstable patients such as ours, we need to balance the importance of a timely diagnosis with the risk of decompensation if the patient leaves the department. Enter bedside cardiac ultrasound, which can assess for right heart strain, which may be present with a saddle pulmonary embolism. Dresden, et al. determined that evidence of right heart strain, RV dilatation and dysfunction seen on point-of-care (POC) echocardiography are very specific (98%) but not sensitive (50%) findings for pulmonary embolism.[12] In our case, the POCUS can aid in the diagnosis of PE but should not determine full management as the patient is at such a high risk; even if the US is negative, a CTA of the chest for PE is indicated. What about the concern for contrast nephropathy? Hinson JS, et al. performed a retrospective cohort study looking at adult patients receiving a CT with serum creatinine levels that were obtained before and after the CT. Primary outcomes looked at creatinine increase of 25% after contrast administration as compared to baseline creatinine. They also looked at the serum creatinine of those who had a CT without contrast and subjects who didn't have a CT. The results showed the probability of acute kidney injury was 6.8% in the contrast group, 8.9% in the non-contrast group, and 8.1% in the no CT group, concluding that IV contrast was not associated with an increased rate of acute kidney injury (AKI).[13] In our patient, the benefits of obtaining the diagnosis of PE greatly outweigh the risks from the administration of contrast.

Section editor comments (Greenwood):

Appreciate the commentary to encourage early echocardiography after cardiac arrest. Common findings include globally reduced myocardial function, pericardial effusion, and regional wall motion abnormalities in the case of coronary occlusion. But the reader must beware of interpreting right ventricular dilation after cardiac arrest as a sign of pulmonary embolism! RV dilation is the first echocardiographic change that occurs in the setting of pressure overload (acute pulmonary hypertension). The pulmonary vascular resistance can increase with hypoxemia, pulmonary edema, arrhythmias, along with many other causes.[14] I agree, a CTPE scan is very appropriate, particularly in this patient who has a high-risk of bleeding after tPA.

Q#5: Should the patient go for immediate cardiac catheterization?

The American Heart Association recommends that patients who have ROSC after cardiac arrest and have ST elevation MI should undergo coronary angiography and that that patients with ROSC who are electrically or hemodynamically unstable without ST elevation MI should be considered for coronary angiography. A systematic review and meta-analysis demonstrated that when taken to the cath lab, 32% of the patients without ST elevation had an acute lesion requiring intervention compared to 71% of those with a STEMI.[15]

Author comments (Weinstock):

This was also discussed in Chapter 1 and is reproduced here:

A 2019 *NEJM* multicenter study randomized 552 post-cardiac arrest without STEMI to undergo immediate coronary angiography vs. angiography which was delayed until after neurologic recovery. They found that at 90 days, 176 of 273 patients (64.5%) in the immediate angiography group were alive and 178 of 265 patients (67.2%) in the delayed angiography group were alive. There were no significant differences in the groups between secondary endpoints such as good cerebral performances, myocardial injury, markers of shock, duration of mechanical ventilation, major bleeding, or neurologic status when discharged from the ICU.[16]

Based on this new data, getting cardiology involved earlier would be helpful; the decision on cardiac catheterization can be individualized, in this case delaying until the patient is stabilized.

The decision for emergency coronary angiography should take into account:

- Consideration of comorbidities
- The condition of the patient
- Shared decision-making with family
- Cardiology consultation

What did the actual provider do?

MDM (10:47): I saw the patient immediately upon arrival and I did palpate good right femoral pulse with the mechanical compressions, and I did turn the machine off, and he maintained his pulse. An ECG was performed which did show atrial fibrillation with rapid ventricular response with a rate of 103 and some evidence of ST depression anteriorly. I do not see evidence of STEMI. The patient had received epinephrine ×3 and sodium bicarbonate and per the paramedics. The initial rhythm was asystole. I did call and speak with the CT tech and told them we would bring the patient over for an emergent CT of the chest to look for pulmonary embolism. He informed me that the patient's creatinine level was 1.8 on the past creatinine level. I do feel the risk versus benefit is in favor of doing the study and the family had not yet arrived, so this was done.

Chapter author comments (Janssen, Hammer):

Upon return of ROSC it is completely appropriate to obtain an initial ECG, and baseline blood work including a cardiac panel. The patient was in atrial fibrillation and the rate, although high, was not unstable. The history of a recent surgical procedure placed this patient at greater risk of pulmonary embolism. Though risky to have the patient leave the ED for a CTA for PE, based on the results of the BP measurement, it is a reasonable next step. We do not recommend awaiting renal function studies prior to performing contrast CT as the benefits far outweigh the risks. Per the study by Hinson, et al. this concern should not even be a question that comes into play.[13] While this study was not a controlled randomized prospective trial, it is the largest well-done study to date.

Author comments (Weinstock):

What happened to the patient? The story continues:

MDM (Physician): At approximately 11:36 the family did arrive, and I was able to speak with them and they told me that the patient actually did not have shortness of breath prior to his arrest but that the patient woke up today confused and they were in the process of trying to arouse him when he became unresponsive. They were talking to 911 on the phone when the patient lost consciousness and so they said the paramedics were there within several minutes. They state the patient did have chest tightness yesterday. The patient does have a history of a heart stent but does not have a history of atrial fibrillation.

Continued ED course: The patient was sent to CT and has just returned as have the labs:

(Labs on next page...)

HEMATOLOGY

WBC	**14.8 (H)**
Hb	**10.3 (L)**
Hematocrit	**34.0 (L)**
Platelets	225

CHEMISTRY

Sodium	**124 (L)**
Potassium	**7.2 (H)**
Chloride	**86 (L)**
CO2	**7 (L)**
Anion Gap	**31.0mmol/L (H)**
Glucose	**219 (H)**
BUN	**94 (H)**
Creatinine	**6.99 (H)**

Est CrCL IBW (mL/min)-RX	8.56mL/min
Calcium Total	8.9
Magnesium	2.7

COAGULATION

Partial Thromboplastin (aPTT)	51.7 Sec
INR	1.34
Prothrombin time (PT)	14.8 Sec
Troponin I	**7.34ng/mL (H)**

MDM (12:32): I just spoke with the radiologist at 1232 who tells me the patient does not have a pulmonary embolism but does have bilateral pleural effusions and cardiomegaly and pulmonary edema consistent with congestive heart failure.

DECISION POINT B – YOU ARE FACED WITH 4 QUESTIONS:

1. **Is the finding of CHF believable based on a CT scan? Is this "flash pulmonary edema" from ischemia?**
2. **The troponin is significantly elevated, should he go to cath *now*?**
3. **How should CHF be managed in a post-arrest patient? What are the etiologies of new onset (flash) CHF?**
4. **How should the elevated potassium be managed? Could this have caused an arrhythmia?**

What does the data show?

Q#1: Is the finding of CHF believable based on a CT scan? Is this "flash pulmonary edema" from ischemia?

CTA of the chest has a high sensitivity for pulmonary edema and CHF but is non-specific. On the other hand, the sensitivity of CTPA for PE is high, around 80%, with specificity around 96%.[17] CTA can also be very sensitive for pericardial effusion and can detect from as little as 50mL of fluid in the pericardium.[18] Although the CTA for PE is negative, it is not surprising that the patient was found to have CHF as surgical procedures can be a "cardiac stress test" for some patients. The stress of the surgery, excessive IV fluid administration and anesthesia can precipitate fluid overload and/or cardiac ischemia. As an outpatient the patient had been treated for hypertension, diabetes, and certainly could have undiagnosed cardiovascular disease. The patient likely had an ischemic event driven by the surgical procedure that precipitated his flash pulmonary edema, which then decompensated to cardiac arrest.

Section editor comments (Greenwood):

Interestingly enough, this was an outpatient TURP, and I wonder if this is a delayed presentation of TURP syndrome. Given his history of chronic kidney disease (CKD), there may have been a delayed clearance of absorbed hyperosmolar molecules used as irrigation, such as glycine, sorbitol, and/or mannitol. He may have "seemed" well after his procedure, but this may have been his trigger for worsening AKI and heart failure. TURP syndrome is described as a cause for acute hyponatremia, heart failure, and renal failure.

Q#2: The troponin is significantly elevated, should he go to cath *now*?

Troponin can be elevated for a number of reasons. The obvious cause is cardiac ischemia. In massive and even submassive pulmonary emboli, troponin will be elevated (at this point ruled out). Other conditions requiring excessive oxygen demand of the cardiac muscle can also raise troponin, for example cardiac arrest.[19] The ECG demonstrating ischemia is a better indicator for catheterization but would be a stronger argument with ST elevation. Regardless, this is an opportunity for discussion with the cardiologist.

Causes of elevated troponin include:[20]

- ACS related
- Acute MI
- Post-PCI
- Open heart surgery

Non-ACS-related:

- End stage renal disease (ESRD)
- Pulmonary embolism (PE)
- Myocarditis/pericarditis
- Aortic dissection
- Chronic heart failure
- Strenuous exercise/ultra-endurance athletes
- Cardiotoxic chemotherapy
- Ablation/cardioversion/defibrillator shocks

- Cardiac infiltrative disorders (ex: amyloidosis)
- Heart transplant
- Cardiac contusion (after trauma)
- Sepsis/critically ill patients

Q#3: How should CHF be managed in a post-arrest patient? What are the etiologies of new onset (flash) CHF?

Cardiac ischemia should always be considered after cardiac arrest associated with CHF and patients with evidence of STEMI on ECG should undergo cardiac catheterization. After the initial assessment, go back to the ABC's:

- **Airway:** Verify that the patient is maintaining an adequate airway.
- **Breathing:** Optimize ventilator settings with the goal of attaining an end tidal CO_2 35–45mm of Hg. Optimize oxygenation by maintaining SPO_2 94–99%.
- **Circulation:** Optimize the blood pressure by maintaining the MAP of greater than 65. Although it seems counterintuitive to administer a fluid bolus to a patient with CHF, a patient with CHF can also be intravascularly depleted. Utilization of bedside US can help aid the decision-making process in real time by checking for IVC compressibility to assist in determining if fluids or vasopressors are necessary. The safest, most readily available vasopressor is norepinephrine (Levophed) at 0.01–1mcg/kg/min to maintain an MAP > 65. Consideration for use of Dopamine can be entertained, but it is not the first choice. These vasopressors can predispose to tachyarrhythmias.[21]

Section editor comments (Greenwood):

Many would argue that dopamine, particularly given it's increased associated mortality in patients with cardiogenic shock[22] should not be used—if ever. Epinephrine infusion may be considered as an "inopressor" in this patient, particularly if in a low cardiac output state.

Hyponatremia can be a common complication of CHF as renin, angiotensin II, and release of endogenous vasopressin can cause hyponatremia. Patients with CHF will present with hypervolemic hyponatremia. Administering IV normal saline may exacerbate the hypervolemia. Using diuretics such as spironolactone and furosemide may increase sodium excretion, thus worsening the hyponatremia. In the event that the hyponatremia results in seizure or altered mental status, the administration of 3% normal saline is recommended.

New onset flash pulmonary edema may be the result of an ischemic cardiac event (MI), hypertensive emergency, acute mitral or aortic regurgitation, arrhythmias, or end stage renal disease.

Q#4: How should the elevated potassium be managed? Could this have caused an arrhythmia?

The potassium is severely elevated. It would be important to know if there were ECG changes consistent with hyperkalemia; however, care should be driven by clinical presentation. To help reduce potassium, several treatment modalities can be utilized including:

- Stabilizers
- Shifters
- Excretors

A patient presenting with hyperkalemia and dysrhythmia should emergently receive calcium to stabilize the cardiac membrane. Preference should be given to calcium chloride over calcium gluconate as it has increased additional bioavailability. Calcium can cause irritation to peripheral veins, so when possible administer through a central line. The calcium chloride works within 5 minutes, and repeat dosing should be administered until there is shortening of the QRS, gaining of the p waves, and improvement of the bradycardia associated with hyperkalemia.[23]

Consideration is then given to the "shifters." Albuterol and insulin drive potassium into the cell, temporarily reducing serum potassium. Albuterol is given 10–20mg in 4mL of NS nebulized over 10 minutes. Insulin is given 10 units IV with 25gm of dextrose to prevent associated hypoglycemia. Sodium bicarb was once thought to aid in the intracellular shift of potassium but has recently been shown to do little for reducing serum potassium,[23] though is beneficial if the pH is < 7. Our patient may have benefited as his pH was 6.7.

Finally, we consider the "excretors." Dialysis is the best treatment and is clearly indicated for this patient. Dialysis will physically remove the potassium and assist in the patient's other metabolic abnormalities. In addition, stooling the potassium will remove it from the body. Kayexalate (sodium polystyrene sulfate) theoretically works to pull potassium from the gut into stool, and is then excreted. The research supporting the use of Kayexalate was extracted from a study in 1961. The study was based on comparing a group treated with sorbitol (control) against those treated with sorbitol with a cation exchange (kayexalate). Both groups had a decrease in their serum potassium within 5 days and there was no statistically significant difference between both groups.[24] Kayexalate has been associated with colonic necrosis, which can be fatal. Based on current practice and evidence, it can no longer be supported for hyperkalemia.

Section editor comments (Greenwood):

Is the blood gas data missing from above? Is this a respiratory or metabolic acidosis? I'm assuming this is a metabolic acidosis, in which case sodium bicarbonate boluses may be of clinical benefit to improve response to vasopressor therapy. The provider should be aware that one "amp" of sodium bicarbonate bolus includes approximately 50mL of 6% sodium chloride. The clinical effects of a hypertonic saline solution are complex including overly aggressive correction of the patient's hyponatremia, and hemodynamic consequences of a hypertonic fluid bolus. If the family has decided to be aggressive in this patient's medical management, early renal replacement therapy should be considered.

What did the actual provider do?

MDM (12:39): I did call and speak with [the cardiologist] about the possibility of an emergent cardiac catheterization however as the patient did not have an initial ventricular fibrillation or ventricular tachycardia rhythm, [they state that] he would not be a candidate for the cath lab. Patient does not have evidence of STEMI on the ECG however the troponin returned significantly elevated. A second ECG will be performed at this time. The patient does have rapid cooling protocol in place however I did ask that they decrease the IV fluids down to KVO as the patient does have pulmonary edema. Additional history was from the family that the patient has had bilateral lower extremity swelling in the last several days.

The patient will be admitted to the intensive care unit and I will speak with the intensivist as well as the hospitalist.

I just did receive a call from the lab with critical values potassium is 7.2. The patient does appear to be in acute renal failure 6.9 as the creatinine level. The patient is profoundly acidotic with a serum bicarbonate level of 7 and his ABG shows a pH of 6.7, PCO_2 37 and PO_2 of 226. He is in extremely critical condition. I did speak with [the cardiologist] who will come in to see the patient. A stat echocardiogram will be done. I did just call and speak with the charge nurse and they will emergently give the patient calcium gluconate, dextrose and insulin and sodium bicarbonate 50 IV. We're obtaining records from [the hospital which performed the TURP].

Chapter author expert commentary: How is the provider doing?
We think the provider is doing well given the complexity of this case. The documentation of the lab results and subsequent treatment was appropriate. Timed notes outlining the clinical course would possibly have cleaned up the chart and further justified the actual event timing as it occurred. We would have liked to see documentation on ECG changes associated with the potassium, in addition to associated ECG changes in response after initiation of treatment for hyperkalemia. Additionally, we would have recommended that nephrology be consulted earlier in the treatment course.

DECISION POINT C – YOU ARE FACED WITH 4 QUESTIONS:

1. **How should IVF bolus be managed with rapid cooling of a patient with CHF or ESRD?**
2. **Should the patient receive dialysis for the hyperkalemia and pulmonary edema?**
3. **How should the vent be managed based on the ABG results?**
4. **How does the severe acidosis change our management?**

Q#1: How should IVF bolus be managed with rapid cooling of a patient with CHF or ESRD?

If the patient is hypotensive and there is concern for fluid overload, bedside US can help in directing a treatment regimen. Inferior vena cava (IVC) compressibility can assist in determining if fluids or vasopressors are required. If the IVC compresses > 50% with inspiration, then the patient is vascularly depleted and requires IV fluids. If the IVC compresses less than this, then vasopressors are the treatment of choice.

Consulting editor comments (Weingart):

As to fluids in the setting of an x-ray that may be consistent with CHF, we need to throw the echo probe on the heart and see what's happening. If the heart is thumping away, then that is probably more representative of acute lung injury and not actually CHF. On the other hand, if the heart is barely pumping, then before you give fluids to the patient, you need to get that heart to generate a good cardiac output with ionotropic support. Check their ionized calcium, and make sure that everything is optimized to get the heart beating; only at that point would I consider fluids. Now if they have external losses of fluid out of their body, for example a patient with horrible diarrhea or they're vomiting, well sure, maybe we need to replete their fluids. But if the fluid is just going to other places—third spacing, it's going to come back and bite you. I am far more stingy with fluids than I was 15 years ago.

Q#2: Should the patient receive dialysis for the hyperkalemia and pulmonary edema?

This patient is a candidate for dialysis. This treatment would not only correct his life-threatening hyperkalemia but will correct for his severe acidosis. Placing a femoral dialysis catheter may be the preferred line of choice. Placing an IJ or subclavian could potentially irritate the myocardium and send the patient into an arrhythmia.

Q#3: How should the vent be managed based on the ABG results?

The patient has primary metabolic acidosis with respiratory acidosis (expected PCO_2 17–21) and an anion gap acidosis. The high anion gap is likely due to a combination of the uremia and lactic acidosis associated with cardiac arrest and hypoperfusion. There has been no documentation of a problem with oxygenation.Ventilator management would include assist control mode and a tidal volume based on ideal body weight x 8–10mL/kg. Attention and consideration should be given to monitoring the patient's status with serial ABG's. The target goal for the PaO_2 would be to titrate the FIO_2 to maintain an SpO_2 of > 94%.[25] $PaCO_2$ directly effects cerebral vasculature after cardiac arrest as a major regulator of cerebral blood flow.[26] Mild permissive hypercarbia is an emerging concept,[25] however, with this patient's acidosis it would likely be optimal to target a range closer to normocarbia (PCO_2 35–45mmHg) rather than even mild hypercarbia. If there is a concern for ARDS (unfortunately, we have no FIO_2 to compare with the PaO_2 to determine this) a volume of 6mL/kg would be preferred. When considering respiratory rate, slight hyperventilation to help with the respiratory acidosis (14–16 breaths), and a PEEP of 5 is preferred. The goal is to optimize the FIO_2 by maintaining the SPO_2 in the 94–99% range to prevent hyperoxia.[27]

Section editor comments (Greenwood):

I will emphasize that our patient should be on lung-protective ventilation settings with TV 6–8cc/kg IBW as he is at high risk for ARDS post arrest. The range of 8–10 is probably too high.

Q#4: How does the severe acidosis change our management?

Our patient is severely acidotic. Sodium bicarbonate administration should be administered as a pH of 6.7 will not allow medications to function optimally. Also, as mentioned above, ABG's will assist in directing management of the vent settings to optimize management of the acidosis.

What did the actual provider do?

MDM (13:02): I did see the patient again and also spoke with the family. The patient does have a living will and is in a critical condition. They would like life sustaining measures to be continued. They would like him to remain at full code which I think is a reasonable decision as he does have potentially reversible problems occurring. The patient has already received calcium and dextrose and insulin and is getting bicarbonate right now. Additionally, nephrology is paged to discuss consideration of emergent dialysis.

MDM (13:10): The patient did just degenerate into cardiac arrest again. The rhythm just prior to this involved severe bradycardia and then asystole. I did go back into the room and chest compressions were done with good pulses with compressions. Patient received epinephrine 1mg IV. He also received the sodium bicarbonate which was done during the code.

At this point he does have a pulse again after about 2 minutes of chest compressions. ECG is repeated showing a wide complex tachycardia with a rate of 136bpm. Nephrology is paged to discuss consideration of emergent dialysis. I did inform the patient's daughter and the two grandchildren of the poor prognosis of the patient.

DECISION POINT D – In light of the wide complex tachycardia, should additional calcium be given? When should the potassium level be repeated?

The question of re-treating the wide complex tachycardia with additional calcium should ultimately be driven by the clinical scenario. We know that elevated potassium causes a clear pattern of electrocardiographic changes, but the reliability of this pattern in unclear. Montaque, et al. completed a retrospective review of the frequency of ECG changes with hyperkalemia. Charts were reviewed in patients admitted with hyperkalemia with a level greater than or equal to 6.0. The results suggested a low sensitivity and specificity for predicting hyperkalemia based on the ECG. Other studies have suggested a specificity between 85–86% and a sensitivity between 34–43%.[23,28] So, while the ECG should not be ignored, the clinical scenario together with the ECG pattern should both be considered in determining the treatment protocol. Calcium acts immediately to stabilize cardiac cell membranes, but has a duration of action of only 30–60 minutes. Likely the potassium should be repeated within that 30-minute time frame,[23] but the reality is that plasma potassium alone is also not an adequate index of when to initiate therapy.

What happened to the patient?

MDM (13:21): I spoke with the nephrologist who is checking his records and is on his way to the hospital. Foley catheter will be placed. Patient will be assessed for consideration of dialysis.

(14:08): I spoke with [the intensivist] who accepts consult and is seeing Pt. now. I spoke with [the hospitalist] who accepts admission. The nephrologist should be here momentarily for consideration of emergent dialysis. I did speak with [the cardiologist] who tells me the emergent echo shows an ejection fraction of 20%, but it is questionable whether this is chronic.

Critical care time: 90 minutes
DIAGNOSIS: Cardiac arrest, acute renal failure, hyperkalemia, unresponsive, acute myocardial infarction, congestive heart failure with pulmonary edema, hyponatremia.

Hospital course:
Pulm/CCM Note: Patient remains sedated on the ventilator. We started him on propofol last evening because his myoclonus was so bad it was becoming disturbing to the family. Currently is on 35mcg/kg/min of propofol. He is requiring high doses of pressors. Currently he is on norepinephrine at 20mcg/min, vasopressin 0.04 units/min, and epinephrine at 4mcg/min. Blood pressure is stable. Is oxygenating well. However, he is requiring 95% FiO_2.

Assessment and plan:

- cardiac arrest
- severe anoxic encephalopathy
- myoclonus
- acute renal failure
- hyperkalemia
- lactic acidemia
- anemia

Communication discussion:

1. We will continue the patient on full mechanical ventilation at this time. His pH has improved. He certainly is not ready for any weaning attempts.
2. We will continue patient on all pressors. He actually has a fairly improved blood pressure. However he is requiring large doses of pressors.
3. The daughter did tell me that the patient has a living will that states he would not want to remain in this state if it came down to it. I don't believe that the patient is going to recover from this. We are awaiting the other two daughters to get into town. We do need to speak to them about moving forward. His renal function is improving with CRRT. We will continue this for now. His potassium is greatly decreased.
4. Continue DVT/GI prophylaxis.
5. We will hold off on starting any type of tube feeds. He is on entirely too many pressors.
6. We'll continue patient on a bicarbonate drip at this time.

Patient outcome: Additional consults included Cardiology and Nephrology. Hypothermia protocol and heparin were started. Cardiology did not feel it was necessary to take him for coronary angiography. The electrolytes normalized, but he required 3 vasopressors to maintain his blood pressure. Neurology was consulted and determined that the prognosis was poor. After family conference the decision was made to change the patient's code status to comfort measures only. He subsequently expired.

Chapter summary:

- Initial treatment for ROSC is **BLEACHO**
  - o **B**lood pressure, systolic > 90mmHg
  - o **L**abs – Obtain post-arrest cardiac labs
  - o **E**CG
  - o **A**irway, definitive airway
  - o **C**O$_2$, end tidal, to maintain CO$_2$ 35–45mmHg
  - o **H**ypothermia protocol
  - o **O**$_2$ sats 94–99%
- It is appropriate to obtain a CTA to look for PE, despite having prior kidney insufficiency, without knowledge of the baseline renal function.
- Treatment for hyperkalemia includes 1) cardiac stabilizers (Calcium), 2) shifters (albuterol/insulin/dextrose), and 3) excretors (dialysis). Kayexalate has no role in the treatment of emergent hyperkalemia.
- Point-of-care US can provide valuable information for resuscitation of ill patients.

References:

1. Frohlich GM, Lyon RM, Sasson C, et al. Out-of-hospital cardiac arrest–Optimal management. Curr Cardiol Rev 2013;9(4):316-24.
2. Pepe PE, Roppolo LP, Fowler RL. Prehospital endotracheal intubation: Elemental or detrimental? Crit Care 2015;19:121.
3. Dell'Anna AM, Lamanna I, Vincent J, et al. How much oxygen in adult cardiac arrest? Crit Care 2014;18(5):555
4. Loubani OM, Green RS. A systematic review of extravasation and local tissue injury from administration of vasopressors through peripheral intravenous catheters and central venous catheters. J Crit Care 2015;653:e.9-17.
5. Cardenas-Garcia J, Schaub KF, Belchikov YG, et al. Safety of peripheral intravenous administration of vasoactive medication. J Hosp Med 2015;10(9):581-5.
6. Kern KB. Optimal treatment of patients surviving out-of-hospital cardiac arrest. JACC Cardiovasc Interv 2012;5(6):597-05.
7. Trzeciak S, Jones AE, Kilgannon JH, et al. Significance of arterial hypotension after resuscitation from cardiac arrest. Crit Care Med 2009;37(11):2895-903.
8. Li H, Wang D, Yu Y, et al. Mechanical versus manual chest compressions for cardiac arrest: A systematic review and meta-analysis. Scand J Trauma Resusc Emerg Med 2016;24:10.
9. Brooks SC, Hassan N, Bingham BL, et al. Mechanical versus manual chest compressions for cardiac arrest. Cochrane Database Syst Rev 2014;2.
10. Das SK, Choupoo NS, Haldar R, et al. Transtracheal ultrasound for verification of endotracheal tube placement: A systematic review and meta-analysis. Can J Anaesth 2015;62(4):413-23.
11. Silvestri S, Ladde JG, Brown JF, et al. Endotracheal tube placement confirmation: 100% sensitivity and specificity with sustained four-phase capnographic waveforms in a cadaveric experimental model. Resuscitation 2017;115:192-8.
12. Dresden S, Mitchell P, Rahimi L, et al. Right ventricular dilatation on bedside echocardiography performed by emergency physicians aids in the diagnosis of pulmonary embolism. Ann Emerg Med 2014;63(1):16-24.
13. Hinson JS, Ehmann ER, Fine DM, et al. Acute kidney injury after intravenous contrast media administration. Ann Emerg Med 2017;69(5):577-86.
14. Wardi G, Blanchard D, Dittrich T, et al. Right ventricle dysfunction and echocardiographic parameters in the first 24h following resuscitation in the post-cardiac arrest patient: A retrospective cohort study. Resuscitation 2016;103:71-4.
15. Millin MG, Comer AC, Nable JV, et al. Patients without ST elevation after return of spontaneous circulation may benefit from emergent percutaneous intervention: A systematic review and meta-analysis. Resuscitation 2016;108:54-60.
16. Lemkes JS, Janssens GN, van der Hoeven NW, et al. Coronary angiography after cardiac arrest without ST-segment elevation. N Engl J Med 2019;380(15):1397-407.
17. Cardinale L, Priola AM, Moretti F, et al. Effectiveness of chest radiography, lung ultrasound and thoracic computed tomography in the diagnosis of congestive heart failure. World J Radiol 2014; 6(6): 230-37.
18. Wong BY, Lee KR, MacArthur RI. Diagnosis of pericardial effusion by computed tomography. Chest 1982;81(2):177-81.
19. Polena S, Shen KH, Mamakos E, et al. Correlation between cardiac enzyme elevation and the

duration of cardiopulmonary resuscitation. Proc West Pharmacol Soc 2005;48:136-8.
20. Korff S, Katus HA, Giannitsis E. Differential diagnosis of elevated troponins. Heart 2006;92(7):987-93. doi:10.1136/hrt.2005.071282
21. Peberdy MA, Callaway, CW, Neumar RW, et al. Part 9: Post cardiac arrest care: 2010 American Heart Association Guidelines for cardiopulmonary resuscitation and emergency cardiovascular care. Circulation 2010;122(18 Suppl 3):S768-86.
22. De backer D, Biston P, Devriendt J, et al. Comparison of dopamine and norepinephrine in the treatment of shock. N Engl J Med 2010;362(9):779-89.
23. Weisberg LS. Management of severe hyperkalemia. Crit Care Med 2008;36(12):3246-51.
24. Flinn RB, Merrill JP, Welzant WR. Treatment of the oliguric patient with a new sodium-exchange resin and sorbitol; A preliminary report. N Engl J Med 1961;264:111-5.
25. Johnson N, Caribom DJ, Gaieski DF. Ventilator management and respiratory care after cardiac arrest: Oxygenation, ventilation, infection, and injury. Chest 2018;153(6):1466-77.
26. Cold GE. Cerebral blood flow in acute head injury. The regulation of cerebral blood flow and metabolism during the acute phase of head injury, and its significance for therapy. Acta Neurochir Suppl 1990;49:1-64.
27. Topjian AA, Berg RA, Taccone FS. Haemodynamic and ventilator management in patients following cardiac arrest, Curr Opin Crit Care 2015;21(3):195-01.
28. Wrenn KD, Slovis CM, Slovis BS. The ability of physicians to predict hyperkalemia from the ECG. Ann Emerg Med 1991;20(11):1229-32.

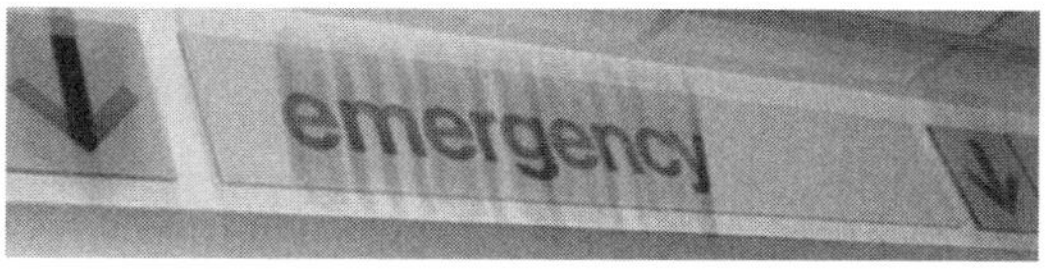

SECTION D – DRUGS & DELIRIUM

Chapter 16: A 52-year-old woman with ESRD and confusion

Gregory J. Eisinger, MD, MSSW
Emergency Medicine and Internal Medicine Attending
Fellow in Pulmonary and Critical Care Medicine
The Ohio State University Wexner Medical Center
Columbus, OH

Daniel R. Martin, MD, MBA, FACEP, FAAEM
Professor and Vice Chair of Education
Director EM IM Residency Program
Department of Emergency Medicine
The Ohio State University Wexner Medical Center
Columbus, OH

Section editor:
Michael Winters, MD, MBA, FACEP, FAAEM
Professor of Emergency Medicine and Medicine
Vice Chair for Clinical and Administrative Affairs
Department of Emergency Medicine
University of Maryland School of Medicine
Baltimore, MD

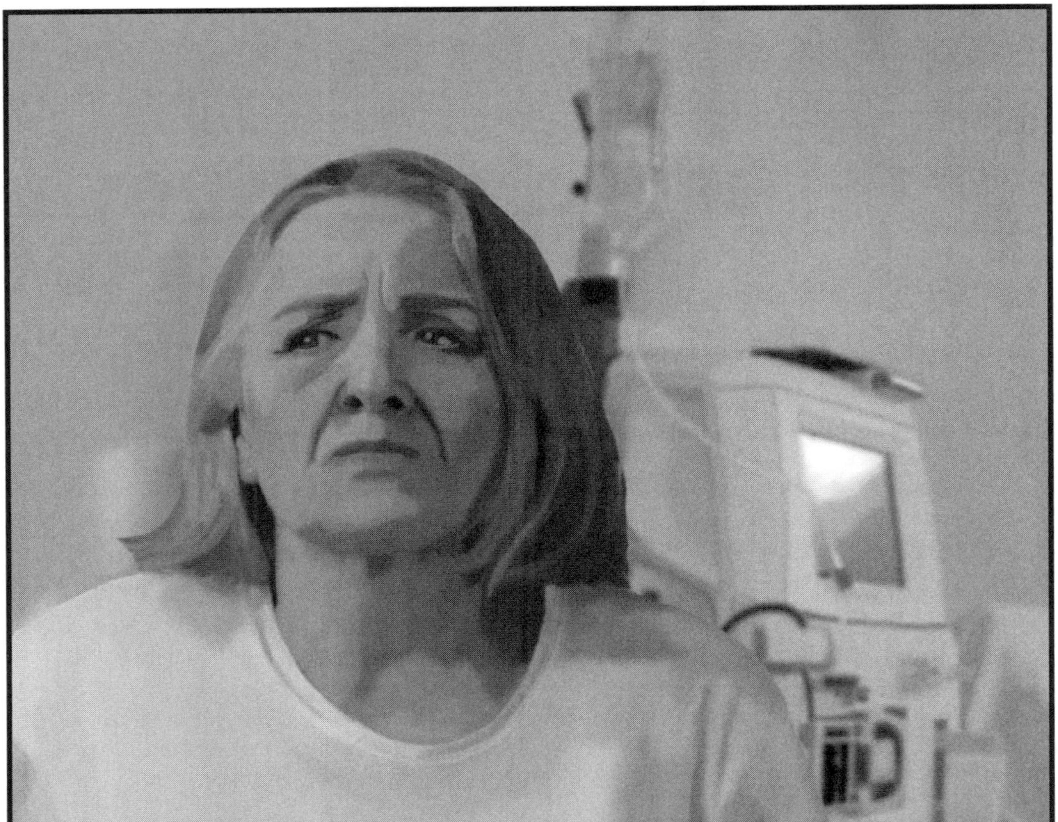

SECTION D/CHAPTER 16

A 52-year-old woman with ESRD and confusion

End-stage renal disease (ESRD) is typically defined by the prolonged need for renal replacement therapy,[1] usually with a glomerular filtration rate (GFR) < 15mL/min/1.73m,[2] and represents the final common pathway of a variety of acute and chronic medical renal diseases. ESRD affects 0.21% of the U.S. population, with an incidence that has continued to rise despite advances in care.[2] Diabetes mellitus remains by far the most common cause, followed by hypertension, with other causes such as glomerulonephritis and polycystic kidney disease occurring much less frequently.[2] 87% of new cases of ESRD are initially managed with hemodialysis (HD), while 10% receive peritoneal dialysis (PD), and less than 3% undergo kidney transplant prior to dialysis initiation.[2]

Few ED shifts pass without encountering this diagnosis; more than 50% of all ESRD patients visit the ED each year with an average of almost three visits per year.[3] Nearly half will require admission, most frequently for complications related to HD access (12.6%), infection (7.8%), congestive heart failure (7.5%), volume overload (1.2%), and hyperkalemia (1.1%).[3] Mortality is startlingly high with a 50% three-year survival from onset of ESRD. Even young patients diagnosed before age 30 will, on average, die before they reach 50.[2] Causes include:

- Cardiovascular (55%)
- Withdrawal from dialysis (17%)
- Infections (11%)
- Malignancy (4%)[2]

Patients who undergo transplant fare better with nearly half the annual death rate and significantly improved quality of life compared with patients on the waitlist.[4] However, transplanted patients come with their own set of complications, including chronic immunosuppression, and are at increased risk for cardiovascular mortality, especially with comorbid diabetes.[5]

INITIAL ED VISIT

HPI (12:52): I did review the previous record. I did see this patient in the past. In the past, I discussed the case with the hospitalist physician and the treatment plan has been made not to administer narcotic medicine, as this may worsen the patient's symptoms. The patient presents today with a severe, constant, mid abdominal aching sensation without radiation that started this morning. No change with food. She has had identical pain in the past. She denies any fever, vomiting, diarrhea. No blood in the urine or stool, dysuria or urinary frequency, vaginal bleeding or discharge. The patient does make urine. Last dialysis was 2 days ago and next scheduled dialysis is tomorrow.

Social history: No smoking or alcohol. Is here with her fiancé. I reviewed the nurse's notes.

PMH:

- End-Stage Renal Disease (ESRD)
- Acute renal failure syndrome
- Gastroparesis
- Diabetes Mellitus, type 2
- Hypertension
- Neuropathy

PSH: caesarian section

Medications: aspirin, insulin, carvedilol, lisinopril, doxazosin, pantoprazole, promethazine, metoclopramide, nitroglycerin, atorvastatin, vitamin B complex (Nephrocaps)

Allergies: shellfish

Social history: no smoking or alcohol

Family history: diabetes, hypertension, kidney disease

Vitals:

Time	Temp (F)	Pulse	Resp	BP	SpO2	Pain
12:49	98.1	103	16	150/106	97% (RA)	9/10

PE:

GA: Alert and oriented X3, well-nourished, well appearing, in no apparent distress

HEAD: Normocephalic; atraumatic.

EYES: PERRL, no scleral icterus.

RESP: Normal chest excursion with respiration; breath sounds clear and equal bilaterally; no wheezes, rhonchi, or rales

CARDIO: Regular rhythm, without murmurs, rub or gallop

ABD: Non-distended; mild to moderate pain with palpation but soft without rigidity, rebound, guarding.

SKIN: Normal for age and race; warm and dry; no apparent lesions

MDM (13:06): Labs ordered including LFTs and lipase and lactate, IV fluids, IV Phenergan. No narcotic medication at this time. Urine testing will be done. ED labs pending.

TESTING:

WBC Count	9.6 thou/mcL
Hemoglobin	**9.3 gm/dL LOW**
Platelet Count	301 thou/mcL
Sodium Level	**134 mMol/L LOW**
Potassium Level	**3.5 mMol/L LOW**
Chloride Level	103 mMol/L
Carbon Dioxide Level	25 mMol/L

Anion Gap	6.0 mMol/L
Glucose Level	**280 mg/dL HI**
BUN	**30 mg/dL HI**
Creatinine	**4.11 mg/dL HI**
Est CrCl IBW (mL/min)-RX	**22.07 mL/min LOW**
Calcium Total	**7.5 mg/dL LOW**
Troponin I	0.03 ng/mL
Glucose POCT-LAB	**469 mg/dL HI**
Lactic Acid Level	1.7 mMol/L
Calcium Total	**8.1 mg/dL LOW**
Alkaline Phosphatase	55 Units/L
ALT/SGPT	23 Units/L
AST/SGOT	34 Units/L
Bilirubin Total	0.9 mg/dL
Bilirubin Direct	0.3 mg/dL
Protein	**5.0 gm/dL LOW**
Albumin Level	**1.6 gm/dL LOW**
Bilirubin Indirect	0.6 mg/dL
Lipase Level	**16 Units/L LOW**

MDM (14:07): I did just check up on the patient and she is feeling better. No further vomiting since she has arrived.

15:46: I did review the patient's final labs which were obtained with a redraw which did not show acute abnormality. The patient will be discharged. She did receive a second dose of intravenous promethazine. Follow-up with primary care in the next 1 or 2 days as well as for dialysis tomorrow as scheduled. I did just see the patient again. She is walking in the hall. Will be discharged.

DIAGNOSIS: abdominal pain, gastroparesis, diabetes with hyperglycemia, anemia, end-stage renal disease
Condition: Improved.
Patient was given the following educational materials: Gastroparesis, Diabetes, Abdominal Pain (Nonspecific)
Follow-up with: [PCP] within 1 to 2 days; [nephrologist] within 1 to 2 days

Chapter author discussion of the intital visit:
Documentation:

It is no secret that we are in the midst of an opioid epidemic. The rate of opioid-related ED visits has doubled in the past 10 years[6] as an estimated 4.3 million Americans currently misuse prescription or illicit narcotics.[7] Despite these frightening statistics, many of these patients are high risk and all deserving of compassion; the first two sentences of the HPI frame the entire encounter with bias and have no place in the HPI. If considerations such as these are to be included, they belong in the medical decision-making section, but even then, be sure to avoid premature closure and remain open to the possibility that even the ostensibly narcotic-seeking patient may be seriously ill.

Though we may become desensitized to abnormal vital signs, they are associated with bad outcomes and are one of the one of the most common abnormalities seen in patients who die within seven days of an ED discharge, present in 83% of cases.[8] In one study of deaths within a week of discharge, tachycardia was the most commonly abnormal vital sign and in every case, it either persisted despite interventions, or was not rechecked prior to discharge.[9] Another study found that heart rate > 101 at discharge was associated with a two-fold increase in the odds of admission within the next seven days.[10]

Secondly, the provider documented that the labs showed "no acute abnormalities." Is this true? Set aside the blood sugar of 469 and consider the hemoglobin. Granted, 9.3g/dL is not jaw-dropping for a patient with ESRD, but is it normal? What if it had been 12g/dL two days prior? Could a bleeding ulcer explain her abdominal pain? This is where the EMR can be your best friend.

If the patient will still be discharged despite abnormal vital signs and labs or unclear diagnosis, it is worthwhile to pursue and document shared decision-making including discussion of the risks and benefits[11] and how it has been shown to be feasible, to decrease healthcare resource utilization, and improve patient satisfaction.[12]

Author comments (Weinstock):

Reviewing and documenting the previous Hb would likely have confirmed anemia of chronic disease, but if it had recently been in the normal range, this may have been a game-changer.

Differential diagnosis for abdominal pain in the ESRD patient		
• gastritis / peptic ulcer disease	• small bowel obstruction	• diabetic ketoacidosis
• hepatitis / cholecystitis	• mesenteric ischemia	• uremia / volume overload
• diverticulitis	• secondary peritonitis	• bacteremia
• pancreatitis	• acute coronary syndrome	• electrolyte disturbances
• appendicitis	• aortic dissection	• heart failure
• UTI / pyelonephritis	• abdominal aortic aneurysm	• nephrolithiasis
• pelvic inflammatory disease	• diabetic gastroparesis	• lower lobe pneumonia

Though there are many possibilities, some of the more frequent and serious deserve extra discussion:

1. Acute coronary syndrome: This patient is certainly at high risk for ACS. Her diabetes is considered a clinical equivalent to coronary artery disease (CAD)[13] and ESRD confers a 10–20 fold increase in risk for cardiovascular death.[14] About 70% of patients on hemodialysis have some form of cardiovascular disease and more than half of them will die from it, typically at a much younger age than matched cohorts.[2] Up to 20% present without Heberden's classic angina pectoris[15] and these patients carry a two-fold increase of in-hospital mortality compared to patients with typical symptoms.[16] Risk factors associated with an atypical presentation include female sex, diabetes mellitus, hypertension, renal failure, older age, nonsmoking status, and late presentation[16]—many of these are present in our patient.

Whereas early generation cardiac biomarkers such as troponin take about 4–6 hours to rise and are poorly sensitive at the time of arrival to the ED,[17] the electrocardiographic changes associated with a current of injury can be seen nearly immediately. Although ECG is an insensitive modality for ACS, it is the pivotal point in the evaluation. Even in the absence of ST elevation or abnormal biomarkers, the ECG may reveal important indicators of myocardial strain such as ST depression or T wave inversions and should be evaluated in conjunction with cardiac enzymes. The troponin in our patient was negative.

Even if we had ordered an ECG, a single negative troponin is still insufficient; even modern troponin assays are only able to achieve a sensitivity of 84% for acute MI within the first 3 hours of symptom onset.[18] Sensitivity for 30-day major adverse cardiac events can be improved to 99% when combined with a clinical decision rule such as the HEART score and a second troponin drawn at a three hour interval.[19] Although high-sensitivity cardiac troponin assays offer up to 99% sensitivity with a single test,[20] they have only recently been approved by the FDA and are not yet available in most U.S. EDs. As such, current guidelines still support a serial troponin approach to evaluation of potential ACS.[21]

Interpretation of elevated troponins in ESRD patients can be challenging since they are often elevated in the absence of myocardial injury. Troponin is renally cleared, but troponin I retains its specificity to a greater degree than troponin T, owing to a shorter elimination half-life.[22] The accepted biomarker criteria for MI is a troponin level greater than the 99th percentile OR a 20% increase for patients whose baseline already exceeds this level.[23] Since our patient's troponin was normal, we are more concerned with sensitivity than specificity.

2. Mesenteric ischemia: All of the CAD risk factors that impact ESRD patients also predispose to mesenteric ischemia, of which 40–50% of cases are caused by arterial embolism,[24] most often resulting from atrial fibrillation which is present in about 20% of HD patients.[2] This is another reason that an ECG documenting sinus origin would be helpful. Arterial thrombosis and non-occlusive arterial ischemia account for another 25–30%[25] and when it comes to atherosclerotic vascular disease, if you've got it somewhere, you've probably got it everywhere. Calciphylaxis (calcific uremic arteriolopathy/CUA), a rare but devastating disorder of calcium and phosphorus metabolism in patients on long-term HD, most often presents with cutaneous ulcers but is another potential cause of intestinal ischemia specific to patients with ESRD.[26,27]

Although the average age of patients presenting with mesenteric ischemia is 69,[24] ESRD accelerates the development of atherosclerotic disease. Was the provider considering this diagnosis when he/she ordered the lactate level? The sensitivity of lactate for mesenteric ischemia is 86%, but it is a finding present after the infarction has developed; a normal lactate does not exclude the disease.[28] This is a difficult diagnosis to make, and of course, you can't order CT angiography on everyone who comes in with abdominal pain. However, with a mortality of 60–80% in the first 24 hours of onset,[25] it is worth considering in patients at high risk, especially those with reported pain out of proportion to their abdominal exam, such as our patient.

3. Secondary peritonitis: Although the vast majority of patients with ESRD undergo HD, those on PD are at risk for peritonitis resulting from the direct communication between the bacteria-laden outside world and the sterile environment of the peritoneal cavity. The incidence is 0.24–1.66 episodes/patient/year,[29] most often caused by skin flora such as *S. aureus* and *S. epidermidis*, followed by gram negatives such as *E. coli* and *Pseudomonas*.[30] Diagnosis is made by collecting a sample of the effluent after a 2-hour dwell time and sending it for cell count and culture. Fluid white blood cell count is typically > 100/μL with > 50% neutrophils and cultures are positive in 80–90% of cases.[31] Treatment is with broad spectrum antibiotics administered intraperitoneal unless the patient has signs of systemic sepsis; removal of the catheter is not required for uncomplicated episodes but is recommended if the patient deteriorates, the effluent does not clear within 5 days, and in the case of recurrence.[31]

Though most patients do well with appropriate treatment, mortality is about 5% per episode and 16% of patients on PD will ultimately die from complications related to this diagnosis.[31] Sclerosing encapsulated peritonitis is a rare but important long-term complication which often results in bowel obstruction and malnutrition and carries a 50% 1-year mortality rate.[32]

4. Urinary tract infection: This provider planned to check a urinalysis (UA) but ultimately discharged the patient without documenting the results. This happens frequently in the ED, especially with patients who make little urine. A UTI certainly could be causing our patient's abdominal pain and vomiting. Although data on the topic is sparse, UTI does appear to occur in oliguric and anuric patients, though admittedly it is more challenging to make the diagnosis since bladder lavage may be required to obtain a specimen.[33] Decreased frequency of micturition leads to urinary stasis which predisposes to infection and may account for why UTI in males is more common in ESRD.[34] ESRD patients do have an unusually high rate of asymptomatic bacteriuria and culture-negative pyuria, decreasing the specificity of a positive UA.[34] However, the relative immunocompromise conferred by impaired clearance of uremic toxins, in combination with the multiple comorbidities associated with ESRD, places these patients at higher risk for invasive and life-threatening infection.[35] Frequent health care encounters results in increased risk of resistant pathogens.[36]

5. Uremia/volume overload: Dialysis replaces two primary functions of the kidney: clearance and ultrafiltration.

- Clearance is partially assessed by the electrolytes and acid-base status but the clearance of uremic toxins is more difficult to assess. Although blood urea nitrogen (BUN) is a surrogate, it is not the urea itself that causes symptomatic uremia, but rather a host of other unmeasured toxic compounds.[37] More than 200 potential offenders have been identified but no single putative toxin or group of toxins appears to be responsible.[37] Azotemia refers to asymptomatic elevation of the BUN—a marker of nitrogen balance that may be related to renal function, intestinal absorption of GI blood loss, or a host of other issues. Uremia is the syndrome of confusion, weakness, fatigue, abdominal pain, pruritis, insulin resistance, decreased RBC survival, platelet dysfunction, increased muscle turnover, and serositis caused by inadequate renal clearance of uremic toxins. The absolute value of BUN correlates inconsistently with symptomatic uremia and therefore the BUN level is not used exclusively as an indication for initiation of dialysis. The mechanism for abdominal pain in uremia is not completely understood; it may be related to serositis of the peritoneum.
- The other component of HD is ultrafiltration, assessed with history and exam. Volume overload can cause abdominal pain due to vascular congestion resulting in bowel wall edema and ascites.

History should include the timing of the last HD session, how much fluid was taken off, and an assessment of recent weight gain. Assess for signs of volume overload on exam, though the physical exam is a notoriously poor predictor of true volume status.[38] Chest x-ray may show signs of pulmonary edema or pleural effusion and bedside ultrasound can be helpful in demonstrating dilation and lack of respiratory variation of the IVC.[39] The serum level of brain natriuretic peptide (BNP) is often ordered, though the metabolism of natriuretic peptides in ESRD has been found to be complex and poorly reliable in this population.[40]

6. Pneumonia: Though lower lobe pneumonias can present with isolated abdominal pain in the pediatric population, this has been rarely reported in adults[41] despite a very old but oft-cited study reporting an 8% incidence.[42] The ED work-up in ESRD should be targeted to the individual differential diagnosis—our patient is not complaining of cough, dyspnea, or sputum production, is not tachypneic or hypoxic and has clear lungs on exam. Without a fever or some respiratory complaint, there is not a clear indication for a chest x-ray to exclude pneumonia as the diagnosis requires clinical symptoms in addition to radiographic findings, and in their absence, the presence of an infiltrate is difficult to interpret and should probably not trigger an order for antibiotics—pneumonia is fairly low on our differential.

7. Gastroparesis: Gastroparesis is a chronic neuromuscular disorder characterized by impaired gastric emptying, resulting in episodes of food intolerance, pain, bloating, and vomiting—the diagnosis given to our patient on discharge. Though commonly seen in diabetes mellitus, it is most often idiopathic and affects women about four times as often as men.[43] It may be suspected in the ED, but a definitive diagnosis is made by radionuclide gastric emptying scintigraphy studies. The first line of treatment consists of lifestyle modification including smaller, more frequent meals, liquid diet, low fat, low fiber, and improved glycemic control.[44] ED management is focused on symptom control with medications such as metoclopramide (the only FDA approved drug) or erythromycin.[43] Haloperidol has also been found to be an effective adjunct.[45] Opioid analgesic medications should be avoided as they may worsen symptoms.[44] Refractory symptoms may be managed with pyloric injection of botulinum toxin, jejunostomy tube placement, or insertion of a gastric pacemaker.[43] Those with significant dehydration, electrolyte abnormalities, or refractory symptoms may require admission.

RETURN ED VISIT (2 days later)

CC (09:41): per RN: altered LOC

HPI: 52 yo woman presents per EMS. Per old records, was here 2 days ago with exacerbation of chronic diabetic gastroparesis and now per EMS who say the family at the apartment found her unresponsive in bed this AM. They went to check on her and she was not able to be aroused. Pt did not feel well yesterday so did not go to dialysis. EMS has checked a BS which was 'low' and were not able to start an IV line. No meds have been given. BP was 70/palp en route. Pt. unable to give any history secondary to her medical condition of being unresponsive. Additional history to be obtained when family arrives.

PMH, PSH, meds, allergies, social history, family history: *see Initial Visit above*

Vitals:

Time	Temp (F)	Pulse	Resp	BP	SpO2	Pain
09:43	97.8	117	12	60/40	91% (4L NC)	N/A

PE:
GA: Unresponsive to verbal and painful stimuli
HEAD: Normocephalic; atraumatic.
EYES: PERRL, no scleral icterus
RESP: Breath sounds decreased with bilateral rhonchi, minimal wheezing symmetric
CARDIO: Regular rhythm, without murmurs, rub or gallop
ABD: Minimally distended, no pain response with palpation, low transverse well healed old surgical scar
SKIN: Mottled, slightly cool; no apparent lesions

ECG: Wide complex tachycardia with rate of 119bpm, nonspecific ST changes

Author comments (Weinstock):

Our patient is unresponsive, profoundly hypotensive, hypoxemic, and tachycardic. Alright, strap on your boots because *this* is why we practice emergency medicine!

DECISION POINT A – YOU ARE FACED WITH 5 QUESTIONS:

1. **Which abnormalities should be addressed first?**
2. **The resident asks about placing an IO—what are the options for access?**
3. **How should we initially manage the wide-complex tachycardia (WCT)?**
4. **How should the hypotension be assessed and addressed?**
5. **What are potential causes of altered mental status and hypotension in patients with ESRD?**

What does the literature say?

Q#1: Which abnormalities should be addressed first?

In the past several years, circulation has risen to become the king of the ABCs. The AHA has revised the canonical ABCs mantra to C-A-Bs and now says hands-only CPR is OK,[46] in fact, intubation may be harmful in cardiac arrest.[47]

Here we have an unresponsive patient with a wide-complex tachycardia (WCT) and a potentially non-perfusing blood pressure: we need to ensure a pulse is present and begin addressing the hypotension. This may not be a cardiac arrest scenario yet, but it will be if we don't get that blood pressure up in a hurry. A recent study looked at the blood pressures of ICU patients just before they succumbed to terminal cardiovascular collapse and found an average critical MAP of 35 ± 11 mmHg, with collapse at even higher pressures in certain populations, such as those with severe aortic stenosis (46 ± 12mmHg).[48] With our patient's current MAP of 47 there is not much room for error—induction medications may worsen hypotension, so we should resuscitate before intubation!

High-flow oxygen or noninvasive positive-pressure ventilation (NIPPV) can be used to temporize her respiratory status and begin preoxygenation while IV access is established. The hypoglycemia can be addressed simultaneously using intramuscular glucagon, which is quickly efficacious in restoring blood sugar levels and consciousness in hypoglycemic patients.[49]

Q#2: The resident asks about placing an IO—what are the options for access?

In a hypotensive patient where time is mortality,[50,51] speed is essential. No matter how skilled a provider is with peripheral IVs or CVC placement, an IO will go in faster. One study found an average time to placement of 2 minutes for IOs versus 8 minutes for CVCs, with a first attempt success rate of 85% versus 60%,[52] with fewer complications and lower cost.[53] The proximal tibia can be accessed faster than the humerus, with higher first attempt success rate, especially in obese patients, and with a much lower rate of dislodgement.[54]

Any medication or fluid that can be given through a central line can be given through an IO. When pressure bags are used to compensate for resistance created by bone spicules, flow rates of over 150mL/min can be achieved,[55] which is slightly higher than what you get with the 16g port of a standard triple lumen central line,[56] though still lower than with a cordis or a 16g peripheral IV. Labs can also be obtained per IO, though certain values such as potassium may be less reliable, and results cannot be trusted in cardiac arrest or after fluids/medications have been infused.[57]

Once a good peripheral IV is established, the urgency for a CVC is decreased. Each site carries its own set of advantages and disadvantages, so the optimal site depends on a combination of patient characteristics and provider comfort. Although ultrasound has unquestionably improved the success rate and incidence of complications for central lines,[58,59] it also takes time to set up and perform. The femoral site has some advantages as it can be cannulated fastest by about a minute[60] and usually does not require the use of ultrasound. It also avoids draping the head of the bed where important monitoring and procedures may be taking place simultaneously and allows for the placement of an arterial line at the same site without relocating your sterile setup. It also avoids the possibility of iatrogenic pneumothorax and can be performed in a supine patient wearing a cervical collar or requiring thoracolumbar spine precautions, or in a semi-recumbent patient whose respiratory status will not allow them to lay flat. Although it may be more challenging when there is a large pannus and the rate of blood stream infection may be slightly higher,[61] we recommend this as the site of choice in most emergent situations.

Consulting editor comments (Weingart):

I recommend using ultrasound every time when placing a femoral line.

Q#3: How should we initially manage the wide-complex tachycardia (WCT)?

Assuming that the patient does in fact have a pulse, the best management here depends on the cause of the WCT. The basic differential includes ventricular tachycardia (VT) and supraventricular tachycardia (SVT) with aberrancy. Aberrant ventricular conduction may be caused by baseline or rate-dependent bundle branch blocks, ventricular pacing, or toxic/metabolic pathology.[62] Note that SVT refers to any tachycardia originating above the AV node and includes sinus tachycardia and atrial fibrillation/flutter, not just atrioventricular nodal re-entry tachycardia (AVNRT) for which the term is often used as a synonym. It is commonly reported that VT is the most common cause of

WCT;[63] as it turns out, this narrative comes from data in cardiac populations and has not held true in the ED population where about 70% of cases are due to aberrant conduction of various SVTs.[62]

Our patient has a history of ESRD and has missed dialysis, which should prompt consideration of hyperkalemia as the cause of her WCT. Besides this clinical history, other findings on the ECG may clue us into this diagnosis. Although VT is defined by a rate > 100 and QRS duration > 120ms, it is usually much faster than that and is rarely wider than 200ms.[64] "REALLY wide-complex tachycardia" is often seen with metabolic or toxicologic etiologies such as hyperkalemia or tricyclic antidepressant toxicity and rarely indicates VT.[64] Be aware that there is no data regarding the diagnostic characteristics of these ECG features. In the absence of a likely alternative explanation, we should still assume that a WCT is VT and treat it as such, especially in a patient with cardiac risk factors.[65] Differentiating VT from SVT with aberrancy is no easy task; while we will not be faulted for "cardioverting first and asking questions later," electricity does not fix a hyperkalemic sine wave rhythm. In addition, antiarrhythmic drugs further block cardiac sodium channels and can cause degeneration into asystole or ventricular fibrillation and death in hyperkalemic patients.[66] In this situation, start by treating for hyperkalemia with IV calcium, while simultaneously setting up to treat for VT if unsuccessful.

Q#4: How should the hypotension be assessed and addressed?

The RUSH exam: <u>R</u>apid <u>U</u>ltrasound in <u>S</u>hock and <u>H</u>ypotension is a point-of-care ultrasound (POCUS) protocol designed to quickly assess the etiology of shock. The exam seeks to differentiate the four causes of shock (hypovolemic, cardiogenic, distributive, and obstructive) through assessment of the "pump" (heart), the "tank" (IVC, peritoneal space, pleural space), and the "pipes" (aorta) by obtaining 14 sonographic views. The skilled operator can use this exam to identify conditions such as tamponade, severe left ventricular dysfunction, right heart strain or lower extremity DVT suggestive of PE, volume overload, sources of infection such as pneumonia, empyema, or SBP, hemoperitoneum, abdominal aortic aneurysm, and pneumothorax. Though the exam is dependent on operator skill level and the diagnostic characteristics of each individual component vary, the overall performance of the exam in identifying the etiology of shock has been excellent. A study in 77 hypotensive ED patients found a sensitivity/specificity of 100%/96.2%, 90%/98%, 90.9%/98.2%, 72.7%/100%, and 63.6%/98% for hypovolemic, cardiogenic, obstructive, distributive, and mixed shock respectively.[67] In addition, the exam is easily learned and can be quickly performed at the bedside by emergency physicians[68] with similar diagnostic accuracy as when performed by radiologists.[67]

Consulting editor comments (Weingart):

The RUSH exam was created by my group in 2006 and has been available since March, 2008 at www.emcrit.org/rush-exam. Another protocol with the same name was published in 2012 at https://emcrit.org/wp-content/uploads/2011/03/New-RUSH-Review-Article1.pdf.

Push-dose pressors: Even with good IV access and pressure bags in place, the hemodynamic response to IV fluids is not immediate and consideration should be given to concomitant initiation of vasopressors to temporize vital organ perfusion while fluid resuscitation is under way.[69] Push-dose pressors (PDP) have been utilized with increasing frequency in the ED for peri-procedural hypotension[70] and for patients in shock as a bridge to vasopressor infusion.[69] Both phenylephrine and epinephrine are stocked in most ED crash carts, though there are no commercially available premixed preparations, so dosing requires mixing at the bedside.[71] Although PDP have been safely used in the OR for decades, a dearth of evidence exists regarding their safety and appropriate use in the ED and concerns have been raised regarding the potential for medication errors.[71,72] Although there is face validity to this approach, there is also no evidence that use of PDP improves outcomes relative to use of IVF or simply waiting for a vasopressor infusion to arrive. There is some evidence that patients who are adequately fluid-resuscitated prior to PDP administration ultimately require less vasopressors.[73]

While phenylephrine is probably fine for most patients, it is a pure alpha-agonist and can cause reflex bradycardia and increased afterload leading to decreased cardiac output in patients with poor left ventricular function.[74] Epinephrine is a more physiologic and balanced inopressor, though its chronotropic effects may exacerbate tachyarrhythmias. The ampules of cardiac epinephrine stocked in crash carts contain doses that should NEVER be given to a patient with a pulse without dilution due to increased risk of cardiovascular complications.[75]

Consulting editor comments (Weingart):

There is no reflex bradycardia in sick patients. Cardiac epinephrine can absolutely be given; the dose is 0.5mL.

Vasopressors: Transition to a pharmacy-prepared infusion should be made as soon as possible. So-called "dirty epinephrine" drips can be mixed at the bedside by injecting an entire 10cc ampule of cardiac epinephrine (1:10,000) into a 1L bag of normal saline to create a 1mcg/cc solution that can be infused wide open (up to about 20cc/min) until the pressor arrives, but this is rarely necessary.[76] There is now little disagreement that norepinephrine should be the first-line vasopressor of choice with only a few exceptions.[77,78] Phenylephrine may help to slow the heart rate in uncontrolled atrial fibrillation[78,79] for patients without significant heart failure. Dopamine may be useful for unstable patients with bradycardia who are at low risk for ventricular arrhythmias, though epinephrine is another option.[77,78] Either vasopressin or epinephrine may be added as a second agent for patients refractory to norepinephrine infusion.[75] Purely inotropic medications such as dobutamine and milrinone should very rarely be used as monotherapy in hypotensive patients, even when cardiogenic shock is suspected, due to their vasodilatory properties.[78] However, when inotropic support is required, dobutamine is the recommended first-line agent.[77] Alternatively, as a balanced inopressor, epinephrine is a reasonable first-line option for hypotensive patients with cardiogenic shock.[80]

Vasopressors through a peripheral line: Though the relative safety of vasopressor administration a peripheral IV line has been largely established in the literature,[81-83] it remains a frequent barrier in clinical practice due to outdated hospital policies, as well as nursing and pharmacy staff comfort level. Initiation of peripheral vasopressors while working on establishing central access is very low risk when compared to the risk of ongoing hypotension, especially when a 20g or larger IV located at or above the antecubital fossa is used. If extravasation does occur, local injection of phentolamine or topical application of nitroglycerin paste can be used to prevent the rare outcome of tissue ischemia.[83]

Q#5: What are potential causes of altered mental status and hypotension in patients with ESRD?

First, we need to differentiate acute versus chronic hypotension as about 5% of ESRD patients are chronically hypotensive and require alpha-agonist medications such as midodrine to maintain their blood pressure either following HD or continuously.[84] The pathophysiology is complex but may involve autonomic dysfunction, vasoplegia due to a chronic hyper catecholaminergic state, overproduction of vasodilators such nitric oxide and adrenomedullin, or heart failure; it is associated with a poor prognosis.[84] Missing even a single dose of midodrine can result in profound hypotension. Of course, our patient was mildly *hypertensive* on presentation 2 days ago and takes several antihypertensive medications, leading us away from the consideration of chronic hypotension.

The prevalence and morbidity of invasive infections in ESRD patients, particularly bacteremia secondary to infected HD lines, places septic shock at the top of the differential for our patient but we should consider other causes as well, including hypovolemia following volume removal during HD. This occurs in 30–40% of HD patients, even when no net ultrafiltration is performed due to the volume shifts associated with filling the dialysis circuit with the patient's blood.[84] Our patient could also have hypovolemic shock simply due to persistent vomiting, given her presentation with symptomatic gastroparesis two days prior. Bleeding is another important cause to consider; ESRD patients typically have normal coagulation studies, but uremic platelet dysfunction can predispose to major bleeding. A rectal exam for gross or occult blood should be documented, especially given her recent visit with abdominal pain and anemia. Intracranial hemorrhage is a potential cause of her altered mental status, so we recommend a CT of the head. Finally, consider bleeding from an AV fistula, which can be severe, though it is typically obvious on exam.

The high risk for cardiovascular disease puts ACS in the mix; our patient's WCT could easily be VT due to an acute MI. Other potential cardiac etiologies include cardiogenic shock precipitated by volume overload after missing dialysis or tamponade due to uremic pericarditis.[85] A quick sonographic evaluation of the chest should be sufficient to rule out these diagnoses.

Medication-related adverse events are another major cause of morbidity due to frequent polypharmacy and altered pharmacokinetics due to impaired renal function. Our patient takes multiple medications that cause hypotension (carvedilol, doxazosin, lisinopril, nitroglycerin). She also takes several QTc-prolonging medications which places her at risk for torsades de pointes as a cause of both the WCT and hypotension. In addition, her hypoglycemia could be a result of insulin overdose due to altered metabolism and lack of renal clearance in ESRD which often results in significantly decreased insulin requirements.[86] Rounding out the list is her history of opioid use which can cause both hypotension and altered mental status, so consider giving Narcan up front, especially since it can be given by other routes if we're still working on an IV.

DECISION POINT A – ***What did the actual provider do?***

(Chart on next page...)

ED course:
09:46: Blood sugar checked and is 27
09:48: Pt. received 2 amps of D50 through a 20g IV left forearm
09:51: Reassessment reveals no improvement in mental status. A 2nd IV is not able to be established
09:52: BP recheck is systolic 62/palp
09:55: 1 amp of cardiac epi is mixed to 10mcg/mL at bedside and 2mL are administered as "push dose"
09:59: SBP 61/palp
10:02: Norepinephrine infusion is ordered

ED course: Monitor shows the patient still has wide-complex tachycardia

Author comments (Weinstock):

Summary/problem list:

- Patient's mental status has not improved with the D50
- She remains hypotensive despite pressors
- Her monitor continues to show a wide-complex tachycardia
- The only IV access being used is a 20g IV left forearm

DECISION POINT B – YOU ARE FACED WITH 4 QUESTIONS:

1. **Is the patient safe to leave the department for head CT?**
2. **With a suspicion of hyperkalemia as a cause of the wide-complex tachycardia, should calcium be given before labs have returned?**
3. **For emergent treatment of hyperkalemia, should we use calcium chloride or calcium gluconate?**
4. **Should the patient be intubated *now*?**

Q#1: Is the patient safe to leave the department for head CT?

One the many unspoken rules in emergency medicine is that unstable patients should not travel to the CT scanner. But is this practice evidence-based? The population in question is by definition "high risk" for imminent decompensation, whether we travel with them or not, but sometimes this information will alter their management. However, the very act of moving a patient can rattle their very tenuous physiology or disrupt our interventions such as dislodgement of an ET tube or loss of IV access. Furthermore, even if that decompensation was bound to occur, it is much more difficult to manage in the cramped and relatively resource-poor setting of the radiology department than in the resuscitation bay.

A recent large multicenter prospective observational study examined 441 episodes of intrahospital transport of critically ill ICU patients and found an 80% overall incidence of adverse events.[87] While a large percentage of these events were relatively minor such as loss of monitor power, disconnected oxygen tubing, and agitation, about a third of patients experienced so-called "critical" events related to vital sign or blood gas abnormalities. However, only one patient was accidentally extubated, and no patients experienced cardiac arrest or death. Unfortunately, this study is limited by the lack of a comparison group of similarly ill patients who did not undergo transport.

A large multicenter French study in 2013 attempted to address this limitation by using a prospective cohort study design.[88] They compared 1659 mechanically ventilated patients who underwent intrahospital transport to a propensity-matched cohort of patients who did not. Complications occurred in 37% of transported patients with an odds ratio of 1.9 (95% CI, 1.7–2.2) compared to the non-transported group, though many of these events were minor. Transportation was associated with longer ICU length of stay but not increased mortality. Several other studies have found much lower rates of critical adverse events, likely due to differing definitions. A 2007 Austrian prospective observational study of 452 intrahospital transports found only 4.2% incidence of critical events and no association with mortality.[89] A 2011 study retrospectively reviewed 3383 patients who were transported by a specialized team and found only 1.7% incidence of adverse events, mostly related to hypotension and hypoxia, with only a single accidental extubation and a single code blue.[90]

These data seem to suggest that when crucial information is needed, it is reasonable to travel to the scanner, but first consider how likely the results are to change your immediate management. If you suspect a ruptured AAA in a hypotensive patient and the vascular surgeon won't activate the OR on the basis of your ultrasound findings until they see the CT scan, then initiate massive transfusion and get them to CT. For many patients though, care can be started to stabilize the patient without undergoing the risks inherent in transport. For our patient, intracranial hemorrhage is much less likely than other diagnoses such as septic shock, ACS, or hyperkalemia. Furthermore, since we are not seeing obvious signs of intracranial hypertension, we are unlikely to change our immediate management even if we did identify a bleed. The safest thing to do here is to focus on resuscitation before travelling to CT.

Q#2: With a suspicion of hyperkalemia as a cause of the wide-complex tachycardia, should calcium be given before labs have returned?

Unfortunately, we do not have the luxury of waiting in a hemodynamically unstable patient. In a recent study of arrhythmias, cardiac arrests, and deaths in hyperkalemic patients, all adverse cardiac events occurred either before (59%) or shortly after (within 36 minutes on average) the potassium level became available.[91] All of these patients had hyperkalemic changes identifiable on their initial ECG that could have been empirically treated an average of 47 minutes before the adverse event.

Most EDs have the ability to rapidly obtain point-of-care potassium values using blood gas analyzers and their use is recommended by the UK Renal Association.[92] Though many physicians distrust their results,[93] potassium values provided by these assays actually differ very little from laboratory values (less than 0.1mmol/L),[94] though variability may be greater in cardiac arrest (mean difference 0.106 mmol/L; 95% CI, -1.182–1.394mmol/L).[95]

The classic progression of ECG changes from peaked T waves to asystole does not reliably occur at particular serum potassium levels.[91] Cases of serum potassium > 10mmol/L with no ECG changes have been reported and cardiac arrest has occurred without so much as a peaked T wave on the preceding ECG.[92] However, when the ECG does suggest hyperkalemia, empiric treatment should be initiated as quickly as possible. While you're putting the pads on the patient and drawing up your antiarrhythmic drug of choice (current evidence favors procainamide for "stable" VT),[65] trying pushing an amp of calcium from the crash cart. This is a quick intervention that is unlikely to harm your patient (even if the hyperkalemia is due to digoxin toxicity, despite the dogma)[96] or significantly delay your ability to deliver a shock. In fact, calcium actually has inotropic and vasopressor properties so it may be helpful even if the patient turns out to be hypokalemic.[97] If you're right, you'll watch the QRS complex narrow in front of your eyes. If not, then you're all set to treat the impending VT.

Q#3: For emergent treatment of hyperkalemia, should we use calcium chloride or calcium gluconate?

The treatment of hyperkalemia consists of 4 steps:

1. Stabilize the plasma membrane of the cardiomyocytes to reduce arrhythmogenicity
2. Shift potassium from the blood into the cells.
3. Eliminate excess potassium from the body.
4. Consider and treat the underlying cause to prevent recurrence.

Calcium:

Hyperkalemia increases myocardial excitability by moving the resting membrane potential closer to the threshold potential for depolarization and slows ventricular conduction.[98] Calcium suppresses arrhythmias primarily by increasing the threshold potential to restore the normal electrical "distance" from the resting potential.[98] It is available in two formulations: calcium chloride and calcium gluconate. The chloride salt is more concentrated, providing 3 times more elemental calcium per unit volume than the gluconate (6.8 vs. 2.26mmol of $Ca2+$ per 10mL of 10% solution). As such, calcium chloride carries a higher risk for tissue necrosis and calcinosis cutis and should be administered via a central line whenever possible.[92] Despite reports to the contrary, calcium gluconate does not require hepatic metabolism to reach an active form; both formulations are equally fast-acting (onset within about 3 minutes) when equivalent doses are provided.[99,100] Though there is relatively limited evidence available, most authors recommend using the chloride salt in the setting of hemodynamic instability.[92,101] The recommended dose is 1g given over 3–5 minutes, with consideration of a second dose after 5 minutes if there is no response.[102] The UK Renal Association guidelines recommend giving calcium for any ECG changes.[92] Other authors also suggest giving it for potassium > 6 mEq/L even in the absence of ECG changes.[102] The half-life is relatively short at 30–60 minutes and the repeat dosing may be necessary if serum potassium levels are not quickly reduced.

IV fluids – LR or NS?

After, cardiac membrane stabilization, proceed to a fluid bolus to:

1. Correct dehydration and metabolic acidosis.
2. Dilute out the potassium concentration.
3. Increase urine output to induce kaliuresis.

However, a recent *Cochrane* review found no studies that have examined the safety and effectiveness of this strategy.[101] This is balanced by the fact that many causes of hyperkalemia are associated with volume overload (e.g., heart failure, missed HD) and may be worsened with the administration of

IV fluids. It is a fallacy that lactated Ringer's (LR) should be avoided due to potassium content. As the 4mEq/L in LR is lower than the patient's potassium level and, more importantly, LR is a mildly alkalinizing solution. Since the majority of total body potassium is contained in the intracellular space, even the small shifts to the extracellular space caused by the hyperchloremic metabolic acidosis induced by normal saline (NS) infusion can worsen hyperkalemia. Three prospective randomized controlled trials have shown LR to have favorable effects on serum potassium relative to NS in patients undergoing renal transplantation.[103-105]

Insulin and dextrose:
Numerous studies have demonstrated the efficacy of insulin in shifting potassium to the intracellular space via upregulation and activation of the Na-K ATPase,[92] in fact, this is why we don't give insulin in DKA until the potassium level returns. The effect is dose-dependent and results in an average reduction in serum potassium about 0.8mEq/L within about an hour and lasting about 2 hours.[92] The obvious downside of using insulin is the risk for hypoglycemia, especially in a patient such as ours who is already hypoglycemic. This risk appears to be especially pronounced in patients with renal impairment,[102] likely owing to altered insulin metabolism. As such, insulin should be given *after* administration of dextrose in all but the profoundly hyperglycemic patient. The recommended dose is 10 units insulin IV plus 25g of 50% dextrose, though more dextrose may be needed in patients at higher risk for hypoglycemia. Several recent studies also suggest that similar potassium lowering effects can be achieved using 5 units of insulin while reducing the risk of hypoglycemia, especially in patients with poor renal function (e.g., LaRue 2017). Some guidelines recommend insulin for any potassium > 5.5mEq/L100 while others suggest waiting until it is > 6.0–6.5mEq/L.[92]

Inhaled beta-2 agonists:
Inhaled beta-2 agonists also decrease serum potassium by activating the Na-K ATPase. Pharmacokinetics are similar to insulin, with an average decrease in potassium of 0.5–0.9mEq/L, peak effect in about 60 minutes, and duration of about 2 hours. However, a small subset of patients may experience a transient increase in potassium, and up to 40% of ESRD patients may not respond.[92] The effect of beta-agonists in combination with insulin is greater than either intervention alone,[92] therefore, beta-agonists should not be used as monotherapy. Guidelines recommend treatment with adjuvant beta-agonists at similar threshold levels of serum potassium as those noted for insulin above. Dose is 10mg, higher than the standard breathing treatment.[92]

Sodium bicarbonate:
The use of sodium bicarbonate in hyperkalemia remains controversial. Theoretically, serum alkalinization drives serum potassium into cells via an H+/K+ exchange pump and increases the kidney's ability to excrete potassium.[106] However, the limited evidence available has largely failed to confirm these benefits. No studies have shown that sodium bicarbonate infusion significantly lowers serum potassium acutely or that it enhances the effects of other interventions.[92] Furthermore, hypertonic sodium bicarbonate ampules may actually worsen serum potassium levels through a phenomenon known as "solute drag" in which serum hypertonicity causes cell crenation, increasing the intracellular potassium concentration and subsequently serum potassium levels as equilibration with the extracellular fluid occurs.[106] A few small studies have suggested that bicarbonate may be effective in decreasing potassium in patients with concurrent metabolic acidosis,[107] though methodological issues limit the ability to draw any robust conclusions. Though more high-quality

randomized studies are needed, the use of sodium bicarbonate is not recommended by most guidelines,[101] except in the case of cardiac arrest, where its effects on serum pH may be beneficial and it is reasonable to try.[92] Other guidelines recommend considering bicarb if the patient is acidotic AND potassium is > 7.5mEq/L or there are ECG changes.

Ion exchange resins:
There are three possible routes for the elimination of potassium from the body:
1. The urine (kaliuresis)
2. The stool (binding resins)
3. The blood (dialysis)

For years, ion exchange resins such as sodium polystyrene sulfonate (SPS) have been the cornerstone of conservative management for patients without dialysis access. In the solvent environment of the GI tract, these insoluble polymers give up their preloaded sodium moieties in exchange for binding potassium from the stool and are then eliminated from the body by defecation.[108] SPS has become part of the canon of medicine despite very little evidence for its safety or efficacy.[108] There are essentially no well-designed controlled trials that show a robust decrease in serum potassium and there have been numerous reports of potentially devastating colonic necrosis, even after the older 70% sorbitol formulations were replaced by 33% sorbitol as mandated by the FDA.[108] For now, most guidelines recommend against its use for the emergent treatment of hyperkalemia.[101,102]

Dialysis:
Hemodialysis is the most important therapy for hyperkalemia in patients with ESRD or anuria. HD removes potassium by diffusion down its concentration gradient across a semipermeable membrane into a dialysate solution. Though HD carries its own risks, it is the only intervention that is quickly and universally effective in reducing serum potassium, by an average of 2mmol/L following a 3-hour session.[102] After equilibration following an HD session, there may be a rebound hyperkalemia. For our patient, there is no doubt that she is going to need emergent HD and we should advocate for it early and emphatically.

Q#4: Should the patient be intubated *now*?
Clearly intubation is on the horizon for this patient. Fortunately, she is currently breathing and has a reasonable O2 saturation, so it is worth spending a few moments trying to create safer intubating conditions. Intubation can be a very dangerous procedure, especially in the setting of difficult peri-intubation physiology[109] which can be summarized by the mnemonic HOP Killers, which stands for hypotension, oxygenation, and pH (acidosis).[110] Though we need to protect the airway, multiple studies have found hypotension to be an independent predictor of death and cardiac arrest following intubation.[111-113] In most situations intubation can be safely postponed using noninvasive interventions while the hemodynamics are addressed. Peri-intubation hypoxemia is also associated with a risk of cardiac arrest and death[113,114] so we also need to do our best to preoxygenate before inducing apnea and creating further desaturation.

De Jong, et al.[115] looked at 1,847 intubations in 64 French ICUs and found a peri-intubation cardiac arrest rate of 2.7%, of note, 28.5% of the cardiac arrest patients failed to achieve return of spontaneous circulation (ROSC) and 73.5% had died at 28 days, as compared with 30.1% in the group that did not suffer cardiac arrest. The authors identified 5 risk factors that independently predicted peri-intubation cardiac arrest:

1. Pre-intubation hypoxemia (OR 4)
2. Failure to preoxygenate (OR 3.6)
3. Pre-intubation SBP < 90mmHg (OR 3.4)
4. Age > 75 (OR 2.3)
5. BMI > 25kg/m^2

Since the first 3 are potentially modifiable, care should be optimized before intubation.

Preoxygenation/denitrogenation is the process of maximizing hemoglobin saturation and dissolved oxygen in the blood and filling the alveoli and anatomic dead space with the highest concentration of oxygen possible in order to provide a reservoir that can passively oxygenate the blood by diffusion and delay desaturation during apnea.[116] Preoxygenation prolongs the safe apnea time providing a buffer to allow for difficult intubation.[117]

The best choice is going to depend on individual patient characteristics, physician and respiratory therapist familiarity, and device availability. Most ED providers will start by reaching for an NRB or the BVM to preoxygenate, but note that commonly available NRB masks do not contain a 1-way valve and thus does not approach 100% FiO_2 as commonly believed, delivering closer to 60–70% FiO_2 when set to 15L/min flow rate.[117] This deficiency can be crucial since the incremental benefit in delaying hemoglobin desaturation is greatest at higher levels of FiO_2 (i.e. the benefit of increasing from 90 to 100% FiO_2 is actually much greater than the benefit of increasing from room air to 90%).[118] However, setting the flow regulator to "flush rate" by continuing to open the valve past the limits of the calibrated notches that typically stop at 15L/min can increase flow to as much as 60L/min and result in an FiO_2 of 90% or greater.[117]

Secondly, most BVMs will deliver little more than room air oxygen unless a tight seal is created on the face AND either the bag is actively squeezed or patient inspires with enough force to open the 1-way inspiratory valve between the oxygen reservoir and the mask.[117] Assisting patient-initiated breaths by squeezing the bag to augment oxygenation is a common practice but in fact only generates about 1–2cm H_2O of positive pressure in the absence of a PEEP valve and likely does not make a difference in a spontaneously breathing patient.[119,120]

Many experts recommend the combination of a nasal cannula set to 15L/min and an NRB mask set to flush rate as the optimal preoxygenation strategy.[121] In addition to providing excellent preoxygenation, this strategy allows you to leave the nasal cannula in place for apneic oxygenation when the NRB is removed to perform the intubation. Contrary to non-evidence-based dogma, patients can indeed tolerate these flow rates through a standard nasal cannula.[122]

Whatever device is chosen, preoxygenation should continue for approximately 3 minutes of normal tidal-volume breathing or 8 vital capacity breaths (about 60 seconds) by a cooperative patient.[116] If SpO_2 > 93–95% is not achieved in this time period, use of noninvasive positive pressure (NIPPV) devices should be considered to account for shunt physiology in which perfused alveoli are not ventilated due to alveolar infiltrates or atelectasis.[117] Multiple studies have demonstrated the effectiveness of NIPPV in improving preintubation SpO_2 and reducing critical desaturation during intubation.[116] NIPPV can be achieved using CPAP or BiPAP devices, the latter of which provides the additional benefit of augmenting ventilation, or a simple PEEP valve affixed to a BVM.

In scenarios where patient agitation or vomiting preclude the use of an occlusive mask, heated humidified high flow nasal cannula devices can be used to deliver up to 100% FiO_2 with approximately 3cm H_2O of CPAP.[123] Despite the face validity and enthusiasm for this approach, several recent large analyses of published trials, including a *Cochrane* review, have failed to show a benefit to HHFNC over conventional oxygen therapy or NIPPV, though both analyses were limited by low quality evidence and heterogeneity of included studies.[124,125]

After preoxygenating we should be prepared to deliver apneic oxygenation to provide the largest reserve in the event of a difficult intubation. Flow of about 250cc/minute of oxygen passively from the alveoli into the bloodstream, balanced with a much lower 8–20cc/minute flow of CO_2 from the blood into the alveoli, results in a slightly subatmospheric alveolar pressure during apnea, creating flow of air from the pharynx into the alveoli.[117] High PAO_2 (in the alveoli) creates high PaO_2; as long as PaO_2 remains above 60mmHg, the hemoglobin will remain saturated. This can be achieved by simply leaving the NC we applied during the preoxygenation period in place and flowing at 15L/min throughout the period of apnea. A classic study showed that in paralyzed surgical patients with normal physiology and adequate preoxygenation, apneic oxygenation via endotracheal tube could maintain $SpO_2 > 90\%$ for up to 100 minutes![126] A 2017 meta-analysis found that apneic oxygenation significantly reduces peri-intubation hypoxemia, cuts the incidence of critical desaturation in half, and actually improves first-pass success rate.[127] Another meta-analysis published the same year showed similar findings as well as a trend towards reduced mortality bordering on statistical significance (RR 0.77; 95% CI 0.59–1.02).[128]

Since no ventilation takes place during the apneic period, pCO_2 rises by 8–16mmHg during the first minute, followed by a linear increase of about 3mmHg/min thereafter.[116] Outside the setting of profound acidosis, this rate of rise during the time it takes to perform endotracheal intubation is unlikely to be of clinical significance.[117] Of course, pausing to deliver manual ventilations during prolonged periods of apnea is indicated in the case of multiple attempts. Whenever manual ventilation via BVM is performed, it is prudent to utilize a PEEP valve to avoid generating high pressures of > 25mmHg which can open the lower esophageal sphincter and lead to aspiration.[117] A facemask connected to a mechanical ventilator or NIPPV devices can also be used to deliver pressure-controlled breaths during apnea.

DECISION POINT B – ***What did the actual provider do?***

11:02: The intern asks, “There’s a hemodialysis catheter in the neck. Can’t we just use it for IV access?”

10:32 – Labs return:
K+ = 8.9
ABG: Ph = 6.87
$PaCO_2$ = 30

ED course: 10:36: BP drops to 50/30

ED course: 10:52: Pt. is intubated with ketamine and rocuronium and placed on vent with settings: Rate 28 and tidal volume 8cc/kg with 100% FiO_2 and 6 of PEEP. Bicarb is pushed during the intubation.

10:58: RUSH exam is done:
Cardiac exam – heart hyperdynamic
IVC midsized and not collapsing
Aorta nl
No free fluid
Lung =windows B lines bilat w good lung slide

We only have 1 IV which is 20g and staff have not been able to get another line.

DECISION POINT C – YOU ARE FACED WITH 5 QUESTIONS:

1. **Which vent settings should be used?**
2. **Can the hemodialysis catheter be used?**
3. **The mental status is still altered, and he remains hypotensive; should antibiotics be administered?**
4. **The sepsis order set comes up on the computer; should he receive 30mL/kg of IVF despite the ESRD?**
5. **Does the patient need emergent dialysis?**

Q#1: Which vent settings should be used?

To describe the ABG as unfavorable for intubation may be a bit of an understatement! Low pH results in impaired myocardial contractility, vasoplegia, and decreased response to catecholamines.[129] Although the precise pH associated with cardiovascular collapse is unknown, there is no doubt that our patient has a critical acidemia.

The modern era of mechanical ventilation has been defined by lung protective ventilatory (LPV) strategies characterized by:

- Lower tidal volumes
- Lower plateau pressures
- Higher PEEP
- Permissive hypercapnia

In the seminal ARMA trial conducted by the ARDSNet group, the use of LPV led to a nearly 10% reduction in mortality compared to traditional ventilation using 12cc/kg IBW in patients with ARDS.[130] The benefits of LPV are thought to be due to a reduction in ventilator induced lung injury (VILI) caused by some combination of volutrauma (overdistention of alveoli), atelectrauma (alveolar collapse), and barotrauma (elevated airway pressures). LPV appears to be so important that even implementing it during the patients' time in the ED may reduce mortality (19.6 vs. 34%), incidence of ARDS, and shorten duration of mechanical ventilation and hospital stay.[131]

Though there is some controversy regarding the generalizability of the ARMA data[132] and the need for low tidal volumes in patients without ARDS,[133] LPV remains the standard initial approach for most mechanically ventilated patients.[77, 134]

For most patients, tidal volume should be set to 6cc/kg and titrated down as necessary to keep plateau pressures < 30cc H_2O. When pre-intubation ventilation is appropriate, the respiratory rate should be set to match the patient's minute ventilation and titrated as needed to a maximum of 35 breaths/minute to keep pH > 7.15 while observing for excessive autoPEEP.[77,130] The initial post-intubation FiO_2 of 100% should be weaned quickly to keep SpO_2 92–96% or PaO_2 > 55.[77,130] PEEP can be empirically set in proportion to the degree of hypoxemia according the ARDSnet protocol.[130]

Despite the advantages of allowing for permissive hypercapnia in favor of lung protection, our patient has another perhaps bigger problem than hypoxemic respiratory failure: profound metabolic and respiratory acidosis. She needs us to provide the respiratory compensation that she is not generating on her own; we should set her to tidal volume to the higher end of the recommended range, perhaps 8cc/kg IBW with an initial rate of 30/min. Keep her on capnography with a target $EtCO_2$ of 20cm H_2O and check a blood gas in 20 minutes to see how we're doing.

Q#2: Can the hemodialysis catheter be used?

The short answer to this question is: YES. This patient is dying in front of you and you can do little more than squeeze her hand and comfort her unless we have IV access. With an emergent situation and a patient with tenuous venous access, the risk/benefit ratio absolutely favors using that line. The longer answer involves thinking about your patient's long-term outcomes in terms of infectious risk and vein preservation. HD patients who dialyze through a CVC already carry a 2–3 fold risk for infection compared to those with a fistula or graft[135] with an incidence of about 16 catheter-related infections per 1000 dialysis days with routine use.[136] Every time that catheter is accessed the risk of infection goes up, especially when it is accessed hastily in a chaotic resuscitation bay. When a line becomes infected, it typically must be removed and replaced, causing trauma to the vein and potential loss of a precious source of venous access. When an HD-dependent patient runs out of veins, they are left with two options: urgent transplantation or hospice care. For this reason, nephrologists go to great lengths to avoid placing indwelling lines in their patients whenever possible, since the veins may become stenosed or thrombosed and unusable for future HD lines or AV fistulae.[137]

When infected lines are changed, it often requires the placement of 2 catheters: first, a temporary line for dialysis until blood cultures clear, then a new tunneled line, further multiplying the opportunities for vein destruction. If an ESRD patient needs central access in the ED, it is worth at least considering whether they would benefit from placement of an HD line rather than a standard triple-lumen catheter. This may be true in the case of a known or strongly suspected infected HD line which will likely require removal, a nonfunctioning HD line or AV fistula, or a patient requiring urgent dialysis who does not yet have HD access. Placing a triple lumen in a patient who is going to need an HD line as soon as he/she hits the ICU may result in potential loss of a vein.

When an HD line does need to be accessed in the ED, it is important to withdraw the anticoagulant catheter-locking solution from the line prior to infusing and to replace it after use. The opportunities for introducing infection can be limited by starting a low infusion rate (TKO) of crystalloid solution so that future access can be obtained via the piggyback port of the IV tubing, rather than through reaccessing the line. Although algorithms exist for the use of a tunneled HD line for urgent venous access,[138] the bottom line is simple and intuitive; if the patient is in trouble, they need access more than they need that dialysis line. Go ahead and use it, being sure to preserve sterile technique—you can apologize later for saving the patient's life!

Q#3: The mental status is still altered, and he remains hypotensive; should antibiotics be administered?

Although the differential for this patient is still quite broad, septic shock firmly tops the list and must be treated empirically until it is ruled out. Though the importance of rapid antibiotic administration continues to be hotly debated,[139] multiple trials have demonstrated that each hour that antibiotics are delayed results in a measurable increase in mortality.[140,141] This finding was recently confirmed by a large multicenter observational trial including nearly 50,000 patients.[142] Current Surviving Sepsis Campaign (SSC) guidelines recommend the administration of IV antibiotics as soon as possible after recognition of sepsis, ideally within the first hour.[77] However, the choice of agent is left up to the clinician depending on the suspected source of infection and most likely pathogen.

For our patient, the source of infection remains unclear at this point. Of course, any patient with an indwelling HD catheter is at risk for bacteremia and endocarditis, including fungal pathogens.[143] Our patient presented 2 days ago with abdominal pain, making it prudent to consider intra-abdominal gram-negative sources such as cholecystitis, cholangitis, pancreatitis, diverticulitis, appendicitis, perforated viscous, and intra-abdominal abscess. More common sources such as pneumonia and urinary tract infection remain on the differential as well. At the very least, this patient needs broad gram-positive and gram-negative coverage, including MRSA and *Pseudomonas*.

Before selecting a drug, review any prior cultures to see if there is a history of MDR infections. In the absence of such data, the initial choice will typically be vancomycin and an antipseudomonal beta-lactam such as piperacillin/tazobactam or cefepime. However, given the severity of her presentation, the high risk for MDR organisms in the ESRD population, and the waning sensitivity of *Pseudomonas* to these common first line agents,[144] it is worth considering double coverage of *Pseudomonas* by adding an agent such as tobramycin, or moving directly to an antipseudomonal carbapenem. Such "combination therapy" approach is supported by the current SSC guidelines.[77]

Given the high incidence and mortality associated with fungemia in patients with indwelling HD lines, the Infectious Disease Society of America (IDSA) also recommends considering empiric fungal coverage with a drug such as caspofungin.[145] Although the recent large double-blind placebo-controlled EMPIRICUS trial failed to show a benefit to empiric antifungal therapy in critically ill non-neutropenic, non-transplanted adults, a trend towards improved mortality was seen in the subgroup with high SOFA scores, suggesting a potential benefit in patients such as ours.[146]

Q#4: The sepsis order set comes up on the computer; should he receive 30mL/kg of IVF despite the ESRD?

If your training was anything like mine, then you were taught that if the question is "hypotension" then the answer is "fluids." This dogma seems to have become engrained in clinical practice as well as multiple sets of guidelines, including the controversial 2015 Centers for Medicare and Medicaid Services (CMS) benchmarks.[147,148] Several studies have shown that ESRD patients tend to be under-resuscitated relative to guidelines when compared to their non-ESRD peers,[149,150] though the impact that this has on patient outcomes is not clear. One group of authors in the nephrology literature suggest that it is reasonable to follow the principals of early goal-directed therapy (EGDT) in ESRD, though with the caveats that excess fluid administration has more significant consequences from both a respiratory and serum tonicity standpoint in the anuric patient[137] and that strict adherence to EGDT is no longer recommended.[77] Similar recommendations for fluid management in ESRD have come from the EM literature,[151] though this was based on the lack of cardiopulmonary complications in ESRD patients who were aggressively resuscitated in a single small retrospective study that was never published.

Recent years have brought an evolving understanding that positive fluid balance is associated with increased mortality in septic shock,[152] especially in patients with AKI and CKD.[153] Cytokine-mediated injury to the endothelial glycocalyx and increased capillary hydrostatic pressure from volume expansion combine to create the capillary-leak syndrome which results in third-spacing of fluids and often ARDS.[154] Increased preload can easily congest the often stunned myocardium of the septic patient.[155] Nonetheless, the current SSC guidelines continue to emphasize early fluid resuscitation as the cornerstone of therapy for septic shock.[77] They recommend an initial 30cc/kg bolus for all-comers regardless of age, comorbidities, or clinical impression of volume status with further fluid management guided by markers of perfusion.[77] The authors do concede, however, that little evidence supports this specific volume.

The fact is that some patients will benefit greatly from fluid resuscitation while others will be harmed. The fundamental purpose of giving exogenous fluids is to improve perfusion by increasing stroke volume.[156] However, only about 50% of hypotensive patients will be "fluid responders" and for those who are not, administration of IV fluids is unlikely to be of benefit and is potentially harmful.[156] At the top of the list of these patients are those with ESRD and CHF. While a gentle fluid challenge is reasonable for most patients, we must be very careful with folks who live on the horizontal portion of the Starling curve, especially if their respiratory status is tenuous or they show signs of cardiogenic shock. Unfortunately identifying fluid responders at the bedside remains challenging.

Multiple studies have shown that physicians are not great at assessing volume status on exam,[157] and we are even worse at determining the more important question of volume responsiveness. Static methods such central venous pressure monitoring, do not take into account important physiologic parameters such as heart-lung interactions and chest wall compliance and have been found to be of no use whatsoever.[156] The passive leg raise is a technique which simulates a fluid bolus by reversibly augmenting preload with about 300cc of blood from the lower extremities (e.g.).[158] When doing so leads to an increase in cardiac output, a patient is considered to be fluid-responsive. However, this technique still requires a method of assessing the change in cardiac output since an increase in blood pressure with the maneuver can simply be a result of sympathetic nervous system discharge due to pain, coughing, or anxiety associated with the change in body position.[159] In the post-Swann-Ganz era, numerous dynamic methods for assessing changes in cardiac output have been studied such as IVC collapsibility index, velocity-time integral at the left ventricular outflow tract, end-tidal CO_2 monitoring, transcutaneous bioimpedance or bioreactance devices, and pulse pressure or stroke volume variation, many of which have shown excellent performance.[160]

However, for many community emergency medicine providers, these methods remain either unavailable or impractical given constraints of time, lack of equipment or sufficient training.

Until some savvy doc finally figures out how to quickly and reliably identify fluid responders, we are often left to rely on the good old history and exam. If a patient is sent in from their 3L ultrafiltration HD session, then assume hypovolemia and be aggressive with fluid boluses. If they haven't been dialyzed in a week, look for signs of cardiogenic shock and consider early vasopressor administration and emergent HD. If no information is available or volume status is unclear, then try giving gentle fluid boluses and closely monitoring the hemodynamic and respiratory response.

In this case, we have a patient with a history of missed dialysis, with findings suggesting volume overload on the RUSH exam, and a tenuous respiratory status. Given that only 50% of all patients with shock will respond to fluids, what are the chances that this patient is going to respond? We recommend starting pressors right away.

Consulting editor comments (Weingart):

Note that fluid-responders have only a temporary response in sepsis, and almost half of this fluid will be gone in 60 minutes.

Q#5: Does the patient need emergent dialysis?

YES. Remember the **A-E-I-O-U** mnemonic for dialysis indications? Our patient meets just a few of those criteria!

Acidosis: pH < 7.1
Electrolytes: Refractory hyperkalemia
Ingestions: Salicylates, lithium, methanol, ethylene glycol
Overload: Volume overload unresponsive to diuresis (ESRD patients on hemodialysis)
Uremia: Symptomatic uremia such as bleeding, encephalopathy, pericarditis

We dodged a bullet when the calcium worked its magic on our patient's cardiomyocytes, but we've only got about an hour or so before we're staring down the barrel of that same gun. We can't give insulin because of our patient's severe hypoglycemia, and albuterol should never be given as monotherapy. The patient probably isn't making urine, so furosemide is out and SPS has no role in the emergent management of hyperkalemia. Some guidelines consider it reasonable to try giving more bicarb in this setting,[102] but the evidence supporting this is weak. In summary, we have no viable medical options to treat this patient's hyperkalemia. Additionally, she has severe metabolic acidosis that needs to be emergently addressed and her volume status precludes doing so using fluid resuscitation or bicarbonate infusion. Finally, I suspect that uremia may be playing a role in her encephalopathy, giving us yet another indication to dialyze.

Although she clearly needs emergent HD, she is not going to tolerate standard intermittent HD due to her hemodynamic instability and is going to require continuous renal replacement therapy (CRRT). CRRT creates an artificial GFR of about 5–20mL/min/1.73m^2 to provide clearance with a lower incidence of volume shifts causing hypotension than intermittent HD. The amount of ultrafiltration performed during CRRT can be dialed in and adjusted moment-to-moment to compensate for hemodynamic changes while attempting to slowly remove fluid. While CRRT is typically going to be initiated and managed in the ICU, it cannot be safely performed using an AV fistula. Though the necessity of this practice has been recently called into question,[161] most centers still require placement of a temporary HD line for CRRT, even for patients with an established and functional AV fistula or graft.

DECISION POINT C – ***What did the actual provider do?***

ED course:
The vasopressors are switched to the hemodialysis catheter
Vasopressin is added
Radial arterial line is put in by resident.

ED course: Antibiotics are started—piperacillin-tazobactam and vancomycin. A brain CT is ordered with chest and abdomen added.

Radiology results:
Head and abd CT both negative.
Chest CT shows multilobar pneumonia.

Diagnosis: hyperkalemic ventricular conduction delay secondary to ESRD, hypoglycemia, septic shock secondary to multilobar pneumonia.

The patient is admitted to the ICU.

Chapter summary:

- ESRD patients are at high risk for major complications and mortality—keep a broad ddx.
- Resuscitate before intubation. If emergent intubation is needed, optimize blood pressure, oxygenation, and acid-base status before pushing drugs.
- Consider metabolic and toxicologic etiologies with a wide-complex tachycardia (QRS duration > 200ms or rate < 120).
- Give calcium for any hyperkalemic ECG changes or K > 6mEq/L. Give insulin, dextrose, and albuterol for the same situations. Kayexalate has no role in the emergent setting. Push for early HD to decrease total body stores of potassium.
- Don't allow patients to stay hypotensive. Fluid challenge and use push-dose pressors as a bridge to a vasopressor infusion.
- Give empiric antibiotics as soon as possible in sepsis, ideally with the first hour of presentation.

References:

1. Agarwal R. Defining end-stage renal disease in clinical trials: A framework for adjudication. Nephrol Dial Transplant 2016;31(6):864-7.
2. United States Renal Data System. 2017 USRDS Annual Data Report: Epidemiology of kidney disease in the United States. Bethesda, MD; 2017. Available at: https://www.usrds.org/2017/view/Default.aspx.

3. Lovasik BP, Zhang R, Hockenberry JM, et al. Emergency department use and hospital admissions among patients with end-stage renal disease in the United States. JAMA Intern Med 2016;176(10):1563-65.
4. Wolfe RA, Ashby VB, Milford EL, et al. Comparison of mortality in all patients on dialysis, patients on dialysis awaiting transplantation, and recipients of a first cadaveric transplant. N Engl J Med 1999;341(23):1725-30.
5. Cosio FG, Hickson LJ, Griffin MD, et al. Patient survival and cardiovascular risk after kidney transplantation: The challenge of diabetes. Am J Transplant 2008;8(3):593-9.
6. Weiss A, Elixhauser A, Barrett M, et al. Opioid-related inpatient stays and emergency department visits by state, 2009-2014. 2017;1-16.
7. Center for Behavioral Health Statistics and Quality. (2016). Key substance use and mental health indicators in the United States: Results from the 2015 National Survey on Drug Use and Health (HHS Publication No. SMA 16-4984, NSDUH Series H-51). Retrieved from https://www.samhsa.gov/data/.
8. Sklar DP, Crandall CS, Loeliger E, et al. Unanticipated death after discharge home from the emergency department. Ann Emerg Med 2007;49(6):735-45.
9. Gabayan GZ, Sun BC, Asch SM, et al. A qualitative analysis of the factors associated with unanticipated short-term death following emergency department discharge. Ann Emerg Med 2012;60(4):S74.
10. Gabayan GZ, Gould MK, Weiss RE, et al. Emergency department vital signs and outcomes after discharge. Acad Emerg Med 2017;24(7):846-54.
11. Grudzen CR, Anderson JR, Carpenter CR, et al. The 2016 Academic Emergency Medicine Consensus Conference - Shared decision making in the emergency department: Development of a policy-relevant patient-centered research agenda.Acad Emerg Med 2016;23(12):1313-9.
12. Flynn D, Knoedler MA, Hess EP, et al. Engaging patients in health care decisions in the emergency department through shared decision-making: A systematic review. Acad Emerg Med 2012;19(8):959-67.
13. Hajar R. Diabetes as coronary artery disease risk equivalent: A historical perspective. Heart Views 2017;18(1):34-7.
14. Foley RN, Parfrey PS, Sarnak MJ. Epidemiology of cardiovascular disease in chronic renal disease. J Am Soc Nephrol 1998;9(12 Suppl):S16-23.
15. Pinto D, Lunet N, Azevedo A. Prevalence and determinants of atypical presentation of acute coronary syndrome. Acta Med Port 2011;24 Suppl 2:307-18.
16. El-Menyar A, Zubaid M, Sulaiman K, et al. Atypical presentation of acute coronary syndrome: A significant independent predictor of in-hospital mortality. J Cardiol 2011;57(2):165-71.
17. Tucker JF, Collins RA, Anderson AJ, et al. Early diagnostic efficiency of cardiac Troponin I and Troponin T for acute myocardial infarction. Acad Emerg Med 1997;4(1):13-21.
18. Keller T, Zeller T, Peetz D, et al. Sensitive troponin I assay in early diagnosis of acute myocardial infarction. N Engl J Med 2009;361(9):868-77.
19. Mahler SA, Miller CD, Hollander JE, et al. Identifying patients for early discharge: Performance of decision rules among patients with acute chest pain. Int J Cardiol 2013;168(2):795-802.
20. Carlton E, Greenslade J, Cullen L, et al. Evaluation of high-sensitivity cardiac Troponin I levels in patients with suspected acute coronary syndrome. JAMA Cardiol 2016;1(4):405-12.
21. Amsterdam EA, Wenger NK, Brindis RG, et al. 2014 AHA/ACC guideline for the management of patients with non-st-elevation acute coronary syndromes: A report of the American College

of Cardiology/American Heart Association task force on practice guidelines. Circulation 2014;130(25):e344-e426.
22. Stacy SR, Suarez-Cuervo C, Berger Z, et al. Role of troponin in patients with chronic kidney disease and suspected acute coronary syndrome: A systematic review. Ann Intern Med 2014;161(7):502-12.
23. Newby LK, Jesse RL, Babb JD, et al. ACCF 2012 expert consensus document on practical clinical considerations in the interpretation of troponin elevations: A report of the American College of Cardiology Foundation task force on clinical expert consensus documents. J Am Coll Cardiol 2012;60(23):2427-63.
24. Alhan E, Usta A, Çekiç A, et al. A study on 107 patients with acute mesenteric ischemia over 30 years. Int J Surg 2012;10(9):510-3.
25. Campion EW, Clair DG, Beach JM. Mesenteric Ischemia. N Engl J Med 2016;374(10):959-68.
26. Pillai UPK, Balabhadrapatruni K, Hothi J, et al. Acute abdominal pain in an end stage renal disease patient. West J Emerg Med 2013;14(2):153.
27. Volpini K, Kinonen C. Abdominal catastrophe in a 43-year-old female with end stage renal disease. Semin Dial 2011;24(1):79-82.
28. Singh M, Long B, Koyfman A. Mesenteric Ischemia. Emerg Med Clin North Am 2017;35(4):879-88.
29. Akoh JA. Peritoneal dialysis associated infections: An update on diagnosis and management. World J Nephrol 2012;1(4):106.
30. Kofteridis DP, Valachis A, Perakis K, et al. Peritoneal dialysis-associated peritonitis: Clinical features and predictors of outcome. Int J Infect Dis 2010;14(6):e489-93.
31. Li PKT, Szeto CC, Piraino B, et al. ISPD peritonitis recommendations: 2016 update on prevention and treatment. Perit Dial Int 2016;36(5):481-508.
32. Brown EA, Bargman J, Van Biesen W, et al. Length of time on peritoneal dialysis and encapsulating peritoneal sclerosis—Position paper for ISPD: 2017 update. Perit Dial Int 2017;37(4):362-74.
33. Rault R. Symptomatic urinary tract infections in patients on maintenance hemodialysis. Nephron 1984;37(2):82-4.
34. Manha F, Mohammed A, Ali K. Urinary tract infection in hemodialysis patients with renal failure. Fac Med Baghdad 2012;54(1):38-41.
35. Naqvi SB, Collins AJ. Infectious complications in chronic kidney disease. Adv Chronic Kidney Dis 2006;13(3):199-04.
36. Wong SSY, Ho PL, Yuen KY. Evolution of antibiotic resistance mechanisms and their relevance to dialysis-related infections. Perit Dial Int 2007;27 Suppl 2:S272-80.
37. Meyer TW, Hostetter TH. Approaches to uremia. J Am Soc Nephrol 2014; 25(10):1-8.
38. Kalantari K, Chang JN, Ronco C, et al. Assessment of intravascular volume status and volume responsiveness in critically ill patients. Kidney Int 2013;83(6):1017-28.
39. Jambeih R, Keddissi JI, Youness HA. IVC measurements in critically ill patients with acute renal failure. Crit Care Res Pract 2017;2017:3598392.
40. Rosner MH. Measuring risk in end-stage renal disease: Is N-terminal pro brain natriuretic peptide a useful marker? Kidney Int 2007;71(6):481-83.
41. Koochak HE, Tabibian E, Dehgolan SR. Abdominal pain as extrapulmonary presentation of pneumonia in an adult: A case report. Acta Med Iran 2017;55(2):131-3.
42. Gauss H. Abdominal pain in pneumonia. Am J Dig Dis 1946;13:73-7.

43. Nagarwala J, Dev S, Markin A. The vomiting patient: Small bowel obstruction, cyclic vomiting, and gastroparesis. Emerg Med Clin North Am 2016;34(2):271-91.
44. Camiller M, Parkman HP, Shafi MA, et al., Gerson L. Clinical guideline: Management of gastroparesis. Am J Gastroenterol 2013;108(1):18-38.
45. Roldan CJ, Chambers KA, Paniagua L, et al. Randomized controlled double-blind trial comparing haloperidol combined with conventional therapy to conventional therapy alone in patients with symptomatic gastroparesis. Acad Emerg Med 2017 Nov;24(11):1307-14.
46. Kleinman ME, Brennan EE, Goldberger ZD, et al. American Heart Association. Web-based integrated guidelines for cardiopulmonary resuscitation and emergency cardiovascular care—Part 5: Adult basic life support and cardiopulmonary resuscitation quality. Circulation 2015;132(18):suppl 2.
47. Andersen LW, Granfeldt A, Callaway CW, et al. Association between tracheal intubation during adult in-hospital cardiac arrest and survival. J Am Med Assoc 2017;317(5):494-06.
48. Brunauer A, Koköfer A, Bataar O, et al. The arterial blood pressure associated with terminal cardiovascular collapse in critically ill patients: A retrospective cohort study. Crit Care 2014;18(6):719.
49. Kedia N. Treatment of severe diabetic hypoglycemia with glucagon: An underutilized therapeutic approach. Diabetes Metab Syndr Obes 2011;4:337-46.
50. Jones AE, Yiannibas V, Johnson C, et al. Emergency department hypotension predicts sudden unexpected in-hospital mortality: A prospective cohort study. Chest 2006;130(4):941-6.
51. Zenati MS, Billiar TR, Townsend RN, et al. A brief episode of hypotension increases mortality in critically ill trauma patients. J Trauma 2002;53(2):232-36.
52. Leidel BA, Kirchhoff C, Bogner V, et al. Comparison of intraosseous versus central venous vascular access in adults under resuscitation in the emergency department with inaccessible peripheral veins. Resuscitation 2012;83(1):40-5.
53. Dolister M, Miller S, Borron S, et al. Intraosseous vascular access is safe, effective and costs less than central venous catheters for patients in the hospital setting. J Vasc Access 2013;14(3):216-24.
54. Santos D, Carron PN, Yersin B, et al. EZ-IO® intraosseous device implementation in a pre-hospital emergency service: A prospective study and review of the literature. Resuscitation 2013;84(4):440-5.
55. Ong MEH, Chan YH, Oh JJ, et al. An observational, prospective study comparing tibial and humeral intraosseous access using the EZ-IO. Am J Emerg Med 2009;27(1):8-15.
56. Reddick AD, Ronald J, Morrison WG. Intravenous fluid resuscitation: Was Poiseuille right? Emerg Med J 2011;28(3):201-2.
57. Petitpas F, Guenezan J, Vendeuvre T, et al. Use of intra-osseous access in adults: A systematic review. Crit Care 2016;20(1):102.
58. Powell JT, Mink JT, Nomura JT, et al. Ultrasound-guidance can reduce adverse events during femoral central venous cannulation. J Emerg Med 2014;46(4):519-24.
59. Leung J, Duffy M, Finckh A. Real-time ultrasonographically-guided internal jugular vein catheterization in the emergency department increases success rates and reduces complications: A randomized, prospective study. Ann Emerg Med 2006;48(5):540-7.
60. Parienti J-J, Mongardon N, Mégarbane B, et al. Intravascular complications of central venous catheterization by insertion site. N Engl J Med 2015;373(13):1220-9.
61. Arvaniti K, Lathyris D, Blot S, Apostolidou-Kiouti F, Koulenti D, Haidich A-B. Cumulative

evidence of randomized controlled and observational studies on catheter-related infection risk of central venous catheter insertion site in ICU patients: A pairwise and network meta-analysis. Crit Care Med 2016:1-12.

62. Brady WJ, Mattu A, Tabas J, et al. The differential diagnosis of wide QRS complex tachycardia. Am J Emerg Med 2017;35(10):1525-9.
63. Steinman RT, Herrera C, Schuger CD, et al. Wide QRS tachycardia in the conscious adult: Ventricular tachycardia is the most frequent cause. J Am Med Assoc 1989;261(7):1013-6.
64. Mattu A. ECG tricks and mimics. Essentials EM Digital Course. 2017; Available at: https://www.essentialsofem.com/course/2017.
65. Al-Khatib SM, Stevenson WG, Ackerman MJ, et al. 2017 AHA/ACC/HRS guideline for management of patients with ventricular arrhythmias and the prevention of sudden cardiac death. Heart Rhythm 2018 Oct;15(10):e190-e252.
66. McLean SA, Paul ID, Spector PS. Lidocaine-induced conduction disturbance in patients with systemic hyperkalemia. Ann Emerg Med 2000;36(6):615-8.
67. Ghane MR, Gharib MH, Ebrahimi A, et al. Accuracy of rapid ultrasound in shock (RUSH) exam for diagnosis of shock in critically Ill patients. Trauma Mon 2015;20(1):1-5.
68. Perera P, Mailhot T, Riley D, et al. The RUSH exam 2012: Rapid ultrasound in shock in the evaluation of the critically Ill patient. Ultrasound Clin 2012;7(2):255-78.
69. Weingart S. Push-dose pressors for immediate blood pressure control. Clin Exp Emerg Med 2015;2(2):131-2.
70. Panchal AR, Satyanarayan A, Bahadir JD, Hays D, Mosier J. Efficacy of Bolus-dose phenylephrine for peri-intubation hypotension. J Emerg Med 2015;49(4):488-94.
71. Holden D, Ramich J, Timm E, et al. Safety considerations and guideline-based safe use recommendations for "Bolus-Dose" vasopressors in the emergency department. Ann Emerg Med 2018 Jan;71(1):83-92.
72. Acquisto NM, Bodkin RP, Johnstone C. Medication errors with push dose pressors in the emergency department and intensive care units. Am J Emerg Med 2017;35(12):1964-5.
73. Schwartz MB, Ferreira JA, Aaronson PM. The impact of push-dose phenylephrine use on subsequent preload expansion in the ED setting. Am J Emerg Med 2016;34(12):2419-22.
74. Yamazaki T, Shimada Y, Taenaka N, et al. Circulatory responses to afterloading with phenylephrine in hyperdynamic sepsis. Crit Care Med 1982;10(7):432-5.
75. Campbell RL, Bellolio MF, Knutson BD, et al. Epinephrine in anaphylaxis: Higher risk of cardiovascular complications and overdose after administration of intravenous bolus epinephrine compared with intramuscular epinephrine. J Allergy Clin Immunol Pract 2015;3(1):76-80.
76. Coralic Z. The Dirty Epi Drip: IV epinephrine when you need it. Acad Life Emerg Med Blog 2013; Available at: https://www.aliem.com/dirtyepi/.
77. Rhodes A, Evans LE, Alhazzani W, et al. Surviving sepsis campaign: International guidelines for management of sepsis and septic shock: 2016. Intensive Care Med 2017;43(3):304-77.
78. Stratton L, Berlin DA, Arbo JE. Vasopressors and inotropes in sepsis. Emerg Med Clin North Am 2017;35(1):75-91.
79. Ng J, Passman RS, Arora R, et al. Paradoxical change in atrial fibrillation dominant frequencies with baroreflex-mediated parasympathetic stimulation with phenylephrine infusion. J Cardiovasc Electrophysiol 2012;23(10):1045-50.
80. Annane D, Vignon P, Renault A, et al. Norepinephrine plus dobutamine versus epinephrine alone for management of septic shock: A randomised trial. Lancet 2007;370(9588):676-84.

81. Loubani OM, Green RS. A systematic review of extravasation and local tissue injury from administration of vasopressors through peripheral intravenous catheters and central venous catheters. J Crit Care 2015;30(3):653.e9-653.e17.
82. Medlej K, Kazzi AA, El Hajj Chehade A, et al. Complications from administration of vasopressors through peripheral venous catheters: An observational study. J Emerg Med 2018 Jan;54(1):47-53.
83. Cardenas-Garcia J, Schaub KF, Belchikov YG, et al. Safety of peripheral intravenous administration of vasoactive medication. J Hosp Med 2015;10(9):581-5.
84. Wanic-Kossowska M, Czekalski S. Hypotension in renal failure patients undergoing dialysis therapy. Pol Arch Med Wewn 2007;117(4):178-83.
85. Bentata Y, Hamdi F, Chemlal A, et al. Uremic pericarditis in patients with end stage renal disease: Prevalence, symptoms and outcome in 2017. Am J Emerg Med 2018;36(3):464-6.
86. Iglesias P, Díez JJ. Insulin therapy in renal disease. Diabetes Obes Metab 2008;10(10):811-23.
87. Jia L, Wang H, Gao Y, et al. High incidence of adverse events during intra-hospital transport of critically ill patients and new related risk factors: A prospective, multicenter study in China. Crit Care 2016;20:12.
88. Schwebel C, Clec'h C, Magne S, et al. Safety of intrahospital transport in ventilated critically ill patients: A multicenter cohort study. Crit Care Med 2013;41(8):1919-28.
89. Lahner D, Nikolic A, Marhofer P, et al. Incidence of complications in intrahospital transport of critically ill patients—Experience in an Austrian university hospital. Wien Klin Wochenschr 2007;119(13-14):412-6.
90. Kue R, Brown P, Ness C, et al. Adverse clinical events during intrahospital transport by a specialized team: A preliminary report. Am J Crit Care 2011;20(2):153-62.
91. Durfey N, Lehnhof B, Bergeson A, et al. Severe hyperkalemia: Can the electrocardiogram risk stratify for short-term adverse events? West J Emerg Med 2017;18(5):963-71.
92. Alfonzo A, Soar J, MacTier R, et al. UK Renal Association clinical practice guidelines: Treatment of acute hyperkalemia in adults. 2014; Available at: https://renal.org/wp-content/uploads/2017/06/hyperkalaemia-guideline-1.pdf.
93. José RJP, Preller J. Near-patient testing of potassium levels using arterial blood gas analysers: Can we trust these results? Emerg Med J 2008;25(8):510-3.
94. Ayhan H, Erdoğan MÖ, Yiğit Y, et al. The reliability of blood gas electrolytes. 2014; doi:10.5152/jaem.2014.06978.
95. Johnston HLM, Murphy R. Agreement between an arterial blood gas analyser and a venous blood analyser in the measurement of potassium in patients in cardiac arrest. Emerg Med J 2005;22(4):269-71.
96. Levine M, Nikkanen H, Pallin DJ. The effects of intravenous calcium in patients with digoxin toxicity. J Emerg Med 2011;40(1):41-6.
97. Hempelmann G, Piepenbrock S, Frerk C SE. Effects of calcium gluconate and calcium chloride on cardiocirculatory parameters in man. Anaesthesist 1978;27(11):516-22.
98. Parham WA, Mehdirad AA, Biermann KM, Fredman CS. Hyperkalemia revisited. Texas Heart Inst J 2006;33(1):40-7.
99. Martin TJ, Kang Y, Robertson KM, et al. Ionization and hemodynamic effects of calcium chloride and calcium gluconate in the absence of hepatic function. Anesthesiology 1990;73(1):62-5.
100. Hayes B. Mythbuster: Calcium gluconate raises serum calcium as quickly as calcium chloride. Acad Life Emerg Med Blog 2013; Available at: https://www.aliem.com/mythbuster-calcium-gluconate-raises-serum-calcium-as-calcium-chloride/.

101. Mahoney BA, Smith WA, Lo D, et al. Emergency interventions for hyperkalaemia. In: Cochrane Database Syst Rev 2005;18(2):CD003235.
102. Ashurst J, Sergent S, Wagner B. Evidence-based management of potassium disorders in the emergency department. Evidence-Based Med Pract 2016;18(11).
103. O'Malley CMN, Frumento RJ, Hardy MA, et al. A randomized, double-blind comparison of lactated ringer 's solution and 0.9% NaCl during renal transplantation. Anesth Analg 2005;100(5):1518-24.
104. Khajavi MR, Etezadi F, Moharari RS, et al. Effects of normal saline vs. lactated ringer's during renal transplantation. Ren Fail 2008;30(5):535-9.
105. Modi MP, Vora KS, Parikh GP, Shah VR. A comparative study of impact of infusion of Ringer's Lactate solution versus normal saline on acid-base balance and serum electrolytes during live related renal transplantation. Saudi J Kidney Dis Transpl 2012;23(1):135-7.
106. Farkas J. Management of severe hyperkalemia in the post-Kayexalate era. EMCrit Blog 2015; https://emcrit.org/pulmcrit/management-of-severe-hyperkalemia-in-the-post-kayexalate-era/. Accessed March 1, 2018.
107. Fraley DS, Adler S. Correction of hyperkalemia by bicarbonate despite constant blood pH. Kidney Int 1977;12(5):354-60.
108. Sterns RH, Rojas M, Bernstein P, et al. Ion-exchange resins for the treatment of hyperkalemia: Are they safe and effective? J Am Soc Nephrol 2010;21(5):733-5.
109. Mosier J, Joshi R, Hypes C, Pacheco G, Valenzuela T, Sakles J. The physiologically difficult airway. West J Emerg Med 2015;16(7):1109-17.
110. Weingart S. The HOP mnemonic and airwayworld.com next week. EMCrit Blog 2012. https://emcrit.org/emcrit/hop-mnemonic/. Accessed January 1, 2017.
111. Schwartz DE, Matthay MA, Cohen NH. Death and other complications of emergency airway management in critically ill adults. A prospective investigation of 297 tracheal intubations. Anesthesiology 1995;82(2):367-76.
112. Kim WY, Kwak MK, Ko BS, et al. Factors associated with the occurrence of cardiac arrest after emergency tracheal intubation in the emergency department. PLoS One 2014;9(11):e112779.
113. Heffner AC, Swords DS, Neale MN, et al. Incidence and factors associated with cardiac arrest complicating emergency airway management. Resuscitation 2013;84(11):1500-4.
114. Mort TC. The incidence and risk factors for cardiac arrest during emergency tracheal intubation: a justification for incorporating the ASA Guidelines in the remote location. J Clin Anesth 2004;16(7):508-16.
115. De Jong A, Rolle A, Molinari N, et al. Cardiac arrest and mortality related to intubation procedure in critically ill adult patients: A multicenter cohort study. Crit Care Med 2018;46(4):532-39.
116. Nimmagadda U, Salem MR, Crystal GJ. Preoxygenation: Physiologic basis, benefits, and potential risks. Anesth and Analg 2017;124:507-17.
117. Weingart SD, Levitan RM. Preoxygenation and prevention of desaturation during emergency airway management. Ann Emerg Med 2012;59(3):165-75.
118. McNamara MJ, Hardman JG. Hypoxaemia during open-airway apnoea: A computational modeling analysis. Anesthesia 2005;60(8):741-6.
119. Driver BE, Klein LR, Carlson K, et al. Preoxygenation with flush rate oxygen: Comparing the nonrebreather mask with the bag-valve mask. Ann of Emerg Med 2018;71(3):381-6.
120. Groombridge C, Chin CW, Hanrahan B, et al. Assessment of common preoxygenation strategies outside of the operating room environment. Acad Emerg Med 2016;23(3):342-6.

121. Weingart S. Preoxygenation, reoxygenation and deoxygenation. 2015; https://emcrit.org/preoxygenation/. Accessed August 1, 2018.
122. Brainard A, Chuang D, Zeng I, et al. A randomized trial on subject tolerance and the adverse effects associated with higher-versus lower-flow oxygen through a standard nasal cannula. Ann Emerg Med 2015;65(4):356-61.
123. Corley A, Caruana LR, Barnett AG, et al. Oxygen delivery through high-flow nasal cannulae increase end-expiratory lung volume and reduce respiratory rate in post-cardiac surgical patients. Br J Anaesth 2011;107(6):998-04.
124. Nedel WL, Deutschendorf C, Moraes Rodrigues Filho E. High-flow nasal cannula in critically ill subjects with or at risk for respiratory failure: A systematic review and meta-analysis. Respir Care 2017;62(1);123-32.
125. Corley A, Rickard CM, Aitken LM, et al. High flow nasal cannulae for respiratory support in adult intensive care patients. Cochrane Database Syst Rev 2017;5(5):CD010172.
126. Frumin MJ, Epstein RM, Cohen G. Apneic oxygenation in man. Anesthesiology 1959;20:789-98.
127. Binks MJ, Holyoak RS, Melhuish TM, et al. Apneic oxygenation during intubation in the emergency department and during retrieval: A systematic review and meta-analysis. Am J Emerg Med 2017;35(10):1542-6.
128. Pavlov I, Medrano S, Weingart S. Apneic oxygenation reduces the incidence of hypoxemia during emergency intubation: A systematic review and meta-analysis. Am J Emerg Med 2017;35(8):1184-9.
129. Kimmoun A, Novy E, Auchet T, et al. Hemodynamic consequences of severe lactic acidosis in shock states: From bench to bedside. Crit Care 2015;19(1):175.
130. Brower RG, Matthay MA, Morris A, et al. Ventilation with lower tidal volumes as compared with traditional tidal volumes for acute lung injury and the acute respiratory distress syndrome. N Engl J Med 2000;342(18):1301-8.
131. Fuller BM, Ferguson IT, Mohr NM, et al. Lung-protective ventilation initiated in the emergency department (LOV-ED): A quasi-experimental, before-after trial. Ann Emerg Med 2017;70(3):406-18.
132. Spiegal R. The case of an ugly truth. EMCrit Blog2. 2017. https://emcrit.org/emnerd/case-ugly-truth/. Accessed September 1, 2018.
133. Simonis FD, Serpa Neto A, Binnekade JM, et al. Effect of a low vs intermediate tidal volume strategy on ventilator-free days in intensive care unit patients without ARDS: A randomized clinical trial. JAMA 2018;320(18):1872-80.
134. Serpa Neto A, Cardoso SO, Manetta JA, et al. Association between use of lung-protective ventilation with lower tidal volumes and clinical outcomes among patients without acute respiratory distress syndrome: A meta-analysis. J Am Med Assoc 2012;308(16):1651-9.
135. Miller LM, Clark E, Dipchand C, et al. Hemodialysis tunneled catheter-related infections. Can J Kidney Heal Dis 2016;3:2054358116669129.
136. Sahli F, Feidjel R, Laalaoui R. Hemodialysis catheter-related infection: Rates, risk factors and pathogens. J Infect Public Health 2017;10(4):403-08.
137. Szamosfalvi B, Yee J. Considerations in the critically ill ESRD patient. Adv Chronic Kidney Dis 2013;20(1):102-9.
138. Manning MA. Use of dialysis access in emergent situations. J Emerg Nurs 2008;34(1):37-40.
139. Sterling SA, Miller WR, Pryor J, et al. The impact of timing of antibiotics on outcomes in

severe sepsis and septic shock. Crit Care Med 2015;43(9):1907-15.
140. Kumar A, Roberts D, Wood KE, et al. Duration of hypotension before initiation of effective antimicrobial therapy is the critical determinant of survival in human septic shock. Crit Care Med 2006;34(6):1589-96.
141. Ferrer R, Martin-Loeches I, Phillips G, et al. Empiric antibiotic treatment reduces mortality in severe sepsis and septic shock from the first hour: Results from a guideline-based performance improvement program. Crit Care Med 2014;42(8):1749-55.
142. Seymour CW, Gesten F, Prescott HC, et al. Time to treatment and mortality during mandated emergency care for sepsis. N Engl J Med 2017;376(23):2235-44.
143. Pyrgos V, Ratanavanich K, Donegan N, et al. Candida bloodstream infections in hemodialysis recipients. Med Mycol 2009;47(5):463-7.
144. Appaneal HJ, Caffrey AR, Jiang L, et al. Antibiotic resistance rates for Pseudomonas aeruginosa clinical respiratory and bloodstream isolates among the Veterans Affairs Healthcare System from 2009 to 2013. Diagn Microbiol Infect Dis 2018;90(4):311-5.
145. Pappas PG, Kauffman CA, Andes DR, et al. Clinical practice guideline for the management of candidiasis: 2016 update by the Infectious Diseases Society of America. Clin Infect Dis 2016;62(4):409-17.
146. Timsit JF, Azoulay E, Schwebel C, et al. Empirical micafungin treatment and survival without invasive fungal infection in adults with ICU-acquired sepsis, candida colonization, and multiple organ failure: The EMPIRICUS randomized clinical trial. JAMA 2016;316(15):1555-64.
147. Centers for Medicare and Medicaid Services (CMS). NQF-endorsed voluntary consensus standards for hospital care. Measure information form: 2015; https://www.nhfca.org/psf/resources/Updates1/SEP-1 Measure Information Form (MIF).pdf.
148. Kalantari A, Mallemat H, Weingart S. Sepsis definitions: The search for gold and what CMS got wrong. West J Emerg Med 2017;18(5):951-6.
149. Lowe KM, Heffner AC, Karvetski CH. Clinical factors and outcomes of dialysis-dependent end-stage renal disease patients with emergency department septic shock. J Emerg Med 2018;54(1):16-24.
150. Abou Dagher G, Harmouche E, Jabbour E, et al. Sepsis in hemodialysis patients. BMC Emerg Med 2015; Available at: https://pubmed.ncbi.nlm.nih.gov/26467100-sepsis-in-hemodialysis-patients/.
151. Long B, Koyfman A, Lee CM. Emergency medicine evaluation and management of the end stage renal disease patient. Am J Emerg Med 2017;35(12):1946-55.
152. Boyd JH, Forbes J, Nakada T, et al. Fluid resuscitation in septic shock: A positive fluid balance and elevated central venous pressure are associated with increased mortality. Crit Care Med 2011;39(2):259-65.
153. Neyra JA, Li X, Canepa-Escaro F, et al. Cumulative fluid balance and mortality in septic patients with or without acute kidney injury and chronic kidney disease. Crit Care Med 2016;44(10):1891-1900.
154. Ratiani L, Gamkrelidze M, Khuchua E, et al. Altered microcirculation in septic shock. Georgian Med News 2015;7-8(244-245):16-24.
155. Walley KR. Deeper understanding of mechanisms contributing to sepsis-induced myocardial dysfunction. Crit Care 2014;18(3):137.
156. Marik PE, Cavallazzi R. Does the central venous pressure predict fluid responsiveness? An updated meta-analysis and a plea for some common sense. Crit Care Med 2013;41(7):1774-81.

157. Wong GC, Ayas NT. Clinical approaches to the diagnosis of acute heart failure. Curr Opin Cardiol 2007;22(3):207-13.
158. Rameau A, de With E, Boerma EC. Passive leg raise testing effectively reduces fluid administration in septic shock after correction of non-compliance to test results. Ann Intensive Care 2017;7(2): doi: 10.1186/s13613-016-0225-6.
159. Ansari BM, Zochios V, Falter F, et al. Physiological controversies and methods used to determine fluid responsiveness: A qualitative systematic review. Anaesthesia 2016;71(1):94-105.
160. Monnet X, Marik PE, Teboul JL. Prediction of fluid responsiveness: an update. Ann Intensive Care 2016;6:111.
161. Al Rifai A, Sukul N, Wonnacott R, et al. Safety of arteriovenous fistulae and grafts for continuous renal replacement therapy: The Michigan experience. Hemodial Int 2018 Jan;22(1):50-5.

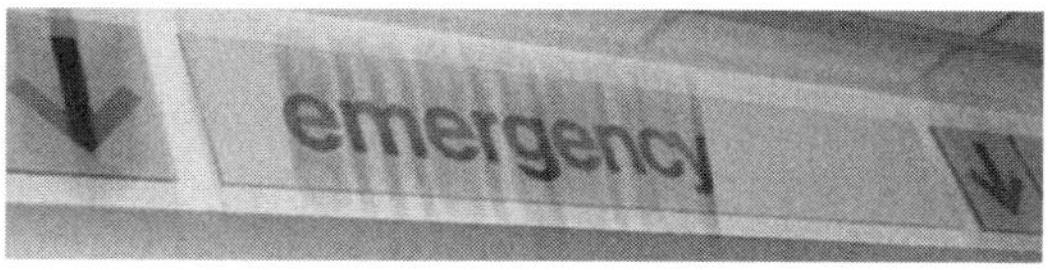

SECTION D – DRUGS & DELIRIUM

Chapter 17: A 48-year-old suicidal man with beta-blocker overdose

Colin G. Kaide, MD, FACEP, FAAEM

Professor of Emergency Medicine
Specialist in Hyperbaric Medicine
Department of Emergency Medicine
The Ohio State University Wexner Medical Center, Columbus, OH

Katherine Hunold Buck, MD

Assistant Professor
Department of Emergency Medicine
The Ohio State University Wexner Medical Center, Columbus, OH

Guest author:

Sean Patrick Nordt, MD, Pharm D, DABAT, FAACT, FAAEM, FACMT

Adjunct Associate Professor of Emergency Medicine
University of California, Irvine
Attending Physician
Department of Emergency Medicine
LAC+USC Medical Center, Los Angeles, CA
Herbert Endowed Professor of Pharmacy
School of Pharmacy and Crean College of Health and Behavioral Sciences
Chapman University, Irvine, California

Section editor:

Michael Winters, MD, MBA, FACEP, FAAEM

Professor
Emergency Medicine and Medicine
Vice Chair for Clinical and Administrative Affairs
Department of Emergency Medicine
University of Maryland School of Medicine, Baltimore, MD

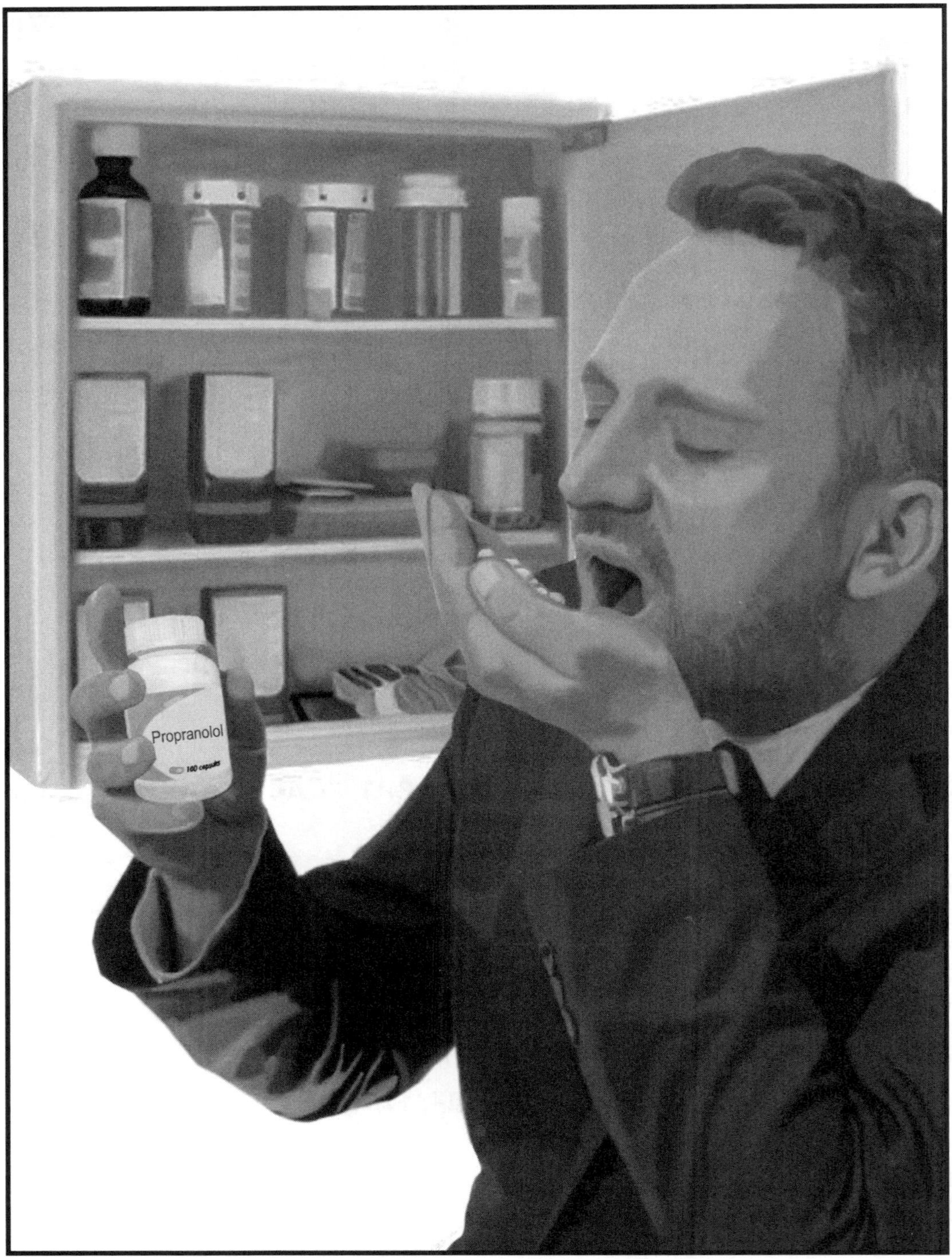
Propranolol
100 capsules

SECTION D/CHAPTER 17

A 48-year-old suicidal man with beta-blocker overdose

The patient's story:
Bob Sitz, a divorced father of three grown children, recently started a new antidepressant medication. He has worked at a convenience store, then a supermarket, and most recently for a lawn service company. Due to monetary and transportation issues he has struggled to obtain his medications but recently found help at a clinic for low-income patients. His adherence to the prescriptions is not perfect and at the end of the month is often left with half-used prescription vials in the back of the medicine cabinet.

When he learns of a non-fatal overdose of his 22-year-old son, his feelings of sadness escalate. He presents to the emergency department with suicidal ideation and is admitted to a psychiatric hospital for 6 days. He is determined by psychiatrist to be safe for discharge and referred for outpatient follow-up.

Less than 24 hours after discharge, he is overwhelmed by feelings of hopelessness. He obtains his partially-used blood pressure medications and impulsively ingests the remaining tablets. He sits down on the tile floor, staring straight ahead. After approximately 90 minutes, he begins to feel dizzy, then short of breath. Panicking, he goes to the bedroom and dials 911.

INITIAL ED VISIT

CC (08:48): Suicidal and Ingestion

HPI: This patient is 48-year-old male with the PMH of depression and HTN who presents with the intentional ingestion of approximately 2.4 grams of propranolol, approximately 40 propranolol long-acting 60 mg tablets (90 min prior to arrival. He denies any coingestants but mentions he was discharged from a psychiatric hospital the day before. He notes that the intent of this overdose was suicide and still actively suicidal but is cooperative with medical treatment. On review of systems he reports dizziness and shortness of breath. He has no prior intentional medication or illicit suicide attempts but has tried to hang himself once before.

NKDA
PMH: Depression, anxiety, suicidal ideation
PSH: Negative

PE:

Vitals:

Time	Temp (F)	Pulse	Resp	BP	SpO2
N/A	97.3	55	16	104/55	98%

CONSTITUTIONAL: He is oriented to person, place, and time. He appears well-developed and well-nourished. Mild diaphoresis but not in extremis. Odd affect, pleasant, smiling.
MOUTH/THROAT: Oropharynx is clear and moist. No oropharyngeal exudate.
NECK: Normal range of motion. No JVD present.
CARDIO: Bradycardia, regular rhythm, peripheral pulses presents, no murmurs, no rubs
PULM/CHEST: Effort normal. No respiratory distress. He has no wheezes. He has no rales.
ABDOMEN: Soft. There is no tenderness.
NEURO: A&O X 3. He exhibits normal muscle tone. Coordination normal. CN2-12 grossly intact. Moving all extremities spontaneously.
SKIN: Slightly cool, diaphoretic, no rash
PSYCH: Thought content normal. Endorses suicidal ideation.

ED COURSE & MDM (09:23): 50 y.o. male with PMH of depression who presents with suspected beta-antagonist poisoning. I reviewed the patient's medical records and noted his allergies, past medical history, and previous visits. The review showed recent discharge from the psychiatric facility.

Chapter author note: We have a patient with a suspected overdose on large beta-antagonist sustained release medication based on history in a suicide attempt. We know that beta-adrenergic antagonists are class II antiarrhythmic agents which decrease the heart rate, contractility, SA/AV nodal conduction, and blood pressure. Acute poisoning presentations may include CNS depression, hypotension, hypoglycemia, and bronchospasm. This patient is manifesting signs and symptoms consistent with acute beta-antagonist poisoning. How should his evaluation and management be started and what is the potential for decompensation? With a minimally symptomatic patient and history of a significant overdose, how fast and intensively should we "mobilize the troops?" What studies should be obtained?

DECISION POINT A – YOU ARE FACED WITH 5 QUESTIONS:

1. **How many people die of a beta-blocker overdose every year?**
2. **Should other ingestions be considered?**
3. **Which studies should be ordered?**
4. **What initial treatments should he receive?**
5. **Which types of poisonings will present well-appearing then decompensate?**

What does the literature say?

Q#1: How many people die of a beta-blocker overdose every year?

In 2015, there were approximately 25,000 poison control center cases involving beta-antagonists, approximately 10,500 of these were single ingestions, i.e., beta-antagonist only.[1] The history may be unreliable as there is a potential for co-ingestants.

Q#2: Should other ingestions be considered?

The differential diagnosis of bradycardia and hypotension in poisoning includes primary cardiac events (heart block, cardiogenic shock sick sinus syndrome), metabolic derangements (hyper/hypocalcemia, hyper/hypokalemia), hypothyroidism, as well as other ingestions including:

- Calcium channel antagonists
- Digoxin or other cardiac glycosides
- Clonidine or other imidazolines
- Cholinergic agents (assess for SLUDGE toxidrome)

In a patient with suspected or reported beta-antagonist poisonings, co-ingestions including acetaminophen and aspirin should be considered and both acetaminophen and salicylate concentrations obtained in intentional poisonings. Specific beta-antagonist drug concentrations should not be obtained.

Q#3: Which studies should be ordered?

Given the wide differential diagnosis and high concern for co-ingestion, the appropriate laboratory work-up is broad and should include:

(Table on next page...)

Test	Possible Findings	Comments
CBC	Low HgB	Concomitant anemia
Chem 10	Look for hyperkalemia, hypokalemia, hypocalcemia, hypoglycemia, hyperglycemia	Calculate anion gap in all poisonings
Hepatic function panel	Elevated transaminases	Baseline if APAP is considered as a possible coingestant or if elevated suggests delayed presentation of APAP poisoning
Acetaminophen level	Elevated levels need to correlate with time post-ingestion. However, acetaminophen Rumack Matthews nomogram can only be used in single acute ingestion not chronic use or multiple acute ingestions.	Common co ingestant
Salicylate level	Elevated level confirms ingestion. Must obtain serial levels as often delayed absorption. Hemodialysis indicated for severe poisonings not level alone.	Usually associated with respiratory alkalosis and metabolic acidosis followed by respiratory acidosis. Sodium bicarbonate infusion may increase urinary excretion but not substitute for hemodialysis. Follow potassium closely. Hemodialysis is definitive therapy.
Drug screen	Limited utility of drugs of abuse screen. Assess for toxidrome. Positive urine toxicology careen does not equate to toxicity just recent exposure eg, within 48 to 72 hours	Consider false positives and negatives eg, methadone and fentanyl are not detected as "opiates" and many positive cross reactivity with amphetamines eg, pseudoephedrine
EKG	Beta antagonists and calcium channel antagonists cause bradycardia, AV blocks, do not generally affect intraventricular conduction eg, sodium channels. However, propranolol can cause sodium channel blockade similar to cyclic antidepressants with wide QRS.	
VBG	Look for acidosis in combination with anion gap. Anion gap acidosis with beta antagonist generally hypoperfusion lactic acidosis. Propranol can cause seizures and increase lactic acid. Consider co ingestants.	**<u>MUDPILES</u>** Methanol, Metformin Uremia DKA Phenformin Isoniazid, Iron Lactic acidosis Ethylene glycol, AKA Salicylate

Q#4: What initial treatments should he receive?

This patient ingested a large amount of sustained release propranolol, and though only minimally symptomatic, we suspect that most of medication may still be in the gut (i.e., not absorbed). Gastric lavage is generally not performed for any acute poisonings and would not be indicated in this patient either, as it has been more than 1 hour since the ingestion and sustained release products are often too big to be removed by endogastric tube. Abdominal x-ray may show presence of sustained release tablets, but a normal x-ray does not exclude their presence.

Our patient is anticipated to become more symptomatic and requires ICU admission. If he worsens and requires intubation, once the airway is secure, we can consider a single dose of activated charcoal 1g/kg.[2] But there is a concern with giving activated charcoal to a patient with an unprotected airway and possible obtundation or seizures, both of which can be seen with propranolol.

As activated charcoal can be complicated by aspiration, the harms and benefits should be weighed, but given that our patient is symptomatic and only a few hours following ingestion, we anticipate that there may be many tablets still in the intestines, so whole bowel irrigation with PEG-ELS (GoLytely®) is indicated as the mainstay of therapy. Before initiating whole bowel irrigation and activated charcoal, intubation should be considered to protect airway, though aspiration may occur even after intubation. PEG-ELS can be administered through NG tube or OG tube at rate of 1 to 2 liters per hour until clear effluent (0.5 liter per hour in pediatric). There is no maximum; it may require many liters and is generally safe as it does not cause major electrolyte shifts.

Establishing good peripheral intravenous access is needed. If unable to place multiple peripheral saline locks, obtain central access for aggressive resuscitation. Our patient also reported this was a suicide attempt; he will need a psychiatric evaluation after medical clearance as well as suicide precautions.

Guest author comments (Nordt):

I agree with the statements above; I would give this patient whole bowel irrigation and activated charcoal.

Q#5: Which types of poisonings will present well-appearing then decompensate?

Many acute poisonings may decompensate after an initial well-appearing presentation. Sustained release-medications, such as ingested in our patient, are intended to be absorbed over many hours and may have a delayed onset of poisoning. For any potential sustained-release acute ingestion such as beta antagonist, calcium channel antagonist, lithium, or valproic acid, admit to a monitored setting for minimum of 24 hours. Aspirin ingestions, including enteric coated (but also immediate release as a result of bezoar formation), often have delayed onset. Iron poisoning can also decompensate after clinical improvement as tablets absorbed from gastrointestinal tract. Cyclic antidepressants can appear well early but often decompensate within hours of ingestion.

Section editor comments (Winters):

This point cannot be overstated; it is critical to be prepared for rapid decompensation. In addition to communicating the plan to bedside staff, I suggest informing other services such as pharmacy about the potential for high-dose insulin or intralipid therapy.

What did the actual provider do?

ED course & MDM (09:23): Differential diagnosis includes beta-blocker overdose, co-ingestion of acetaminophen/salicylates, other household poisons. Plan for CBC, chem 7, LFTs, lipase, EKG. Activated charcoal 100g is given.

The physician did appropriately consider that the patient may have co-ingested other medications and they did obtain acetaminophen and salicylate levels. Note that:

- Beta-antagonists may present with hypotension and bradycardia and hypoglycemia although hypoglycemia is more common in pediatric patients with beta-antagonist poisoning.
- Calcium channel antagonists present with hypotension and bradycardia and hyperglycemia.
- Clonidine presents with hypotension and bradycardia with opioid toxidrome. This may respond to naloxone but results variable.
- Digoxin and other cardiac glycosides present with hypotension and bradycardia and often hyperkalemia following acute poisonings.

What happened next?

Vitals:

Time	Temp	Pulse	Resp	Syst	Diast	O2 sat (RA)	Weight
09:57	N/A	44	26	88	40	93	72kg

ED course (09:59): The patient is on the monitor and bradycardia worsens which cause the alarm bells to ring. The patient is becoming more confused. The patient's blood pressure is low. A bolus of 1L of normal saline is started with atropine 0.5mg intravenously with minimal response. A decision to intubate is made and this occurs without difficulty. The patient is given a second bolus of 1L lactated Ringer's solution and an epinephrine infusion is started at a rate of 4mcg/min, then titrated up. In addition, glucagon 5mg IV followed by an infusion of 5mg an hour is begun. Calcium gluconate 3g is given intravenously.

Author comments (Weinstock):

The vital signs have been rechecked, and the patient is now bradycardiac and hypotensive. We are at:

DECISION POINT B – YOU ARE FACED WITH 3 QUESTIONS:

1. **The patient is now symptomatic—did we wait too long?**
2. **How should the management proceed?**
3. **If the patient becomes more bradycardiac, should pacing be employed?**

Q#1: The patient is now symptomatic—did we wait too long?

This patient had reported a large-quantity beta-blocker ingestion, so we need to anticipate the potential for decompensation. The patient was intubated, and activated charcoal and whole bowel irrigation were ordered. Based on the history, many toxicologists would anticipate decompensation, would intubate early, and initiate whole bowel irrigation. As there are now signs of decompensation, the patient is being treated aggressively with multiple therapies including IV fluids, atropine, vasopressors, glucagon and calcium gluconate.

Q#2: How should the management proceed?

Many of the therapies used in treating beta-antagonist and calcium channel antagonist poisoning have transient beneficial effects. However, multiple approaches are often needed.

- Glucagon: May enhance myocardial contractility, increase heart rate, and increase AV conduction. Treat with a bolus of 5mg (50–150mcg/kg in pediatric patients) every 5 minutes until patient responds, with a maximum dose of 15mg. Response can be profound but is temporary, so a drip should be started at 2–5mg/hr (70mcg/kg/hr) but can go as high as 10 to 15mg/hr, though there is currently no established maximum dose. Glucagon will often cause nausea, so consider administering an anti-emetic.

- Atropine: Atropine 0.5–1mg IV (0.02mg/kg in pediatrics) can be tried for symptomatic bradycardia. Studies found that 5 of 17 patients had some effect from atropine, but 2 of these patients also received agents with a chronotropic effect. It is reasonable to try atropine for bradycardia but consider moving quickly to other agents if no or minimal response is seen.[3]

- Catecholamines: Epinephrine often is used as it has both alpha- and beta-agonist properties. Start epinephrine infusion at 1 mcg/minute and titrate to maintain a systolic blood pressure greater than 100 and a heart rate greater than 50. The dose should be escalated rapidly if no initial response is seen.[4,5] Norepinephrine or phenylephrine can also be used but these are more specific alpha-agonists. Often, both epinephrine and norepinephrine infusions are used.

- Calcium: The initial bolus should be *calcium gluconate.* The initial bolus should also be 3g or 60mg/kg up to 3g, followed by a continuous infusion. Calcium chloride provides 3 times more calcium per gram than does calcium gluconate but requires a central line. Similar to previous agents, without the bolus, the effect will be short-lived and doses much higher than normal may be required.[6]

- High-dose insulin: Insulin has positive inotropic effects and has been reported to be beneficial in both beta-antagonist and calcium channel antagonist poisonings. The doses are high and require close monitoring of glucose and potassium. High dose insulin is generally recommended in patients refractory to intravenous fluids, atropine and glucagon. The usual initial dose is a bolus of 1unit/kg of regular human insulin along with 0.5g/kg of dextrose, followed by a continuous infusion of 1unit/kg/h. A continuous dextrose infusion (e.g., D10W), beginning at 0.5g/kg/h should also be started. Glucose should be monitored every 15 to 30 minutes until stable and then every 1 to 2 hours and titrated to maintain the blood glucose between 100 and 250mg/dL. If patients do not respond, the infusion can be titrated to 10units/kg/h. Note that if the blood glucose is greater than 300mg/dL, the dextrose bolus is not necessary.[7]

- Sodium bicarbonate: Sodium channel blockade is not expected with most beta receptor antagonists, although may be seen. Propranolol, in particular, has the potential to cause sodium channel blockade and QRS widening. QRS widening > 120ms should be treated with IV bicarbonate (1–2mEq/kg IV bolus every 3–5 minutes) until QRS is < 120ms. If a widened QRS is seen, consider a co-ingestion of a sodium channel blockade agent such as a cyclic antidepressant.

Consulting editor comments (Weingart):

Agree that these patients will actually need a dextrose infusion in most cases.

Q#3: If the patient becomes more bradycardiac, should pacing be employed?

Cardiac pacing may be effective in some patients but usually has variable benefit due to decreased intracellular calcium stores. Often there is capture but limited inotropy. Patients may require higher voltages than typically used for transcutaneous pacing. Pacing may capture and improve heart rate but does not always improve the hypotension. As a result, pacing can be one of many interventions, but certainly not the only intervention; often, the hypotension is refractory. Isoproterenol, a beta-agonist, is not generally recommended as has been shown to be less effective than epinephrine. More recently, ECMO is being considered in poisonings, but experience is limited.

Section editor comments (Winters):

While high-dose insulin or intralipid therapy will be the focus in the critically ill patient with a beta-blocker overdose, select patients may eventually require transvenous pacing. Consider placing the appropriate central venous access before the patient decompensates as it may be more challenging to place the appropriately sized catheter when the patient is moribund or in cardiac arrest.

What did the actual provider do?

ED course (10:37): Pt becomes bradycardiac and receives atropine 0.5 mg x 2 with minimal to no improvement. BP drops to 68/palp and he now has decreased level of consciousness. He is given a 5mg bolus of glucagon followed by an infusion of 5 mg an hour and then given 3 grams of calcium gluconate with improvement of blood pressure and heart rate for approximately 20 minutes. An epinephrine infusion is started with blood pressure increasing to 95/45 and heart rate increasing to 56bpm.

As you are entering the orders in the computer, you look up to see the patient's nurse, with the charge nurse just behind, a worried look on her face.

"Have you called poison control?" she asks, with a touch of accusation in her voice?

"Not yet," you respond. "I just hung up with pharmacy. They are sending down a medication which may help."

Was this the appropriate course of action?

Patients with symptomatic beta-blocker poisoning must be treated aggressively. This is the time to "go big or go home." The appropriate intervention at this point is to use all of the treatments discussed above—glucagon, catecholamines, calcium, atropine and high-dose insulin. The doses are higher than typically given, so pre-emptive communication to prevent delays is essential. In our case, the physician started some of those interventions, but not all—perhaps poison control could have been contacted earlier? The recommendation is that the emergency physician should initiate resuscitation with the above therapies and have a nurse or other staff call poison control center or toxicology consult as soon as possible. Beta-antagonist poisonings can decompensate quickly and require multiple and large amounts of various medications, which requires working closely with pharmacy. A delay in calling poison control or a toxicologist can result in poor outcomes and open the provider to medical-legal risk.

DECISION POINT C – YOU ARE FACED WITH 2 QUESTIONS:

1. **The BP is now 68 and you are concerned about possible arrest. What do you do next?**
2. **Is there a role for intralipids or dialysis in a beta-blocker overdose?**

Q#1: The BP is now 68 and you are concerned about possible arrest. What do you do next?

For the patient who decompensates after initial stabilization following beta-antagonist poisoning, there are two major considerations:

- Continued absorption from gastrointestinal tract of medication (e.g., sustained release) or
- Decreased effectiveness of therapies

But it is often a combination of both. The above therapies in beta-antagonist poisoning often have limited benefit. The goal is to rapidly reassess potential etiologies and aggressively resuscitate. At this point, we recommend a 1L bolus of lactated Ringers, an additional 3 to 6 grams of calcium gluconate to increase the glucagon infusion, increase insulin infusion, increase epinephrine infusion, and increase or add norepinephrine infusion. Consider an additional dose of activated charcoal and continue GoLytely® once stabilized. Consider consulting for possible aortic balloon pump or ECMO if available.

Guest author comments (Nordt):

With the hypotensive beta-blocker patient, my "go to" is an epinephrine drip. It gives you cardiac squeeze and peripheral vasoconstriction. Agree with the atropine, but it is not commonly helpful. Glucagon for a beta-blocker overdose is a much higher dose that that used for an esophageal obstruction, so make sure to give anti-emetic. Regarding calcium, it can be helpful, but it is transient and may give you a false sense of security.

What did the actual provider do?

MDM (11:14): Intravenous lipid emulsion (Intralipid 20%) was given by intravenous bolus at a dose of 100 mL with a bolus and drip and concern of impending cardiopulmonary arrest. High dose insulin was ordered.

Twenty minutes later, the nurse goes to recheck the vitals and finds the blood pressure improved at 103/69 with a pulse of 52. The insulin has not yet arrived from pharmacy and a decision is made to hold at bedside while determining if the improvement is transient or will persist.

One hour later, the vitals have held, and the patient is admitted to the MICU.

Impression: 1. Beta-blocker poisoning. 2. Suicidal ideation.

Disposition: Patient admitted to the MICU and was maintained on a glucagon drip with an Intralipid infusion. High-dose insulin was not needed. The patient remained stable and the drips were stopped the next morning.

Hospital course: Patient was admitted to the MICU. Aggressive measures were continued and patient returned to baseline over the next 24 hours. All medications were tapered off. He was evaluated by psychiatry after medically stable and it was determined that he would benefit from inpatient psychiatric treatment.

Q#2: Is there a role for intralipids or dialysis in a beta-blocker overdose?

1. Intravenous lipid emulsion (Intralipid®) has been used in beta-antagonist poisonings. Though the literature in animals is not clear,[8] a number of case reports in humans have reported to be beneficial in peri-arrest patients.[9-11] Intravenous lipid emulsion can act as a "lipid sink" for lipophilic medications such as propranolol. Intravenous lipid emulsion also may act as a myocyte substrate and increase intracellular calcium. There are some potential adverse events with intravenous lipid emulsion and at this time should be considered as "lipid rescue" to be given if code anticipated. The vast experience with intravenous lipid emulsion is with local anesthetic systemic poisoning (e.g., bupivacaine); the routine administration of intravenous lipid emulsion "early" in poisonings is not supported by the current literature or professional societies.[12] High dose insulin therapy and aggressive vasopressors are strongly recommended before intravenous lipid emulsion. The dose and duration of intravenous lipid emulsion therapy is controversial. Often a 1.5mL/kg to maximum of 100mL is recommended of 20% Intralipid® over 2 to 3 minutes. If minimal or no response this dose can be repeated. A continuous infusion can be considered following bolus dose at 0.25mL/kg/min over 30 to 60 minutes with the total dose not to exceed 10 to 12mL/kg.[13] There is some risk, as intravenous lipid emulsion may have some adverse effects including iatrogenic injury, interference with both laboratory and drug concentration analysis and may decrease effectiveness of ECMO and resuscitation medications.[12, 14-18] We recommend consulting poison control center or toxicologist before considering intravenous lipid emulsion.

2. Though dialysis may be effective for some beta-antagonist poisonings (e.g., acebutolol, atenolol, nadolol, and sotalol), the major limitation is hypotension. Often symptomatic patients are too hypotensive for hemodialysis to be used, and if they are not severely symptomatic, there is not a need for hemodialysis. Of note, dialysis is not indicated in calcium channel poisoning.

Guest author comments (Nordt):

The fat globules in intralipid trap in the drugs, in particular the lipophilic drugs such as propranolol. It should be reserved for patients with impending arrest. There are animal models as well as some case reports showing efficacy, but there are no great trials showing a mortality benefit.

Bonus: Nightmare scenario – While the patient awaits a MICU bed, the patient again begins to decompensate.

Ensure all ordered medications are being administered and that we are not "waiting for it to come down from pharmacy." The doses of medications given in beta-blocker poisonings are significantly higher than "normal" doses, and nursing staff and pharmacists may not be aware or may have changed the order after drug mapping or pharmacist discussion, including glucagon, calcium, insulin, and vasopressors. For the patient who decompensates after initial stabilization following beta antagonist poisoning, as previously discussed, two major considerations are made: continued absorption or coingestant of another medication. The decreased effectiveness of therapies is common as there is often a transient benefit. The goal is to rapidly reassess potential etiologies and aggressively resuscitate.

Summary: A beta-blocker poisoning can be challenging due to the delay of onset and severity and duration of toxicity. These poisonings are often resource and staff intensive. Frequently assess for worsening toxicity and anticipate the potential for decompensation. Even in stable patients, start to assemble the appropriate treatments as the medications (and quantities needed) may not be stocked; be ready to be very aggressive. With early, directed intervention, these patients may have good outcomes.

References:

1. Mowry JB, Spyker DA, Brooks DE, et al. 2015 Annual Report of the American Association of Poison Control Centers' National Poison Data System (NPDS): 33rd annual report. Clin Toxicol (Phila) 2016;54(10):924-1109.
2. Chyka PA, Seger D, Krenzelok EP, et al. American Academy of Clinical Toxicology; European Association of Poisons Centres and Clinical Toxicologists. Position paper: Single-dose activated charcoal. Clin Toxicol (Phila) 2005;43(2):61-87.
3. Weinstein RS. Recognition and management of poisoning with beta-adrenergic blocking agents. Ann Emerg Med 1984;13(12):1123-31.
4. Chimienti M, Previtail M, Medicia A, et al. Acute verapamil poisoning: successful treatment with epinephrine. Clin Cardiol 1982;5(3):219-22.
5. Shepherd G. Treatment of poisoning caused by beta-adrenergic and calcium-channel blockers. Am J Health Syst Pharm 2006;63(19):1828-35.
6. Newton CR, Delgado JH, Gomez HF. Calcium and beta receptor antagonist overdose: a review and update of pharmacological principles and management. Semin Respir Crit Care Med 2002;23(1):19-25.
7. Hoffman RS, Howland MA, Lewin AN, et al. eds. Goldfrank's toxicologic emergencies. 10th ed. New York, NY: McGraw Hill, 2015.
8. Harvey M, Cave G, Lahner D, et al. Insulin versus lipid emulsion in a rabbit model of severe propranolol toxicity: A pilot study. Crit Care Res Pract 2011; 2011:361737.
9. Jovic-Stosic J, Gligic B, Putic V, Brajkovic G, Spasic R. Severe propranolol and ethanol overdose with wide complex tachycardia treated with intravenous lipid emulsion: a case report. Clin Toxicol (Phila). 2011;49(5):426-30.
10. Escajeda JT, Katz KD, Rittenberger JC. Successful treatment of metoprolol-induced cardiac

arrest with high-dose insulin, lipid emulsion, and ECMO. Am J Emerg Med 2015;33(8):1111.e1-4.
11. Le Fevre P, Gosling M, Acharya K, et al. Dramatic resuscitation with intralipid in an epinephrine unresponsive cardiac arrest following overdose of amitriptyline and propranolol. BMJ Case Rep 2017.
12. Gosselin S, Hoegberg LC, Hoffman RS, et al. Evidence-based recommendations on the use of intravenous lipid emulsion in poisoning. Clin Toxicol 2016;54(10):899-23.
13. Olson KR, Anderson NL, Benowitz PD, et al. eds. Poisoning and drug overdose. 7th ed.. New York, NY: McGraw Hill, 2018.
14. Grunbaum AM, Gilfix BM, Hoffman RS, et al. Review of the effect of intravenous lipid emulsion on laboratory analyses. Clin Tox 2016;54(2):92-02.
15. Hiller DB, Gergorio GD, Ripper R, et al. Epinephrine impairs lipid resuscitation from bupivacaine overdose: A threshold effect. Anesthesiology 2009;111(3):498-05.
16. Cao D, Heard K, Foran M, et al. Intravenous lipid emulsion in the emergency department: A systematic review of recent literature. J Emerg Med 2015;48(3):387-97.
17. Lee HM, Archer JR, Dargan PL, et al. What are the adverse effects associated with the combined use of intravenous lipid emulsion and extracorporeal membrane oxygenation in the poisoned patient? Clin Toxicol 2015;53(3):145-50.
18. Levine M, Skolnik AB, Ruha AM, et al. Complications following antidotal use of intravenous lipid emulsion therapy. J Med Toxicol 2014;10:10-14.

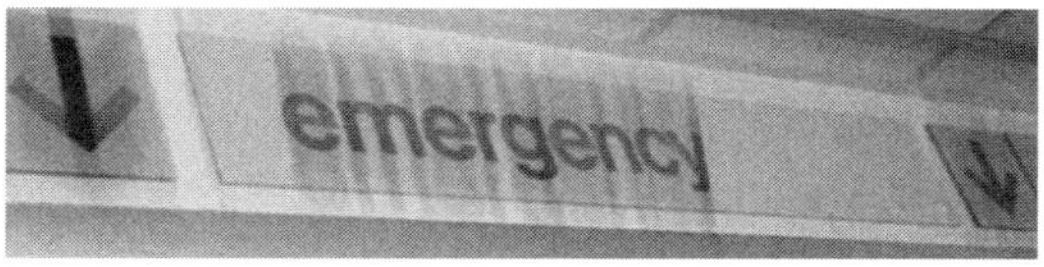

SECTION D – DRUGS & DELIRIUM

Chapter 18: A 32-year-old man with hemorrhoids and heroin

Daniel Z. Adams, MD
Critical Care Medicine Fellow
Department of Pulmonology and Critical Care Medicine
Washington University/Barnes-Jewish Hospital
St. Louis, MO

Jennifer Yee, DO, FAAEM
Clinical Assistant Professor
Emergency Medicine Simulation Director
Department of Emergency Medicine
The Ohio State University Wexner Medical Center
Columbus, OH

Section editor:
Michael Winters, MD, MBA, FACEP, FAAEM
Professor
Emergency Medicine and Medicine
Vice Chair for Clinical and Administrative Affairs
Department of Emergency Medicine
University of Maryland School of Medicine
Baltimore, MD

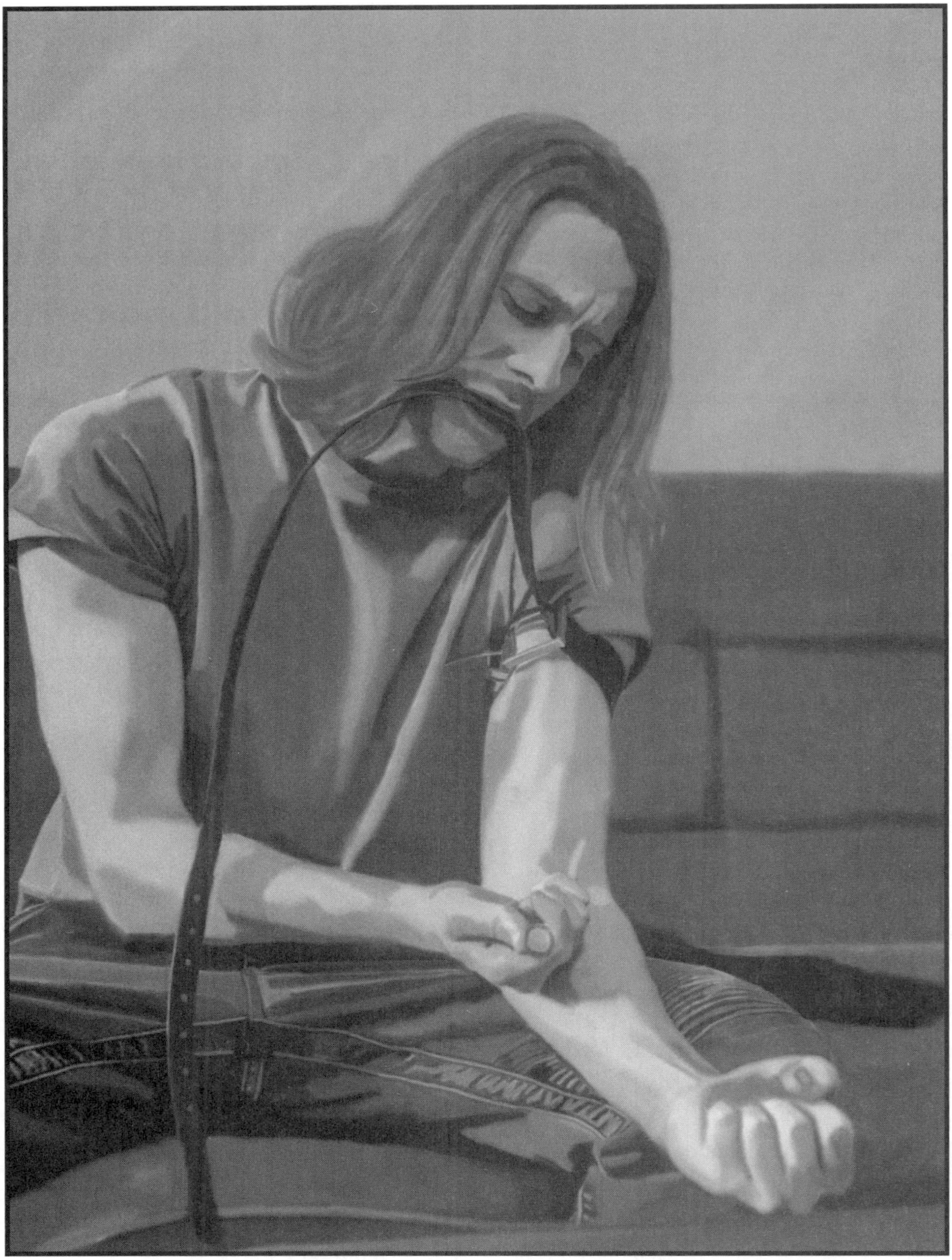

SECTION D/CHAPTER 18

A 32-year-old man with hemorrhoids and heroin

There has been a staggering increase in opiate use in the United States since the late 1990s, with deaths reaching epidemic proportions.[1] From 1999 to 2015, the total number of opioid overdose deaths quadrupled from 8,050 to 33,091, representing an increase in heroin supply and the introduction of synthetic opiates to the United States market.[2] One of many challenges to emergency department (ED) providers is knowing when an opiate is appropriate for acute pain management, as opiate prescribing patterns can lead to dependence and significant downstream effects.[3] Furthermore, ED providers must be able to identify sequelae of drug use or dependence, such as cellulitis and endocarditis. The opiate demanding patient presents another potential problem, as bias may impede an accurate diagnosis.

Patients presenting with multiple complaints can also be challenging, leading to misdiagnosis or mismanagement. Our patient presents with two chief complaints: hemorrhoid pain and syncope. In this instance, the provider focuses on the patient's request for pain medication in light of his known history of opiate abuse and overlooks the potentially more serious complaint of "syncope." While syncope itself accounts for approximately 1% of all ED visits, the admission rate is high (over 50%), and a missed diagnosis can be devastating.[4] The following case highlights the challenges and pitfalls of multiple complaints and potential biases of perceived drug-seeking behavior.

INITIAL ED VISIT

CC (10/10/2016 @22:03): Syncope

HPI: The patient is here with hemorrhoid pain and syncope.

The patient has a history of anxiety. He also has a history of syncope. He has passed out for 5 times in the last year and a half but has passed out several times prior to that. Most of the time when he passes out, he feels lightheaded and is out for a few seconds. Had syncope for up to 20 minutes in the past. He has had chest pain prior to syncope in the past but has not today. When asked about his workup for syncope in the past, his girlfriend answers because the patient is focused on his hemorrhoid at this point.

The patient was sitting in a chair smoking a cigarette. He suddenly felt very hot. He stood up and felt lightheaded. He then passed out for anywhere from a few seconds to a couple of minutes. He had no confusion afterwards. He realized what had happened right away. He had no hemorrhoid pain prior to passing out but did after waking up.

Patient has not been straining recently. He has chronic problems with his hemorrhoids that occasionally bleed. He has had no change in this recently. His hemorrhoid pain is uncontrolled. It is constant severe pain that is worse with movement or palpation. There are no relieving factors. It does not radiate. He denies abdominal pain, nausea or vomiting. Urination has been normal. No black stools. No fevers. He has been eating and drinking well.

He denies any chest pain or shortness of breath today. No vision changes, trouble talking or swallowing, numbness or focal weakness. No headache or neck pain.

When he passes out, he usually goes to [an outside hospital]. His friend thinks that he has had a CAT scan of his chest in the past. He does not have a primary care doctor and doesn't like to follow up though he does see a cardiologist every 6 months.

The patient apparently overdosed on Sunday and was in the emergency department then. He apparently has been supplementing his heroin and opiate addiction with his Suboxone films. He is not enrolled in counseling. He is not exactly honest with the information that he is presenting today.

No fever, rhinorrhea, cough, cp, sob, abd pain, n/v/d, blood in the stool/urine, rash, HA, vision change, numbness or weakness, difficulty speaking.

Social history: + tob, No EtOH

NKDA
Medications: Suboxone

PMH:
Active
- Asystole
- Cocaine abuse
- Marijuana abuse
- Opiate dependence
- Personality disorder
- Syncope

Resolved
- Arrhythmia
- Pacemaker catheter, device

Surgical history: Pacemaker catheter
Family history: No family history items have been selected or recorded

PE:
Vital Signs

23:17 EDT	Pain Score	10
	Pain Location Site #1	Rectal
	Pain Characteristics Site #1	Burning
22:07 EDT	Temperature	98.5 Degrees F NML
	Temperature Route	Oral
	Pulse Rate	80 BPM NML
	Respiratory Rate	18 Br PM NML
	Pulse Oximetry	100 % NML
	Oxygen Delivery	Room air
	Systolic BP	120 mm Hg NML
	Diastolic BP	80 mm Hg NML
	Weight Lb	220 lbs

PE:
CONSTITUTIONAL: Alert and oriented appropriately, thin. very anxious. Eye contact is fair. Occasionally writhing and moaning in bed. No evidence of respiratory distress.
EYES: PERRL, no scleral icterus. Conj are pink
NECK: Trachea is midline. Voice is normal. Supple
RESP: Normal chest excursion with respiration; breath sounds clear and equal bilaterally; no wheezes, rhonchi, or rales
CARDIO: Normal S1, S2. Regular rate and rhythm, without murmurs
ABD: Non-distended; non-tender, soft, without rigidity, rebound or guarding. Normal BS. No masses or organomegaly
BACK: No CVA, midline or paraspinal muscle tenderness.
SKIN: Normal for age and race; warm and dry; no apparent lesions
EXTREM: Well perfused w/o cyanosis or edema. MOE x 4 easily. 2+ radial and DP pulses equal bilat.
NEURO: Patient is alert and oriented times three. Cranial nerves III-XII are intact. Sensory and motor functions are intact. Strength is 5/5 for flexion and extension in all 4 extremities (abd/add at the shoulders). Patellar DTR's are equal and intact. Finger to nose testing is equal and normal bilaterally. Pronator testing shows no drift. Grips are equal bilaterally. No clonus.
RECTAL: Large protruding hemorrhoids noted that are purplish in color. Very tender. No active bleeding. No perirectal tenderness.

TESTING: EKG - reviewed by me

PROCEDURE: Pacer interrogation - nothing acute; PAT in August but no asystole or concerning rhythms per d/w tech.

MDM:
10/11/2016–01:08 - s/w [the EP cardiologist] about presentation and pacer interrogation.

This patient's management is very challenging. He obviously has uncontrolled mental illness in the form of his personality disorder and anxiety. This is complicated by his polysubstance abuse and his deceptive behavior. He is not being honest with people around him trying to help him. He is simply wanting to get high and is likely treating his mental illness with medications. He also has very poor insight into his dual diagnosis of addiction and mental illness.

I spent some time talking with his girlfriend. She was very honest with him and said that she was not going to lie to cover for him. I talked with her therefore out in the hallway because I wanted her to be able to give me more information. The patient has been using Suboxone to supplement his withdrawal and his need to get high on the days basically can't get drugs. He persisted in asking for medication here and clearly has no understanding of how his behavior is affecting both his addiction and mental illness. He is making very poor choices and despite several efforts by me to try and get him to understand, he is refusing to do so.

In talking with his girlfriend, the patient has been very good at victimizing himself and manipulating her, making her feel guilty about his life choices and disease processes. He is choosing to manage in an unhealthy way. I did talk with the social worker and asked him to give her some resources for support groups in counseling.

I declined giving the patient opiates further here after I was able to uncover some of his more significant problems through [a record from a different outside hospital] as well as our old electronic medical record.

I talked with the patient about supportive care, recommendations for follow-up and returning if worse or any new symptoms/concerns. The patient seems unconcerned by his syncopal episodes but is extremely concerned about his hemorrhoids and [wants] surgery right now or sometime today to get rid of them. He is obviously extremely poor candidate for surgery partly because of his ongoing opioid use and polysubstance abuse in conjunction with his poorly controlled mental illness. Pain management for him postop is going to be extremely difficult.

The patient was disappointed with but eventually agreeable to the plan of care with no further questions. The patient's girlfriend was agreeable to drive him home. The patient had actually asked her to drive him somewhere to get some drugs but she declined.

Results review: Lab results: Lab

WBC Count	**17.6thou/mcL HI**
Hemoglobin	15.4gm/dL
Platelet Count	187thou/mcL
Sodium Level	141mMol/L

10/10/2015 23:24 EDT

	Potassium Level	**3.5 mMol/L LOW**
	Chloride Level	104mMol/L
	Carbon Dioxide Level	29mMol/L
	Anion Gap	8.0mMol/L
	Glucose Level	84mg/dL
	BUN	13mg/dL
	Creatinine	0.95mg/dL
	Calcium Total	8.9mg/dL
10/10/2015 23:08 EDT	Troponin I POCT	0.01ng/mL

Impression and Plan
DIAGNOSIS:

1. acute syncope with history of syncope status post pacemaker placement for asystole
2. history of polysubstance misuse: cocaine, marijuana
3. history of opiate and nicotine dependence
4. recent initiation of Suboxone therapy
5. history of personality disorder and anxiety with acute exacerbations

Plan
Condition: Stable.
Disposition: Discharged: to home.
Prescriptions: Tucks 50% rectal pad, Proctofoam, MiraLax oral powder, Colace
Instructions: Drug Abuse and Addiction-SportsMed, Generalized Anxiety Disorder, Hemorrhoids
Follow-up with primary care and cardiology within 3–4 days

Discussion points:
Syncope:
When a patient presents with syncope, they are providing us with a symptom, not a diagnosis. The definition of syncope is a transient loss of consciousness due to global cerebral hypoperfusion.[5,6] By definition, the event is self-limited and recovery is rapid. Presyncope represents transient hypoperfusion, often preceded by prodromal symptoms of dizziness, lightheadedness, sweating, palpitations, nausea, and vision changes, but without loss of consciousness. Importantly, presyncope and syncope share similar mechanisms (loss of adequate perfusion of the entire cerebral cortex or reticular activating system) and similar diagnostic evaluations.[6] In contrast to syncope, patients presenting with presyncope tend to be slightly younger (age 56 vs. 59), have less comorbidities associated with serious outcomes, and have half as many serious outcomes (5% versus 10%). However, providers should not be reassured, as serious outcomes, such as death and dysrhythmia, still occur in 2.6% of patients with presyncope compared to 5% in those presenting with syncope.[6,7] In a study by by Thiruganasambandamoorthy, et al. of 780 patients presenting to the ED with presyncope, 5.1% experienced a serious outcome at 30-day follow-up, including 2 deaths of unknown cause (0.3%), 24 cardiovascular-related events (e.g., atrial fibrillation, myocardial infarction, supraventricular tachycardia) (3.1%), and 14 non-cardiac events (e.g., anemia, hemorrhage, sepsis) (1.8%).[7]

When patients describe episodes with atypical features, such as a prolonged period of unconsciousness, confusion, or focal neurologic complaints, a non-syncopal cause should be considered. Initial management should focus on those with a time-critical diagnosis, such as loss of consciousness from significant blood loss or a potentially fatal dysrhythmia or a seizure. In the hemodynamically stable patient with completely resolved symptoms, we should define the event further with history and physical exam supplement.

Syncope differential diagnosis:
The differential diagnosis for syncope is broad. Causes of syncope (Table 1) are grouped into 4 major categories that can be recalled by the pneumonic "OSCaR:"

Orthostatic syncope
Structural cardiopulmonary disease
Cardiac dysrhythmias
Reflex syncope (aka neurally-mediated reflex syncope)

A fifth category ("unknown") is sometimes included, as upwards of 50% of patients presenting with syncope have no discernible etiology.[8,9]

(Table on next page...)

Table 1. Causes of syncope

Category	Definition	Etiologies
Orthostatic Syncope	Drop in systolic blood pressure >20 mmHg or tachycardia >20 beats per minute with supine to sitting or standing positioning	**Dehydration**, **autonomic dysfunction** (i.e. multiple system atrophy, Parkinson's disease with autonomic failure, diabetes, amyloidosis, spinal cord injuries, etc.), **hemorrhage** (i.e. aortic aneurysm, ruptured ectopic pregnancy), **drug induced** (i.e. alcohol, anticholinergics, vasodilators, diuretics, etc.)
Structural Cardiopulmonary Disease	Structural heart disease leading to reduced cardiac output	**Valvular heart disease** (i.e. aortic stenosis, mitral stenosis, prosthetic valve dysfunction), **acute coronary syndrome**, **cardiomyopathy** (i.e. ischemic, dilated or restrictive), **congenital** (i.e. hypertrophic cardiomyopathy), **cardiac tamponade**, **pulmonary embolism**, **aortic dissection**, **pulmonary hypertension**, **subclavian steal syndrome**
Cardiac Dysrhythmias	Dysrhythmia of any cause leading to transient *global* hypoperfusion	**Bradycardia** (sick sinus syndrome, heart block, pacemaker failure), **tachycardia** (supraventricular, ventricular), **drug induced** (i.e. beta-blockers, calcium channel blockers, etc.), **Brugada syndrome**, **prolonged QTc, Arrhythmogenic right ventricular cardiomyopathy (ARVC)**
Reflex Syncope	Neurally mediated increase in vagal tone leading to inappropriate vasodilation and/or bradycardia with associated hypotension	**Vasovagal** (pain, fear, emotional distress, coughing, sneezing, micturition, postprandial, etc.), **carotid sinus hypersensitivity**

Atypical presentations with associated symptoms such as headache, chest pain, persistent altered mentation, or focal neurologic complaints should prompt work-up of non-syncopal etiologies, such as seizure, TIA, stroke, subarachnoid hemorrhage, subdural/epidural hemorrhage, toxic/metabolic syndromes, or psychogenic etiologies.

Patients with cardiogenic syncope are at the greatest risk for death, though patients without an identifiable cause for their syncope are still a significant risk of death, with a reported multivariableadjusted hazard ratio of 1.32 in one study.[10] Of note, a significant number of patients initially diagnosed with epilepsy are later found to have underlying cardiogenic syncope.[11] Cerebral hypoxia can cause myoclonic jerks, which may be visually indistinguishable from seizure activity and lead to an incorrect diagnosis.

Work-up of the syncopal patient—What does ACEP recommend?
The American College of Emergency Physicians' (ACEP) clinical policy on syncope recommends that low-risk patients have a thorough history and physical exam with a standard 12-lead ECG.[12] They provide a level C recommendation for laboratory testing and imaging only in situations dictated by findings on history and physical examination. Examples include the following:

- Did a severe headache precede the syncopal event? If so, consider subarachnoid hemorrhage.
- Does the patient appear postictal? Consider seizure.
- Did the patient have associated chest pain, shortness of breath, and/or a history of heart disease? Consider structural heart conditions such as decompensated congestive heart failure or symptomatic aortic stenosis.
- Was there recent surgery with complaints of shortness of breath? Consider pulmonary embolism.
- Is there melena, bright red blood in their stool, or history of anemia? Consider acute blood loss.

Most concerning, however, are patients without prodromal symptoms that might differentiate them from reflex-mediated syncope. Syncope without a prodrome is concerning for dysrhythmia, which is less often the etiology in those presenting with presyncope.[13]

Special populations—Patients and symptoms associated with increased risk:
Older age in combination with a history of cardiac disease is an independent predictor for an adverse outcome, though some literature suggests that age > 65 alone does not predict adverse outcomes in patients without risk factors.[13,14] The utility of using any specific age as a cutoff to determine who requires further evaluation is not recommended. Interestingly, of the risk stratification tools available (San Francisco Syncope Rule (SFSR), Evaluation of Guidelines in Syncope Study (EGSYS), the Risk Stratification of Syncope in the Emergency Department (ROSE) score, Osservatorio Epidermiologico sulla Sincope del Lazio (OESIL) score, etc.), only the OESIL score uses age > 65 to predict risk.

The focus should be on the historical and exam clues that warn of a high-risk patient: *older age, history of cardiovascular disease, syncope without a prodrome, abnormal ECG findings, exam findings consistent with heart failure, anemia and/or positive fecal occult blood test, chest pain and syncope, and hypoxemia.*

The most powerful predictors of adverse outcome from greatest to least are: *palpitations preceding syncope, syncope during effort, heart disease, evidence of bleeding, syncope while supine, absence of symptoms preceding syncope, age, and trauma related to syncope.*[15]

Clinical decision tools:
When initially reported in the literature, there was great hope for the SFSR, as it was simple and seemed logical, but it has not been able to be externally validated. Saccilotto, et al. performed a

systematic review of 12 studies and found a pooled estimate of sensitivity of 87% and specificity of 52% in predicting short-term serious outcomes. The most common cause of false-negative classification was from cardiac dysrhythmia.[16] Schladenhaufen, et al. reported that both sensitivity and specificity were lower in patients aged 65 years and older (76.5% and 36.8% respectively).[17]

Interestingly, the ROSE rule includes evaluation of the brain natriuretic peptide (BNP) concentration in the evaluation of syncope. If $\geq$ 300pg/mL, it was a major independent predictor of serious outcome and death 1 month after initial presentation. Costantino, et al, evaluated the use of a 6-hour delta NT-proBNP in 18 patients with syncope secondary to underlying dysrhythmia (ventricular tachycardia (VT) or ventricular fibrillation (VF)) vs. 15 patients with vasovagal syncope with tilt-table testing. The 6-hour change was significantly elevated in those with syncope caused by dysrhythmia, with a median increase of 32% in the ventricular tachycardia/ventricular fibrillation group vs. the vasovagal patients.[18]

Lastly, Costantino, et al. used a meta-analysis to externally validate syncope prediction tools (SFSR, OESIL, and EGSYS) compared to clinical judgement, finding that these prediction tools did not have better sensitivity, specificity, or prognostic yield compared to clinical judgment to predict short-term serious outcome.[19]

In summary, no score is perfect, so we are left to focus on historical clues, physical exam findings combined with an ECG, and directed work-up. Of note, syncope without a prodrome deserves special attention.

What ECG findings are concerning?

Patients presenting to the ED with syncope should receive an ECG.[12, 20-22] While the overall diagnostic yield is reportedly low, patients with a cardiogenic syncope are at high risk, and the test is inexpensive. Concerning features include any non-sinus rhythm or any left bundle conduction problem, including left bundle branch block (LBBB), left anterior fascicular block (LAFB), left posterior fascicular block (LPFB) or QRS widening.[21] Interestingly, the simple ECG criteria from the San Francisco Syncope Rule (i.e. new ECG changes from prior or any non-sinus rhythm on ECG) may predict which patients are at risk for poor cardiac outcome.[21] Other rhythm disturbances to consider include conduction delays, such as type II second degree atrioventricular block or third degree atrioventricular (AV) block, presence of Q waves, ST segment abnormalities, or prolonged QT interval.[21] Common rhythm disturbances associated with syncope are listed in Table 2 and Table 3.[20, 22]

(Tables on next page...)

Table 2. ECG rhythm disturbances associated with syncope

Concerning ECG Findings
Asymptomatic and inappropriate sinus bradycardia (<40-50 bpm) or sinus pauses >3 seconds
LBBB
LPFB
Bifasicular block (either LBBB or right bundle branch block with LAFB or LPFB)
Type II second degree AV block
Prolonged QRS (>0.12s)
Ventricular tachycardia or paroxysmal supraventricular tachycardia with rapid ventricular rate
Acquired long QT

Table 3. ECG patterns of inherited causes of syncope

Etiology	**ECG Findings**
Pre-excitation syndromes (Wolff Parkinson White Syndrome, Lown-Ganong-Levine Syndrome)	Short PR (<120 ms), +/- wide QRS (>120 ms), +/- slurred upstroke of the QRS complex (delta wave)
Hypertrophic Cardiomyopathy (HCM)	Left ventricular hypertrophy with deep, narrow (<40 ms) Q waves in the lateral > inferior leads, rarely giant T wave inversions in precordial leads (associated with apical HCM)
Arrhythmogenic Right Ventricular Cardiomyopathy (AVRC)	Right precordial T wave inversions, terminal notching of the QRS (epsilon wave), localized QRS widening (leads V1-3) with prolonged S-wave upstroke
Brugada Syndrome	Coved or saddleback-type ST-segment elevation in two or more right precordial leads in the setting of a structurally normal heart
Long QT Syndrome (LQTS)	QTc ≥500 ms without an alternative etiology, long QTc interval in the presence of a history of syncope +/- family history of sudden cardiac death <30 years or family member diagnosed with LQTS
Short QT Syndrome (SQTS)	QTc ≤330 ms or QTc <360 ms with a family history of cardiac arrest, syncope or sudden cardiac death at age <40 years or family member with a diagnosis of SQTS
Catecholaminergic Polymorphic Ventricular Tachycardia (CPVT)	Normal resting ECG, adrenergic (i.e. physical exercise, emotional distress) induced bidirectional and polymorphic ventricular tachycardia

BOUNCEBACK ED VISIT (9 days later)

Nursing CC (01:46): Cardiac-Resp Arrest

HPI: I reviewed the nurses notes. I met patient in room upon arrival of EMS. Pt. arrives in full cardiopulmonary arrest. Pt. was found unresponsive and EMS was called. No bystander CPR. Pt. found unresponsive and pulseless by EMS. Pt. received full ACLS care without successful resuscitation. No history able to be obtained from patient

History obtained from EMS and the girlfriend. Girlfriend reports he was normal at 12:15 AM and at 12:45, a half hour later, he was in the bathroom she heard a door slam and she found him lying there unconscious with heroin by him and a needle and he was blue. She called EMS. EMS reported that the patient was pulseless but they did see pacer spikes on the monitor and he does have a pacemaker per girlfriend for a cardiac arrhythmia as a child. They did obtain IO access and placed an ET tube with direct and indirect visualization and waveform capnography. They report bilateral breath sounds and easy bagging. Patient did receive multiple medicines during the arrest including IO and intranasal Narcan. Patient received several doses of epinephrine. Patient had a blood sugar in the 30s and received D50 and had a recheck of the blood sugars of 110. Patient also received bicarbonate.

ROS: Unable to obtain due to unresponsiveness

PE:
CONSTITUTIONAL: Unresponsive; pt. receiving chest compressions and BVM to ET tube; no spontaneous movements or respirations noted
ENT: Blood through nares and ET tube
HEAD: Atraumatic
EYES: Pupils unresponsive
MOUTH: ET tube noted
LUNGS: No spontaneous respirations; breath sounds equal with BVM
CARDIO: No heart tones
ABD: Non-distended; soft
SKIN: Cool; no obvious rash
NEURO: GCS 3; unresponsive; no movement of extremities

Consulting editor comments (Weingart):

Are people really listening for heart sounds during a code?

Author comments (Weinstock):

Our patient is intubated and unresponsive after epinephrine, Narcan and bicarbonate. As chest compressions continue, the staff looks at you for direction. We are in the footsteps of the emergency physician. We are at:

DECISION POINT A – YOU ARE FACED WITH 5 QUESTIONS:

1. **Which aspects of the patient's care require immediate assessment and confirmation?**
2. **What does the blood at the nares signify?**
3. **The medics gave Narcan—is this helpful in an intubated patient?**
4. **Why was the patient hypoglycemic?**
5. **How does management of a code differ in patients with a pacemaker or implantable cardiac defibrillator (ICD)?**

What does the literature say?

Q#1: Which aspects of the patient's care require immediate assessment and confirmation?

Airway and ventilation:

With our patient, it was noted that EMS found the patient in asystole. They performed endotracheal intubation (ETI) with tube confirmation by direct visualization, waveform capnography, bilateral breath sounds, and "easy bagging." Was intubation a good idea, and which of these confirmatory measures reassures us that we have a definitive airway?

For patients with in-hospital cardiac arrest, ETI at any time during the first 15 minutes of resuscitation compared with no intubation is associated with worse outcomes, defined as decreased survival to hospital discharge (16.3% vs. 19.4%, RR 0.84)[23] A similar finding is reported in the pediatric literature.[24]

Similarly, data from out-of-hospital cardiac arrest would support the use of a supraglottic airway compared to ETI, with evidence of increased rates of return of spontaneous circulation (ROSC), survival to hospital admission, and neurologically intact survival favoring the former. A study from 2015 that showed prehospital supraglottic airway placement demonstrated increased rates of return of spontaneous circulation (ROSC), survival to hospital admission, and neurologically intact survival in contrast to ETI.[25] A more recent study by Jeong, et al. reported decreased survival in out-of-hospital cardiac arrest patients receiving any advanced airway (including ETI and supraglottic airway (SGA)) (OR 0.51) compared to basic airway management, including head-tilt, chin lift or any variation thereof with a bag valve mask with or without a nasopharyngeal airway or oropharyngeal airway (OR 0.64).[26]

Consulting editor comments (Weingart):

All of the literature is hopelessly confounded by the other things that happen during the intubation and by what happens to the respiratory rate as a result of intubation, so to state it this way without those provisos doesn't make a whole lot of sense. There is nothing to indicate that intubation that kept the respiratory rate the same and didn't stop chest compressions would be anything except a neutral or beneficial intervention.

Author comments (Weinstock):

Chest compressions should not be delayed or stopped to intubate a patient who is being adequately ventilated with bag-valve-mask or supraglottic airway.

Upon arrival to the emergency department, ACLS should be continued, beginning with a brief rhythm and pulse check. Placement of prehospital airways must then be confirmed. If a supraglottic airway is in place and working effectively, we recommend keeping it in place through resuscitation and then replacing with an endotracheal tube when ROSC is obtained and the patient is stabilized.

Consulting editor comments (Weingart):

This is predicated on confirmation with continuous waveform ETCO2, without which neither BVM nor SGA is acceptable.

Confirming endotracheal tube placement can be done in a number of ways, but no single method has 100% sensitivity. Direct visualization of the tube going through the cords is predictive of good placement, but this cannot be relied upon as a sole measure. Neither can other physical exam findings, such as adequate chest rise, tube condensation during ventilation, or auscultation of bilateral breath sounds.[27-30]

Colorimetric end-tidal carbon dioxide (ETCO2) detection for correct endotracheal tube placement has been used for years with great success but should be used as an adjunct and not primary indicator, with a false-negative failure rate of 7% (tube appropriately in the trachea but capnography would indicate it is in the esophagus) and a false-positive rate of 3% (tube in the esophagus but capnography would indicate it is in the trachea).[30] Lastly, ultrasound has been used to check placement but should be a confirmatory adjunct and not used exclusively in any instance.[31, 32]

Consulting editor comments (Weingart):

Waveform end-tidal CO2 is perfect if used properly for confirming intubation during chest compressions. Note that if the patient is deceased, there may still be a waveform with esophageal intubation; however, after approximately 6 ventilations, there will no longer be a waveform. The only time waveform is not acceptable is if the ET tube is obstructed with emesis, blood, or secretions in which case other forms of confirmation should be used. Ultrasound is not a reliable method to confirm tube placement as it is fraught with interpreter variability; I don't trust it. I would only use US when end-tidal CO2 fails or if waveform is not available.

Circulation and vascular access:

Once airway placement has been confirmed and we are adequately ventilating the patient, we need to ensure vascular access. In this case, EMS placed an intraosseous (IO) line. IO placement is fast, reliable, and almost anything can be given through it, including vasopressors. In both children and adults in cardiac arrest or severe shock without readily available peripheral intravenous access, the recommended next step is to place an IO line.[33] In both of these populations, success rates by EMS and hospital providers are high and placement is faster than attempts at peripheral or central access.[34-37] Sites of insertion include the proximal tibia, medial malleolus, proximal humerus, ileum, and distal femur.[38]

When the IO is placed, confirmation of correct placement can be performed by aspiration of bone marrow, visualization of blood in the stylet, firm placement of the needle in bone, and the ability to easily flush or administer fluids in a continuous fashion without evidence of tissue extravasation. A "squeeze test" has been described in which compressing the soft tissues around the site will lead to decreased flow rates if the IO is in the soft tissue or has gone through both cortices.[39] This is probably most useful in obese patients where it can be difficult to detect extravasation. When in doubt, place a second IO and use the one you know is functional.

When fluids are administered through the IO, they should be done so with a pressure bag or infusion pump to overcome the resistance of emissary veins in the intramedullary cavity.[40] Anticipate absolute flow rates for volume expansion equivalent to a 21-gauge peripheral IV, though flow rates may vary depending on site. When giving push-dose medications, flush the IO cannula before and after each use. Intraosseous medication doses are equivalent to intravenous dosing.

Absolute contraindications to IO placement include ipsilateral fracture or vascular injury. Relative contraindications include overlying cellulitis, burns, osteomyelitis, osteogenesis imperfecta or osteoporosis, and patients with right-to-left cardiac shunts which may predispose them to systemic complications of cerebral fat or bone-marrow emboli. While we would avoid IO placement in the aforementioned situations, in the crashing or arresting patient without reasonable vascular alternatives, any vascular access is better than no access.

Adequate CPR:

With confirmation of ETT placement and vascular access being performed simultaneously, we need to ensure that adequate CPR is being provided. Many EMS agencies are now using automated devices, albeit with mixed results.[41-43] Our goal with compressions is to provide adequate coronary perfusion pressure (CPP), which is associated with ROSC.[44-47] As the coronaries fill during diastole, CPP is defined as the difference between the diastolic aortic pressure and right atrial end diastolic pressure. Repeated studies have shown that targeting a CPP of > 15mmHg is associated with improvement in ROSC and potentially improved neurological outcomes, at least in swine models.

If the resources are available, placement of an arterial line with a goal systolic pressure of 100mmHg and diastolic pressure of 40mmHg ensures adequate coronary filling during compressions. Otherwise, we are left with some older methods, such as palpating a femoral pulse. But does a palpable femoral pulse equate to adequate compressions? The question may have been inadvertently answered by Hilty, et al. when they looked at use of real-time ultrasound guidance for placement of femoral lines during CPR. The "palpable pulses" they noted in the landmark approach group were actually venous in origin about half of the time![48] While we should be hesitant to draw conclusions from a single study, consider the use of other methods to determine CPR quality, such as waveform capnography.

With adequate chest compressions, blood is circulating in a manner that allows for offloading of CO_2 at the level of the alveoli. We can detect this quantitatively using waveform end-tidal capnography, and return value equates to cardiac output and, thus, coronary perfusion pressure.[49] Our goal should be for an end-tidal CO_2 ($ETCO_2$) measurement of at least 10–20mmHg during CPR, which is associated with ROSC. That said, a higher $ETCO_2$ goal is suggested in a study by Hartmann, et al, in which the mean $ETCO_2$ in patients with ROSC was 25.8mmHg versus 13.1mmHg without ROSC.[50] Dropping $ETCO_2$ measurements (<10 mmHg) can indicate compressor fatigue. An abrupt and sustained rise of $ETCO_2$ indicates ROSC, and at 20 minutes the $ETCO_2$ value can have prognostic significance.[51] If at 20 minutes the $ETCO_2$ measurement is < 10mmHg, the chance of survival is abysmal, though ETCO2 values should not be used exclusively when deciding to call the code. Given heterogeneous findings in multiple studies, other prognostic indicators should be used adjunctively.[52, 53]

Adjuncts and "cutting edge" techniques:
Point-of-care ultrasound (POCUS) has been used for nearly a decade in cardiac arrest. It can help rule out mechanical causes for the arrest (e.g. tension pneumothorax, pericardial tamponade, massive pulmonary embolism), particularly if the presenting rhythm is pulseless electrical activity (PEA). However, it should not impede chest compressions. In a study by Huis In 't Veld, et al. they showed that the use of POCUS during cardiac arrest led to increased duration of pulse checks, and multiple studies have shown the deleterious effects on patient outcomes with interruptions during CPR.[54]

While ultrasound findings during cardiac arrest may provide prognostic information, cardiac standstill does not translate to non-survival in all instances. That said, its overall utility is defined in a meta-analysis by Tsou, et al. where they found that spontaneous cardiac movement on bedside ultrasound had a sensitivity of 95% and specificity of 80% in predicting ROSC, with a positive likelihood ratio of 4.8 and negative likelihood ratio of 0.06.[55] Transesophageal echo is an evolving diagnostic tool that can be used during an arrest. It can be left in place during the resuscitation to monitor ongoing chest compression quality as well as diagnosing other causes for the arrest, including aortic dissection and massive pulmonary embolism.[56]

A "cutting edge" approach to monitor adequacy of chest compressions is cerebral oximetry, which uses near-infrared spectroscopy to assess regional cerebral oxygenation (rSO_2) in the frontal lobe of the brain.[57] Like ETCO2 monitoring, it has been used to predict ROSC, determine adequacy of chest compressions and used as a prognostic tool for survival and neurological outcomes, though more study is needed.

While initial circulation, airway, and breathing assessment and confirmation are crucial, we recommend simultaneously obtaining a point-of-care blood glucose (C-A-B-G)—when we did this in our patient, it was low.

Q#2: What does the blood at the nares signify?
Minimal information is given on the physical examination of the patient's presentation to the ED other than "blood through the nares and ET tube." Blood coming through the nares could mean that a traumatic attempt at nasotracheal intubation could have taken place, although this is no longer common prehospital practice. Other considerations include coagulopathy (e.g. disseminated intravascular coagulation, medication side-effects, or supratherapeutic anticoagulation) and posterior epistaxis that can lead to hemorrhagic shock if not identified early.

More interestingly, it was noted that blood was present in the endotracheal tube, which might be more meaningful. First, acute noncardiogenic pulmonary edema is a known complication of both heroin and naloxone use. Albeit rare, patients with heroin-induced acute pulmonary edema may require intubation for hypoxia.[58] Naloxone administration itself has also been associated with pulmonary edema through multiple mechanisms, including an acute increase in sympathetic tone leading to an abrupt rise in pulmonary pressure, capillary leak related to histamine release within lung tissue, and an increase in negative inspiratory force in the presence of an upper airway obstruction (e.g. secretions, mucus plugging, a closed glottis, opioid-induced glottis laxity) leading to negative pressure pulmonary edema.[59, 60] Finally, pulmonary edema is a frequent manifestation during or shortly after prolonged CPR. The mechanism is likely related to increases in pulmonary arterial pressures with chest compressions, and the development is predicted by both total duration of CPR and the initial pCO_2 level.[61] The presence and severity of pulmonary edema during cardiac arrest correlate with worsening mortality and neurologic outcomes.

Q#3: The medics gave Narcan—is this helpful in an intubated patient?

Naloxone rapidly reverses respiratory and CNS depression related to opiate toxicity. There are no significant harmful effects when administered to patients who are not opiate-intoxicated or dependent, but administration may induce withdrawal in those who are opiate-dependent. These withdrawal symptoms are rarely life-threatening. While pulmonary edema has been described with naloxone use, it may also be precipitated by use of intravenous opiates, making the definitive cause difficult to ascertain.

These authors agree with the 2015 AHA guidelines and recommend administering naloxone to opiate-associated life-threatening emergencies.[62] No specific recommendation can be made regarding the use of naloxone for patients in cardiac arrest, and precedence should be given to acute resuscitative efforts. With ongoing resuscitative efforts, it may be administered if there is suspicion of opiate overdose. Note that patient's use of carfentanil may require significantly larger doses of naloxone for reversal.

Q#4: Why was the patient hypoglycemic?

It was noted that during the arrest the patient's blood glucose was low, requiring dextrose. Hypoglycemia is a well-known cause of cardiac arrest, mostly likely secondary to neuroglycopenia and the resultant sympathoadrenal response that can lead to fatal dysrhythmias.[63] This, however, is most often seen in insulin-dependent diabetics that experience sudden nocturnal death without a clear cause but postulated to be related to excess insulin administration and resultant severe hypoglycemia. ECG changes associated with hypoglycemia include PR interval shortening, ST segment depression, T wave flattening, and QTc prolongation.[64]

Interestingly, a recent article by Peng, et al. looked at the impact of dextrose administration during in-hospital cardiac arrest and noted an association with decreased chance of survival and good neurological outcome, but an increased chance of ROSC. It is unknown if this applies to out-of-hospital cardiac arrest as well, and it was a single retrospective study.[65] Whether our patient's hypoglycemia was causal is uncertain; it is more probable that it was secondary. Furthermore, methadone itself may be associated with hypoglycemia, and administration of naloxone can reverse this effect.[66]

Q#5: How does management of a code differ in patients with a pacemaker or implantable cardiac defibrillator (ICD)?

Pacemakers are composed of the pacemaker pulse generator and the intracardiac leads. The more commonly seen dual chamber pacemakers have 2 leads (one in the right atrium and one in the right ventricle), while single chamber pacemakers have a single lead, which is usually placed in the right ventricle. A universal language has been developed to describe the function of these devices, with the first 3 positions of the 5 being the most important to understand for the emergency physician. They can be remembered by the pneumonic "PaSeR:" pacing, sensing, and response[67] (Table 4). The remaining 4th and 5th positions represent programmability and anti-tachycardia function. The device can pace and sense the ventricle (V), atrium (A), both (D), or none (O), and the subsequent pacemaker response is either inhibition (I), triggering (T), dual (inhibit and trigger) (D), or none (O).

Table 4. NASPE/BPEG Generic Code for Antibradycardia Pacing (67-68)

Position	I	II	III	IV	V
Function	Chamber **paced**	Chamber **sensed**	**Response** to sensing	Programmability	Anti-tachycardia function
	V = ventricle A = atrium D = both (atrium and ventricle) O = none	V = ventricle A = atrium D = both (atrium and ventricle) O = none	I = inhibit T = trigger D = dual (trigger and inhibit) O = none	O = none P = simple programmable M = multiprogrammable C = communicating R = rate responsive	O = none P = packing S = shock D = dual

As an example, with dual chamber (DDD) pacing, the system can pace, sense, and either trigger or inhibit both the atrium and the ventricle. In such a patient in normal sinus rhythm at a rate faster than the pacemaker lower limit and with normal AV conduction that is faster than the programmed AV interval, the pacemaker will be completely inhibited by sensing the native impulses and the normal sinus rhythm will march through. However, other scenarios exist. If the patient simply has sinus bradycardia but normal AV conduction, the atrium will be paced with sensing of the native QRS complex that follows that inhibits the pacemaker from pacing the ventricle. In the same patient, if there is sinus bradycardia and delayed AV conduction, both the atrium and ventricle will be paced based on the bradycardia and conduction delay in an attempt to maintain the lower rate limit set by the pacemaker and maintain the set AV interval. Lastly, if the problem is simply AV conduction delay or absent AV conduction, the atrial impulse will be sensed and inhibit pacing of the atrium but the lack of a sensed ventricular depolarization at the set AV interval will lead to ventricular pacing. Many alternative pacing modes exist, but a basic understanding of the mode and what is happening with regards to the chamber(s) paced, sensed, and the response to sensing the native beat is important.

The three described categories of pacemaker malfunction include failure to pace, failure to sense, and failure to capture.[67]

A. Failure to pace occurs when the pacemaker fails to trigger a myocardial depolarization. The ECG will show no pacemaker activity and only the native rhythm will be seen. This may be from lead misplacement, a fractured lead, lead migration, a dead battery or failure of the pulse generator or device component.

B. Failure to sense can occur with under-sensing and over-sensing.

1. Under-sensing occurs when the device is not correctly interpreting the native rhythm or

myocardial depolarization, leading to asynchronous pacing. The ECG will show too many or inappropriate pacemaker spikes (i.e. inappropriate pacing after a native QRS). Causes include lead misplacement, lead fracture, lead migration, a low sensing threshold (native beats are not recognized and so the device triggers), myocardial scarring, electrolyte disturbances, or battery failure.

2. Over-sensing is the result of inappropriate inhibition of a pacing stimulus when any electrical signal that has sufficient amplitude and frequency is encountered. The ECG might show a sinus rhythm with an inappropriately dropped pacemaker impulse followed by a prolonged asystolic pause. Causes include physiologic signals (e.g., peaked T waves in hyperkalemia) and non-physiologic signals in which electrical signals are misinterpreted as native beats (e.g. electromagnetic interference). Other causes include lead fracture or insulation break.

C. Failure to capture occurs when the pacemaker fires an impulse, but it is insufficient to depolarize the myocardium. The ECG will show pacemaker spikes but no cardiac response to the impulse is seen. Causes include lead misplacement, lead fracture, lead migration, myocardial scarring, or low energy impulses below depolarization threshold (e.g., a dying battery). Of note, both electrolyte abnormalities and supratherapeutic drug levels of antidysrhythmic medications can elevate the myocardial pacing threshold leading to failure to capture.

Implantable cardiac defibrillators (ICDs), on the other hand, are used for primary or secondary prevention of fatal cardiac dysrhythmia and sudden cardiac death, most commonly the result of ventricular fibrillation and ventricular tachycardia.[69] Similar to pacemakers, the ICD is composed of pacing and sensing electrodes (usually in a single ventricular lead), defibrillation electrodes, and a pulse generator. Functions include documentation of tachydysrhythmias and remote monitoring capabilities, anti-tachycardia pacing, bradycardia pacing, cardioversion or defibrillation. Patients with an ICD most often present to the ED for ICD defibrillation or series of defibrillations as well as other unrelated reasons that might be associated with the condition for which the ICD was placed (e.g. worsening heart failure symptoms, chest pain, etc.). When patients undergo multiple defibrillations, a determination should be made as to whether the defibrillations are appropriate or inappropriate.

Pacemaker dysfunction in the critically ill patient:
For the patient in extremis or arrest, management of pacemaker malfunction starts with standard ACLS guidelines. If the patient is symptomatically bradycardic, pacer pads should be placed, but not directly over the pacemaker. However, transcutaneous pacing may be inadequate, necessitating the conversion to transvenous pacing.

- In cases of over-sensing resulting in inappropriate inhibition and bradycardic rhythms, place a magnet over the device, which reverts it to asynchronous pacing at a fixed rate.
- Less frequently encountered, pacemaker-mediated tachycardia can be seen when an endless feedback loop of ventricular discharges is initiated by a premature ventricular contraction (PVC) or paced ventricular depolarization in patients with dual-chamber pacemakers. In this instance, the PVC or paced ventricular depolarization is received by the atria in a retrograde fashion. Atrial sensing then triggers ventricular depolarization, and an endless feedback loop is created at a rate upwards of the upper limit that the pacemaker is set. Setting a magnet over the

device to put it into asynchronous pacing mode is an option in management, as are overdrive pacing, electrical cardioversion, and medications to break the reentrant loop by increasing the AV nodal refractory period (i.e. adenosine, beta-blockade, calcium channel blockade).

- A more serious issue is the patient who presents with a "runaway pacemaker," which occurs when the pulse generator's central processing unit paces the patient inappropriately at a rate that exceeds the programmed threshold, differentiating it from pace-maker mediated tachycardia. This was more commonly seen in older generation pacemakers. Management options are few, though use of a magnet has been successful, as has opening of the pacemaker pocket and disconnecting the pacemaker leads, typically performed by cardiology. If the patient is pacemaker-dependent, the pacing unit can be removed, and the associated electrodes connected to an external pacing device.[70]

ICD issues:

A single ICD defibrillation without persistent or severe symptoms does not necessarily mandate an ED visit, as these patients can be seen on an urgent outpatient basis with their cardiologist for device interrogation.[71] As with the evaluation of pacemaker malfunctioning, consider an ECG, electrolytes, device interrogation, and CXR. If the patient is asymptomatic and there was a single defibrillation with normal test results, patients can undergo interrogation in the ED or be discharged for early follow-up with their cardiologist.[67] Cardiac biomarkers should only be checked in selected patients with symptoms concerning for acute coronary syndrome, as defibrillation itself can cause an elevated troponin.

Patients who have received multiple defibrillations should have the ICD interrogated.

- Inappropriate defibrillations are often delivered in the event of hemodynamically insignificant supraventricular tachycardias (SVTs). If there are ongoing defibrillations, medical management to treat the SVT should be initiated. If unsuccessful, a magnet placed over the ICD will terminate the defibrillation function while preserving its pacemaker function depending on the device. However, in some instances the ICD may need to be reprogrammed once the magnet is removed.[67]
- If a ventricular dysrhythmia is the cause, the defibrillation attempts are likely appropriate. In such circumstances, initiate medical therapies aimed at terminating the dysrhythmia, place pads as you would if a pacemaker were present, and initiate ACLS.

In our patient in full arrest with a known pacemaker, ACLS was delivered as any patient. Unique considerations include:

- Defibrillation pads are placed in an anterior-posterior fashion and never directly over the cardiac device. Defibrillation may reset older pacemakers, but this is less common with newer devices.
- It is appropriate to deliver external shocks per ACLS guidelines for VF and pulseless VT, as lead displacement, fracture, or other device malfunction may prevent the patient's device from delivering adequate defibrillations. A magnet should not be used to prevent ICD defibrillation when they are appropriate.[67]
- In a patient presenting early (several days) after placement of an ICD or pacemaker, consider tension pneumothorax. Pericardial tamponade may present as an early or late cause of PEA arrest, and perforation of the myocardium leading to a hemorrhagic pericardial effusion and tamponade can occur at any time.[67, 72]

What did the actual provider do?

MDM (02:13): 32-year-old presents in full pulmonary arrest. On initial pulse check patient was in PEA and had pacer spikes. I did confirm bilateral breath sounds. Patient bagged easily. We did obtain IV access. Patient initially received another epinephrine 1mg IVP. We did recheck the blood sugar. Patient did receive bicarbonate. My suspicion was this was a respiratory arrest.

Author comments (Weinstock):

Despite your efforts, the patient remains asystolic. We are running out of options. We are at:

DECISION POINT B – YOU ARE FACED WITH 4 QUESTIONS:

1. **Our interventions have been unsuccessful; where do we go from here?**
2. **Does the lack of cardiac activity on ED US portend prognosis?**
3. **Is it helpful to speak with family/friends *during* the code, or should the code be called and then family/friends informed?**
4. **Which cutting edge interventions can be attempted?**

Q#1: Our interventions have been unsuccessful; where do we go from here?

Reviewing the documentation, EMS received an unresponsive patient at around 1245 with institution of ACLS. The initial rhythm was asystole vs. pulseless electrical activity (PEA), and he received "multiple rounds of epinephrine" prior to arrival at 0146. The next decision-making point is at 0213, nearly 90 minutes after the initial down time. Pulse checks were attempted, and the patient was in PEA with pacer spikes, breath sounds were heard to confirm endotracheal tube placement, and intravenous access with administration of sodium bicarbonate was performed. The presumed cause of the arrest is respiratory, which seems to be on point. Should the code be called?

The Universal Termination of Resuscitation (TOR) Guideline for adult patients with presumed cardiac etiology for their arrest was originally developed in 2002 for guidance of BLS providers to determine which patients should be transported to the hospital.The original study reported a sensitivity of 100% in identifying survivors and 100% negative predictive value for identifying non-survivors, suggesting that resuscitation can be discontinued if the cardiac arrest was unwitnessed by emergency medical services personnel, the patient did not obtain ROSC despite attempted resuscitation (defined as four 2-minute intervals of CPR), and no shocks were delivered prior to transport (non-shockable rhythm). The rule was prospectively validated for both BLS and ACLS providers in OHCA by Morrison, et al. with a specificity of 100%, a positive predictive value of 100%, and a significant reduction in transport rate by EMS.[74]

In a more recent study by Drennan, et al. they found that survival to hospital discharge in patients that met Universal TOR Guideline criteria for termination (arrest unwitnessed by EMS providers, no ROSC despite attempted resuscitation, no shocks delivered) was only 0.7% vs. 3.0% for those who met criteria for transport.[73] They concluded that the sole use of the absence or presence of pre-hospital ROSC to identify potential survivors is unfounded. Patients should continue to be transported if at any time the patient has any of the following: a shockable rhythm, the arrest is witnessed, or ROSC occurs. In our patient, one could argue that the patient may not have required transport given that the arrest was unwitnessed, there was no ROSC despite attempts at adequate CPR, and no shockable rhythm was present.

Once the patient is in the ED, when can we decide to end resuscitative efforts? First, obtaining historical factors that might indicate the cause of the arrest, underlying comorbid conditions, and the circumstances of the arrest should be obtained to help guide the resuscitation. Second, trying to clarify code status is highly important, but this information can be difficult to obtain if not present on patient arrival. Lastly, patient historical factors used in conjunction with other measures (i.e. $ETCO_2$ monitoring, bedside ultrasound, etc.) should be considered before resuscitative efforts are terminated.[52, 53, 75] More drastic measures, such as institution of extracorporeal life support (ECLS), may be considered for patients with refractory ventricular dysrhythmias (and other indications) on a case-by-case basis.[76] In some instances, prolonged CPR might improve survival, specifically those with PEA and asystole.[77, 78]

Q#2: Does the lack of cardiac activity on ED US portend prognosis?

Though ultrasound is an adjunctive tool for prognostication in cardiac arrest, it is not, by itself, a perfect instrument. A study by Gaspari, et al. found that the rate of ROSC was over 50% if there was cardiac activity on initial cardiac ultrasound vs. 14.1% if no activity was documented.[79] That said, the rate of survival to hospital discharge remained abysmal, with a survival rate of only 3.8% in those patients with cardiac activity on ultrasound. They did note, however, that their reported rate of overall survival was greater than previously reported studies, likely owing to identification of secondary causes for the arrest (i.e. pericardiocentesis for tamponade or thrombolysis for pulmonary embolism). The cohort of patients who had an identifiable cause for their arrest had improved survival (15.4% vs. 1.3%). Importantly, nearly 10% of patients thought to have asystole had cardiac activity on ultrasound, comparable to other studies.

How about PEA arrest? Gaspari, et al. also assessed patients receiving at least 1 round of ACLS in those who presented with PEA, finding only 0.6% of those without cardiac activity by ultrasound survived to hospital discharge vs. 3.8% of those with cardiac activity.[79] The study excluded those with a shockable rhythm, had ROSC, or had termination of resuscitative efforts immediately after the ultrasound. More specifically, in patients with asystole and lack of cardiac activity on ultrasound, the sensitivity was 90% and positive predictive value for non-survival to hospital discharge was 99%.

Cutting edge: On the forefront of cardiac arrest management is the use of transesophageal echocardiography (TEE). In a proof of concept article by Blaivas, six cases were presented in which TEE led to a change in management in each case (i.e. diagnosis of aortic dissection, thrombus, etc.).[80] Use of TEE provides better image resolution to diagnose causes for the arrest, allows assessment for adequacy of compressions, and helps guide hemodynamic management.[81]

Take home: While US can identify alternative etiologies causative to the arrest, termination of resuscitative efforts should include other factors, such as medical comorbidities and events leading up to the arrest. If the initial rhythm is asystole and there is no cardiac activity on US, the prognosis is extremely poor.[82, 83]

Q#3: Is it helpful to speak with family/friends *during* the code, or should the code be called and then family/friends informed?

The decision to include family members during a code is complex; whereas, most studies report no difference in patient outcomes, some report a deleterious effect of family presence.[84-88] The positive or negative impact on family members has also been variable, though most studies point towards benefits for families.[86-88] The problem with these studies is that most rely on opinion surveys of families and health professionals. A reasonable approach is to develop a policy that allows family the option to be present during the resuscitation. This should include trained support staff who are able to explain activities taking place during the resuscitation, provide emotional/spiritual support, and answer questions.

Q#4: Which cutting edge interventions can be attempted?

Thrombolytics in cardiac arrest:

In general, patients with undifferentiated cardiac arrest *without* suspected pulmonary embolism are unlikely to benefit from administration of thrombolytics, and their use cannot be recommended.[89,90] That said, benefit can be seen in the select population presenting with a high likelihood of massive pulmonary embolism (PE) as the cause of their arrest.

The diagnosis of massive PE as the cause of a patient's cardiac arrest can be very difficult. The most common presenting rhythm is described as PEA, followed by asystole, and least commonly ventricular fibrillation.[91] To help make the diagnosis, one must rely on historical features of the presentation. Bedside ultrasound can be highly useful, looking for the presence of right ventricular dilation, cardiac thrombus, or proximal femoral DVT. Reported benefit is defined primarily in case reports and series, but we agree with the 2015 AHA guidelines and the evidence is compelling enough to use it on a case-by case-basis when massive PE is the known or suspected culprit for the arrest.[62, 92] Most commonly, a *50mg intravenous bolus dose of alteplase* is given over 2 minutes, and a repeat dose can be given after another 15 minutes if ROSC is not achieved. Alternatively, a single weight-based dose of tenecteplase can be given. After administration of a thrombolytic, it has been *recommended to allow another 15 to 30 minutes of ongoing chest compressions before considering further attempts at ROSC futile.*

In a study by Sharifi, et al. the authors reported ROSC occurred between 2 to 15 minutes after administration of tissue plasminogen activator (t-PA) in 22 of 23 patients with PEA arrest due to massive PE.[92] Of the initial 23 patients, 20 were still alive at follow-up and there were no reported major bleeding complications. Of note, the time from initiation of CPR to administration of t-PA in their study was 6.5 +/-2.1 minutes. These results are in stark contrast to a study by Abu-Laban, et al. that looked prospectively at 233 patients with PEA arrest of unknown or presumed cardiovascular cause given t-PA or placebo.[89] The rate of ROSC and survival were similar in both groups, and no beneficial effect of thrombolysis was noted.

Automatic compression devices:

There are two types available on the market: a load-distributing band that circumferentially squeezes the chest and a piston-based system that compresses the chest in an anteroposterior plane. The thought behind their utilization is that it theoretically allows providers to focus on other interventions, minimize chest compression interruptions, and removes the risk of compressor fatigue.

However, the data is mixed, and their use is probably best left to situations in which the clinical setting makes it difficult to perform quality or prolonged CPR.[93-95]

Extracorporeal life support (ECLS):
To date, study heterogeneity has made it difficult to define absolute indications and contraindications for ECLS as well as associated outcomes. However, in a systematic review of the literature of ECLS use in refractory cardiac arrest, the reported survival rate was 22%, with 13% having a good neurological recovery.[96] In a meta-analysis by Ouweneel, et al. use of ECLS increased 30-day survival by 13%, with a number needed to treat (NNT) of 7.7.[97] They also noted a higher rate of favorable neurological outcome at 30 days, with an absolute risk difference of 14% and NNT of 7.1. The overall indications for implementation of ECLS are broad, including respiratory failure, bridge to transplantation, refractory cardiogenic shock, massive PE, and cardiac arrest. In all instances, and especially in patients with cardiac arrest, patient selection is absolutely critical, with attention to factors that preclude an exit strategy (i.e. recovery, placement of a durable left ventricular assist device, etc.). Some general considerations and contraindications for those presenting with cardiac arrest include patients with an unrecoverable heart or are not a candidate for transplant or ventricular assist device support, metastatic malignancy, suspected aortic dissection, severe brain injury, unwitnessed cardiac arrest, or severe underlying comorbidities. Such patients are unlikely to meaningfully benefit from ECLS. Favorable outcomes have been associated with sustained VF/VT, younger age, witnessed arrest, implementation of bystander CPR, time from OHCA to ECLS, and diagnosis of acute coronary syndrome.[98] In the case we describe, the patient was in PEA arrest with a prolonged downtime, and he would be a very poor candidate for ECLS.

Interposed mid-abdominal compressions (IAC-CPR):
Two-compressor CPR using interposed mid-abdominal compressions during application of external chest compressions has been described. By and large, most of the studies looking at efficacy of this technique have been in animals with mixed results. However, a few in-hospital studies reported an increased rate of ROSC and possible survival benefit.[99,100] That said, the technique remains unproven and we would not start using this technique without further studies to prove that it enhances patient outcomes.

What did the actual provider do?

MDM (02:33): Bedside US shows complete cardiac standstill with no motion.

ED course: The resus is not going well, and staff now is giving the indication that they have other patients to care for and want to stop the code. You order another round of epi, and the charge nurse says, "Do you *really* think that will be helpful?" In your mind, you know that it will not, but the girlfriend is at bedside and the patient is young. Is it time to call the code? You arrive at decision point C:

DECISION POINT C – YOU ARE FACED WITH 3 QUESTIONS:

1. **What is the next step?**
2. **Is there a role for ED extracorporeal life support (ECLS)?**
3. **Can we call the code *now*?**

Q#1: What is the next step?

Before calling a code of a patient in PEA arrest, run through the traditional **"H's"** (hypovolemia, hypoxia, hydrogen ion (acidosis), hypo/hyperkalemia, hypoglycemia, hypothermia) and **"T's"** (toxins, tamponade (pericardial), tension pneumothorax, thrombosis (coronary, pulmonary), trauma). We agree with the provider's decision to recheck the patient's blood glucose level after dextrose administration, as hypoglycemia is an easily treatable cause of altered mental status and even cardiac arrest.

Regarding epinephrine, early use in those with an initial shockable rhythm may be associated with harm. In a study by Andersen, et al. early administration of epinephrine in patients with an initial shockable rhythm (within 2 minutes of the *first* attempted defibrillation) was associated with decreased odds of survival to hospital discharge, decreased odds of ROSC, and decreased survival to hospital discharge with a good functional outcome.[101] Most of our patients, however, present by EMS and are given epinephrine prior to arrival.

So, what benefit do we get with epinephrine? The data is poor, with most studies showing improved ROSC, but either no difference or worse impact on overall survival to discharge or good neurological outcomes regardless of the presenting rhythm.[102, 103] Some data suggests that the dosing intervals for epinephrine should be lengthened as it provides improved survival, at least for in-hospital cardiac arrest.[104] This ultimately may lead us to a time when we titrate our vasopressor use in cardiac arrest to target coronary perfusion pressure. Until then, however, we recommend the standard epinephrine dosing in cardiac arrest as per ACLS guidelines, realizing that this could potentially change in the future. The same goes for utilization of other ACLS medications, such as amiodarone and lidocaine, as none have been shown to improve long-term patient outcomes.

What about patients in refractory VT/VF? Besides standard ACLS guideline management, the use of double sequential defibrillation has been suggested as a means of managing refractory VT/VF. Multiple case reports have demonstrated ROSC only after double sequential defibrillation was applied, theoretically by enhancing the amount of energy delivered.[105, 106] Similarly, esmolol has been used successfully in refractory VT/VF to obtain sustained ROSC, as has its use in conjunction with double sequential defibrillation with some success.[107, 108]

Q#2: Is there a role for ED extracorporeal life support (ECLS)?

ECLS is best implemented at centers with high volume and adequate resources, but prehospital mobile units have also been described.[109] General indications for ECLS can be divided into three main categories: cardiac support, respiratory support, other.[110-112]

(Tables on next page...)

Table 5. Indications for ECLS

Indications
Cardiac support
Refractory cardiac arrest*
Refractory cardiogenic shock
Massive pulmonary embolism with cardiogenic shock
Bridge to cardiac transplant or ventricular assist device
Respiratory support
Severe hypoxemic respiratory failure
Severe hypercapnic respiratory failure
Bridge to lung transplant
Other
Profound hypothermia
Drug intoxication

** Refractory cardiac arrest has been defined as the absence of ROSC despite adequate CPR for > 10 minutes*

In the ED, there is sparse literature for patient selection. Prior studies have focused on inclusion and exclusion criteria and are listed in Table 6.[113-114]

Table 6. General inclusion and exclusion criteria for initiation for ECLS

Inclusion criteria	Exclusion criteria
Refractory cardiopulmonary arrest*	Initial rhythm asystole
Refractory cardiogenic shock	Initial non-shockable rhythm
	No CPR within 10 minutes of the arrest
	EMS transport time >10 minutes
	Total arrest time >60 minutes
	Non-cardiac origin of arrest (e.g. sepsis, trauma, etc.)
	Pre-existing severe neurological disease (e.g. stroke, dementia, etc.)
	Advanced age >75

**Typically, VT/VF as the presenting rhythm or initial shockable rhythm*

Placing a patient on ECLS who has an irreversible cause for their arrest or is past the point of salvage can lead to difficult ethical scenarios, especially in those without the hope for recovery or eligible for more advanced therapies (e.g. ventricular assist device) as an exit strategy. In the case presented, we would not consider this patient an ECLS candidate based on multiple factors, including his initial non-shockable rhythm and the prolonged duration of CPR.

Q#3: Can we call the code *now*?

The decision to terminate CPR is difficult and is highly variable depending on the scenario. Unfortunately, there are no evidence-based guidelines regarding when to terminate, and unvalidated rules such as terminating CPR if the patient is asystolic for more than 20 minutes in the absence of a reversible cause excludes some patients who would otherwise survive.

Regarding OHCA, American Heart Association Guidelines recommend termination of resuscitation if all of the following criteria are met:[115]

- Arrest not witnessed by emergency medical services personnel
- No return of spontaneous circulation prior to transport
- No AED shock was delivered prior to transport

Once the patient arrives to the hospital with ongoing resuscitative efforts, getting a thorough history of the patient's baseline functionality, medical comorbidities, and events leading up to the arrest can provide us with prognostic information. Factors associated with a failure to survive to discharge include advanced age, malignancy, poor baseline neurologic or functional status, baseline renal failure, pneumonia, acute stroke, septicemia, respiratory insufficiency, and major trauma.[116] Factors associated with survival include witnessed arrest, initial shockable rhythm, ROSC within 10 minutes of CPR, and proper CPR administration (i.e. compression rate, compression depth, full recoil of the chest with compressions, minimization of interruptions of chest compressions, avoidance of excessive ventilation, etc.).

However, none of the aforementioned factors can independently guide the termination decision.

The European Resuscitation Council Guidelines for Resuscitation state that providers should consider withholding or withdrawing CPR in the following scenarios:[117]

- The safety of the provider can no longer be sufficiently assured.
- There is obvious mortal injury or irreversible death.
- A valid and relevant advance directive becomes available.
- There is other strong evidence that further CPR would be against the patient's values and preferences or is considered "futile."
- Asystole for more than 20 minutes despite ongoing advanced life support in the absence of a reversible cause.

The document discusses prior studies looking at predictors of a poor outcome, including advanced age, presence of organ failure, malignancy, and admission from a nursing home with a low cerebral performance score. Better outcomes are associated with lack of comorbidities, presence of a shockable rhythm, and myocardial infarction, indicating a reversible cause. The authors specifically state that decisions to end resuscitative efforts should not be made on a single variable, such as patient age, and that resuscitation should be continued as long as VT/VF persists.

The American Heart Association Guideline is similarly vague overall, but it does mention the use of $ETCO_2$ as potentially helpful in determining futility. In particular, in intubated patients, failure to achieve an $ETCO_2 > 10$mmHg by waveform capnography after 20 minutes of high-quality CPR can be used as a component in a multimodal approach to terminating resuscitative efforts. Torke, et al. proposed the mnemonic CEASE (clinical features, effectiveness, ask, stop, explain) to help incorporate all the factors that should be considered.[116] When resuscitative efforts are prolonged or deemed futile, the decision to terminate resuscitative efforts should be made by the physician. It is unacceptable to place this decision on a grieving family.

Poor long-term neurological outcomes, defined as cerebral performance score 3–5 at 6 months, are associated with advanced age, arrest occurring at home, initial rhythm other than VF/VT, longer duration of CPR, treatment with epinephrine, absence of corneal and pupillary reflexes, a GCS motor score of 1, lower pH and arterial $PaCO_2 < 4.5$kPa (33mmHg)[118] Age does have a significant impact on overall outcomes, as previously discussed. This is partially related to pre-existing comorbidities, and younger patients are more likely to have reversible cause of arrest, including congenital conditions leading to a shockable dysrhythmia. Pediatric patients are more likely to have a respiratory cause to their arrest. In the end, the decision to terminate resuscitation should be as objective as possible. While younger age may make us more determined to continue resuscitative efforts for a longer duration, age by itself should not be used independently to continue or cease ongoing resuscitative efforts.

MDM (02:51): After several rounds of CPR pulse checks epinephrine bicarbonate and a cardiac standstill the code was deemed futile and the code was called. Time of death 02:47.

Critical Care Time: 31 minutes of critical care time. this included the entire code multiple meds and discussing with girlfriend and family.

Procedure: Bedside cardiac ultrasound showed no cardiac activity.

Diagnosis: Cardiac arrest, heroin overdose.

The code is called—what now? While heroin overdose is certainly a possibility in this instance, answers are best left to those handling the post-mortem autopsy if requested by the family. As with all deaths in the ED, the best course of action is to approach the family with sympathy and empathy rather than speculation and accusation. Sit with the family. Answer questions while avoiding medical jargon. Offer religious support when appropriate and ask if they would like to see their loved one. Offer to make calls to other family members and update the primary care physician. While this may take some time, it can make all the difference.

Chapter summary: While increasing numbers of patients with opiate-related illnesses and drug-seeking behaviors are presenting to our EDs, that does not preclude other illness in addicted patients. Multiple complaints should be addressed in turn. Special consideration should be paid to potential sequelae of illicit drug use, including febrile patients who may have a wide array of both unrelated and related underlying serious bacterial infections. Resuscitative efforts should keep in mind all potential etiologies for an arrest, both related and unrelated to opiates. We should not allow a patient's addiction history to cloud our judgment into the diagnostic evaluation, and instead, treat these populations with sincerity, empathy, and thoughtfulness.

References:

1. Rudd RA, Aleshire N, Zibbell JE, et al. Increases in drug and opioid overdose deaths -United States, 2000-2014. MMWR Morb Mortal Wkly Rep 2016;64(50-51):1378-82.
2. O'Donnell JK, Gladden RM, Seth P. Trends in deaths involving heroin and synthetic opioids excluding methadone, and law enforcement drug product reports, by Census Region - United

States, 2006-2015. MMWR Morb Mortal Wkly Rep 2017;66(34):897-903.
3. Barnett ML, Olenski AR, Jena AB. Opioid-prescribing patterns of emergency physicians and risk of long-term use. N Engl J Med 2017;376(19):1896.
4. Patel PR, Quinn JV. Syncope: A review of emergency department management and disposition. Clin Exp Emerg Med 2015;2(2):67-74.
5. Walsh K, Hoffmayer K, Hamdan MH. Syncope: Diagnosis and management. Curr Probl Cardiol 2015;40(2):51-86.
6. Quinn JV. Syncope and presyncope: Same mechanism, causes, and concern. Ann Emerg Med 2015;65(3):277-8.
7. Thiruganasambandamoorthy V, Stiell I, Wells GA, et al. Outcomes in presyncope patients: A prospective cohort study. Ann Emerg Med 2015;65(3):268-76.
8. Quinn JV. Yield of diagnostic tests in evaluating syncopal episodes in older patients -Invited commentary. Arch Intern Med 2009;169(14):1305-6.
9. Patel PR, Quinn JV. Syncope: A review of emergency department management and disposition. Clin Exp Emerg Med 2015;2(2):67-74.
10. Soteriades ES, Evans JC, Larson MG, et al. Incidence and prognosis of syncope. N Engl J Med 2002;347(12):878-85.
11. Zaidi A, Clough P, Cooper P, et al. Misdiagnosis of epilepsy: Many seizure-like attacks have a cardiovascular cause. J Am Coll Cardiol 2000;36(1):181-4.
12. Huff JS, Decker, WW, Quinn JV, et al. Clinical policy: Critical issues in the evaluation and management of adult patients presenting to the emergency department with syncope. Ann Emerg Med 2007;49(4):431-44.
13. Krahn AD, Klein GJ, Yee R, et al. Predictive value of presyncope in patients monitored for assessment of syncope. Am Heart J 2001;141(5):817-21.
14. Grossman SA, Chiu D, Lipsitz L, et al. Can elderly patients without risk factors be discharged home when presenting to the emergency department with syncope? Arch Gerontol Geriatr 2014;58(1):110-4.
15. D'Ascenzo F, Biondi-Zoccai G, Reed MJ. Incidence, etiology and predictors of adverse outcomes in 43,315 patients presenting to the emergency department with syncope: An international meta-analysis. Int J Cardiol 2013;167(1):57-62.
16. Saccilotto RT, Nickel CH, Bucher HC, et al. San Francisco Syncope Rule to predict short-term serious outcomes: A systematic review. CMAJ 2011 Oct 18;183(15):E1116-26.
17. Schladenhaufen R, Feilinger S, Pollack M, et al. Application of San Francisco Syncope Rule in elderly ED patients. Am J Emerg Med 2008;26(7):773-8.
18. Costantino G, Solbiati M, Casazza G, et al. Usefulness of n-terminal pro-b-type natriuretic peptide increases as a marker for cardiac arrhythmia in patients with syncope. Am J Cardiol 2014;113(1):98-102.
19. Costantino G, Casazza G, Reed M, et al. Syncope risk stratification tools versus clinical judgment: An individual patient data meta-analysis. Am J Med 2014;127(11):1126.e13-25.
20. Task Force for the Diagnosis and Management of Syncope, European Society of Cardiology (ESC), European Heart Rhythm Association (EHRA), Heart Failure Association (HFA), Heart Rhythm Society (HRS), Moya A, Sutton R, Ammirati F, et al. Guidelines for the diagnosis and management of syncope (version 2009). Eur Heart J 2009;30(21):2631
21. Quinn J, McDermott D. Electrocardiogram findings in emergency department patients with syncope. Ann Emerg Med 2011;18(7):714.

22. Shen WK, SHeldon RS, Benditt DG, et al. 2017 ACC/AHA/HRS Guideline for the evaluation and management of patients with syncope: A report of the American College of Cardiology/American Heart Association task force on clinical practice guidelines, and the Heart Rhythm Society. J Am Coll Cardiol 2017;70(5):e39-e110.
23. Andersen LW, Grandfeldt A, Callaway CW, et al. Association between tracheal intubation during adult in-hospital cardiac arrest and survival. JAMA 2017;317(5):494-06.
24. Andersen LW, Raymond TT, Berg RA, et al. Association between tracheal intubation during pediatric in-hospital cardiac arrest and survival. JAMA 2016;316(17):1786-97.
25. Jeong S, Ahn KO, Shin SD. The role of prehospital advanced airway management on outcomes for out-of-hospital cardiac arrest patients: A meta-analysis. Am J Emerg Med 2016;34(11):2101-6.
26. Hasegawa K, Hiraide A, Chang Y, Brown DF. Association of prehospital advanced airway management with neurologic outcome and survival in patients with out-of-hospital cardiac arrest. JAMA 2013;309(3):257-66.
27. Bair AE, Smith D, Lichty L. Intubation confirmation techniques associated with unrecognized non-tracheal intubations by pre-hospital providers. J Emerg Med 2005;28(4):403.
28. Grmec S. Comparison of three different methods to confirm tracheal tube placement in emergency intubation. Intensive Care Med 2002;28(6):701-04.
29. Bozeman WP, Hexter D, Liang HK, et al. Esophageal detector device versus detection of end-tidal carbon dioxide level in emergency intubation. Ann Emerg Med 1996;27(5):595-9.
30. Li J. Capnography alone is imperfect for endotracheal tube placement confirmation during emergency intubation. J Emerg Med 2001;20(3):223-9.
31. Das SK, Choupoo NS, Haldar R, et al. Transtracheal ultrasound for verification of endotracheal tube placement: A systematic review and meta-analysis. Can J Anaesth 2015;62(4):413-23.
32. Adi O, Chuan TW, Rishya M. A feasibility study on bedside upper airway ultrasonography compared to waveform capnography for verifying endotracheal tube location after intubation. Crit Ultrasound J 2013;5(1):7.
33. Luck RP, Haines C, Mull CC. Intraosseous access. J Emerg Med 2010;39(4):468-75.
34. Banerjee S, Singhi SC, Singh S, et al. The intraosseous route is a suitable alternative to intravenous route for fluid resuscitation in severely dehydrated children. Indian Pediatr 1994;31(12):1511.
35. Glaeser PW, Hellmich TR, Szewczuga D, et al. Five-year experience in prehospital intraosseous infusions in children and adults. Ann Emerg Med 1993;22(7):1119-24.
36. Reades R, Studnek JR, Vandeventer S, et al. Intraosseous versus vascular access during out-of-hospital cardiac arrest: A randomized controlled trial. Ann Emerg Med 2011;58(6):509-16.
37. Leidel BA, Kirchhoff C, Bogner V, et al. Is the intraosseous access route fast and efficacious compared to conventional central venous catheterization in adult patients under resuscitation in the emergency department? A prospective observational pilot study. Patient Saf Surg 2009;3(1):24.
38. Lewis GC. Critical skills and procedures in emergency medicine: vascular access skills and procedures. Emerg Med Clin North Am 2013;31(1):59-86.
39. Miller L, Kramer GC, Bolleter S. Rescue access made easy. JEMS 2005;30(10):suppl 8.

40. Hodge D 3rd. Intraosseous infusions: A review. Pediatr Emerg Care 1985;1(4):215-8.
41. Hallstrom A, Rea TD, Sayre MR, et al. Manual chest compression vs use of an automated chest compression device during resuscitation following out-of-hospital cardiac arrest: A randomized trial. JAMA 2006;295(22):2620-8.
42. Hock Ong ME, Fook-Chong S, Annaturai A, et al. Improved neurologically intact survival with the use of an automated, load-distributing band chest compression device for cardiac arrest presenting to the emergency department. Crit Care 2012;16(4):R144.
43. Brooks SC, Hassan N, Bigham BL, et al. Mechanical versus manual chest compressions for cardiac arrest. Cochrane Database Syst Rev 2014;(2):CD007260.
44. Paradis NA, Martin GB, Rivers EP, et al. Coronary perfusion pressure and the return of spontaneous circulation in human cardiopulmonary resuscitation. JAMA 1990;263(8):1106-13.
45. Reynolds JC, Salcido DD, Menegazzi JJ. Coronary perfusion pressure and return of spontaneous circulation after prolonged cardiac arrest. Prehosp Emerg Care 2010;14(1):78-84.
46. Sutton RM, Friess SH, Naim, et al. Patient-centric blood pressure-targeted cardiopulmonary resuscitation improves survival from cardiac arrest. Am J Respir Crit Care Med 2014;190(11):1255-62.
47. Naim YM, Sutton RM, Friess SH, et al. Blood pressure and coronary perfusion pressure-targeted cardiopulmonary resuscitation improves 24-hour survival from ventricular fibrillation cardiac arrest. Crit Care Med 2016;44(11):e1111-e17.
48. Hilty WM, Hudson PA, Levitt MA, et al. Real-time ultrasound-guided femoral vein catheterization during cardiopulmonary resuscitation. Ann Emerg Med 1997;29(3):331-6
49. Pernat A, Weil MH, Sun S, et al. Stroke volumes and end-tidal carbon dioxide generated by precordial compressions during ventricular fibrillation. Crit Care Med 2003;31(6)1819-23.
50. Hartmann SM, Farris RW, Di Gennaro JL, Robers JS. Systematic review and meta-analysis of end-tidal carbon dioxide values associated with return of spontaneous circulation during cardiopulmonary resuscitation. J Intensive Care Med 2015;30(7):426-35.
51. Pokorna M, Necas E, Kratochvil J, et al. A sudden increase in partial pressure end-tidal carbon dioxide (P(ET)CO(2) at the moment of return of spontaneous circulation. J Emerg Med 2010;38(5):614-21.
52. RL Levine, MA Wayne, CL Miller. End-tidal carbon dioxide and outcome of out of hospital cardiac arrest. N Engl J Med 1997;337(5):301-6.
53. Touma O, Davies M. The prognostic value of end tidal carbon dioxide during cardiac arrest: a systematic review. Resuscitation 2013;84(11):1470-9.
54. Huis In 't Veld MA, Allison MG, Bbostick DS, et al. Ultrasound use during cardiopulmonary resuscitation is associated with delays in chest compressions. Resuscitation 2017;119:95-8.
55. Tsou PY, Kurbedin J, Chen YS, et al. Accuracy of point-of-care focused echocardiography in predicting outcome of resuscitation in cardiac arrest patients: A systematic review and meta-analysis. Resuscitation 2017;114:92-9.
56. Blaivas M. Transesophageal echocardiography during cardiopulmonary arrest in the emergency department. Resuscitation 2008;78(2):135-40.
57. Singer AJ, Nguyen RT, Ravishankar ST, et al. Cerebral oximetry versus end tidal CO2 in predicting ROSC after cardiac arrest. Am J Emerg Med 2018;36(3):403-07.

58. Sporer KA, Dorn E. Heroin-related noncardiogenic pulmonary edema: A case series. Chest 2001;120(5):1628-32.
59. Horng HC, Ho MT, Huang CH, et al. Negative pressure pulmonary edema following naloxone administration in patients with fentanyl-induced respiratory depression. Acta Anaesthesiol Taiwan 2010;48(3):155-7.
60. Lemyze M, Mallat J. Understanding negative pressure pulmonary edema. Intensive Care Med 2014;40(8):1140-3.
61. Kang DH, Kim J, Rhee JE, et al. The risk factors and prognostic implications of acute pulmonary edema in resuscitated cardiac arrest patients. Clin Exp Emerg Med 2015;2(2):110-6.
62. Lavonas EJ, Drennan IR, Gabrielli A, et al. Part 10: Special circumstances of resuscitation: 2015 American Heart Association guidelines update for cardiopulmonary resuscitation and emergency cardiovascular care. Circulation 2015;132(18 suppl 2):S501-S18.
63. Reno CM, Daphna-Iken D, Chen YS, et al. Severe hypoglycemia-induced lethal cardiac arrhythmias are mediated by sympathoadrenal activation. Diabetes 2013;62(10):3570-81.
64. Sanon VP, Sanon S, Kanakia R, et al. Hypoglycemia from a cardiologist's perspective. Clin Cardiol 2014;37(8):499-04.
65. Peng TJ, Andersen LW, Saindon BZ, et al. The administration of dextrose during in-hospital cardiac arrest is associated with increased mortality and neurologic morbidity. Crit Care 2015;19:160.
66. Faskowitz AJ, Kramskiy VN, Pasternak GW. Methadone-induced hypoglycemia. Cell Mol Neurobiol 2013;33(4):537-42.
67. Allison MG, Mallemat HA. Emergency care of patients with pacemakers and defibrillators. Emerg Med Clin North Am 2015;33(3):653-7.
68. Bernstein AD, Daubert JC, Fletcher RD, et al. The revised NASPE/BPEG generic code for antibradycardia, adaptive-rate, and multisite pacing. North American Society of Pacing and Electrophysiology/British Pacing and Electrophysiology Group. Pacing Clin Electrophysiol 2002;25:260-4.
69. Russo AM, Stainback RF, Bailey SR, et al.ACCF/HRS/AHA/ASE/HFSA/SCAI/SCCT/SCMR 2013 appropriate use criteria for implantable cardioverter-defibrillators and cardiac resynchronization therapy: A report of the American College of Cardiology Foundation appropriate use criteria task force, Heart Rhythm Society, American Heart Association, American Society of Echocardiography, Heart Failure Society of America, Society for Cardiovascular Angiography and Interventions, Society of Cardiovascular Computed Tomography, and Society for Cardiovascular Magnetic Resonance. J Am Coll Cardiol 2013;61(12):1318-68.
70. Makaryus AN, Patrick C, Maccaro P. A rare case of "runaway" pacemaker in a modern CPU-controlled pacemaker. Pacing Clin Electrophysiol 2005;28(9):993-6.
71. Braunschweig F, Boriani G, Bauer A, et al. Management of patients receiving implantable cardiac defibrillator shocks: recommendations for acute and long-term patient management. Europace 2010;12:1673-90.
72. Pavia S, Wilkoff B. The management of surgical complications of pacemaker and implantable cardioverter-defibrillators. Curr Opin Cardiol 2001;16(1):66-71.
73. Morrison LJ, Verbeek PR, Zhan C, et al. Validation of universal prehospital termination of resuscitation clinical prediction rule for advanced and basic life support providers. Resuscitation 2009;80(3):324-8.

74. Drennan IR, Case E, Verbeek PR, et al. A comparison of the universal TOR Guideline to the absence of prehospital ROSC and duration of resuscitation in predicting futility from out-of-hospital cardiac arrest. Resuscitation 2017;111:96-02.
75. Kodali BS, Urman RD. Capnography during cardiopulmonary resuscitation: Current evidence and future directions. J Emerg Trauma Shock 2014;7(4):332-40.
76. Siao FY, Chiu CC, Chiu CW, et al. Managing cardiac arrest with refractory ventricular fibrillation in the emergency department: Conventional cardiopulmonary resuscitation versus extracorporeal cardiopulmonary resuscitation. Resuscitation 2015 Jul;92:70-6.
77. Youness H, Al Halabi T, Hussein H, et al. Review and outcome of prolonged cardiopulmonary resuscitation. Crit Care Res Pract 2016;2016:7384649.
78. Goldberger ZD, Chan PS, Berg RA, et al. Duration of resuscitation efforts and subsequent survival after in-hospital cardiac arrest. Lancet 2012;380(9852):1473-81.
79. Gaspari R, Weekes A, Adhikari S, et al. Emergency department point-of-care ultrasound in out-of-hospital and in-ED cardiac arrest. Resuscitation 2016;109:33-9.
80. Blaivas M. Transesophageal echocardiography during cardiopulmonary arrest in the emergency department. Resuscitation 2008;78(2):135-40.
81. Arntfield R, Pace J, Hewak M, Thompson D. Focused transesophageal echocardiography by emergency physicians is feasible and clinically influential: Observational results from a novel ultrasound program. J Emerg Med 2016;50(2):286-94.
82. Tsou PY, Kurbedin J, Chen YS, et al. Accuracy of point-of-care focused echocardiography in predicting outcome of resuscitation in cardiac arrest patients: A systematic review and meta-analysis. Resuscitation 2017;114:92-9.
83. Kim HB, Suh JY, Choi JH, et al. Can serial focused echocardiographic evaluation in life support (FEEL) predict resuscitation outcome or termination of resuscitation (TOR)? A pilot study. Resuscitation 2016;101:21-6.
84. Fernandez R, Compton S, Jones KA, et al. The presence of a family witness impacts physician performance during simulated medical codes. Crit Care Med 2009;37(6):1956-60.
85. Brasel KJ, Entwistle JW 3rd, Sade RM. Should family presence be allowed during cardiopulmonary resuscitation? Ann Thorac Surg 2016;102(5):1438-43.
86. Goldberger ZD, Nallamothu BK, Nichol G, et al. Policies allowing family presence during resuscitation and patterns of care during in-hospital cardiac arrest. Circ Cardiovasc Qual Outcomes 2015;8(3):226-34.
87. Jabre P, Belpomme V, Azoulay E, et al. Family presence during cardiopulmonary resuscitation. N Engl J Med 2013;368(11):1009-18.
88. Jabre P, Tazarourte K, Azoulay E, et al. Offering the opportunity for family to be present during cardiopulmonary resuscitation: 1-year assessment. Intensive Care Med 2014;40(7):981-7.
89. Abu-Laban RB, Christenson JM, Innes GD, et al. Tissue plasminogen activator in cardiac arrest with pulseless electrical activity. N Engl J Med 2002;346(20):1522.
90. Bottiger BW, Arntz HR, Chamberlain DA, et al. Thrombolysis during resuscitation for out-of-hospital cardiac arrest. N Engl J Med 2008;359(25):2651-62.
91. Kurkciyan I, Meron G, Sterz F, et al. Pulmonary embolism as a cause of cardiac arrest: Presentation and outcome. Arch Intern Med 2000;160(10):1529-35.
92. Sharifi M, Berger J, Beeston P, et al. Pulseless electrical activity in pulmonary embolism treated with thrombolysis (from the "PEAPETT" study). Am J Emerg Med 2016;34(10):1963.

93. Rubertsson S, Lindgren E, Smekal D, et al. Mechanical chest compressions and simultaneous defibrillation vs conventional cardiopulmonary resuscitation in out-of-hospital cardiac arrest: the LINC randomized trial. JAMA 2014;311(1):53-61.
94. Wik L, Olsen JA, Persse D, et al. Manual vs. integrated automatic load-distributing band CPR with qual survival after out of hospital cardiac arrest. The randomized CIRC trial. Resuscitation 2014;85(6):741-8.
95. Perkins GD, Lall R, Quinn T, et al. Mechanical versus manual chest compressions for out-of-hospital cardiac arrest (PARAMEDIC): A pragmatic, cluster randomized controlled trial. Lancet 2015;385(9972):947-55.
96. Ortega-Deballon I, Hornby L, Shemie SD, et al. Extracorporeal resuscitation for refractory out-of-hospital cardiac arrest in adults: A systematic review of international practices and outcomes. Resuscitation 2016;101:12-20.
97. Ouweneel DM, Schotborgh JV, Limpens J, et al. Extracorporeal life support during cardiac arrest and cardiogenic shock: A systematic review and meta-analysis. Intensive Care Med 2016;42(12):1922.
98. Tan BK. Extracorporeal membrane oxygenation in cardiac arrest. Singapore Med J 2017;58(7):446-8.
99. Sack JB, Kesselbrenner MB, Jarrad A. Interposed abdominal compression-cardiopulmonary resuscitation and resuscitation outcome during asystole and electromechanical dissociation. Circulation 1992;86(6):1692-700.
100. Sack JB, Kesselbrenner MB, Bregman D. Survival from in-hospital cardiac arrest with interposed abdominal counterpulsation during cardiopulmonary resuscitation. JAMA 1992;267(3):379-85.
101. Andersen LW, Kurth T, Chase M, et al. Early administration of epinephrine (adrenaline) in patients with cardiac arrest with initial shockable rhythm in hospital: Propensity score matched analysis. BMJ 2016;353:i1577.
102. Hagihara A, Hasegawa M, Abe T, et al. Prehospital epinephrine use and survival among patients with out-of-hospital cardiac arrest. JAMA 2012;307(11):1161-8.
103. Lin S, Callaway CW, Shah PS, et al. Adrenaline for out-of-hospital cardiac arrest resuscitation: A systematic review and meta-analysis of randomized controlled trials. Resuscitation 2014;85(6):732-40.
104. Warren SA, Huszti E, Bradley SM, et al. Adrenaline (epinephrine) dosing period and survival after in-hospital cardiac arrest: A retrospective review of prospectively collected data. Resuscitation 2014;85(3):350-8.
105. Merlin MA, Tagore A, Bauter R, et al. A case series of double sequence defibrillation. Prehosp Emerg Care 2016;20(4):550-3.
106. Cortez E, Krebs W, Davis J, et al. Use of double sequential external defibrillation for refractory ventricular fibrillation during out-of-hospital cardiac arrest. Resuscitation 2016;108:82-6.
107. Lee YH, Lee KJ, Min YH, et al. Refractory ventricular fibrillation treated with esmolol. Resuscitation 2016;107:150-5.
108. Boehm KM, Keyes DC, Mader LE, Moccia JM. First report of survival in refractory ventricular fibrillation after dual-axis defibrillation and esmolol administration. West J Emerg Med 2016;17(6):762-5.
109. Shah AS. Mobile extracorporeal membrane oxygenation: Lead, follow, or get out of the way. J Thorac Cardiovasc Surg 2017;153(6):1369-70.

110. Makdisi G, Wang I. Extra corporeal membrane oxygenation (ECMO) review of a lifesaving technology. J Thorac Dis 2015;7(7):E166-76.
111. ELSO guidelines for ECMO centers (updated March 2014). Available at: https://www.elso.org/Portals/0/IGD/Archive/FileManager/faf3f6a3c7cusersshyerdocumentselsoguidelinesecmocentersv1.8.pdf (Accessed on December 25, 2017).
112. Debaty G, Babaz V, Durand M, et al. Prognostic factors for extracorporeal cardiopulmonary resuscitation recipients following out-of-hospital refractory cardiac arrest. A systematic review and meta-analysis. Resuscitation 2017;112:1-10.
113. Bellezzo JM, Shinar Z, Davis DP, et al. Emergency physician-initiated extracorporeal cardiopulmonary resuscitation. Resuscitation 2012;83(8):966-70.
114. Sakamoto T, Morimura N, Nagao K, et al. Extracorporeal cardiopulmonary resuscitation versus conventional cardiopulmonary resuscitation in adults with out-of-hospital cardiac arrest: a prospective observational study. Resuscitation 2014;85(6):762-8.
115. Mancini ME, Diekema DS, et al. Part 3: Ethical Issues: 2015 American Heart Association guidelines update for cardiopulmonary resuscitation and emergency cardiovascular care. Circulation 2015;132(18 Suppl 2):S383-96.
116. Torke AM, Bledsoe P, Wocial LD, et al. CEASE: A guide for clinicians on how to stop resuscitation efforts. Ann Am Thorac Soc 2015;12(3):440-5.
117. Bossaert LL, Perkins GD, Askitopoulou, et al. European Resuscitation Council guidelines for resuscitation 2015 Section 11. The ethics of resuscitation and end-of-life decisions. Resuscitation 2015;95:302-11.
118. Martinell L, Nielsen N, Herlitz J, et al. Early predictors of poor outcome after out-of-hospital cardiac arrest. Crit Care 2017;21(1):96.

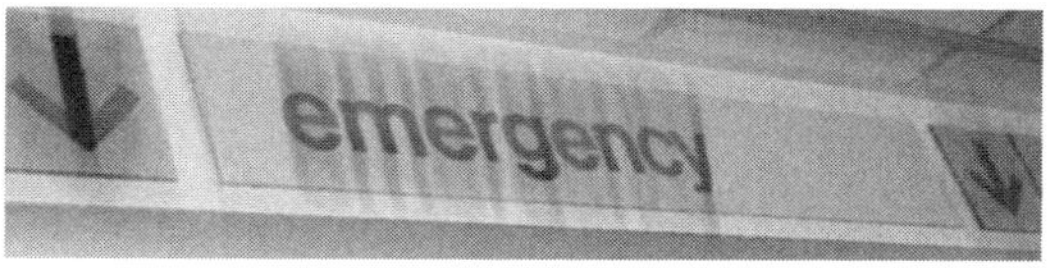

SECTION D – DRUGS & DELIRIUM

Chapter 19: A 52-year-old alcoholic man with chest pain

Heath Jolliff, DO
Program Director Adena Emergency Residency
Double boarded Emergency Medicine and Toxicology
Chillicothe, OH

Robert Sim Culley IV, DO
Attending Emergency Physician
Riverside Tappahannock Hospital
Spotsylvania Regional Medical Center
Fredericksburg, VA

Julie Lynn Hughett, MSN, CNL, CCRN
Nurse practitioner
Mt. Carmel Health Systems
Columbus, OH

Section editor:
Michael Winters, MD, MBA, FACEP, FAAEM
Professor
Emergency Medicine and Medicine
Vice Chair for Clinical and Administrative Affairs
Department of Emergency Medicine
University of Maryland School of Medicine
Baltimore, MD

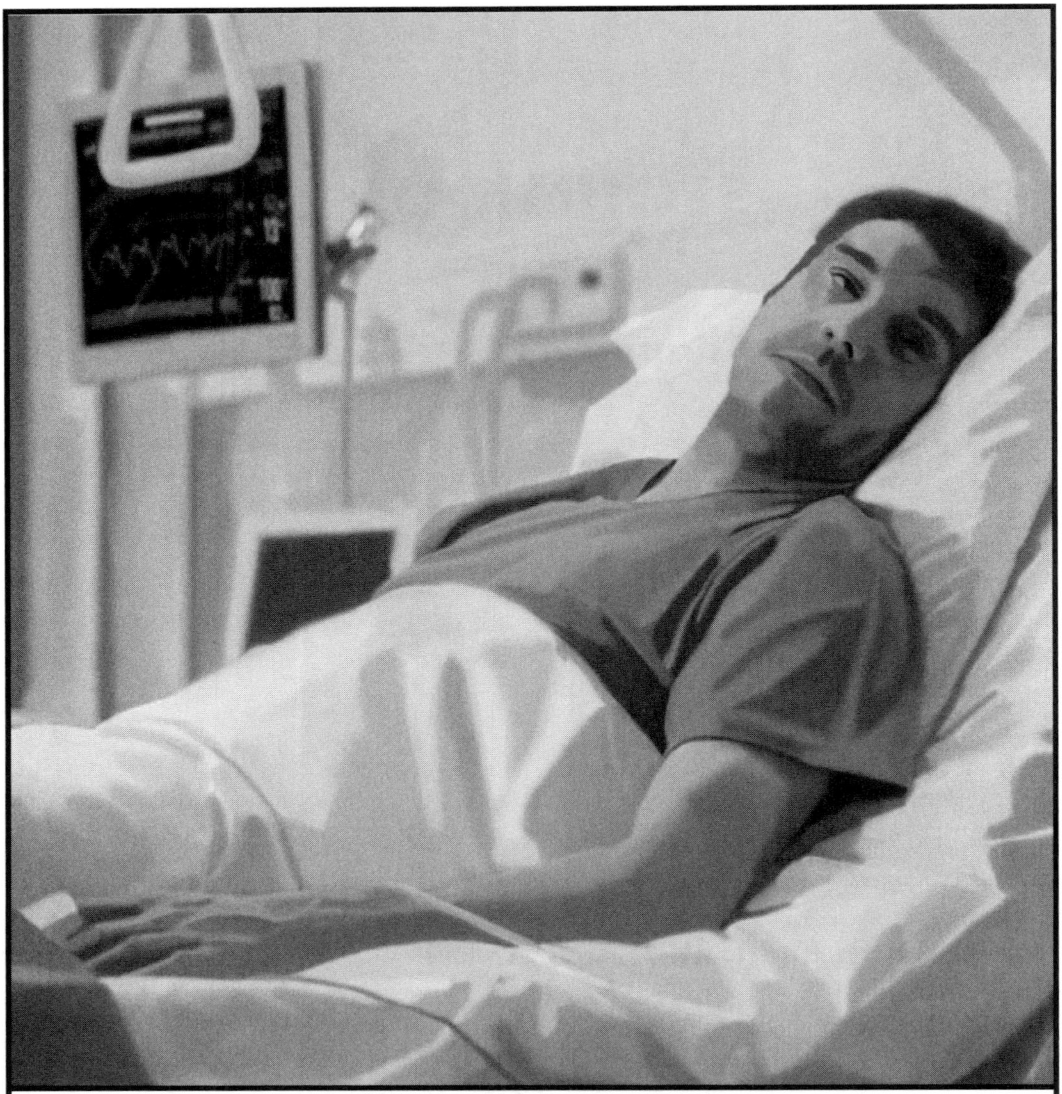

"I'M STARTING TO SEE PURPLE ELEPHANTS."

SECTION D/CHAPTER 19

A 52-year-old alcoholic man with chest pain

The patient's story:
Matt Eberling is a 52-year-old man with three adult children, separated from his wife for the last five years. He currently lives with his brother, staying in a spare room which was sectioned off the garage. He has not worked in years.

Matt has used alcohol and drugs through much of his life, starting in adolescence. Despite his health problems including coronary artery disease, congestive heart failure (CHF), and the recent placement of an AICD, he continues to struggle with cocaine and alcohol.

On June 30 he is admitted for shortness of breath and bilateral leg swelling. Labs on admission are significant for hypoalbuminemia, hypokalemia, hypomagnesemia, anemia, azotemia, and BALg/dL. He is discharged the next morning with a diagnosis of CHF exacerbation, deconditioning, and medication noncompliance with recommendations to stop drinking and to take his furosemide as scheduled.

Several weeks later his symptoms begin to return including leg swelling to the point of pain with ambulation. When he tells his brother's wife that he has chest pain, she dials 911.

ED BOUNCEBACK

HPI (09:25): The patient is a 52 y/o AAM with a PMH significant for COPD, CAD, AICD placement, HTN, anxiety, CHF, polysubstance abuse including cocaine, and chronic alcoholism. He drinks 1 to 2 pints of moonshine daily. He presents today with a chief complaint of chest pain which began this morning and is sharp and constant. He initially stated this was new onset but further history reveals he has had similar pain in the past. He has minimal associated shortness of breath, but is unable to say if this is exertional as he has been in bed the last day or so. No radiation to the back. No pleuritic aspect. He has bilateral leg swelling and pain is improved after his hospital discharge almost 3 weeks ago, but has now returned. He sleeps on 3 pillows. No fever, vomiting, blood in the urine or stool, bruising, respiratory symptoms. He feels anxious.

Allergies: Codeine
Social history: + smoking, + alcohol, + cocaine – has not used for "a minute"
Family history: CAD, CVA
PMH: COPD, CAD, AICD placement, HTN
Medications: Metoprolol, furosemide, nitroglycerine, lisinopril, potassium, buspirone

PSH: Hernia, AICD, GSW

PE:

Vitals:

Time	Temp	Pulse	Resp	BP: Syst	BP: Diast	Sat
	98.2 (F)	123	22	167	92	93% (RA)

GA: Alert, speaking normally, extremities slightly tremulous
EYES: PER
CV: RRR wo m/r/g
RESP: CTAB wo wheezes, rales, rhonchi
ABD: Soft and non-tender throughout, abdominal striae, no r/r/g
SKIN: Normal except for facial telangiectasias and palmar erythema, no vesicles

TESTING (11:32):
CXR: Hyperexpanded lung fields secondary to COPD, no acute process
ECG: Sinus tachycardia with nonspecific ST changes
Labs: Point of care troponin negative 0.00

MDM (11:47): The patient was recently here and discharged so at this point we will admit and a second troponin is due to be checked in 2 hours. He does have a BNP level pending. Other labs pending. Cardio will be consulted. Awaiting call back from hospitalist.

IMPRESSION (10:43): Chest pain r/o MI, cocaine use, alcoholism

Section editor comments (Winters):

Though minor, the cardiovascular exam states "RRR" but the heart rate is documented at 123 beats per minute which is clearly tachycardic. From a medicolegal perspective, this can give the impression that the provider may not be attentive to documentation. In addition, there is no documentation of an extremity exam in a patient reporting bilateral lower extremity swelling.

Author comments (Weinstock):

Seems like an open and shut case... except... You sit down in front of the computer and call the hospitalist who says, "We are getting slammed. The hospital is full and there are 19 surgeries scheduled, so any bed which opens up will already be taken. I just don't know... You said he uses coke. What did the urine tox show?"
"How about the alcohol level?" she asks.
"Pending," you fib, and quickly click the order for an alcohol level and urine tox.
"Call me back when the second trop returns," she replies, hanging up before you have a chance to respond.

"Oh well, it won't matter anyway," you think, "we have 12 holding patients down here anyway. There is no way this guy is going to get a bed before the end of my shift."

ED course:
Additional labs return:

WBC count = 12.3 (H)
Hb = 9.2gm/dL (L)
Plt = 92thou/mcL (L)

Sodium = 128mmol/L (L)
Potassium = 3.1 (L)
Creatinine = 1.51 (H)
Bicarbonate = 21mmol/L (L)
Creatinine = 1.5mg/dL (H)
Glucose 151 (H)

INR = 1.50
Albumin=1.8 (L)
Magnesium=1.4 (L)

Repeat troponin – 0.00
BNP = 236

Author comments (Weinstock):

You are faced with a "stable" patient with a "chest pain r/o MI" admission. The troponin is negative, and the BNP is only minimally elevated, but not to the point where you have increased concern for a CHF exacerbation. You pick up the phone to call the hospitalist back, but anticipating resistance, entertain second thoughts. Trying to buy time you ask that the ECG be repeated, but it is identical. A recheck of the patient confirms that he has now had almost seven hours of constant pain. Does he really need to be admitted? What will be gained?

Why is this case in a critical care book? Well, stay tuned, one problem with holding patients in the ED is that they will get worse...

DECISION POINT A – YOU ARE FACED WITH 4 QUESTIONS:

1. **Does the history of cocaine use change the evaluation and management of patients with chest pain?**
2. **What is the utility of urine toxicology and blood alcohol screening in a known alcoholic and cocaine user?**
3. **Which physical exam and lab findings may be present in alcoholic patients?**
4. **Is admission indicated? What are the risks and benefits of admission?**

What does the literature say?

Q#1: Does the history of cocaine use change the evaluation and management of patients with chest pain?

Cocaine is a sympathomimetic drug that has known adverse effects on the cardiovascular system, with associated coronary and peripheral vasoconstriction and vasospasm, myocardial infarction, cardiac dysrhythmias, cardiac myopathies, accelerated atherosclerosis, and increased risk of aortic dissection.[1,2]

Our patient could be having acute chest pain due to vasospasm from recent use, though the history does not correlate with the timing, making it difficult to differentiate between association and causation. We do know that cocaine users have accelerated atherosclerosis; in addition, our patient does have a history of coronary artery disease, making his presentation more concerning.

Does the history of cocaine use increase his risk of acute coronary syndrome? On the surface, the easy answer is "yes," however, a retrospective study examined 363, 143 hospital admissions for chest pain and cocaine abuse between 2001 to 2012, with a mean age of 45 years, with 6.7% undergoing cardiac catheterizations. The surprising finding was that the rate of adverse events was low, in fact much lower than the average patient presenting to the ED with chest pain; acute MI frequency was 0.69%, in hospital mortality was 0.09%, and 0.22 underwent PCI.[3,4]

Author comments (Weinstock):

Will admission for evaluation of acute coronary syndrome (ACS) after a negative ED evaluation help this patient? If we say that his history is moderately concerning for ACS, we can calculate a HEART score of 5 (H=1, E=1, A=1, R=2, T=0).[5] However, his risk of an adverse cardiac event while hospitalized is low,[6] and there are risks to hospitalization,[7] not the least of which is alcohol withdrawal.

Q#2: What is the utility of urine toxicology and blood alcohol screening in a known alcoholic and cocaine user?

The urine drug of abuse screening test is *qualitative*, meaning that its results are positive or negative and do not give a specific drug level. In contradistinction, quantitative drug testing, such as a serum ethanol level, gives a specific level of the drug. A urine drug test can tell the clinician what drugs are present, but it does not tell the clinician if they are causing impairment. For example, the urine metabolites of many drugs may be detected longer than the drug remains in a person's blood stream and therefore beyond any period of potential impairment. Most drug screens include cannabinoid metabolites (marijuana), cocaine metabolites, opiate metabolites, amphetamines and phencyclidine. In addition, there are many false positive and false negatives associated with urine drug screening.

Urine drug of abuse screening in the Emergency Department is not likely to impact a clinician's management of the patient and should not be routinely ordered.[8]

With our patient's known risk factors of CAD and history of cocaine abuse, there is little utility in obtaining a screening test to only confirm that the patient has used cocaine in the past. The urine drug screen tests for the non-active metabolite benzoylecgonine, not cocaine itself; it may be present 3–5 days after cocaine use, which is well after the intoxicating effects have subsided.[9,10]

The hospitalist also asked for a blood alcohol level. In chronic alcoholics, it is thought that patients with a positive blood alcohol level may be protected from alcohol withdrawal symptoms. However, data are lacking to confirm this due to wide individual variability in alcohol metabolism.[11] Our patient was subsequently found to have an elevated alcohol level in the ED of 0.29g% (290mg/dL), though he was "alert, speaking normally" without any clear signs of intoxication documented. His baseline alcohol is unknown and therefore this "high" alcohol level may not be high for him and may not be protective in preventing withdrawal. Alcohol withdrawal can begin at any level; it is the decline in the level, usually within 6–8 hours of the last drink that causes the withdrawal.[12] Protocols to treat alcohol withdrawal are based upon signs and symptoms and not a blood alcohol level.[13]

Section editor comments (Winters):

This point cannot be overstated. Patients can still develop signs and symptoms of acute alcohol withdrawal even in the presence of a detectable alcohol level in the serum. Consider placing patients with alcohol history on withdrawal precautions early in their ED course. Once alcohol withdrawal symptoms begin, it may be very difficult to treat.

Q#3: Which physical exam and lab findings may be present in alcoholic patients?

- **Exam:** Findings include jaundice, spider hemangiomas and telangiectasias on the face or upper extremities. The abdomen may demonstrate ascites or caput medusa (painless, swollen blood vessels around the umbilicus), which can reflect collateral blood flow due to hepatic congestion. The extremities may have peripheral edema. The neurologic exam may reveal a resting tremor, alteration of mentation, or other signs of active intoxication such as ataxia and slurred speech.
- **Labs:** CBC may show mild anemia and thrombocytopenia. A chemistry may reveal hyponatremia and low albumin. Laboratory testing may reveal elevations in transaminases (AST > 2 times the ALT is common), elevated GGT and bilirubin. Coagulation testing will commonly demonstrate an elevation in PT and INR in the chronic alcoholic with liver damage.

Our patient has been experiencing bilateral lower extremity swelling thought to be from CHF, but could also be from his alcoholism, given the common finding of hypoalbuminemia. On exam, he is slightly tremulous and is found to have facial telangiectasias. Laboratory testing suggests chronic alcohol use with a hemoglobin of 9.2g/dL, platelet count of 92thou/mcL, sodium of 128mmol/L, albumin of 1.8, and INR of 1.50.

Q#4: Is admission indicated? What are the risks and benefits of admission?

The physician's concern was for ACS, but another consideration, especially for a patient who had been in bed for several days and with tachycardia is pulmonary embolism (PE), but application of the Wells Criteria[14] shows 1.5 points for the tachycardia but no other findings consistent with PE. He has a 1.3% risk of PE, revealing him to be a low risk patient; he should not be further evaluated for PE. Of note, the pulmonary embolism rule out criteria (PERC) rule cannot be used to exclude PE as he is tachycardic.[15]

Concern includes the patient's elevated risk of a major adverse cardiac event (MACE) as well as his tachycardia, hypertension, and hyperthermia, due to unknown etiology. These authors feel the patient should be admitted.

DECISION POINT A – ***What did the actual provider do?***

ED course (15:20): The hospitalist accepts the Pt. for admission. I was asked by the nurse to reassess the Pt and he is now slightly confused, tachypneic, and diaphoretic. Asks for something for his "nerves."

Vitals:

Time	Temp	Pulse	Resp	BP: Syst	BP: Diast	Sat
15:14	N/A	141	24	172	98	94% (RA)

DECISION POINT B – YOU ARE FACED WITH 3 QUESTIONS:

1. **What are the symptoms and signs of alcohol withdrawal and DT's?**
2. **What is The Clinical Institute Withdrawal Assessment of Alcohol Scale (CIWA-Ar) protocol?**
3. **Does the presence of alcohol withdrawal mandate an ICU admission?**

What does the literature say?

Q#1: What are the symptoms and signs of alcohol withdrawal and DT's?

Alcohol is a central nervous system (CNS) depressant due to its activation of the gamma-aminobutyric acid (GABA) receptors which in turn activates the inhibitory tone associated with these receptors. N-methyl-d-aspartate (NMDA) receptors are also activated by alcohol, and in chronic alcohol abuse they undergo a conformational change and subsequent up-regulation. When the chronic alcohol user discontinues alcohol suddenly, the inhibitory tone activated by the GABA receptors is reduced and the now up-regulated NMDA receptors cause pronounced excitatory effects on the CNS. This mechanism is the basis of treatment, as benzodiazepines are GABA agonists, which increase the inhibitory tone that was lost; they are the mainstay of alcohol withdrawal and delirium tremens (DT) management.

Withdrawal symptoms can vary in severity with symptoms typically beginning between 6–8 hours after the last drink. Signs and symptoms may include tachycardia, hypertension, anxiety, tremulousness, increased body temperature, nausea, vomiting, headache, diaphoresis.[8] Alcoholic hallucinations typically begin 12–24 hours after the last drink and may include auditory, visual and tactile hallucinations. These same patients maintain normal sensorium and are not altered.[9,16] Withdrawal seizures may appear 12–48 hours after the last drink and are often generalized tonic-clonic seizures that are short in duration with a brief postictal period.[11,17] Delirium tremens are alcohol withdrawal symptoms and altered mental status, which may manifest up to 3 days after initial withdrawal symptoms begin and include a disturbance in cognition combined with alcohol withdrawal symptoms. However, delirium can begin in as little as 8 hours after the last drink.[16,18]

Q#2: What is The Clinical Institute Withdrawal Assessment of Alcohol Scale (CIWA-Ar) protocol?

The CIWA-Ar protocol has been validated and is the best way to document the patient's symptoms and guide their therapy.[18] The scale scores the following items from 0 (no symptoms) to 7 (most severe symptoms). The last item, "orientation and clouding of sensorium," is scaled 0 to 4.

The entire scale ranges from 0–67. Scores less than 8 demonstrate mild alcohol withdrawal, 8–15 demonstrate moderate withdrawal, and more than 15 demonstrating severe alcohol withdrawal:[18]

- Nausea or vomiting
- Tremor
- Paroxysmal sweats
- Anxiety
- Tactile disturbances
- Auditory disturbances
- Visual disturbances
- Headache, sensation of headband
- Agitation

Orientation and clouding of sensorium:

- Mild symptoms: Patients rarely need medical intervention to control symptoms and are often safe to be discharged home.[18]
- Moderate symptoms: Patients will likely benefit from benzodiazepine therapy as withdrawal symptoms progress.[12]
- Severe symptoms: Patients often require admission to the intensive care unit (ICU) given the risk of decompensation, complications, and higher care needs.

Benzodiazepine dosing:

Numerous studies have failed to show a superior benzodiazepine.[11,16,18]

- Diazepam (IV) can begin with 10mg; onset is 1–5 minutes, with repeat dosing every 5–10 minutes.
- Lorazepam IV can begin with 2mg with onset at 5–20 minutes and repeat dosing every 15–20 minutes.
- Midazolam (IV) can begin with 2mg with an onset of 2–5 minutes and repeat dosing every 5–10 minutes.

Repeat and escalated dosing is often required; some advocate for repeating the same dose 2–3 times, then doubling the dose.[16] An illustrative example would be, three 2mg doses of lorazepam during the initial hour of treatment, then, if still symptomatic doubling the dose and considering repeating.

Given the high doses of benzodiazepines, the provider should remain cognizant of respiratory suppression and monitor with pulse oximetry and/or continuous waveform capnography. Benzodiazepines should not be withheld for alcohol withdrawal symptoms simply because the provider is unfamiliar with administering high doses of BDZs.

Medications for refractory withdrawal symptoms:

In severe or refractory alcohol withdrawal, propofol may be efficacious because it has a rapid onset and ease of titration but may require control of the airway. Phenobarbital acts on the same receptors and can have synergistic effects with benzodiazepines. Although difficult to titrate due to a long half-life, barbiturates are just as effective as benzodiazepines.[19] As with propofol, the patient's airway will need to be controlled and the patient will need to be admitted to the ICU.

Anti-psychotics have been used for agitation. However, but caution is needed as they do not act on GABA or NMDA receptors; therefore, the etiology of the symptoms is not being treated. Additionally, there is concern about prolongation of the QT interval and a lowering of the seizure threshold. Finally, antiepileptic agents and alpha-2 agonists (Dexmedetomidine) have demonstrated benefit to patients with alcohol withdrawal symptoms, but overall, they have either been not well-studied or have demonstrated no clear benefit over benzodiazepines.[20,21]

We recommend that because of the known benefits of benzodiazepines as well as the low cost, they remain the mainstay of management of alcohol withdrawal symptoms. Currently, it is not recommended to use antipsychotics, antiepileptics, or alpha-2 agonists.

Section editor comments (Winters):

When administering benzodiazepines for acute alcohol withdrawal, it may be tempting to initiate a continuous infusion rather than repeated bolus doses. A few small studies have examined this question and found less intubations, a shorter duration of mechanical ventilation, and a shorter ICU length of stay with the intermittent bolus dosing approach.[22] Ketamine may also be considered in the treatment of complicated alcohol withdrawal that fails to respond to benzodiazepines. However, the literature on ketamine for this indication is scant and it cannot be routinely recommended. Phenobarbital and propofol are the next best options for patients who fail to respond to benzodiazepines.

Q#3: Does the presence of alcohol withdrawal mandate an ICU admission?

Our patient has become newly confused, tachypneic, and diaphoretic; though we were lucky to have been made aware of his decompensation by the nurse, this situation illustrates the importance of re-examination.

At initial presentation, we can infer a CIWA score of 3 including points for anxiety and tremors. After the re-evaluation of the patient, we can infer a score of 14 points for tremor, sweating, anxiety, agitation, and disorientation. But first, consideration should be given to diagnoses which could be confused with alcohol withdrawal:

- Electrolyte abnormalities including hypoglycemia/hyperglycemia (DKA), hyponatremia, hypomagnesemia
- Toxic alcohol ingestions including ethylene glycol, methanol, isopropyl alcohol
- Co-ingestion of other substances including sympathomimetics, stimulants, antihistamines
- Head injury including epidural, subdural, subarachnoid hemorrhage
- Sepsis
- Wernicke's encephalopathy

With our lab evaluation and exam, we have been able to exclude many of these possibilities.

Consulting editor comments (Weingart):

The seizure in alcohol withdrawal is a weird thing because often these patients are not in florid withdrawal; maybe it's just been awhile since their last drink. They seize, and they're immediately awake again. This happens all the time, and we think, "Oh, they must be faking," then we consider, "Oh, no, they're a heavy alcoholic," and then we say, "OK, it's probably real." The rule we had from Bellevue Toxicology Center in New York City is if they seize, they get admitted, but these patients are fairly benign. I think they need to get admitted and watched in the hospital or a detoxification unit, but they generally just need a little bit of oral or IV benzodiazepine and they usually do fine.

DECISION POINT B – The ED course: ***What did the actual provider do?***

MDM (16:19): Ativan 2mg IVP, Pt. placed on cardiac monitor and pulse ox. Pt. is now lethargic and difficult to arouse with a heart rate of 151bpm. He is mumbling incoherently. Orders for Thiamine 100mg IM, folate 1mg PO, and Ativan 1mg IVP.

ED course: Overhead code called for room #19. Pt. found to be seizing.

DECISION POINT C – YOU ARE FACED WITH 2 QUESTIONS:

1. **Does the patient meet criteria for DT's?**
2. **How are alcohol withdrawal seizures/DT's treated? What "cutting edge" approaches can be tried for refractory seizure activity?**

What does the literature say?

Q#1: Does the patient meet criteria for DT's?

The change in mental status leads to the concern of the patient developing delirium tremens. Previous citations note a 35% mortality, with the potential to affect the 20% of men and 10% of women with an alcohol-abuse disorder.[18] Though the mortality of hospitalized patients has plummeted, currently at 1–4% mortality of hospitalized patients, it remains high on our differential.[12]

Using the DSM-5 criteria for withdrawal delirium, our patient does demonstrate behavior and signs consistent with acute alcohol withdrawal and delirium. He has a recent cessation of heavy and prolonged alcohol use, autonomic hyperactivity, nausea, psychomotor agitation, anxiety, disturbances in awareness without evidence of other neurocognitive disorders. The "Prediction of Alcohol Withdrawal Severity Scale" is a screening tool; if the score is greater than or equal to 4 (out of 10) this demonstrates a 100% sensitivity and specificity for developing moderate or severe alcohol withdrawal symptoms.[23,24]

Our physician did recognize the acute alcohol withdrawal and administered thiamine, folate, and a repeat dose of Ativan at 1mg IV, but the major concern is the dosing. With no response to 2mg Ativan given, the dose should be escalated. Though we are hesitant to administer sedating medications to sedated patients, the etiology is the key; our patient is altered from the withdrawal. With the onset of seizures, our patient certainly does meet criteria for a diagnosis of DT's.

Consulting editor comments (Weingart):

So, with our "seizure and now normal" patient, we ignore the seizure and reassess their level of withdrawal, predicated on the fact that they're neurologically intact. But with the DT's, they're sick; they're hallucinating, their mental status is bad, and they have incredibly hyperdynamic sympathomimetic vital signs. But when they get to that point, you missed the point. We can classify these patients into DT's/severe alcohol withdrawal because the treatment for them is the same.

Q#2: How are alcohol withdrawal seizures/DT's treated? What "cutting edge" approaches can be tried for refractory seizure activity?

The initial approach to managing DT's will be similar to that of alcohol withdrawal. The major treatment goals are to control agitation, to decrease the risk of recurrent seizures and to decrease the risk of subsequent injury and death.

The mainstay of pharmacologic treatment are benzodiazepines. Benzodiazepines are effective in preventing seizures and reducing the re-occurrences of seizures in alcohol withdrawal patients.[25,26] One study demonstrated a decline in recurrent alcohol withdrawal seizures from 24% to 3% with a single dose of intravenous lorazepam.[27]

Evidence does not suggest that one benzodiazepine is superior. Suggested adult dosing guidance:

- Diazepam 5–20mg IV every 5–10 minutes
- Lorazepam 2–4mg IV every 15–20 minutes
- Midazolam 4–8mg IV every 5 minutes

Symptom-triggered bolus dosing of benzodiazepines appears to be more beneficial than continuous infusions.[28]

Benzodiazepine-resistant seizures:

Re-evaluate the patient's vital signs, overall clinical condition and potential need for intubation. As some patients have low endogenous levels of GABA, when high doses of benzodiazepines do not work, barbiturates may be a useful addition. Phenobarbital in doses of 130–260mg IV every 15–20 minutes until symptom control is an option.[29] Barbiturates have the potential for over-sedation and hypotension and should be used with these caveats in mind. Propofol and dexmedetomidine have been used in refractory DT's but no large prospective trials have been done to be able to recommend these at this time.[30] Unless the patient has a structural CNS lesion, typical anticonvulsants should be avoided and may make DT's worse.[31] Antipsychotics should also be avoided, as they can lower the seizure threshold.[32]

Consulting editor comments (Weingart):

In the spectrum of DT's and severe alcohol withdrawal, we can use a benzos strategy. That's what I used to do, and it requires an enormous dose of benzodiazepine. It's far beyond what most people are comfortable with unless they manage these commonly. When we previously used diazepam, we would give 10 IV, which is insufficient, and then double to 20, and then double to 40, then 80, then 160. In fact, you've gotten rapidly up to 300 or 400 milligrams of benzodiazepines. The point is, you need enormous doses that make your pharmacy hate you and your nurses fear for your sanity. If we fail with that, we would either give them barbiturates such as phenobarb, or we would intubate them and put them on propofol. What I move to is a phenobarb first strategy in these patients. It is more effective in my experience and that of the EMCrit team and Farkas. For these patients go to the website to find the doses and understand that this is not industry standard. Using heavy benzodiazepines is the current industry standard.

If you're going to use barbiturates, make sure you've confirmed it with your entire group and make it a protocol, because if an individual physician decides to use an alternative, that's where things become problematic. But if you sit down with your group, the toxicologist and perhaps the ICU staff and say, "We've looked at the literature and developed a protocol." Then you're protected when you do things that are new and cutting edge.

ED course: ***What did the actual provider do?***

The patient is given 5mg versed and started on a fosphenytoin drip and intubated.

Hospital course:

Tube feeds were initiated on July 20th. On July 26th he was extubated to 6L NC and on the 27th he failed the bedside swallow evaluation and was made NPO. A Dobbhoff NG was placed with tube feeds at 70mL/hour. On July 29th, he experienced severe respiratory distress due to suspicion of aspiration pneumonia and sepsis and was reintubated. Another Dobbhoff was placed after intubation and the KUB showed placement in fundus of stomach with colonic distention. WBC's spiked and he was diagnosed with nosocomial *C. Diff.* August 13th tube feeds were coming from the patient's mouth; second occurrence of aspiration. After multiple attempts to wean the patient from the ventilator the patient's father consented to tracheostomy and peg tube placement. He was discharged to an LTAC on August 19th, ventilator dependent, alert to self only, able to follow simple, one step commands, and NPO except tube feeds.

Final diagnosis:

- Severe alcohol withdrawal
- Malnutrition
- Respiratory failure s/p aspiration
- Nosocomial *C. Diff.*
- Encephalopathy with permanent cognitive impairment

Summary:

1. Urine drug screens do not demonstrate active intoxication and exhibit a large number of false positives.
2. A positive blood alcohol level does NOT exclude that a patient is undergoing acute alcohol withdrawal.
3. Benzodiazepines are the mainstay of treatment of alcohol withdrawal and delirium.
4. The CIWA score has demonstrated an objective and consistent measurement of a patient's withdrawal signs and symptoms. Reassessment is important as withdrawal is a dynamic process.
5. Consider phenobarbital and propofol for patients with acute alcohol withdrawal refractory to treatment with benzodiazepines.

References:

1. Schwartz B, Rezkalla S, Kloner R. Cardiovascular effects of cocaine. Circulation 2010; 122(24): 2558-69.
2. Maraj S, Figueredo MD, Vincent M, et al. Cocaine and the heart. Cardiology Faculty Papers 2010;16.
3. Singh V, Rodriguez AP, Thakkar B, et al. Hospital admissions for chest pain associated with cocaine use in the United States. Am J Med 2017;130(6):688-98.
4. Faranoff AC, Rymer JA, Goldstein SA, et al. Does this patient with chest pain have acute coronary syndrome? The rational clinical examination systematic review. JAMA 2015;314(18):1955-65.
5. Backus BE, Six AJ, Kelder JC, et al. A prospective validation of the HEART score for chest pain patients at the emergency department. Int J of Cardiol 2013;168(3):2153-58.
6. Weinstock MB, Weingart S, Orth F, et al. Risk for clinically relevant adverse cardiac events in patients with chest pain at hospital admission. JAMA Intern Med 2015;175(7):1207-12.
7. James JT. A new, evidence-based estimate of patient harms associated with hospital care. J Patient Saf 2013;9(3):122-8.
8. Tenenbein M. Do you really need that emergency drug screen? Clin Toxicol (Phila) 2009;47(4):286-91.
9. Kosten TR, O'Connor PG. Management of drug and alcohol withdrawal. N Engl J Med 2003;348(18):1786-95.
10. American College of Toxicology. Interpretation of urine analysis for cocaine metabolites. J Med Toxicol 2015;11(1): 153-54.
11. Long D, Long B, Koyfman A. The emergency medicine management of severe alcohol withdrawal. Am J of Emerg Med 2017;35(7):1005-11.
12. Schuckit M.A.: Recognition and management of withdrawal delirium (delirium tremens). N Engl J Med 2014; 371(22):2109-13.
13. Sullivan JT, Sykora K, Schneiderman J, et al. Assessment of alcohol withdrawal: The revised clinical institute withdrawal assessment for alcohol scale (CIWA-Ar). Br J Addict 1989;84(11):1353-7.
14. Wells PS, Anderson DR, Rodger M, et al. Excluding pulmonary embolism at the bedside without diagnostic imaging: Management of patients with suspected pulmonary embolism presenting to the emergency department by using a simple clinical model anddimer. Ann

Intern Med 2001;135(2):98-107.
15. Kline JA, Mitchell AM, Kabrhel, et al. Clinical criteria to prevent unnecessary diagnostic testing in emergency department patients with suspected pulmonary embolism. J Thromb Haemost 2004;2(8):1247-55.
16. Tsuang JW, Irwin MR, Smith TL, et al. Characteristics of men with alcoholic hallucinosis. Addiction 1994;89(1):73-8.
17. Schmidt KJ, Doshi MR, Holzhausen JM, et al. Treatment of severe alcohol withdrawal. Ann Pharmacother 2016;50(5):389-01.
18. Victor M, Brausch C. The role of abstinence in the genesis of alcoholic epilepsy. Epilepsia 1967;8(1):1-20.
19. Jesse S, Brathen G, Ferrara M. Alcohol withdrawal syndrome: mechanisms, manifestations, and management. Acta Neurol Scand 2017; 135(1):4-16.
20. Rosenson J, Clements C, Simon B, et al. Phenobarbital for acute alcohol withdrawal: a prospective randomized double-blind placebo-controlled study. J Emerg Med 2013; 44(3): 592-98. E2.
21. Minozzi S, Amato L, Vecchi S, Davoli M. Anticonvulsants for alcohol withdrawal. Cochrane Database Syst Rev 2010;(3):CD005064.
22. Ferreira JA, Wieruszewski PM, Cunningham DW, et al. Approach to the complicated alcohol withdrawal patient. J Intensive Care Med 2017;32(1):3-14.
23. Maldonado, JR, Sher Y, Ashouri JF, et al. The "Prediction of Alcohol Withdrawal Severity Scale" (PAWSS): systematic literature review and pilot study of a new scale for the prediction of complicated alcohol withdrawal syndrome. Alcohol 2014;48(4):375-90.
24. Wood E, Albarqouni L, Tkachuk S, et al. Will this hospitalized patient develop severe alcohol withdrawal syndrome? The rational clinical examination systematic review. JAMA 2018;320(8):825-33.
25. Amato L, Minozzi S, Davoli M. Efficacy and safety of pharmacological interventions for the treatment of the alcohol withdrawal syndrome. Cochrane Database Syst Rev 2011;(6):CD008537.
26. Schaefer TJ, Hafner JW. Are benzodiazepines effective for alcohol withdrawal? Ann Emerg Med 2013;62(1);34-5.
27. D'Onofrio G, Rathley NK, Ulrich AS, et al. Lorazepam for the prevention of recurrent seizures related to alcohol. N Engl J Med 1999;340(20):915-9.
28. Ungur LA, Neuner B, Johns S, et al. Prevention and therapy of alcohol withdrawal on intensive care units: Systematic review of controlled trials. Alcohol Clin Exp Res 2013:37(4):675-86.
29. Hendey GW, Dery RA, Barnes RL, et al. A prospective, randomized, trial of phenobarbital versus benzodiazepines for acute alcohol withdrawal. Am J Emerg Med 2011;29(4):382-5.
30. Mueller SW, Preslaski CR, Kiser TH, et al. A randomized, double-blind, placebo-controlled dose range study of dexmedetomidine as adjunctive therapy for alcohol withdrawal. Crit Care Med 2014;42(5):1131-39.
31. Rathlev NK, D'Onofrio G, Fish SS, et al. Lack of efficacy of phenytoin in the prevention of recurrent alcohol-related seizures. Ann Emerg Med 1994;23(3):513-8.
32. Dixit D, Endicott J, Burry L, et al. Management of acute alcohol withdrawal syndrome in critically ill patients. Pharmacotherapy 2016;36(7):797-822.

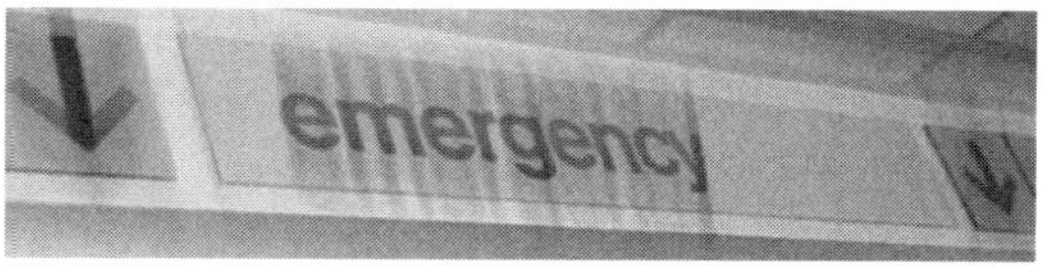

SECTION D – DRUGS & DELIRIUM

Chapter 20: A 35-year-old diabetic man with lower back pain

Matthew DeLaney, MD, FACEP, FAAEM
Associate Professor/Associate Residency Program Director
Department of Emergency Medicine
University of Alabama at Birmingham
Birmingham, AL

Doug Poe, DO
Attending Emergency Physician
Holzer Health System
Gallipolis, OH

Kim Wilcox-White, DO, MS
Adjunct Clinical Assistant Professor
Emergency Medicine
Medicine Section
Ohio University Heritage College of Osteopathic Medicine
Athens, OH

Section editor:
Michael Winters, MD, MBA, FACEP, FAAEM
Professor
Emergency Medicine
Medicine
Vice Chair for Clinical and Administrative Affairs
Department of Emergency Medicine
University of Maryland School of Medicine, Baltimore, MD

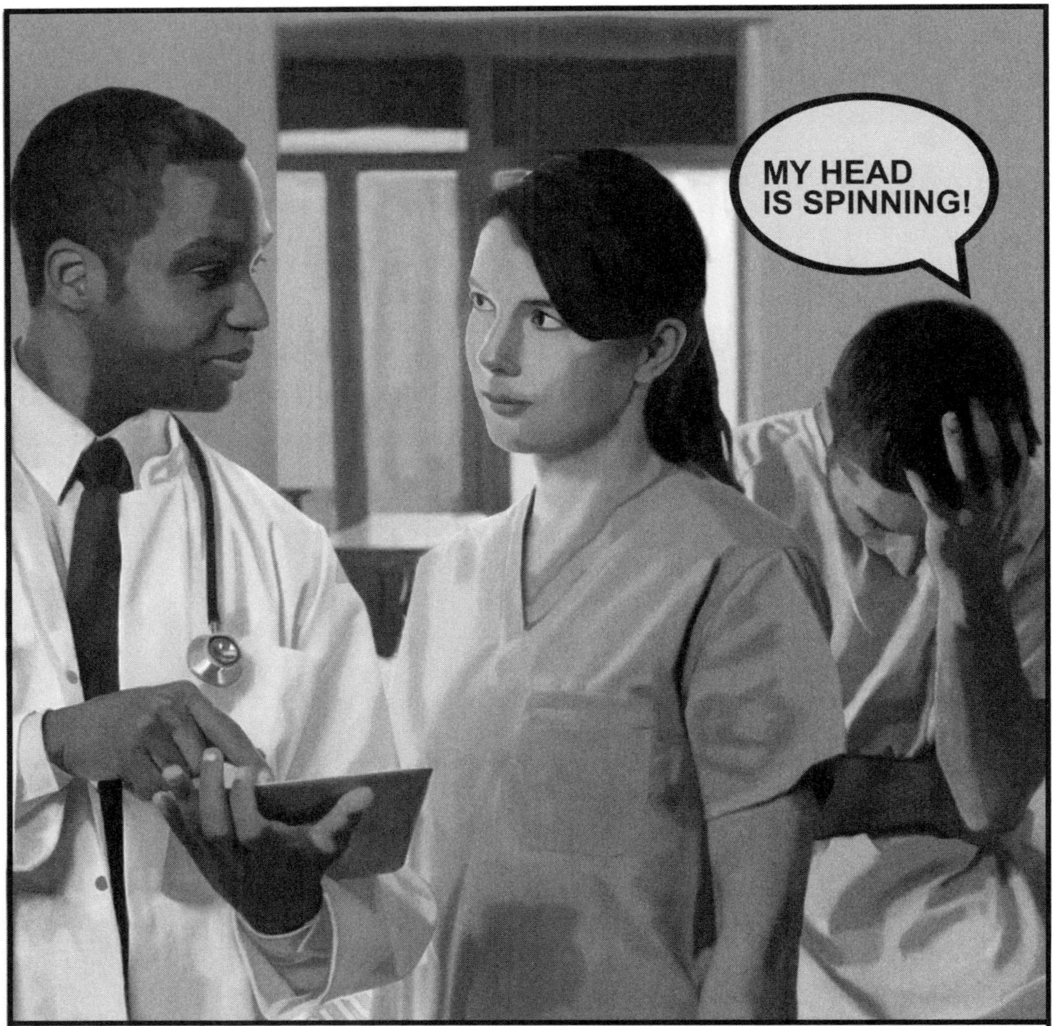

"THIS GUY WAS DISCHARGED A FEW WEEKS AGO."

SECTION D/CHAPTER 20

A 35-year-old diabetic man with lower back pain

While bounceback visits to the emergency department (ED) are not necessarily associated with worse patient outcomes, providers need to step back and consider the factors that contributed to the return, which is often multifactorial and related to suboptimal medical care in ~7% of cases.[1] Less commonly discussed are ED visits after a recent hospital discharge. In a retrospective evaluation of over 15,000 patients who were discharged from the hospital, Rising, et al. found that 23.6% of patients returned to the ED within 1 year and 46% of returning patients were admitted, a rate well above the national average.[2]

INITIAL ED VISIT (2/8/17)

HPI: 35-year-old diabetic man states he developed some lower thoracic back pain has gotten progressively worse. Started 1 hour ago and constant and first episode. Location is LS spine and lower thoracic spine. It is a severe and aching pain without radiation and worse with movement. No injury that he knows of. Denies numbness, weakness, incontinence of bowel/bladder.

PMH: Diabetes, hyperlipidemia, hypertension
Medications: Byetta, insulin, Wellbutrin, Lexapro, lisinopril, Lyrica, zocor, metoprolol
Social History: Current every day smoker, occ alcohol, drug use: none

PE:

Vitals:

Time	Temp (F)	Pulse	Resp	BP	O2 Sat
14:09	100 (H)	119	22	133/68	95% (RA)

GA: No limitations, alert
RESP: Normal lung sounds bilaterally
CARDIO: Present: regular rate, normal rhythm, normal heart sounds
ABDOMINAL: Present: soft, Non-Tender. Absent: tenderness, distention, guarding, rebound, rigidity
EXTREMITIES: Present: normal inspection, full ROM. Absent: tenderness, pedal edema
NEUROVASCULAR/TENDON: Absent: motor deficit, sensory deficit, tendon deficit
GAIT: antalgic
BACK: Present: paraspinal tenderness
NEURO: Present: alert, oriented X3

PSYCH: Present: normal affect, normal mood

X-ray: Lumbar and thoracic x-rays are negative. Thoracic: Multilevel degenerative changes as well as multilevel chronic anterior wedging and multilevel Schmorl's nodes appear stable from prior chest x-rays. There is also stable mild accentuated kyphosis to the lower thoracic spine. Possibility for Scheuermann's disease is raised. If there is persistent clinical concern MRI may be of use for further evaluation.

MRI thoracic/lumbar: Small central disc protrusion at L3–L4. No significant stenosis or nerve root compression is detected. Small central disc protrusion at T7–8 resulting in effacement of the ventral portion of the thoracic cord.

MDM: Patient has pain localizes to the lower thoracic spine. Worse with movement worse with the Valsalva. Labs show WBC 8.2, lytes and creat WNL, glucose 159mg/dL (70–99), ESR 43 (0–10), MRI of the thoracic spine shows a T7-8 disc herniation at the putting pressure on the thecal sac. His symptoms are consistent with that disc herniation. We will send him to see the spine surgeon.

Diagnosis: Thoracic back pain

Aftercare instructions (16:14): Rest, ice or heat to sore area as needed. Follow up with your Primary Care Provider on Monday. Call for a time to be seen. Call [the orthopedist] per the number provided to you as well. Let them know that you have already had an MRI. Return for fever, weakness, trouble breathing, any other concerns or if worse in any way. Rx oxycodone/acetaminophen #15 and cyclobenzaprine 10mg #30.

Discussion: Our patient's back pain seems straightforward; it hurts with range of motion and there is paraspinal tenderness. While there is no preceding trauma, he doesn't report any high-risk features to suggest an ominous cause. Despite what seems like a benign sounding story, the provider ordered an MRI. This is curious. Was this based on the recommendation from the thoracic spine radiology report or did the provider have additional concerns or suspicions that weren't detailed in the note? And why were labs ordered for a simple lumbosacral strain?

Risk management/patient safety concerns include:

- Minimal review of systems; no questions about fever (epidural abscess), weight loss (malignancy), dysuria/frequency (UTI/pyelo), abdominal pain (pancreatitis, ulcer, perforation) or flank pain (ureterolithiasis).
- No history elicited of similar episodes or discussion of past ED visits.
- There was mild but unexplained tachycardia.
- A minimal physician exam of the back.
- No neuro exam of the back.
- Lack of explanation of lab testing for an uncomplicated LS strain.
- Discharge instructions that recommended follow-up with a spine surgeon for what is read as a small disc protrusion.

Based on the documentation, it seems like we don't have a really good feel for what transpired during this ED encounter…

Author comments (Weinstock):

We are not transcriptionists… we are *historians.* Subsequent providers (or attorneys) should be able to read the note and picture the nature of the interaction, the exam findings, as well as thought process (MDM) of the provider. Unfortunately, this documentation does not really give us (the readers) a good idea of the encounter or what was concerning (and reassuring) to the provider.

Section editor comments (Winters):

Red flags include the tachycardia, discussed above, but we also do not have a good explanation from the provider as to the nature of the tachypnea; a respiratory rate of 22bpm. Pay attention to tachypnea, as it is one of the vital sign abnormalities indicative of critical illness. Equally as important, there do not appear to be repeat vital signs demonstrating resolution of tachycardia or tachypnea prior to discharge.

ED BOUNCEBACK (4 days later, visit #2) 2/12/17

ED physician HPI: Patient with hx of DM, hyperlipidemia, asthma, HTN, mood disorder, hx PE who presents emergency room with several days of non-radiating moderate chest pain which is constant burning and aching. The pain started in the anterior aspect of his chest radiating around to his back with a feeling of shortness of breath. Has also been feeling ill with fevers and chills. He has not taken his temperature at home. Denying nausea vomiting or diarrhea headache or vision change. Denied any other cough congestion-like symptoms. He does have a history of IV drug abuse in the past but he has not used in several years. He has been taking his medications properly. He is a poorly controlled diabetic.

Vitals:

Time	Temp (F)	Pulse	Resp	BP	O2 Sat
	99.6	123	22	116/93	96

PE: Lungs are clear heart is regular but tachycardic.

CV: No murmurs auscultated on my examination. Abdomen soft no pulsatile lesions. He is alert and oriented ×3. His oral mucosa is very dry and cracking. No other acute infectious pathology noted.

MDM (02:00): Patient presentation is concerning for possible dehydration as well as DKA based on increased respirations heart rate and generalized malaise. IV fluids, labs pending.

MDM (03:41): His evaluation included imaging and laboratory analysis which showed an elevated d-dimer and CRP in the setting of tachycardia which prompted a CT angiogram of the chest. He was found to have bilateral pulmonary nodules with cavitation concerning for septic emboli. Vancomycin started. Pt. admitted.

Diagnosis: Septic pulmonary emboli, sepsis

Hospital course: [The patient] is a 35-year-old male was admitted for bacteremia and septic emboli in lungs. Patient was treated with antibiotics, blood cultures repeated for several times until negative. After treatment, the tachycardia improved, shortness of breath and chest pain have resolved. Patient has bilateral pleural effusions – ID thinks they will resolve after antibiotic treatment. Sat 95% on room air. Will continue antibiotics for 4 weeks.

Hospital discharge diagnosis: Sepsis, back pain, chest pain, hyponatremia, septic embolism, diabetes mellitus, hepatitis C – new diagnosis.

ED BOUNCEBACK (1 day after hospital discharge, visit #3) 2/18/17

Summary: The patient was evaluated for a chief complaint of back pain by the PA-C and vital signs did show a patient afebrile with a normal BP, but a pulse of 117bpm. Results from the inpatient hospitalization including a normal MRI were reviewed. The patient was already taking IV nafcillin at home for the septic emboli in the lungs and bacteremia. No controlled substances were prescribed. It was documented that the patient related that his heart rate is always fast.

Diagnosis: Back Pain/Injury

Chapter author discussion: While the patient's presentation during his initial ED visit seemed routine, when he returned 1 day after discharge for treatment of septic pulmonary emboli, he is anything but low risk. While he has a negative ROS, he is tachycardic and still has significant risk of complications. While there is a chronic component to his back pain, he is still high risk and warrants a good discussion in the MDM.

ED BOUNCEBACK (3 days after hospital discharge, visit #4) 3/7/17

CC: Dizzy

HPI: Patient presents roughly 3 weeks after discharge via EMS with a chief complaint of vertiginous dizziness and "not feeling myself." He reported that he had previously been hospitalized for a "bloodstream infection" and that he had been sent home with a PICC line and IV antibiotics. He felt dizzy today whenever he was standing up at home. He states they do not know what caused the infection and he wonders if it is because he had cut the skin and he is diabetic. EMS reports he was diaphoretic during transit. He currently complains of back pain. No fevers at home that he is aware of.

PMHx: DM2, HLD, HTN, Asthma, Former IVDU

PSurgHx: Cholecystectomy
Social Hx: Occasional EtOH, Smoker, Former IVDU – reports last use > 1 year ago

PE:

Vitals:

Time	Temp (F)	Pulse	Resp	BP	O2 Sat (RA)
12:52	99.7	131	16	186/84	97%

GA: Alert, appears anxious
HEENT: Normocephalic, Atraumatic, PERLA, EOMI
CV: Tachycardic, regular rhythm w/o m/r/g
RESP: Diminished lung sounds bilaterally, No wheezing/rhonchi
ABDOMINAL: Soft, nontender
BACK: thoracic and lumbar TTP
EXTREMITIES: RUE PICC line w/o induration or erythema
NEURO: Alert

Author comments (Weinstock):

On his fourth visit, we see a patient with a history of IVDU who has worsening tachycardia, diaphoresis (per EMS), and multiple ED visits and a recent hospitalization for septic pulmonary emboli. We are at our first decision point:

DECISION POINT A – YOU ARE FACED W ITH 3 QUESTIONS:

1. **What are the diagnostic possibilities in an IV drug user (IVDU) with dizziness?**
2. **What are possible sites of infection to consider in IV drug users (IVDU)?**
3. **Is our patient septic?**

What does the literature say?

Q#1: What are the diagnostic possibilities in an IV drug user (IVDU) with dizziness?

As rates of IVDU have increased over the past 15 years, the incidence of related infectious endocarditis has nearly doubled and various embolic phenomena that were once rarely seen are now being diagnosed routinely in EDs across the country.[3] While some patients may present with a history and exam consistent with a benign cause of peripheral vertigo, in patients with a history of IVDU the risk of occult endocarditis shouldn't be underestimated.

Though the possibilities for dizziness is broad, when evaluating a patient with a history of IVDU, embolic sequelae from underlying endocarditis moves up in the differential; embolic events may occur in up to 50% of cases of bacterial endocarditis. Cerebral emboli occur in up to 20% of cases of endocarditis.[4] Neurologic complications including abscess, stroke, arteritis, and cerebritis can occur in the setting of IVDU and may present with a similarly broad range of symptoms.

Classic features that are used to distinguish between peripheral and central causes of dizziness should be used with caution in the setting of IVDU. Our patient has a significant risk of endocarditis and septic phenomena; unless there is a clearcut explanation for his dizziness, the lack of historical or clinical features does not reliably reduce the likelihood of a central cause of vertigo.

Q#2: What are possible sites of infection to consider in IV drug users (IVDU)?

Cellulitis and underlying abscess are common with high rates of deep space infections, necrotizing fasciitis, and myonecrosis. While the extent of these soft tissue infections may not be fully appreciated on bedside exam, there is often ample clinical evidence to identify the presence of an underlying infection.[5]

1. **Endocarditis:** Infective endocarditis (IE) is the most common infectious complication related to IVDU and often presents with an atypical clinical picture. While IE can affect any of the valves in the heart, most frequently it is right-sided endocarditis with up to 70% having tricuspid valve involvement.[6] The physiology is somewhat unclear, but it is possibly due to damage from particulate matter found in injected substances.

   Patients with tricuspid valve IE often do not have an appreciable heart murmur and up to 20% may not report fever or malaise. Despite this subclinical picture, these patients have high rates of adverse events, with septic pulmonary emboli occurring in up to 75% of patients with tricuspid IE. As with our patient, the risk of septic embolism is not limited to the pulmonary circulation; some studies have reported rates of distant septic emboli has high as 85% of the time.[7]
2. **Pulmonary Complications:** With septic pulmonary emboli, many patients will report shortness of breath and chest pain; up to 85% of cases have abnormal findings on chest x-ray. Less commonly patients will develop localized pulmonary abscesses which can cause pleural effusions. The presence of these parapneumonic effusions can create a nidus of infection; about 8% of patients with septic pulmonary emboli will develop an empyema.[8]
3. **Spinal Epidural Abscess (SEA):** The etiology of these abscesses is somewhat unclear and can develop from either direct embolism through a persistent right to left anatomic defect or from underlying bacteremia. Clinically, the diagnosis of SEA is difficult, and studies have shown a high rate of diagnostic delay, with only 2% having the classic triad of fever, spine pain, and a neurologic deficit on initial presentation.[9]
4. **HIV/Hepatitis:** Overall the risk of obtaining hepatitis C is much higher than with HIV with 3–10% rate of infection per needlestick reported for hepatitis compared to 0.3% with HIV. This results in staggering rates of disease with an 80% estimated prevalence of hepatitis C reported among injection drug users worldwide.[10]

Section editor comments (Winters):

The majority of SEAs occur via hematogenous spread. High rates of diagnostic delay are common. Importantly, most patients with an SEA will be afebrile upon initial presentation and have a normal neurologic exam, and up to 40% will not have leukocytosis.

Q#3: Is our patient septic?

On presentation our patient does not meet the criteria to be categorized as septic per the Sepsis-3 criteria proposed by Singer, et al. Additionally, while chest x-ray reveals a potential source of infection, he has 0 out of 3 potential prognostic qSOFA criteria (respiratory rate ≥ 22/min, altered mentation, systolic blood pressure < 100mmHg). The patient has mild tachycardia and is found to have leukocytosis but initially shows no signs of significant organ dysfunction. Previous definitions of sepsis incorporating the use of SIRS criteria in the setting of a likely infection would have considered this patient to have sepsis; however the most recent guidelines stop short of making the diagnosis of sepsis, and he does not have septic shock.[11]

Consulting editor comments (Weingart):

A word on elevated lactate levels; some clinicians conflate elevated lactate as fluid depletion—and the two are completely unrelated. If your patient is hypovolemic, and their tissues are not getting oxygen delivered to them, then sure, try giving some fluids. But, we're not in 2001 anymore. We should have some secondary evidence that dehydration is occurring—if we throw on the ultrasound probe and we have an empty heart and the IVC is completely collapsing and the patient had a history of dysentery for the past two weeks, yep, it's fluid depletion. But if our patient is fluid replete and their lactate is high, don't just give extra fluid solely as a result of the lactate value.

To review, an elevated lactate is due to an increased hormonal milieu of inflammation, due to the patient's sugar metabolism being shunted anaerobically, even though there is still oxygen available. We should be careful to eliminate the confounders including albuterol, illicit drug use, alcohol. And yet we have all our treatments predicated on that last case. A patient who is so volume down, with such a low cardiac output, that there's not oxygen being delivered to their tissues. Don't give fluid solely as a result of an elevated lactate.

What did the actual provider do?

MDM (13:14): Plan for patient is an ECG, chest x-ray as well as basic labs as well as blood cultures, lactate for sepsis workup. Patient is tachycardic here, and we will give IV fluids and some analgesics for pain. Reviewed his previous admission which shows bacteremia with MSSA. He had an echo at that time which was negative. He did have a CTA concerning for septic emboli. Patient has been on nafcillin since discharge. ECG was found to be nonischemic.

Radiology interpretation - CXR impressions:
Left pleural effusion left mid and lower lung airspace disease increased since the prior study. Symmetric pulmonary edema or pneumonia could have this appearance.

(Figure on next page...)

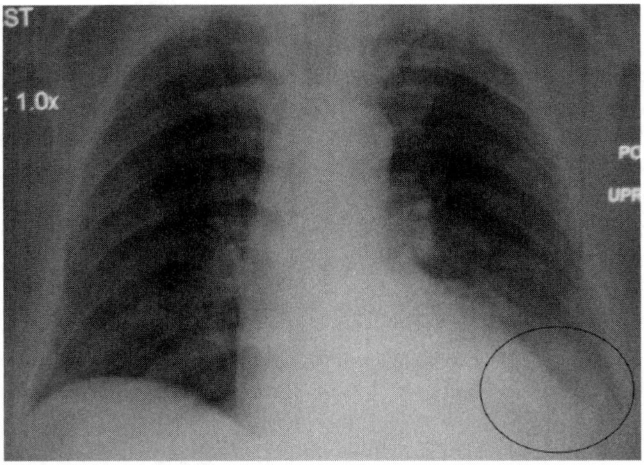

DECISION POINT B – YOU ARE FACED WITH 3 QUESTIONS:

1. **Our patient has a left-sided effusion. Is it true that "the sun never sets on a parapneumonic effusion?"**
2. **Is a chest CT indicated or is the CXR adequate?**
3. **Which antibiotics should be started?**

What does the literature say?

Q#1: Our patient has a left-sided effusion. Is it true that "the sun never sets on a parapneumonic effusion?"

A thoracentesis can provide a fluid sample to differentiate between a transudative or exudative effusion as well as providing infectious source control. In the case of a large effusion/empyema, it can help decrease the physiologic dead space caused by compression of the lung and may improve the patients' respiratory mechanics. Consideration for emergent thoracentesis should be given to patients in respiratory distress secondary to an underlying pleural fluid collection.

For patients who are not in extremis, the decision to perform a thoracentesis is based largely on the likelihood of the patient having an underlying complicated effusion or empyema. The American College of Chest Physicians recommend performing a thoracentesis on any patient with a parapneumonic effusion that meets one of the following criteria:[12]

- Non-loculated but layers > 25mm on lateral decubitus film or CT scan.
- Loculated effusion.
- Associated with thickened parietal pleura on CT scan (associated with increased rate of empyema).

The adage "the sun should never set on a parapneumonic effusion" was first introduced in 1989 journal article in *Chest* and emphasizes the time-sensitive nature of this condition.[13] Since the term was first introduced, studies have demonstrated a wide variety of approaches to management. Patients with an uncomplicated effusion generally improve with antibiotics while those with complicated effusions or empyemas need urgent drainage and often require subsequent surgical interventions.[14]

Q#2: Is a chest CT indicated or is the CXR adequate?

While there is some diagnostic uncertainty in the initial radiology report, the chest x-ray is clearly abnormal. While a CT scan may give some increased diagnostic clarity by providing details that could suggest the presence of an empyema over a complicated effusion, in our case the clinical picture and initial x-ray should give the provider enough information to manage the patient.

Q#3: Which antibiotics should be started?

With a recent hospitalization and an indwelling central line, our patient is at risk for healthcare-associated pathogens including MRSA.[15] He is taking antibiotics, so blood cultures may not offer much diagnostic clarity. Broad-spectrum antibiotics such as Vancomycin and Piperacillin/Tazobactam would be reasonable empiric first line agents.

Section editor comments (Winters):

Be sure to dose vancomycin appropriately based on the patient's weight. One gram of vancomycin is insufficient for many patients with sepsis.

What did the actual provider do?

MDM: At this time the patient meets SIRS criteria. Lactate and blood cultures were drawn in addition to standard labs. IV fluids were initiated for resuscitation. I consulted ID for input given his concerning chest x-ray. They noted that he had been seen a few days before and had imaging of his spine performed at that time. The radiology report was reviewed showing no acute abnormalities of his spine; however, there was a noted left-sided loculated effusion concerning for an empyema.

ED course (13:29):

Lab	**Result**	**Range/Units**
WBC	**13.5 H**	**(4.3-11.1) K/mcL**
Hgb	**12.0 L**	**(12.9-16.9) g/dL**
Plt Count	389	(140-400) K/mcL
Sodium	**129 L**	**(136-145)mEq/L**
Potassium	3.7	(3.5-4.5)mEq/L
Chloride	**97 L**	**(98-109)mEq/L**
Carbon Dioxide	21	(19-29)mEq/L
BUN	10	(8-26)mg/dL
Creatinine	0.87	(0.72-1.25)mg/dL
Glucose	**162 H**	**(70-99)mg/dL**
Lactic Acid	**2.2 H**	**(0.5-2.2)mmol/L**

PE:

Vitals:

Time	**Temp (F)**	**Pulse**	**Resp**	**BP**	**O2 Sat (RA)**
13:58		**128**	**24**	**96/68**	**91% 6L NC**

Returning to the room, you see that the nurse has placed a nasal cannula. The patient is now tachypneic with a respiratory rate of 24 with clammy skin. He asks for oxygen, saying, "Doc, I just can't seem to catch my breath."

DECISION POINT C – YOU ARE FACED WITH 3 QUESTIONS:

1. **Should BiPAP be started or would nasal cannula/NRB be a better starting point?**
2. **Would monitoring with capnography be better than simply pulse ox? Does this change in sepsis/infected patients?**
3. **Is a lactate over 2 and less than 4 predictive of morbidity/mortality?**

What does the literature say?

Q#1: Should BiPAP be started or would nasal cannula/NRB be a better starting point?

With a significant effusion or empyema, our patient is at a high risk of respiratory failure, and with him continuing to decompensate, BiPAP is a good initial choice to assist with ventilation. Given his significant pleural fluid collection, he was likely experiencing physiologic dead space, and PPV offers the potential mitigating effect of increased PEEP compared to NRB which essentially just increases his FiO_2. While an NRB mask may be a reasonable starting point, as he is showing signs of hypoxia and respiratory distress despite a nasal cannula, these authors recommend placement of BiPAP at this time.

Q#2: Would monitoring with capnography be better than simply pulse ox? Does this change in sepsis/infected patients?

End-tidal capnography to measure carbon dioxide concentration ($ETCO_2$) is used in a wide variety of settings and has been shown to have an inverse relationship with both levels of lactate and overall mortality. Hunter, et al. found that $ETCO_2$ had similar performance characteristics compared to lactate when used to predict overall mortality in patients with suspected sepsis.[16] When used in a pre-hospital setting, $ETCO_2 < 25$mmHg outperformed traditional SIRS criteria in terms of identifying patients with sepsis.[17] In the ED there is limited data to suggest that $ETCO_2$ outperforms typical monitors such as pulse oximetry. Theoretically $ETCO_2$ could be used to monitor a patient's degree of acidosis during the course of their stay, but to date we have little evidence to guide such interventions.

Q#3: Is a lactate over 2 and less than 4 predictive of morbidity/mortality?

Under normal aerobic conditions cells utilize oxidative phosphorylation to produce ATP, but under anaerobic conditions such as tissue ischemia, lactic acid forms. Traditionally lactate has been evaluated as a marker for end-organ dysfunction with increased rates of morbidity and mortality occurring with levels greater than or equal to 4. More recently lactate levels less than 4 but greater than 2 have shown to have a similar association with adverse outcomes.

In a cohort study of 830 patients admitted from the ED with severe sepsis, Mikkelsen, et al. found that both initial lactates in the ED were associated with overall patient mortality. In patients with high (> 4) lactates there was an increased risk of mortality (OR = 4.87, $p = 0.001$). A similar increase in mortality was seen in the "intermediate" range lactates (2–3.9) but the findings were not statistically significant (OR = 3.27, $p = 0.022$).[18] In a recent systematic review, Singh, et al.

found that patients with intermediate lactate levels high rates of decompensation with 23% developing subsequent shock. In addition, the overall short-term mortality (in-hospital, 28-day, 30-day) rate was 15%.[19] While patients with intermediate range lactates may have a rather benign clinical appearance, these patients have a significant risk of decompensation. Our patient's lactate was 2.2, but a mortality of 15% is approximately double that of a STEMI patient!

Author comments (Weinstock):

Scott has a slightly different take on lactate between 2 and 4:

Consulting editor comments (Weingart):

I've never been impressed with this 2 to 4 range. All of the big trials on sepsis use a lactate greater than 4. That was the cut-off for "something is probably going on with this patient." And if you can't justify a reason, like they had a ton of albuterol, then you need to look into it; this is the "cryptic" or "occult" sepsis patient that we classically describe—and I still believe in that.

How about an initial lactate of 5? Here I'm going to do some investigation; something is going on. Now, I might find out that the patient was using a lot of cocaine, and then I can write in the chart, "I believe this patient's lactate is from their drug use," but I still want to see it clear. If they are continuing to use cocaine in front of you in the ED, then they should get better (caution with the mesenteric ischemia patient from the "cardiac/vascular" section).

The lactate, which is minimally elevated, for example 2.3, needs to be addressed somehow, but I don't necessarily think we need to always see it come down.

MDM (14:06): The patient is placed on BiPAP and his sat increased to 96%, with resulting decrease in the respiratory rate. After speaking with infectious disease, I consulted cardiothoracic surgery given his prior findings of an empyema on his thoracic lumbar CT scan. They agreed that we should re-image his chest to fully delineate the possible empyema.

Chest CT 03/01/17 14:57:

1. There is a new, small to moderate loculated left pleural effusion which contains several foci of gas. Findings are consistent with empyema.
2. Previously identified bilateral septic emboli have decreased in size. Areas of central cavitation have resolved.

MDM: The patient was admitted to the hospitalist service with a diagnosis of sepsis secondary to empyema with infectious disease and cardiothoracic surgery consultations. Based on his improved hemodynamics, CT surgery will not take the patient to the OR emergently.

Diagnosis: Empyema, sepsis, IVDU.

Hospital course: The patient was admitted to the hospitalist service in serious but stable condition. Infectious disease and cardiothoracic surgery were consulted. The patient underwent a left thoracostomy and decortication with cardiothoracic surgery. He spent several more days in the inpatient setting due to acute kidney injury. Nephrology had to be consulted with a multifactorial etiology of his renal insufficiency attributed to sepsis as well as nephrotoxic agents used during his hospital stay. His renal function improved, and he was discharged with continued IV antibiotics with close follow-up with cardiothoracic surgery and ID.

Teaching points:

- Patients with a history of IVDU have a significant risk of a vast number of complications. From localized infections to distant septic emboli, providers need to maintain a broad differential.
- When a patient has a parapneumonic effusion, the critical decision point involves determining if there is a complicated effusion or underlying empyema. These patients need urgent source control and will often need a surgical intervention.
- Patients with a significant underlying infection may not appear ill; intermediate range lactates (2–3.9) may predict an increased risk of decompensation.

References:

1. Cheng J, Shroff A, Khan N, et al. Emergency department return visits resulting in admission: Do they reflect quality of care? Am J Med Qual 2016;31(6):541-51.
2. Rising KL, White LF, Fernandez WG, et al. Emergency department visits after hospital discharge: a missing part of the equation. Ann Emerg Med 2013;62(2):145-50.
3. Wurcel AG, Anderson JE, Chui KK, et al. Increasing infectious endocarditis admissions among young people who inject drugs. Open Forum Infect Dis 2016;3(3):ofw157.
4. Baddour LM, Wilson WR, Bayer AS, et al. Infective endocarditis: Diagnosis, antimicrobial therapy, and management of complications: A statement for healthcare professionals from the Committee on Rheumatic Fever, Endocarditis, and Kawasaki Disease, Council on Cardiovascular Disease in the Young, and the Councils on Clinical Cardiology, Stroke, and Cardiovascular Surgery and Anesthesia, American Heart Association: endorsed by the Infectious Diseases Society of America. Circulation 2005;111(23):e394-434.
5. Mittapalli D, Velineni R, Rae N, et al. Necrotizing soft tissue infections in intravenous drug users: a vascular surgical emergency. Eur J Vasc Endovasc Surg 2015;49(5):593-9.
6. Dressler FA, Roberts WC. Infective endocarditis in opiate addicts: Analysis of 80 cases studied at necropsy. Am J Cardiol 1989;63(17):1240-57.
7. Ruotsalainen E, Sammalkorpi K, Laine J, et al. Clinical manifestations and outcome in Staphylococcus aureus endocarditis among injection drug users and nonaddicts: A prospective study of 74 patients. BMC Infect Dis 2006;6:137.
8. Ye R, Zhao L, Wang C, et al. Clinical characteristics of septic pulmonary embolism in adults: A systematic review. Respir Med 2014;108(1):1-8.
9. Davis DP, Salazar A, Chan TC, et al. Prospective evaluation of a clinical decision guideline to diagnose spinal epidural abscess in patients who present to the emergency department with spine pain. J Neurosurg Spine 2011;14(6):765-70.
10. Nelson PK, Mathers BM, Cowie B, et al. Global epidemiology of hepatitis B and hepatitis C in people who inject drugs: Results of systematic reviews. Lancet 2011;378(9791):571-83.

11. Singer M, Deutschman CS, Seymour CW, et al. The Third International Consensus Definitions for Sepsis and Septic Shock (Sepsis-3). JAMA 2016;315(8):801-10.
12. Colice GL, Curtis A, Deslauriers J, et al. Medical and surgical treatment of parapneumonic effusions: An evidence-based guideline. Chest 2000;118(4):1158-71.
13. Sahn SA, Light RW. The sun should never set on a parapneumonic effusion. Chest 1989;95(5):945-7.
14. Wurnig PN, Wittmer V, Pridun NS, et al. Video-assisted thoracic surgery for pleural empyema. Ann Thorac Surg 2006;81(1):309-13.
15. Maskell NA, Batt S, Hedley EL, et al. The bacteriology of pleural infection by genetic and standard methods and its mortality significance. Am J Respir Crit Care Med 2006;174(7):817-23.
16. Hunter CL, Silvestri S, Dean M, et al. End-tidal carbon dioxide is associated with mortality and lactate in patients with suspected sepsis. Am J Emerg Med 2013;31(1):64-71.
17. Hunter CL, Silvestri S, Ralls G, et al. A prehospital screening tool utilizing end-tidal carbon dioxide predicts sepsis and severe sepsis. Am J Emerg Med 2016;34(5):813-9.
18. Mikkelsen ME, Miltiades AN, Gaieski DF, et al. Serum lactate is associated with mortality in severe sepsis independent of organ failure and shock. Crit Care Med 2009;37(5):1670-7.
19. Singh M, Koyfman A. What is the prognostic value of intermediate lactate level elevations in emergency department patients with suspected infection? Ann Emerg Med 2016;67(5):643-4.

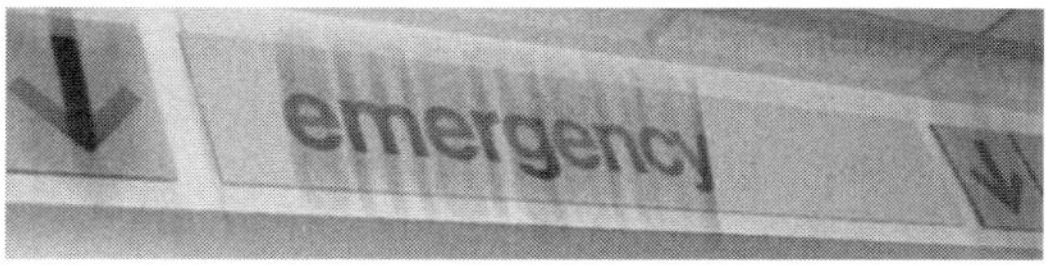

SECTION E – NEURO & SEPSIS

Chapter 21: A 50-year-old woman with flank pain

Michael B. Weinstock, MD

Associate Program Director, Adena Emergency Medicine Residency
Director of Medical Education and Research, Adena Health System, Chillicothe, OH
Professor of Emergency Medicine, Adjunct
The Ohio State University Wexner Medical Center, Columbus, OH

Bryan D. Hayes, PharmD, DABAT, FAACT, FASHP

Assistant Professor of Emergency Medicine, Harvard Medical School
Attending Pharmacist, Emergency Medicine & Toxicology
Massachusetts General Hospital, Boston, MA

Katherine Mayer, MD, FACEP

Assistant Professor, Department of Emergency Medicine
Division of Pulmonary Medicine
University of Colorado Anschutz Medical Campus, Aurora, CO

Karina Reyner Pauly, MD

Associate Professor of Medicine
Texas A&M College of Medicine, Department of Emergency Medicine
Baylor University Medical Center, Dallas, TX

Alan C. Heffner, MD

Co-Director of Critical Care, ECMO Medical Director
Pulmonary and Critical Care Consultants
Department of Internal Medicine and Department of Emergency Medicine
Carolinas Medical Center, UNC School of Medicine – Charlotte Campus, Charlotte, NC

Section editor:

Tiffany M. Osborn, MD, MPH

Professor of Surgery and Emergency Medicine Surgical
Trauma Critical Care
Department of Surgery
Washington University, St. Louis, MO

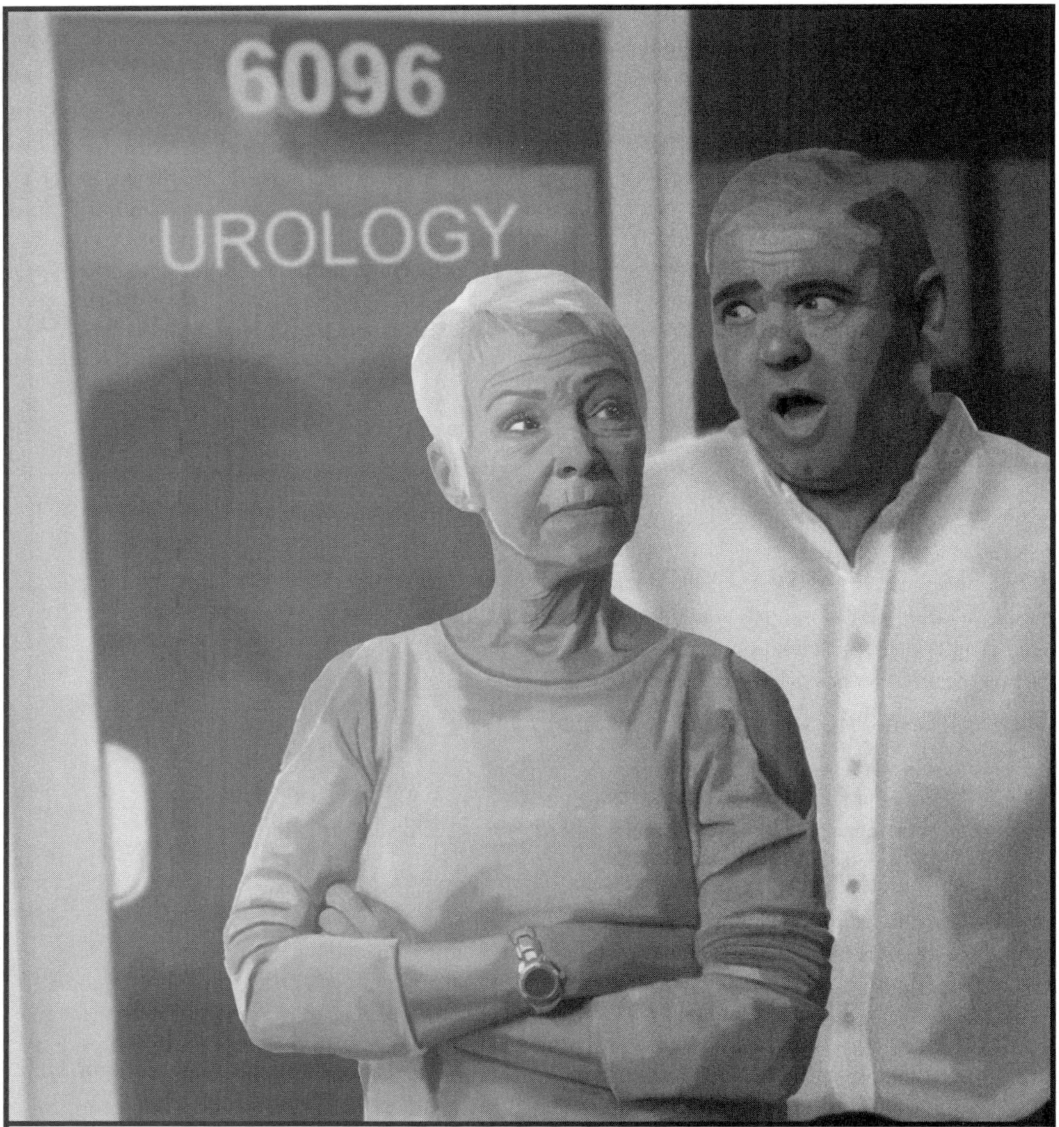

"HONEY, YOU SEEM CONFUSED.
I'LL BET IT'S FROM THE PAIN PILLS."

SECTION E / CHAPTER 21

A 50-year-old woman with flank pain

Flank pain in adults is common with 1.3 million ED visits per year;[1] this is not surprising as "kidney stones" occur in up to 8.8% of the population.[2] The differential diagnosis for acute flank pain ranges from benign etiologies such as a muscular strain or zoster to more serious pathology including malignancy or a ruptured abdominal aortic aneurysm (AAA).[3]

The evaluation is easy, right? Just order a CT scan which will "automatically" exclude the bad stuff, including AAA, cancer, small bowel obstruction (SBO), perforated viscus, retrocecal appendix, pancreatitis… and, if we are lucky, it will "rule-in" a ureteral stone, giving us a quick diagnosis and disposition. Well, not so fast! There are a few questions remaining:

1. Can we avoid CT imaging by clinically diagnosing ureteral colic?
2. When imaging for a stone, how often are we surprised by a life-threatening etiology?
3. Does size and location of ureteral stone predict the chance of spontaneous expulsion?
4. Does medical expulsion therapy work?
5. Are labs helpful for uncomplicated ureterolithiasis?
6. The nightmare scenario: How do patients with seemingly uncomplicated ureteral stones go bad… and how are they managed if this occurs?

Buckle your seatbelt as we put *you* in the footsteps of the EM provider at the initial visit and keep you there until the bounceback. Spoiler alert: Our patient returns 2 days later, crashing soon after hitting the emergency department double-bay doors.

INITIAL ED VISIT

HPI: The patient is a 51-year-old woman with no significant past medical history who presents with right flank pain. She reports that she woke up 2½ hours ago, with sudden onset right flank pain. She had some mild nausea but after attempting to drink water she had an episode of vomiting, nonbloody, nonbilious. She denies chest pain or pressure, shortness of breath, abdominal pain, diarrhea or bloody stools, dysuria, increased urinary frequency, or hematuria. She has no history of kidney stones or pyelonephritis.

Allergies: PCN
Social history: No smoking or alcohol
Family history: See HPI
ROS: All other systems reviewed and are negative except as noted. Nursing triage notes were reviewed

PMH: Migraine headaches
PSH: Knee, breast biopsy

PE:

Vitals:

Temp (F)	Pulse	Resp	Syst	Diast	Sat	Pain
98.2	70	16	132	86	99% (RA)	9/10

GA: A&OX3, appears very uncomfortable
EYES: PERRL
CV: RRR without m/r/g. Normal heart sounds. Good capillary refill. No peripheral edema
RESP: CTAB, no wheezes, rales, rhonchi. Good chest excursion
ABD: Soft and NT throughout, Murphy's sign negative, without r/r/g [rigidity/rebound/guarding]
BACK: No CVAT
SKIN: Normal without petechiae, vesicles, erythema

Urinalysis:
Appearance: Cloudy
Specific gravity 1.011
pH: 7.0
Glucose: Neg
Ketones: 5mg/dl
Blood: 100/ul
Leukocyte esterase: 100/ul
Nitrite: Neg
Protein: 15mg/dl
WBC: 0–5
RBC: 25–50
Squam epi: Occasional
Bacteria: Few

TESTING: Noncontrast helical CT scan abdomen/pelvis: 6mm obstructing right ureteral stone at the mid aspect of the ureter.

MDM: She received morphine and ondansetron. Her records have been reviewed. There is no evidence of associated urinary infection with only 0–5 white blood cells, however I have sent urine for culture since she has leukocyte esterase. I suspect this is related to inflammation from the stone. Will discharge to home with Flomax, Naprosyn, Norco, Phenergan, and MiraLAX. Repeat exam benign, she is much more comfortable after morphine, but still having some discomfort, so will order Norco PO prior to discharge.

IMPRESSION: Ureteral calculus, left

PLAN: Urine strainer, f/u with urology in 3–4 days

Seems straightforward. The management is seemingly open and shut and quite well done—most of us would correctly also send this patient right home. But there is a "game changer" question which was not asked... a question that if answered in the affirmative, would have completely changed the disposition and likely the outcome.

Documentation and patient safety issues:

1. It may seem nit-picky, but how do you wake up with a "sudden onset" of flank pain? Did the pain wake her from sleep or did the pain start suddenly after she woke up, as is typical with a ureteral stone? When deciding whether a patient has pyelonephritis, a ureteral stone, or another etiology, a well-defined onset may be helpful.
2. Medical decision-making (MDM): Part 1 – The provider did a nice job of addressing an abnormality in the lab results: the WBCs found in the urine. This is an important risk management/patient safety technique; specifically addressing unexpected findings discovered during the evaluation. The explanation (ureteral inflammation) sounds reasonable (though may have been a guess and not literature-based), but the provider was left with some concern, so a urine culture was ordered.
3. Medical decision-making (MDM): Part 2 – When deciding on a disposition, we employ an age-old technique; risk stratification. Are we comfortable sending home a patient where we are 95% certain of the diagnosis, or do we strive for 99%? Much of this depends on the diagnosis we are considering. We may be comfortable with a 1% risk of missing an Achilles tendon rupture, but not a 1% risk of missing a ruptured AAA or a subarachnoid hemorrhage. When life-threatening entities are possible, we need to have a fail-safe strategy to catch the atypical presentation; the patient must know when and why to return. It is clear this provider considered infection, and while it may have been reasonable to discharge the patient without antibiotics, why not engage the patient/family with a discussion of unlikely but possible diagnoses remaining... and document the discussion in the "medical decision making" section? This is better for patient safety and more legally protective than simply printing the pre-scripted "aftercare instructions."[4,5]
4. The "game changer" question: "Have you had a fever?" Arguably the most important question in a patient with a confirmed ureteral stone; if this question had been answered in the affirmative, without other explanation for the increased temperature, the possibility of an "infected stone"would have been increased and the management would have likely been different. There was a notation made that the few urine WBCs seen could have been from ureteral irritation due to the stone, indicating the provider considered the possibility of infection. There was good documentation as to other symptoms including a detailed review of symptoms (ROS) stating: "She denies chest pain or pressure, shortness of breath, abdominal pain, diarrhea or bloody stools, dysuria, increased urinary frequency, or hematuria." Infection was considered, but the provider did not inquire about an age-old hallmark of infection—fever.

Section editor comments (Osborn):

Agree that this is a good question to ask. There are various possible responses from "no" to "I felt hot" to "it was 102 degrees at home" [and I took acetaminophen just prior to arrival]. Though our patient was afebrile in the ED, with concern for infection, would a second set of vital signs have been helpful?

What about the work-up? Seems routine and reasonable. We evaluate patients with back pain, flank pain, and "kidney stone" every day; the following is a review of the evaluation and management of flank pain and ureteral stones. More on ultrasound with the bounceback visit...

1. Is it possible to avoid CT imaging by clinically diagnosing ureteral colic?

The classic teaching is that a ureteral stone presents with a sudden onset of sharp and severe, "colicky" pain radiating to the unilateral groin/testicle (in a patient doing a "kidney stone dance"). Pyelonephritis, conversely, presents as a gradual onset of dull and constant flank/back pain with infectious urinary symptoms including dysuria, urinary frequency, and/or urgency.

But allow us to throw a wrench in this "classic" thinking. Consider a patient with a radiographically diagnosed stone who is leaving the ED after their hydromorphone and ondansetron; the only "dance" they are doing is one of joy because their pain is controlled. They still have a stone, but they no longer are exhibiting the "classic" symptoms—why? The severe pain which brought them to the ED was likely from a stone that was *moving* down the ureter. A stationary stone is more difficult to differentiate from pyelo, as there may be no pain or constant and mild pain.

Moore, et al. derived a clinical decision rule, the STONE score, by using a retrospective derivation of 1,040 patients who had a "flank pain protocol" CT to predict the presence of uncomplicated ureteral stones. They then used a prospective validation of 491 patients in whom "the clinician intended to obtain a CT scan for kidney stone." They found the 5 factors most predictive of a ureteral stone included.

1. Male sex
2. Short duration of pain (< 6 hours)
3. Non-black race
4. Presence of nausea or vomiting
5. Microscopic hematuria[3]

They used pilot data and previous studies to estimate that about 50% of CT scans for flank pain would have a ureteral stone. If all 5 findings were present, then a ureteral stone was identified 88.6% (validation set) to 89.6% (derivation set) of the time. But more importantly, the group most likely to have a stone was least likely (< 2%) to have an alternative important cause of their symptoms.[3] So how good is a clinical diagnosis of a stone? Pretty good if the patient presents classically, but in an elderly patient or with an atypical presentation… not good enough. The most interesting findings of the study were the rate of alternative diagnoses.

2. When imaging for a stone, how often are we surprised by a life-threatening etiology?

In many ways, the best utility of a CT scan in patients with flank pain is not to *rule-in* ureteral stones, but to *rule-out* serious alternative diagnoses. Balancing perceived patient expectations of imaging with the potential harm of radiation is difficult, but a conversation using a "shared-decision making" (SDM)[6] model may decrease the use of CT scans. The SDM conversation needs to be between two *reasonable alternative* approaches; for example, a 70-year-old with severe flank pain and no history of stones is not the time to improve your "through-put" numbers!

Combining the derivation and validation set performed by Moore, et al. (above) yielded 1,531 total patients; there was a serious diagnosis in a small, but significant number of patients:

Diverticulitis	10 (0.65%)
Appendicitis	9 (0.59%)
Malignancy	5 (0.32%)
Cholecystitis	3 (0.19%)
Bowel obstruction	2 (0.13%)
Perforated viscus	1 (0.065%)
Abdominal aortic aneurysm (AAA)	1 (0.07%)
Pancreatitis	1 (0.07%)
Total serious alternative diagnoses (note that there were other diagnoses in the total including ovarian pathology, colitis, pneumonia, etc) = 48 (3.1%)[3]	

Adapted from Moore CL, Bomann S, Daniels B. Derivation and validation of a clinical prediction rule for uncomplicated ureteral stone--the STONE score: retrospective and prospective observational cohort studies. BMJ. 2014 Mar 26. 348:g2191.

These findings are similar to an examination of 950 patients by Luchs, et al. who had a CT performed for renal colic, identifying 7% alternative diagnoses (which decreased to 5.6% if ovarian cysts were excluded).[7]

Rapp, et al. examined 613 patients undergoing non-contrast CT scan for flank pain and found if there was presence of all four "Vstone" criteria (flank pain, hematuria, nausea/vomiting, and prior stone) a ureteral stone was present 59% of the time, but the presence of flank pain alone, only yielded 6% ureteral stone disease.[8]

Bottom line: Whereas the different studies describe ureteral stone findings (flank pain, hematuria, short-duration pain), the most interesting findings are the rate of alternative diagnoses such as malignancy or AAA, which range between 3–7%.

3. Does size and location of ureteral calculi predict the probability of spontaneous passage?

Coll, et al. looked at 850 patients and found that 115/172 ureteral stones passed spontaneously and 57 required a urologic intervention.

- Stones 1mm in diameter passed spontaneously 87% of the time.
- Stones 2–4mm passed 76% of the time.
- Stones 5–7mm passed 60% of the time.
- Stones larger than 9mm passed 25% of the time.

Location mattered too, with spontaneous passage of 79% of stones at the ureterovesical junction, 60% of mid-ureteral stones, and 48% in the proximal ureter.[9]

Bottom line: Even for large, proximal stones, if the pain is controlled, it is worth waiting for spontaneous explusion.

4. What about medical expulsion therapy (MET)?

Pickard, et al. performed a meta-analysis of previous randomized controlled trials randomly assigning 1136 participants to tamsulosin (378), nifedipine (304), or placebo (379). They found no difference in stone expulsion between the 3 groups but there were more adverse events reported in the nifedipine group (3 patients with symptoms of diarrhea, vomiting, headache, chest pain, difficulty breathing) and the placebo group (1 patient with headache, dizziness and chronic abdominal pain).[10]

Just when this large meta-analysis would seem to put this issue to rest, along comes another systematic review and meta-analysis of 8 randomized, double-blind, controlled trials including 1,384 patients by Wang, et al. in Annals of Emergency Medicine. This study stratified stones by size and found that for stones measuring 5–10mm, there was an increased rate of stone passage with tamsulosin with a number needed to treat (NNT) of 5, but with the group < 4–5mm, there was no benefit. There were no significant adverse effects of dizziness or hypotension in either group.[11]

Similar results were reported with 403 patients in a double-blind, placebo-controlled, randomized, multicenter trial by Furyk, et al. finding a NNT of 4.5 in a prespecified group for stones 5–10mm.[12] A 2018 *Cochrane Review* had similar results.[13]

Bottom line: There was an NNT of 5 for MET in patients whose stone was 5–10mm in size.

5. Should labs have been obtained? Does the absence of hematuria exclude the possibility of ureterolithiasis?

WBC count:

An elevated WBC count may be deceptive due to stress demargination of circulating leukocytes and is generally unhelpful. Tintinalli recommends against obtaining a WBC count with uncomplicated ureteral colic.[14]

Renal function:

One older study suggested that patients who are stone formers have decreased renal function, but this was not in patients currently with a ureteral stone.[15] A more recent study of 384 stone formers vs. 457 controls found that the rise in serum creatinine is transient and minimal, with a baseline creatinine of 0.84mg/dL before the stone event compared to 0.97mg/dL at the stone event, returning to baseline at the first visit post-stone.[16] This data argues against obtaining serum labs for uncomplicated stones.

Urinalysis:

Blood:

The urinalysis (UA) is arguably the most useful test, although the absence of hematuria does not exclude ureterolithiasis. One retrospective study of 140 patients presenting with ureteral stones found 14.5% to have no hematuria on their UA.[17] Bove, et al. examined 267 consecutive patients with flank pain and found that 11% of patients with stones did not have the presence of blood or RBCs.[18] Luchs, et al. had similar findings after examining 950 patients with CT done for renal colic, of which 587 (62%) had a ureteral stone. Of these patients, only 84% had hematuria.[7]

So, blood is sometimes helpful, but lack of blood cannot exclude the presence of a stone, leading us to arguably the most important laboratory finding…presence of a concurrent infection.

Infection:
Our patient had a urinalysis notable for positive leukocyte esterase activity in the absence of leukocytes on urine microscopy (0–5 WBCs/HPF) and negative urinary nitrite testing. Is this predictive of an infection? Positive leukocyte esterase activity is 77–86% sensitive, but only 54% specific for culture-positive urinary infection.[19,20] Is the specificity high enough that our patient should have been managed with antibiotics and drainage or more investigation including serum labs, lactate, and repeat exam and vital sign assessment?

Our patient's nitrite was negative, seemingly reassuring, until we realize that the sensitivity is low at 45–60%, but if present, the specificity is high at 85–98%.[20] Although not suitable for our patient, it is helpful to use both tests together as the predictive value of combined nitrite and leukocyte esterase for a negative urine culture is 95%.[19]

Without clinical signs of infection, we are not alleging that antibiotics were indicated at the initial visit, but (broken record alert), it would have been nice to know about fever…

6. The nightmare scenario: How do patients with seemingly uncomplicated ureteral stones go bad…and how are they managed if this occurs?

An "infected stone" is treated with respect by experienced emergency providers as these patients can deteriorate quickly. Acute urinary obstruction complicated by septic shock is associated with mortality approximating 30%.[21]

Putting it all together:
This case would have been handled in a similar way by most emergency providers; a routine stone, a routine discharge… but there was an unexpected lab abnormality (leukocyte esterase and a few WBCs) that should prompt consideration and explanation within the medical decision-making documentation. How confident was the provider that "ureteral irritation" caused the abnormality? They were comprehensive in ordering a urine culture, which may be interpreted as at least some degree of clinical concern. Did the patient understand that there was possible infection and that a culture was ordered? If so, it would have been nice to see the conversation documented and aftercare instructions personalized to recommend returning for signs of infection including fever, chills, dizziness, weakness, increased pain, or confusion?

Look, it's not that big of a deal, right? Leukocyte esterase is sensitive, but not specific. Still… wouldn't you feel more comfortable with this additional data, documentation and discharge instructions in place?

ED BOUNCEBACK

Though the patient is straining her urine, she does not catch a stone. A urology appointment is scheduled for Tuesday morning, 2 days after ED discharge. But on the morning of the appointment, her husband notices that she is not acting "exactly right." Her symptoms are nonspecific, so he does not bring her back to the ED. Her urine has turned into a dark brown color. The urology appointment is scheduled for 10 a.m., but just before they leave home for the appointment, the patient begins to vomit.

ED VIST #2 (2 days after the initial ED visit)

CC (15:27): Confusion

HPI (15:42): The patient is a 51-year-old female with no past medical history presents from her urologist office where she was being seen for known left ureteral stone. Patient began having pain approximately 2 days ago and was seen in the ED at that time. She was found to have a 6mm obstructing left ureteral stone. Since that time urine culture have been sent and has been growing Enterobacter aerogens and Klebsiella. Patient is accompanied by her husband who provides most of the history as the patient is very confused at this time. He states that she began having confusion last night with slurred speech and difficulty walking. He called the ED this morning and was asked to bring her back in, but since they had the urology appointment a few hours later, he chose to take her there. Upon presenting to the urologist office given her confusion she was sent to the ER. Husband reports that she has had decreased oral input, decreased urinary output as well as nausea and vomiting. Patient has been very fatigued and husband initially contributed this to her pain medication, however she has not taken that in 2 days. Patient has had chills but no documented fevers.

Vitals:

Time	Temp (F)	Rt	Pulse	Resp	Syst	Diast	O2 sat (RA)
15:31	70	Oral	112	22	81	55	92

Pain	Weight
10/10	72kg

CONSTITUTIONAL: She is lethargic, moderate distress, oriented to person only, Speech is slurred and difficult to understand when she tries to speak
HEENT: Mouth and pharynx are clear, but membranes are tacky
NECK: Supple; no adenopathy or JVD
LUNGS: CTAB
CHEST: She is tender over the anterior chest wall
CARDIO: Tachy but regular rate and rhythm, nl. S1 S2
ABD: Soft but there is tenderness in the LLQ
SKIN: Mottling of the hands and fingertips

MDM (15:45): 50-year-old female with known 6 centimeters obstructing stone in left ureteral stone presents with confusion and lethargy since last night. Urine culture from 2/27 growing Enterobacter aerogens and Klebsiella.

ED course (16:02): Soon after completing the orders the nurse finds you, "Doctor, can you please reassess the patient in room 4?" You understand the concern; the patient's blood pressure has dropped to 72/51. Checking back in on the patient, she is more confused, and combative. Her husband is at the bedside, doing his best to keep her under control.
We are at:

DECISION POINT A – YOU ARE FACED WITH 4 QUESTIONS:

1. **What's the diagnosis? She is hypotensive and altered. Are we able to diagnosis septic shock and just send her up to the ICU?**
2. **Is a cephalosporin or a quinolone enough, or are broader spectrum antibiotics indicated?**
3. **You have ordered a 2L bolus; how long should you wait to see if the pressure improves?**
4. **Should she leave the department to get another CT scan to confirm the presence and location of the ureteral obstruction?**

What does the literature say?

Q#1: What's the diagnosis? She is hypotensive and altered. Are we able to diagnose septic shock and just send her up to the ICU?

In 2016, the Sepsis-3 investigators revised the definition of sepsis, stating that sepsis should be defined as "life-threatening organ dysfunction caused by a dysregulated host response to infection." Septic shock is a subset of sepsis, which occurs when "underlying circulatory and cellular/metabolic abnormalities are profound enough to substantially increase mortality." The task force believed that these new definitions were improvements compared to the former approach using 2 or more SIRS criteria to identify infected patients at high risk of adverse outcome.

Patients with a qSOFA (Quick sequential organ failure assessment) score of 2 or greater have a significantly increased risk of an ICU stay of 3 days or longer and an in-hospital mortality > 10%. This tool should be used to assess patients at risk for organ dysfunction.

qSOFA criteria:

1. Respiratory rate > 22/min
2. Altered mentation
3. Systolic blood pressure < 100mmHg

Sepsis-3 defines septic shock based on:

1. Vasopressor requirement to maintain mean arterial pressure (MAP) of 65mmHg after adequate fluid resuscitation -and-
2. Serum lactate greater than 2mmol/L (> 18mg/dL)

Patients defined by these criteria have mortality rate > 40%.[22] But caution with only using the Sepsis 3 definition. A study of 470 patients by Sterling, et al. found that of patients who met the old definition (but not the Sepsis 3 definition), there was still a 14% mortality in this group, and when a quantitative resuscitation protocol was used, there was significant mortality benefit.[23]

So, does our patient have septic shock? She is febrile with altered level of consciousness and hypotension—even before the lactate level returns, and without "getting in the weeds" with the definitions, the answer is an unequivocal yes! Additionally, she has all 3 of the qSOFA criteria, indicating her risk of mortality is high. Preparing for admission to the ICU at this point will depend on your hospital protocol, but several important treatments need to be started immediately.

Section editor comments (Osborn):

Do not give hospitals or intensivists an out while awaiting additional testing; a patient with BPs of 70's/30's does not need to wait for a lactate to get a definition of septic shock prior to initiating ICU admission. A note of caution on using Sepsis-3 definitions:

1. Across the globe, only one EM medical professional organization signed onto the Sepsis-3 definitions—it was rejected by all other EM organizations to which it was sent.
2. The Centers for Medicare and Medicaid Services (CMS) does not recognize Sepsis-3.
3. Quality organizations (Vizient, etc.) do not recognize the Sepsis-3 definitions

If you use Sepsis-3 to categorize sepsis, no matter how good your care is, it will be seen as worse based on the mortality index. The definitions right now are a mess and likely to continue to evolve.

Consulting editor comments (Weingart):

This question shouldn't have to be coming up; why do we even need these definitions of sepsis? The main reason is so that we can bill and so that government can regulate clinical care and pretend that we can lump everything into algorithmic approaches. That is opposed to treating each patient individually and deciding based on their unique presentation whether or not they're septic. So, by even asking the question, we are failing ourselves as physicians.

If we are forced to use definitions, which ones are good? Sepsis 3.0 was an attempt, at least, to justify a really sick cohort. If you look at their definition of septic shock, it required both resistant hypotension and resistant lactate elevation. That might not catch every single septic shock patient, but what it will do is to confirm that when we do identify septic shock, it is clearly septic shock!

I did like it for that reason; if we're going to compare ourselves, it was a group that everyone could agree was really sick. The problem with most of these definitions is that if you want to make your hospital look good, what you do is you take patients that aren't that ill and lump them into these groups of sick patients because then your mortality looks great; and that always upset me.

The sepsis-3.0 definition at least meant any hospital comparing their patients to another hospital had a pretty fair comparison.

I wish this entire thing would just go away and we could go back to actually being doctors and treating our patients.

Section editor comments (Osborn):

Six hours is the national average ED length of stay for critically ill patients.

The provider should recognize that this patient is severely ill and should have a 30mL/kg IVF bolus, blood cultures, appropriate antibiotics and definitive therapy/source control pursued as quickly as possible. This should be balanced against keeping a patient in the ED too long, as there is a higher in-hospital and ICU mortality in patients boarding for greater than 6 hours.[24]

Q#2: Is a cephalosporin or a quinolone enough, or are broader spectrum antibiotics indicated?

Per the Surviving Sepsis Campaign (SSC) updated response to new bundles, the following should occur within 3 hours of presentation (time of triage in the ED):

1. Measure lactate level
2. Obtain blood cultures prior to administration of antibiotics
3. Administer broad spectrum antibiotics
4. Administer 30mL/kg crystalloid[25]

Recommended antibiotic administration initiation is as fast as possible and within 1 hour of septic shock recognition. Antimicrobial selections should provide activity against the likely pathogens based on the patient's source of infection.[26] For community-acquired urinary tract infection, coverage against *E. coli*, other gram negative pathogens and *Enterococcus* are important, but in this case we have cultures results, making a streamlined approach to antibiotics easier. Absent the prior cultures or other data pinpointing the infection source or anticipated pathogens, a broad-spectrum approach with piperacillin-tazobactam or cefepime PLUS vancomycin is a reasonable combination for many patients with severe infection, as inappropriate initial antibiotics are associated with higher mortality. One additional point to consider is the order of antimicrobials when IV access limits initiation of both agents simultaneously. Beta-lactam agents are generally recommended to be started first based on broad antimicrobial activity and brief administration times, compared to vancomycin.

Even with appropriate antimicrobial support, urinary obstruction represents a critical target to achieve source infection control (see Decision Point B, below).

Section editor comments (Osborn):

There are frequent misconceptions that vancomycin is a broad-spectrum antibiotic, and that it should be given first or that one cannot administer 2 IV antibiotics at the same time. Vancomycin generally takes about 1–1.5 hours to administer, so administering that first could constitue a delay in administering the antibiotic most likely to cover the offending bacteria in the setting of shock, in this case the piperacillin-tazobactam.

Q#3: You have ordered a 2L bolus; how long should you wait to see if the pressure improves?

An initial bolus of 30mL/kg crystalloid IVF is recommended, with the understanding that more fluids may be required in some patients. The fluids should be administered rapidly via straight intravenous tubing and pressure bags rather than an IV pump rate of 999mL/hour. Without an adequate response to IVF, consideration should be given to pressors.[26]

Q#4: Should she leave the department to get another CT scan to confirm the presence and location of the ureteral obstruction?

The clinician should be cautious in sending such a critically ill patient to the radiology suite for a CT scan without some stabilization, unless the information will dictate an immediate new intervention. In the interim, bedside exam should exclude other sources of infection and management should be initiated for the likely etiology of septic shock; a urinary infection complicated by ureteral obstruction.

Bedside ultrasound can be used to confirm the presence of unilateral hydronephrosis and may identify focal abscess. A study by Riddell, et al. showed 82% sensitivity of a positive ED ultrasound finding of either hydronephrosis or visualized stones.[27] Another study in over 300 patients comparing EP performance of ultrasound to CT found that hydronephrosis had a positive predictive value (PPV) of 88% for ureteral stone on CT, and lack of hydronephrosis made a stone > 5mm less likely.[28]

DECISION POINT A – ***What did the actual provider do?***

ED course (15:50): Upon recognizing clinical sepsis, the provider orders labs including a CBC, BMP, urine, lactate level and an IVF bolus totaling 30mL/kg, per a sepsis treatment order set. As diagnostic studies are ordered, the provider places a STAT order for Ceftriaxone 1gm IV.

The story continues:
(16:29): Initial labs results:

WBC count = 15.1 (H)
Hb = 12.4 gm/dL
Plt = 118 thou/mcl (L)
Sodium = 126 mmol/L (L)
Bicarbonate = 18
Creatinine = 5.5 mg/dL (H)
Lactate = 5.8 (H)

Looking up, you see the nurse.

"Do we have urine yet?"

"We have asked twice, but she is not cooperating. Also, we have a bit of a problem. She is crawling out of bed. We have a tech and her husband trying to keep her from falling. I need something to calm her down."

"OK," you respond confidently, "Please give Ativan 2mg IV. I'll put the order in right now."

Hearing silence, you look up to see her staring back at you. After an awkward pause, she asks, "Won't that make her pressure worse?" The 2 liters we gave did nothing. Her BP is still in the low 70s.

(16:32): You order another 2L (for a total of 4L) of IVF. It is infused quickly and a recheck shows no change in the BP.

(17:08): You ask the nurse to set up materials for a central line so pressors can be started. You "glove and gown" and set up all the materials. Despite receiving 50mcg of Fentanyl, and 4 staff holding the patient down, you are not able to keep her under adequate control to safely place a femoral central line. With sweat leaching through your gown, you abandon the attempt and return to the drawing board.

Author note: You are back in the shoes of the emergency provider… at decision point B.

DECISION POINT B – YOU ARE FACED WITH 4 QUESTIONS:

1. **What is the best approach for sedation in a hypotensive patient?**
2. **If the patient cannot be sedated, is intubation indicated?**
3. **Is it time for pressors? Can they be started through a peripheral line?**
4. **Who should be called first, urology for stent placement or interventional radiology for a nephrostomy tube?**

What does the literature say?

Q#1: What is the best approach for sedation in a hypotensive patient?

While a wide range of options is available for sedating combative ED patients, selecting a safe and effective agent can be challenging in the presence of hemodynamic compromise. The ideal sedative has a rapid onset of action, minimal cardiovascular compromise, is easily titratable, short-acting, with minimal interaction with other drugs.[29] Sounds simple right? Consider this approach:

1. Choose medications that have a low chance of decreasing blood pressure such as ketamine or etomidate (low dose) or haloperidol.
2. Start with a low dose and see if sedation is adequate and how it affects the blood pressure, maintaining the option to administer more.
3. Be prepared to use a fluid bolus or pressors (consider "push-dose" pressors with phenylephrine or epinephrine) if there is a significant drop in the blood pressure. Bolus dosing of vasopressors, or push-dose pressors, has been successfully used perioperatively and is well described in the anesthesia literature. While there are no ED-specific national guidelines on their use, some have advocated for their implementation given their ease of use and ability to temporize precipitous drops in blood pressure.[30]
4. In patients who are hypotensive before intubation, plan proactively to add norepinephrine before giving the sedative. There may still be a need for temporary push-dose pressors, but there will at least be a baseline vasopressor infusion running already that can be titrated rapidly. In other words, don't rely solely on push-dose pressors in a patient who is already hypotensive and will likely worsen after intubation. Start the vasopressor infusion early.

Section editor comments (Osborn):

Of note, the benefit of haloperidol, ketamine or etomidate in this situation is sedation without respiratory depression. Lorazepam may cause respiratory depression and worsening acidosis.

Consulting editor comments (Weingart):

There are sedation agents that are blood pressure neutral, or blood pressure bolstering. If you have to get immediate control of a situation and the patient is hypotensive, just give them ketamine. And then, while the ketamine dissociation is occurring, you can place a central line, if necessary. Note that droperidol is available again; it has no blood pressure effects, and it will give instantaneous control of the situation. Can we use benzos? Absolutely. But beware, if the patient's agitation is supporting their blood pressure, the benzodiazepine may take away their endogenous catecholamines and things may get much worse. I'd be reluctant to do that without use of a vasopressor. Fix their blood pressure, and then you're more than free to give benzodiazepines.

A word on push-dose pressors. If you are using as a temporizing measure while the nursing staff is getting a vasopressor drip prepared, that is fine, but I would not give continuous rounds of push-dose pressors; I've never supported that. Push-dose is the immediate temporizing measure to allow you the time to get a drip going with a pump.

Author comments (Weinstock):

There are a lot of podcasts detailing an approach to self-mixing meds to then administer by push-dose... but there are pre-mixed syringes available. Like everything in medicine, conditions and procedures which we see and perform commonly allow for expertise, but if we are not doing things frequently, we are prone to error.

Consulting editor comments (Weingart):

If your institution will buy you pre-mixed, then that is a safer way to go. There has been a spate of ED pharmacologist literature showing mixing errors. We have two breeds of emergency physicians; the incredibly detail-oriented resuscitation docs, and the docs who do not do this frequently and leave medication administration to the nurse; these docs shouldn't be mixing.

A note on pushing cardiac epinephrine; it is a peri-code temporizing measure. I don't push one tenth of a cardic epi syringe, I push a half a cc. All of the cardiac epis are graduated at the level of a half cc. That is 50 micrograms; that is a very reasonable dose. You still may overshoot, but you will not overshoot to "bursting blood vessels in the head" levels, and it'll get the job done on a patient who is about to code. So, if the pressure is 40/20, looking like death, by all means take out the cardiac epi and push half a cc. But never push a full amp of cardiac epinephrine on a patient with a pulse.

Q#2: If the patient cannot be sedated, is intubation indicated?

Intubating critically ill patients is rife with risk, as demonstrated by Heffner, et al.; ED emergency intubation carries a peri-procedure cardiac arrest (CA) rate of 3% among normotensive patients, which jumps to 12% among patients with systemic hypotension at the time of induction. Not surprisingly, the mortality was significantly higher in those patients who had a CA (82%) vs. those who did not (24%).[31] These findings are similar to findings from Schwartz, et al. who examined 297 intubations of hypotensive patients, finding a 15% mortality.[32]

OK. Got it. Intubating a hypotensive, septic patient is risky, but do we have a choice? Not only does this agitated patient represent a risk to herself and to staff, but she will emergently need drainage of the obstructed ureter, which will require sedation and perhaps paralysis. If she is not able to be adequately sedated for a central line, certainly she will not sit still for a nephrostomy tube or ureteral stent.

Q#3: Is it time for pressors? Can they be started through a peripheral line?

Per the SCC guidelines, if a patient remains hypotensive after the initial fluid bolus and if they are "fluid responsive," additional fluid boluses may be given. The initial vasopressor of choice is norepinephrine, and this should be titrated to mean arterial pressure (MAP) > 65mmHg.

For our patient, initiating pressor support with norepinephrine would be advisable, especially as the patient remained hypotensive after the 2nd 2L IVF bolus. But we don't have a central line… should we wait? The main concern with administering pressors through a peripheral line is extravasation and tissue ischemia from intense local vasoconstriction. On the other hand, waiting for placement of a central line may delay care in critical patients, as well as expose the patient to the increased risk of placing a central line in the first place.

In 2014 Loubani, et al. attempted to determine the safety of administering pressors through a peripheral intravenous access. In a systematic review of 85 articles they found 270 patients which met inclusion criteria. The mean duration of infusion was 55 hours, and over 85% of the lines were distal to the antecubital vein. They concluded that "short term" administration (< 2 hours) of vasopressor infusions via proximal, well-placed peripheral IVs is unlikely to cause local tissue injury."[33]

In 2015 Cardenas-Garcia, et al. performed an original investigation with almost 3 times the number of patients. They examined 734 patients, ages 72 +/- 15 years who received vasoactive medication 783 times via peripheral IV access including norepinephrine (n=506), dopamine (n=101) and phenylephrine (n=176) for a duration of 49 +/- 22 hours. They found that extravasation occurred 19 times (2%), which was treated in their study with local phentolamine injection and application of local nitroglycerine paste. They found no tissue injury. And to make matters even better, only 13% of patients eventually required central access.[34]

With the patient agitated, confused and hypotensive, she needs additional fluids as well as norepinephrine; we recommend avoiding a delay in care by trying again for a central line, and instead infusing through a large-bore antecubital peripheral line. If her pressure improves, additional sedation may be attempted with ketamine or haloperidol and if unsuccessful intubation can be considered—we have done so much, but there is arguably the most important intervention for sepsis care which has not yet been completed—source control.

Consulting editor comments (Weingart):

If you have a patient exsanguinating, well that's a relatively tough scenario, but in this case, just fix the hypotension. That is the answer. And then you can use whatever you want to sedate them. So, how do you fix the hypotension? Well, you put them on vasopressors. "Oh, well I don't have a central line." I don't care. Even in places that don't have a protocol for peripheral pressors on the floors, put them on peripheral norepinephrine. We have three trials now demonstrating safety. Get them temporized, and then take all the time in the world to put in your central line when you have a sedated, non-hypotensive patient. To wait for a central line in the face of hypotension is maybe the worst thing you can do for these patients. They will deteriorate, you're now under a time pressure to do a procedure that requires meticulous, slow careful attention to detail. And you are limited in how you can sedate the patient; put them on peripheral norepinephrine and then give whatever you want.

Q#4: Who should be called first, urology for stent placement or interventional radiology for a nephrostomy tube?

Let's cut to the chase—this patient has pus under pressure, due to urinary obstruction, and needs it drained as soon as possible. The specific intervention should be individualized by institution and available resources. There is a paucity of data to declare a single best intervention.

Mokhmalji, et al. looked at 40 patients who had stone-induced hydronephrosis and found the success rate of percutaneous nephrostomy drainage was 100% with *decreased* radiation exposure and decreased analgesics compared to a ureteral stent, which had 80% success.[35]

Pearle, et al. randomized 42 patients with concomitant obstruction and urinary tract infection, defined by temperature greater than 38° C and/or WBC count greater than 17,000), to either percutaneous nephrostomy or ureteral stent and found 1 failure in the nephrostomy group, decreased procedural and fluoroscopy time in the stent group, and a similar "time to normal temperature," "time to normal WBC count" and hospital length of stay between groups. They concluded that "neither modality demonstrated superiority in promoting a more rapid recovery after drainage." Ureteral stent placement was more costly.[36]

Cristoph, et al. agreed with Mokhmalji that both interventions had similar clinical efficacy[37] as did the Canadian Urological Association (2015), concluding these recommendations for infected ureteral stones:

1. Obstructing stones with infection require emergent drainage.
2. Nephrostomy tube and stent have equivalent outcomes and choice should be based on availability of resources.
3. Broad-spectrum antibiotics should be started early.
4. Definitive stone management should be delayed until decompression and antibiotics have been administered.[38]

Consulting editor comments (Weingart):

With an obstructing infected stone, the first thing needed is source control; there's no doubt about that. The decision between options is situation and institution-dependent and best arranged in advance so you are not talking to multiple specialists at 3 AM—you need to force it to happen because these patients are sick and can't wait until morning. A delay goes against all our rules of source control and sepsis.

Now, just as a bonus, be aware that your job is not yet over as these patients have a tendency to get super sick after the drainage happens; this is incredibly common. They get their percutaneous nephrostomy tube, and then they acutely decompensate for a couple hours as there's a huge release of inflammatory hormones. I don't know exactly why; I just know it happens. So, if your plan was, well they'll be much better after they get their procedure and "I'll just get them a floor bed," this will fail. They either need an ICU, or to stay in the ED and be watched until better, then they can go up to the floor.

DECISION POINT B – ***What did the actual provider do?***

MDM (16:52): The urine has returned, showing specific gravity of 1.046, blood, leukocyte esterase (75/UL), WBC 3,352. RBC 791, and moderate bacteria. The patient remains hypotensive with a BP of 70s/50s despite 5L IVF.

MDM (17:08): Despite 5 L of normal saline fluid, the patient remains hypotensive. We attempted to get a central line, but patient became delirious and combative. After attempts to restrain her with 50mcg fentanyl she was still confused which seemed to be secondary to encephalopathy from septic shock.

ED course:
(17:54): Norepinephrine at 7mcg/min through a peripheral 18g IV.
(18:33): The decision was made to place a nephrostomy tube in the interventional radiology suite after intubation and "likely placement of a CVC."

The story continues: With the continued IV fluids and the norepinephrine, the patient's blood pressure improves to 100/60. The provider tells the staff that they will proceed with intubation. We are at:

DECISION POINT C – YOU ARE FACED WITH 4 QUESTIONS:

1. **Which medications should be used for rapid sequence intubation (RSI) in a hypotensive septic patient?**
2. **Why do some patients "crash" after intubation?**
3. **Which ventilator setting should be used after intubation of a septic patient?**
4. **My septic patient is intubated, now what?**

What does the literature say?

Q#1: Which medications should be used for rapid sequence intubation (RSI) in a hypotensive septic patient?

Wow, now we have a bear in a hornet's nest. Our goal is to make patients safer without causing harm, but the mortality of intubating a septic patient is high. Which sedatives are optimal in a hypotensive shock patient?

Stollings, et al. reviewed the Medline® database from 1966–2013 and published a comprehensive review of medications used with rapid sequence intubation (RSI).[39] Not surprisingly, they confirmed that most induction agents can cause or exacerbate hypotension. Here is some more detailed information on two medications commonly used for sedation/induction in RSI:

Etomidate:
Class/action: Sedative-hypnotic
Dose: 0.2mg/kg–0.6mg/kg
Recommended dose in patients with hypotension is 0.1–0.2mg/kg, and not the standard 0.3mg/kg Use of adjusted body weight with morbid obesity is also recommended.
Metabolism: Hepatic
Advantages: Minimal hemodynamic effects, decreases ICP, no histamine release, quick onset of action, short duration of action.
Disadvantages: May induce suppression of cortisol and aldosterone (see Jabre study below).
Note: Myoclonus occurs 22–63% of the time but is typically short-lived and is clinically inconsequential, especially when combined with a neuromuscular blocker.

Ketamine:
Class/action: Causes intense amnesia secondary to dissociative effects and has analgesic properties
Dose: 1–2mg/kg (typically 100mg)
Metabolism: Hepatic
Advantages: Exerts sympathomimetic effects including increases in heart rate, blood pressure, and cardiac output. Contrary to initial reports, does not increase ICP.
Disadvantages: May result in decreased cardiac output in patients with severe heart failure, may rarely increase oral secretions (making intubation more difficult), and can be associated with emergence delirium, nightmares and hallucinations.

What happens when these drugs are compared head-to-head? Jabre, et al. examined etomidate and ketamine for RSI in a multi-center, randomized, single-blind trial. They examined 655 patients requiring sedation for RSI randomized to receive a single dose of etomidate 0.3mg/kg (328 patients) or ketamine 2mg/kg (327 patients). After exclusions, they analyzed 234 patients in the etomidate group and 235 in the ketamine group with a primary study endpoint of the maximum sequential organ failure assessment (SOFA) during the first 3 days of ICU admission. The percentage of patients with a decreased serum cortisol was higher in the etomidate group, but there were no serious adverse events with either drug.[40]

Conclusion: All induction agents can exacerbate hypotension, but both etomidate and ketamine are best choices. Dose reduction to half the typical induction agent dose is also recommended and is often adequate for sedation.

Q#2: Why do some patients "crash" after intubation?

Why is a potentially life-saving intervention, intubation, risky? Rapid sequence intubation (RSI) induces complicated physiologic changes. Sympatholysis from induction agents and conversion to positive pressure breathing negatively impact cardiac venous return. As such, pre-intubation fluid optimization should always be considered prior to RSI, even in patients who are not in shock.

In addition, our septic patient with lactic acidosis is attempting to compensate via increased respiratory rate. They are blowing off CO_2 in an attempt to correct acid/base status. As their disease progresses, despite the interventions of the emergency provider, intubation may become necessary, but respiratory compensation is halted with RSI, which can worsen acidosis. Is there a way to make this critical intervention safer? In addition to the previous comments about RSI hypnotic selection and dosing and preinduction fluid optimization, patients with high minute ventilation requirements prior to intubation often require peri-RSI ventilation and attention to initial ventilator settings to compensate for metabolic acidosis

Weingart, et al. describe a process of "delayed-sequence intubation" where 62 patients at high risk for immediate intubation (primarily because of hypoxemia) were enrolled in a prospective, observational, multi-center trial. The patients received a dissociative dose of ketamine, then either high-flow oxygen with a non-rebreather mask or noninvasive positive pressure ventilation (NIPPV). They found that oxygen saturations increased from a mean of 89.9–98.8% afterward, and there were no complications observed in the patients receiving delayed sequence intubation.[41]

Whereas, their hypoxemic patient population was not the same as our hypotensive septic patient, the goal should be to stabilize the patient prior to intubation with fluid resuscitation, antibiotics, pressors (if needed), and ensuring adequate oxygenation—this is exactly what occurred in our patient… eventually.

Q#3: Which ventilator setting should be used after intubation of a septic patient?

A broad stroke approach utilizes these recommendations:

- Tidal volume: Initial target should be 6mL/kg of predicted body weight,42 though other authors recommend 8mL/kg.[43]
- Don't wait for the ICU staff to do it—what begins in the ED matters. In a 2017 study, Fuller, et al. found that ventilator settings initiated in the emergency department impact clinical outcomes in patients with ARDS.[44]
- Mode: Volume-assist mode.[43]
- Initial respiratory rate: 15–16 breaths/min although a rate of 30–40 breaths/min is acceptable to achieve $PaCO_2$ goals.[43]
- FiO_2 should be rapidly titrated to 30–40%, if tolerated by patient, with a positive end-expiratory pressure (PEEP) of 5cm H_2O. If the patient is hypoxemic, evaluate the patient for ARDS (definition being PaO_2/FiO_2 ratio of < 300 with non cardiogenic pulmonary edema and a PEEP > 5) [ARDSnet].
- Goal plateau pressure < 30cm H_2O.[42,43]

An arterial or venous blood gas should be drawn 20–30 minutes after intubation to allow titration of ventilator settings.[43] Using the VBG in combination with the pulse oximeter is a viable alternative to obtaining an ABG,[45] understanding that patients in shock with poor perfusion may have a VBG that is not reliably predictive of arterial gas exchange.

Q#4: My septic patient is intubated, now what?

Redux to our problem from above, our patient is now intubated but remains hypotensive. We are still between a rock and a hard place; it is cruel to have a patient intubated without sedation, but we don't want our sedative therapy to make the patient's blood pressure worse.

The Surviving Sepsis Campaign (SSC) 2016 guidelines recommended the following possible approaches for sedation and analgesia of intubated patients:[42]

- Sedation should be targeted to specific titration end-points (as opposed to using continuous or intermittent sedation). This approach should reduce the duration of mechanical ventilation and the ICU stay. Possible approaches to minimizing sedation include:
    - "Nurse-directed" protocols with a sedation scale
    - Intermittent as opposed to continuous sedation
    - Daily sedation interruption[46]
- Midazolam (or benzos) are not recommended by the SCCM sedation guidelines, instead propofol or dexmedetomidine are preferred. Ketamine is another option. If a benzo is required, midazolam q 1hr prn might be a better approach.
- Consider use of opioids alone (without any sedatives) as this may result in decreased duration of mechanical ventilation.

DECISION POINT C – ***What did the actual provider do?***

MDM (18:04):

- I have attempted to place a femoral CVC; however, patient was too combative for successful placement. The patient was intubated for septic shock delirium and airway protection and also prior to interventional radiology for nephrostomy tube placement for her obstructing stone.
- The patient was given etomidate 15mg and succinylcholine 100mg and then intubated with a GlideScope with a 7.0 endotracheal tube. The tube was initially placed at 22cm, but CXR showed the tube to be at the level of the carina, so was withdrawn to 20cm and a repeat CXR demonstrated good position. Post-intubation sedation was propofol.
- The patient was initially placed on assist mode ventilation, rate of 14, tidal volume 500cc, PEEP 5 and FiO2 100%, but the FiO2 was quickly decreased to 40%.

ED course (18:56): The patient was transferred to the interventional radiology (IR) suite for placement of a nephrostomy tube. When the tube was placed, it returned a copious amount of purulent material.

What was the patient outcome?

The ICU course was initially rocky, with the patient requiring the addition of vasopressin to maintain a mean arterial pressure (MAP) of 65. She remained in the ICU for 3 days then was moved to the floor and eventually discharged.

Final hospital impression:

- Septic shock and severe sepsis
- Urinary infection
- Obstructing ureteral stone
- Acute kidney injury
- *Enterobacter* bacteremia

Debrief:

Care was well done, but there were some areas for possible improvement:

1. Initial history should have determined presence of infectious symptoms, specifically presence of fever.
2. Discharge instructions from the first visit should detail reasons to return, specifically fever or confusion.
3. At the second visit, the diagnosis was recognized quickly, and appropriate care was initiated, but arrangements for source control (nephrostomy tube or stent) should have been started simultaneously.
4. While the goal of starting a central line was acceptable, it should have been recognized that with her amount of agitation, it was going to be difficult. A surgeon would not take a patient to the OR without adequate anesthesia… in our patient, pressors could have been started through a peripheral line, then sedation administered.
5. Sedative agents which could have been tried before Ativan were ketamine or haloperidol.
6. Kudos to the doctor for adequate resuscitation before intubation, this was well done and decreased her peri-intubation risk significantly

Chapter summary:

- Midstream urine is a poor predictor of infected pelvic urine, especially if there is a completely obstructing stone.
- Nitrite is specific for a UTI, but not sensitive. Leukocyte esterase is sensitive, but not specific.
- Patients with a ureteral stone should be assessed for a possible infection with questions directed for symptoms such as chills, dizziness, confusion, and signs of tachycardia, tachypnea, hypotension, confusion… as well as fever.
- The combination of a ureteral stone and sepsis is a true urologic emergency that requires prompt drainage either with a nephrostomy tube or ureteral stent, whichever is most readily available.
- Hypotensive patients have a high peri-intubation risk. Resuscitate before intubation and use induction agents least likely to exacerbate hypotension.
- Engaging the patient and family with the discharge planning process will increase the chance that they will return if symptoms worsen, change, or don't improve. Inform patients who are being discharged with an uncomplicated ureteral stone to return for any infectious symptoms.

References:

1. Foster G, Stocks C, Borofsky MS. Emergency department visits and hospital admissions for kidney stone disease, 2009: Statistical Brief #139. 2012 Jul. In: Healthcare Cost and Utilization Project (HCUP) Statistical Briefs. Available at https://www.hcup-us.ahrq.gov/reports/statbriefs/statbriefs.jsp. Rockville (MD): Agency for Healthcare Research and Quality (US); 2006 Feb. Available at: https://www.ncbi.nlm. nih.gov/books/NBK100827/
2. Assimos D, Krambeck A, Miller NL, et al. Surgical management of stones: American Urological Association/Endourological Society guideline Part 1. J Urol 2016;196(4):1153–60.
3. Moore CL, Bomann S, Daniels B, et al. Derivation and validation of a clinical prediction rule for uncomplicated ureteral stone—the STONE score: Retrospective and prospective observational cohort studies. BMJ 2014. 348:g2191.
4. Engel K, Buckley BA, Forth VE, et al. Patient understanding of emergency department discharge instructions: where are knowledge deficits greatest? Acad Emerg Med 2012;19(9):E1035–44.
5. Lawrence LM, Jenkins CA, Zhou C, et al. The effect of diagnosis-specific computerized discharge instructions on 72-hour return visits to the pediatric emergency department. Pediatr Emerg Care 2009;25(11):733–8.
6. Hess EP, Grudzen CR, Thomson R, et al. Shared decision-making in the emergency department: respecting patient autonomy when seconds count. Acad Emerg Med 2015;22(7):856–64.
7. Luchs JS, Katz DS, Lane MJ, et al. Utility of hematuria testing in patients with suspected renal colic: correlation with unenhanced helical CT results. Urology 2002;59(6):839–42.
8. Rapp DE, Wood NL, Bassignani M, et al. Clinical variables and stone detection in patients with flank pain. Can J Urol 2016;23(5):8441–45.
9. Coll DM, Varanelli MJ, Smith RC. Relationship of spontaneous passage of ureteral calculi to stone size and location as revealed by unenhanced helical CT. AJR Am J Roentgenol 2002;178(1):101–3.
10. Pickard R, Starr K, MacLennan G, et al. Medical expulsive therapy in adults with ureteric colic: A multicentre, randomised, placebo-controlled trial. Lancet 2015;386(9991):341–9.
11. Wang R, Smith-Bindman R, Whitaker E, et al. Effect of tamsulosin on stone passage for uereteral stones: A systematic review and meta-analysis. Ann Emerg Med 2017;69(3):353–61.e3.
12. Furyk JS, Chu K, Banks C, et al. Distal ureteric stones and tamsulosin: A double-blind, placebo-controlled, randomized, multicenter trial. Ann Emerg Med 2016;67(1):86–95.
13. Campschroer T, Zhu X, Vernooij RWM, et al. Alpha-blockers as medical expulsive therapy for ureteral stones. Cochrane Database Syst Rev 2018;4:CD008509.
14. Tintinalli JE, ed. Emergency medicine, a comprehensive study guide. 5th ed. New York, NY: McGraw Hill, 2000.
15. Worcester EM, Parks JH, Evan AP, et al. Renal function in patients with nephrolithiasis. J Urol 2006;176(2):600–3.
16. Haley WE, Enders FT, Vaughan LE, et al. Kidney function after the first kidney stone event. Mayo Clinic Proceed 2016;91(12):1744–52.
17. Press SM, Smith AD, et al. Incidence of negative hematuria in patients with acute urinary lithiasis presenting to the emergency room with flank pain. Urology 1995;45(5):753–7.
18. Bove P, Kaplan D, Dalrymple N, et al. Reexamining the value of hematuria testing in patients with acute flank pain. J Urol 1999;162(3 Pt1):685–7.
19. Rehmani R. Accuracy of urine dipstick to predict urinary tract infections in an emergency

department. J Ayub Med Coll Abbottabad 2004;16(1):4–7.
20. Deville WL, Yzermans JC, van Duijn NP, et al. The urine dipstick test useful to rule out infections. A meta-analysis of the accuracy. BMC Urol 2004;4:4.
21. Reyner K, Heffner AC, Karvetski CH. Urinary obstruction is an important complicating factor in patients with septic shock due to urinary infection. Am J Emerg Med 2016;34(4):694–6.
22. Singer M, Deutschman CS, Seymour CW, et al. The third international consensus definitions for sepsis and septic shock (Sepsis-3). JAMA 2016;315(8):801–10.
23. Sterling SA, Puskarich MA, Glass AF, et al. The impact of the Sepsis-3 Septic shock definition on previously defined septic shock patients. Crit Care Med 2017;45(9):1436–42.
24. Chaltin DB, Trzeciak S, Likourezos A, et al. Impact of delayed transfer of critically ill patients from the emergency department to the intensive care unit. Crit Care Med 2007;35(6):1477–83.
25. Surviving sepsis campaign: Updated bundles in response to new evidence. https://emcrit.org/wp-content/uploads/2015/04/SSC_Bundle.pdf
26. Riddell J, Case A, Wopat R, et al. Sensitivity of emergency bedside ultrasound to detect hydronephrosis in patients with computed tomography-proven stones. West J Emerg Med 2014;15(1):96–100.
27. Leo MM, Langlois BK, Pare JR, et al. Ultrasound vs. computed tomography for severity of hydronephrosis and its importance in renal colic. West J Emerg Med 2017;18(4):559-68.
28. Brusco L. Choice of sedation for critically ill patients: A rational approach. Adv Stud Med 2002;2(9):343–9.
29. Weingart S. Push-dose pressors for immediate blood pressure control. Clin Exp Emerg Med 2015;2(2):131–32.
30. Heffner AC, Swords DS, Neale MN, et al, Incidence and factors associated with cardiac arrest complicating emergency airway management. Resuscitation 2013;84(11):1500–4.
31. Schwartz DE, Matthay MA, Cohen NH, et al, Death and other complications of emergency airway management in critically ill adults. A prospective investigation of 297 tracheal intubations. Anesthesiology 1995;82(2):367–76.
32. Loubani OM, Green RS. A systematic review of extravasation and local tissue injury from administration of vasopressors through peripheral intravenous catheters and central venous catheters. J Crit Care 2015;30(3)653.e9–17.
33. Cardenas-Garcia J, Schaub KF, Belchikov YG, et al. Safety of peripheral intravenous administration of vasoactive medication. J Hosp Med 2015;10(9):581–5.
34. Mokhmalji H, Braun PM, Martinez Portillo FJ, et al. Percutaneous nephrostomy versus ureteral stents for diversion of hydronephrosis caused by stones: a prospective, randomized clinical trial. J Urol 2001;165(4):1088–92.
35. Pearle MS, Pierce HL, Miller GL, et al. Optimal method of urgent decompression of the collecting system for obstruction and infection due to ureteral calculi. J Urol 1998;160(4):1260–4.
36. Christoph F, Weikert S, Muller M, et al. How sepsic is urosepsis? Clinical course of infected hydronephrosis and therapeutic strategies. World J Urol 2005;23(4):243–7.
37. Ordon M, Andonian S, Blew B, et al. CUA Guideline: Management of ureteral calculi. Can Urol Assoc J 2015;9(11–12):E837.
38. Stollings JL, Diedrich DA, Oyen LJ, et al. Rapid-sequence intubation: a review of the process and considerations when choosing medications. Ann Pharmacother 2014;48(1):62–76.
39. Jabre P, Combes X, Lapostolle F, et al. Etomidate versus ketamine for rapid sequence intubation

in acutely ill patients: A multicentre randomised controlled trial. Lancet 2009;374(9686):293–300.

40. Weingart SD, Trueger NS, Wong N, et al. Delayed sequence intubation: A prospective observational trial. Ann Emerg Med 2015;65(4):349–55.
41. Rhodes A, Evans L, Alhazzani W, et al. Surviving Sepsis Campaign: International Guidelines for Management of Sepsis and Septic Shock: 2016. Crit Care Med 2017;45(3):486–552.
42. Weingart SD. Managing initial mechanical ventilation in the emergency department. Ann Emerg Med 2016;68(5):614–7.
43. Fuller BM, Ferguson IT, Mohr NM, et al. A quasi-experimental, before-after trial examining the impact of an emergency department mechanical ventilator protocol on clinical outcomes and lung-protective ventilation in acute respiratory distress syndrome. Crit Care Med 2017;45(4):645–52.
44. Zeserson E, Goodgame B, Hess JD, et al. Correlation of venous blood gas and pulse oximetry with arterial blood gas in the undifferentiated critically ill patient. 2018;33(3):176–81.
45. Kress JP, Pohlman AS, O'Connor MF, et al. Daily interruption of sedative infusions in critically ill patients undergoing mechanical ventilation. New Engl J Med 2000;342(20):1471–7.

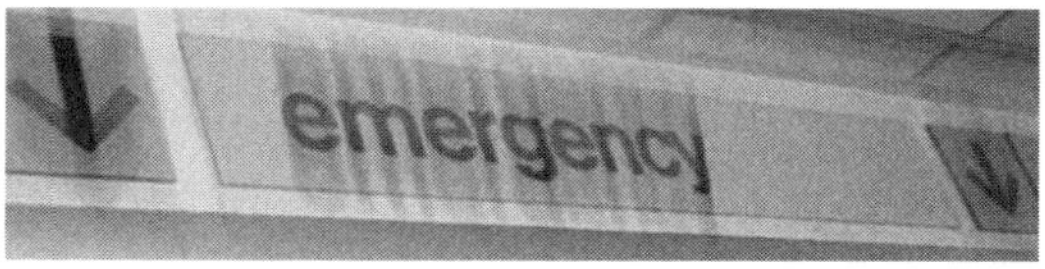

SECTION E – NEURO & SEPSIS

Chapter 22: A 53-year-old man with atrial fibrillation and palpitations

Crystal Ives Tallman, MD
Assistant Clinical Professor
Emergency Medicine
Department of Emergency Medicine
UCSF Fresno
Fresno, CA

Jessica Mason, MD
Assistant Clinical Professor
Emergency Medicine
Department of Emergency Medicine
UCSF Fresno
Fresno, CA

Leann Mainis, MD
Attending Physician
Vituity, Sutter Delta Medical Center
Antioch, CA

Section editor:
Tiffany M. Osborn, MD, MPH
Professor of Surgery and Emergency Medicine
Surgical/Trauma Critical Care
Department of Surgery
Washington University
St. Louis, MO

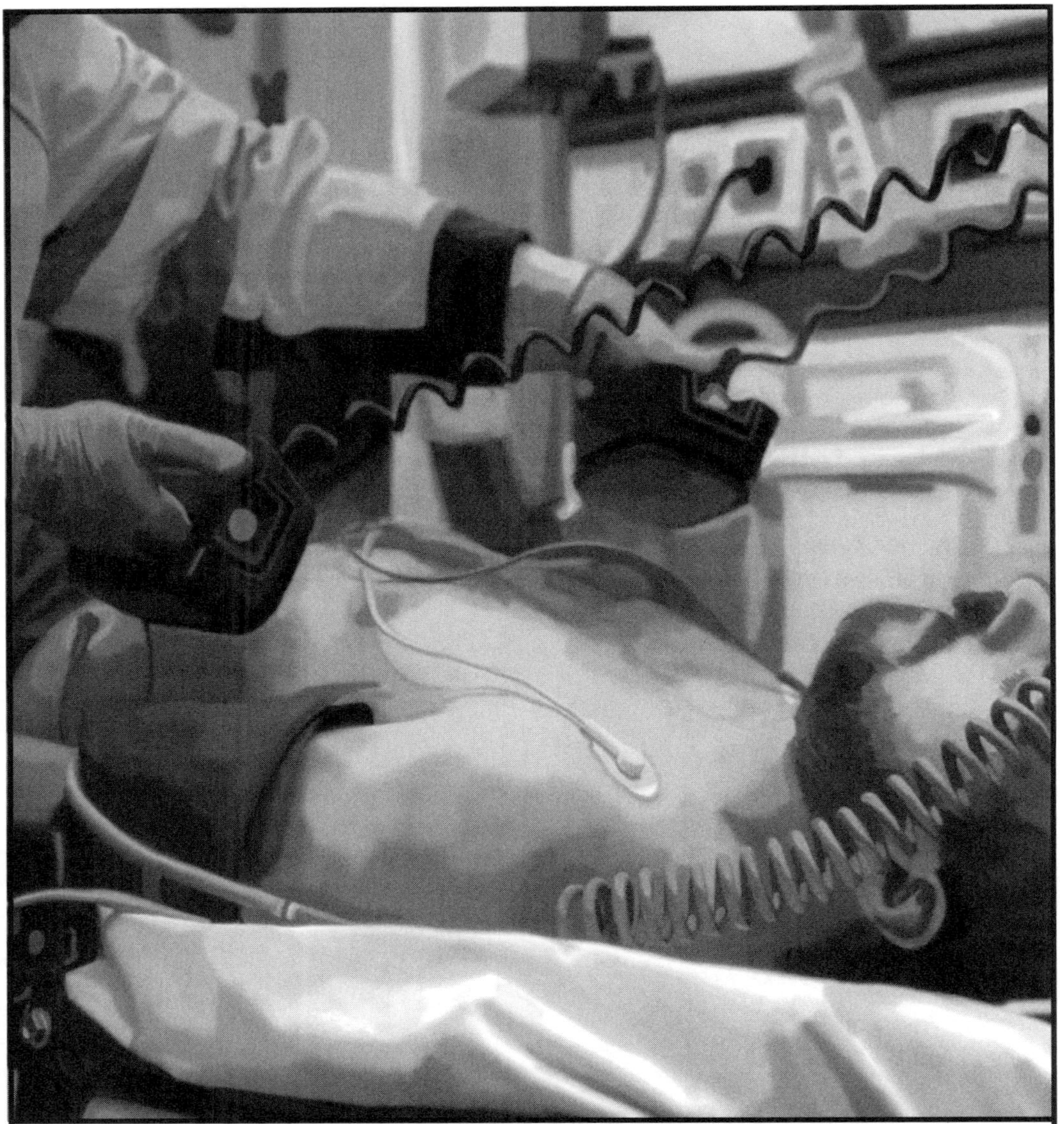

"ALL CLEAR, SHOCK!"

SECTION E / CHAPTER 22

A 53-year-old man with atrial fibrillation and palpitations

"The Shocking Effects of A-fib"

INITIAL ED VISIT

HPI: The patient is a 53-year-old male with past medical history of SVT and atrial fibrillation who presents to the emergency department with chief complaint of palpitations and lightheadedness starting 1 hour prior to arrival. The patient states that he noted a sudden onset of palpitations while at rest. He had similar symptoms 3 years prior and was evaluated in the emergency department and started on metoprolol which he is currently not taking. He denies any chest pain or shortness of breath. He endorses methamphetamine use 2 days ago. He has not followed with a cardiologist.

On EMS arrival states the patient's heart rate was 250bpm and the patient was hypotensive, he was emergently cardioverted in the field.

Medical history:
No known allergies
PMH: SVT, Atrial fibrillation
PSH: Denies pertinent previous surgery
SH: Methamphetamine use, occasional alcohol use
FAMHX: Denies pertinent family history
Medications: Reviewed. Pertinent are: metoprolol (patient has not been taking)

ROS:
CONSTITUTIONAL: No fever, no chills, no unanticipated weight loss, no fatigue
EYES: No acuity change
RESP: No shortness of breath, no cough, no wheezing, no hemoptysis
CV: POS palpitations, no orthopnea
GI: No nausea, no vomiting, no diarrhea. No abdominal pain, no melena, no anorexia
GU: No dysuria, no hematuria, no urinary urgency, no frequency
MUSC: No bone pain. No joint pain. No acute trauma
NEURO: No syncope, no headache, no focal weakness, no seizure
PSYCH: No suicidal ideation, no anxiety
INTEG: No skin lesions, no rash

PE:

Vitals:

BP	HR	RR	SpO_2	Pain
115/70 mmHg	67 bpm	18	99%	0/10

CONSTITUTIONAL: Well-hydrated, no acute distress
PSYCH: A&Ox3, appropriate
EYES: Pupils equal, round and reactive to light, normal conjunctiva
HENT: Moist mucous membranes, no stridor
NECK: Supple, range of motion without difficulty, no masses, thyromegaly, jugular venous distension
RESP: Normal respiratory effort, clear to auscultation, no wheezing, no rales or rhonchi
CV: Regular rate and regular rhythm, no murmurs, rubs or gallops. Symmetric pulses – 2+ radial
ABD: Soft, non-tender and non-distended, normoactive bowel sounds
NEURO: Cranial nerves grossly intact, normal sensory, normal motor, normal speech
MS: All four extremities unremarkable, no peripheral edema
SKIN: warm/dry, no rashes/lesions

EKGS:

1. **10:20** atrial fibrillation, rate 156 bpm, no acute ischemic changes
2. **10:23** Normal sinus rhythm, rate 95 bpm, slight non-specific ST depressions, diffuse

CXR: No acute disease

Labs:
CBC and Chem 10 normal
Troponin < 0.030
BNP 328
TSH 2.180
Magnesium 2.0
Phosphorus 2.5
Urine toxicology: amphetamine positive

ED COURSE: 11:00 Academic cardiology team consulted, discussed case with fellow on call. Recommendation was start rivaroxaban and have patient follow up in cardiology clinic this week.

RECHECK: 11:51 patient re-evaluated, feels better. Feels comfortable going home.

MDM: 53-year-old male here with atrial fibrillation. The patient was hypotensive and cardioverted by EMS. On my evaluation, the patient's rhythm is normal sinus and he feels better.
I considered ischemia, no elevation of troponin or chest pain. TSH within normal limits.

Electrolytes OK, mildly low phosphorus, repleted in the ED. BNP is slightly elevated but no evidence of clinically significant heart failure. Discussed with cardiology fellow on call, will start rivaroxaban and have patient follow up in cardiology clinic this week. Discussed with case manager who felt this follow up would be possible. Patient was agreeable with plan of care, discussed risks of anticoagulation and appropriate precautions as well as return precautions. Discussed importance of discontinuing amphetamine use.

IMPRESSION:
Atrial fibrillation
Amphetamine use

PLAN/Rx:
Rivaroxaban x 4 weeks
Follow-up in cardiology clinic

Condition at Disposition: Improved

Case commentary:

Anatomy of the case: What was the initial rhythm?

There are some serious questions with this presentation, namely a heart rate reported by EMS of 250bpm. EMS was concerned for SVT, but did not document a rhythm strip, raising suspicion for other tachyarrhythmias. We expect heart rates with SVT to be around 160–200, and atrial fibrillation (A-fib) with rapid ventricular response to be around 120–170, though rates up to 300 can also occur.[2] Heart rates above 300 should raise suspicion for an accessory pathway.[1,2] A heart rate of 250bpm is possible with A-fib, but other rhythms should be considered.

There are two possible explanations:

- Either the documented heart rate was simply wrong. -or-
- The initial rhythm was not SVT and an alternative tachyarrhythmia was present.

Either way, the patient was emergently cardioverted in the field, by means that were not documented (chemical vs. electrical and what was the amount of energy?). It is also unclear if the patient was successfully converted to sinus rhythm because the initial ECG in the ED is documented as A-fib with a rate of 156.

Was the cardioversion indicated?

The answer is a resounding "yes!" The patient was in an unstable tachyarrhythmia with hemodynamic compromise. Not only was cardioversion appropriate, but it was also the safest therapy given the possibility for an excitatory accessory pathway. [1-4]

When the patient arrives in the emergency department (ED) he is documented as being in A-fib and then spontaneously converts to sinus rhythm 3 minutes later. The fibrillating atria predispose the patient to clot formation, and with conversion to sinus rhythm, a clot is more likely to embolize. While there are many concerning outcomes with thromboembolism, we are particularly concerned for the risk of stroke. Regardless of the method for conversion to sinus rhythm—electrical, chemical, or spontaneous—the patient is still at risk for thromboembolism and the need for initiation of anticoagulation should be assessed.[3-5]

Section editor comments (Osborn):

This is a very important point that should be highlighted—many people seem to falsely think that chemical cardioversion is safer than electrical—excellent!

The patient has a known history of atrial fibrillation, but it is unknown if it is chronic, paroxysmal, or perhaps just an isolated event. He was prescribed metoprolol and has been noncompliant. Additionally, he uses methamphetamine; needless to say, there are multiple reasons for his A-fib!

Which A-fib patients should be cardioverted?

Consideration of cardioversion weighs the risk of thromboembolism (in particular stroke) against the benefits of rapid conversion to sinus rhythm. There are 3 groups of patients who we should consider for cardioversion:

- those that are unstable.
- those with onset of less than 48 hours.
- those that are already effectively anticoagulated.

Unstable: Patients who are unstable should be cardioverted.[5] It seems like a simple statement, except for the word "unstable," because providers may interpret this differently. Patients who are hypotensive, altered, or hypoxic are easy to classify as unstable. However, there is a broad spectrum of hypotension, altered mental status, and hypoxia, and hard cut points are difficult to determine and vary by clinical situation. For our patient, who is tachycardic and hypotensive pre-hospital, cardioversion was appropriate.

Less than 48 hours of symptoms: Though the exact time frame since onset of symptoms is not clear, the best current evidence suggests that 48 hours is a safe window.[6-9] However, limited data suggest that clots may develop as early as 12 hours after onset of A-fib.[10] For now, the 48-hour time window appears to be accepted as safe by most providers.

Currently anticoagulated: A-fib patients, anticoagulated for at least 3 weeks, can also be cardioverted since their risk of thromboembolism is mitigated.[4] Patients on warfarin should have therapeutic INR values *consistently* over the past 3 weeks, not just on the day they present to the ED.[5] Patients who miss doses are not appropriately anticoagulated.

Patients not appropriate for cardioversion should be rate controlled, which is most commonly done with calcium channel or beta blockade or, less commonly, with digoxin.[5] Diltiazem is a reasonable first option, since it has the benefit of titration when administered by continuous infusion and decreases heart rate more rapidly than metoprolol.[11,12]

How do you cardiovert?

Cardioversion can either be electrical or chemical. A well-studied approach to chemical cardioversion is the Ottawa Aggressive Protocol in which 1g of procainamide is given over 1 hour, which successfully cardioverted about 60% of patients.[13] This comes with risk of hypotension and QT prolongation, so close monitoring is required. Those who failed chemical cardioversion were then electrically cardioverted.

Electrical cardioversion can be attempted with 120–200J and the energy increased if initial attempts are ineffective.[2] There is limited evidence to suggest that pad placement in the anterior-posterior orientation, as opposed to anterolateral orientation, is more effective; however, this study was done with low numbers and in patients with persistent A-fib at an electrophysiology lab.[14]

Anticoagulation:
Whether the patient is cardioverted or rate controlled, the EP should assess need for anticoagulation as patients with A-fib are nearly 5 times more likely to have a stroke,[15] but the risk of major bleeding needs to be considered. When a patient is high risk for stroke and low risk for bleeding, anticoagulation is clearly favored, but marginal cases can be difficult.

The CHADS2 score helps risk stratify who should be anticoagulated, with a score of 2 or higher generally being recommended for anticoagulation, and a score of 0 not recommended for anticoagulation.[5] However, uncertainty remains about the low risk CHADS2 patients with a score of 1. For low risk patients many providers use the CHADS2-VASC score to reclassify patients as high vs. low risk.[16]

We also have scores to assess bleeding risk, including the HAS-BLED score and the ATRIA Bleeding Risk Score.[17,18] Unfortunately, several features on these scores are also risk factors for stroke, so a patient who is high risk for one is likely to be high risk for the other!

In our case the patient's CHADS2 score is 0, but this score still carries a 1.9% per year risk of thromboembolic event.[19] Despite the low risk score, anticoagulation was still recommended after discussion with the consulting cardiologist.

ED BOUNCEBACK (1 day later)

HPI (17:45): The patient a 53 y.o. male who presents to the ED with AMS, last seen normal at 16:40. Patient was found in the bathroom with his small child, altered. He was not speaking, appeared confused. Family called EMS and when EMS arrived, he was sliding down a wall. He seemed to have right leg weakness. Currently, patient is not following commands nor is speaking.

Of note, patient was just discharged yesterday from the hospital after an episode of atrial fibrillation with RVR that was cardioverted in the field due to hypotension. Patient was started on Rivaroxaban per cardiology. Per EMS, he is not compliant with medications.

PMH: No change from previous visit except addition of rivaroxaban
ROS: unable to assess – nonverbal

PE:

Vitals (17:47):

Time	Temp (F)	Rt	Pulse	Resp	Syst Diast	O2	O2%
17:47	97.2	0	77	20	149/83	100	ra

GA: Blank stare. Not following commands
HEAD: Normocephalic, atraumatic
EYES: Normal sclera
MOUTH: Clear oropharynx, moist mucous membranes
NECK: Supple
CV: RRR, no murmurs appreciated
RESP: Clear to auscultation bilaterally
ABD: Soft, nontender, nondistended
GU: Guaiac neg. External hemorrhoid noted
NEURO: Glasgow coma scale 10. R facial droop. Complete aphasia. Moving all extremities but difficult to assess as not following commands. NIHSS = 12
SKIN: Warm, dry
PULSES: 2+ radial bilaterally

EKG (18:00): NSR at 82. No ST/T changes
POC glucose 232

Chapter author note: Your heart increases a beat; our patient is not only high risk, but he was in the ED yesterday, sent home on rivaroxaban. His presentation is certainly consistent with a cerebrovascular accident (CVA), but the only focality is a facial droop and he is so altered it is difficult to make a bedside diagnosis based on the exam. Complicating matters, he has a history of drug use and A-fib. As he looks up with a blank stare, you look up to see the staff awaiting orders. You are in the footsteps of the emergency physician at the bedside. We are at:

DECISION POINT A – YOU ARE FACED WITH 4 QUESTIONS:

1. **When a patient presents with a possible stroke, what techniques can facilitate rapid assessment and diagnosis?**
2. **Which are the most important questions to ask possible stroke patients?**
3. **Is our patient a candidate for thrombolysis? When and how should BP be lowered?**
4. **What is the frequency of stroke mimics, and is there a significant risk of bleeding if thrombolytics are administered to these patients?**

What does the literature say?

Q#1: When a patient presents with a possible stroke, which techniques can facilitate rapid assessment and diagnosis?

The mantra “time is brain” was termed to convey the magnitude of a stroke. To facilitate rapid assessment, some institutions have gone to a “checklist” model. A study from Australia showed that a protocol-driven model leads to more rapid treatment, more patients treated within 3 hours, and more contraindications to thrombolytics caught prior to administration.[20] In another study from Australia, an acute stroke team was implemented consisting of a neurologist, radiologist, and internal medicine team. They accompanied the patient to the computed tomography (CT) scanner and administered tissue plasminogen activator (tPA) once they returned to the ED, which resulted in twice as many people receiving tPA within the window.[21] Implementing a stroke team may be one way to facilitate rapid assessment and treatment of potential stroke patients.

Q#2: Which are the most important questions to ask possible stroke patients?

The key to current stroke assessment is to stratify if a patient is a candidate for thrombolysis or thrombectomy. To determine this, a systematic series of questions must be asked with the most important being "what was the time of onset?" Thrombolysis is only approved for 3 hours (at most 4.5 hours) after onset of symptoms.[22,23] Another approach is to ask about the time "last seen normal" as family may not be able to accurately define when the symptoms started, especially if the patient woke up with the symptoms.[1] A recent review article investigating whether "wake up strokes" (WUS) could be candidates for thrombolysis found the current data lacking; however, there are ongoing trials that may better answer this question.[24] As we will later discuss, these WUS patients may still be candidates for intervention if they have large vessel occlusion (LVO).

The next step is to assess for contraindications to tPA, realizing that even if a patient has a contraindication to systemic tPA, they may remain a candidate for mechanical thrombectomy.

The major contraindications for tPA include:

- Intracranial hemorrhage (ICH)
- History of ICH, AVM, brain neoplasm, or aneurysm
- Severe uncontrollable hypertension with SBP >180mmHg and DBP > 120mmHg) after administration of antihypertensives in the ED
- Evidence of head trauma or history of stroke in the last 3 months
- Coagulopathy
- Active internal bleeding
- Abnormal blood glucose (less than 50mg/dL or greater than 400mg/dL)[22,25-27]

Q#3: Is our patient a candidate for thrombolysis? When and how should BP be lowered?

Absolute contraindications:

Although a history of ICH, AVM, neoplasm or aneurysm in the setting of an acute stroke is considered high risk, a few studies have looked at the use of tPA in these patients. These studies concluded there was no increased risk of ICH in patients with a history of previous ICH or coiled SAH, but further study is needed because the number of patients in each study was small.[22,28,29]

- Our patient has no history of brain pathology precluding thrombolysis.

Blood pressure should be below 185/110mmHg to reduce the risk of hemorrhagic conversion, as higher blood pressures are directly correlated with worse outcomes.[26,27] If a patient has extreme hypertension, it is recommended to carefully lower blood pressure before administration of tPA. The American Heart Association (AHA) recommends labetalol (10–20mg IV with one repeat dose if needed), nicardipine (5mg/hr drip titrating up to 15mg/hr), or clevidipine (1–2mg/hr titrating up to 21mg/hr) until the patient's blood pressure is below 185/110mmHg. Hydralazine can also be considered but is not first line. Blood pressure should be maintained < 180/105mmHg for the first 24 hours after tPA.[27]

Section editor comments (Osborn):

Of these drugs, if a drip is required, my choice is clevidipine due to the fast (seconds) onset and metabolism. Although nicardipine has a short half-life, when on a drip, it can last for hours after being turned off.

Consulting editor comments (Weingart):

Regarding blood pressure lowering, the only agent we should use is nicardipine. I don't recommend labetalol because it rarely will get the BP down. Now if you are rich and have clevidipine at your hospital, it is very efficacious.

With nicardipine, if you go by the manufacturer's recommendation on increasing doses, it'll be an hour before we reach our target, but if we have a very aggressive up-titration nicardipine, we can get their blood pressure down in less than 10 minutes; I think that's a reasonable time course. If you want to go even faster, we can bolus nicardipine. This is in the literature; anesthesia has done it forever. Give .25 milligrams of the nicardipine and repeat every 2 or 3 minutes. Now, no one's done the study, but someone should; this is low-hanging fruit. This is what I do quite frequently, but if you don't feel comfortable with that, just titrate up quicker.

Now the key with nicardipine, the one real pearl, is that once you get them to the target blood pressure, you can't leave the nicardipine at that dose. For example, if you did a rapid up-titration, and you're at 12.5mg/hour and their SBP is 180mmHg, you need to immediately drop that dose down to 3mg/hour. Otherwise they will plummet. We should think of the initial up-titration as our loading dose, and then you drop them down to 3mg/hour, which will be our maintenance dose. If you get them to 15mg/hour, and leave them there, they will become profoundly hypotensive.

In patients not receiving thrombolysis, blood pressure should not be lowered acutely due to the risk of worsening cerebral ischemia. The brain loses capacity to autoregulate blood flow in tissue injured by ischemia and can suffer further from hypoperfusion if blood pressure is lowered too rapidly. Guidelines recommend withholding blood pressure medications in these patients unless systolic pressure is > 220 or diastolic > 120mmHg and limiting the overall decrease in blood pressure by 15% in the first 24 hours.[27,30-32]

- Our patient's blood pressure is 149/83—he did not have extreme hypertension, so this was not a risk.

Evidence of head trauma is a contraindication due to concern for diffuse axonal injury and cerebral contusions, which may lead to ICH, though data regarding this are limited.[22,26] Recent stroke is cited as a contraindication for tPA due to concern for ICH, but these patients were excluded from the initial NINDs study, and no formal study has been done to assess risk of bleeding in a patient with a recent CVA.[33] In one case study, a 90-year-old male received a reduced dose of tPA 4 days after the initial dose for repeat symptoms; he did not have a bad outcome.[34] These authors would not recommend tPA in patients with recent stroke until further data support this practice.

- Assuming the head CT does not show ICH, he will still be eligible for thrombolytics.

Coagulopathy and active internal bleeding lead to increased risk of post-tPA bleeding and poor outcomes. Coagulopathy is typically due to an oral anticoagulant or antiplatelet but can result from liver cirrhosis, inherited coagulopathies, or others. The AHA states that an INR > 1.7 or PT > 15 is an absolute contraindication to tPA .[27] One meta-analysis showed that there is a 4 times greater risk of ICH for patients taking warfarin, regardless of INR, as long as they took their medication the day of or day before the stroke.[26]

- Our patient had been prescribed rivaroxaban the day before; however, it does not seem that he has started the medication. The risk for ICH with the new anticoagulants (such as rivaroxaban, dabigatran, and apixaban) have not been sufficiently studied and a quantitative level is not able to be obtained in the ED, but it can be assumed that, like warfarin, they would also lead to an increased risk of ICH.[26]

Hypoglycemia and hyperglycemia are considered contraindications to tPA. Hypoglycemia is a known stroke mimic, and rapid correction with IV dextrose is indicated.[26] The AHA recommends treatment and re-evaluation of symptoms prior to tPA.[26] Hyperglycemia can also mimic stroke-like symptoms but typically the patient is not altered. Hyperglycemia in a known diabetic can be worsened in the setting of CVA, making differentiation difficult. In one study of tPA given despite contraindications, a small subset of patients had a glucose of < 50mg/dL or > 400mg/dL, and none developed ICH.[35]

- Our patient's glucose was normal.

Relative contraindications:

Relative contraindications to thrombolysis include minor or rapidly improving symptoms, major surgery or serious non-head trauma in the last 2 weeks, history of GI or urinary hemorrhage in last 3 weeks, seizure at stroke onset, recent arterial puncture at non-compressible site, post-myocardial infarction (MI) pericarditis, and pregnancy. Although the following aren't technically relative contraindications, age > 80-years-old, history of prior CVA and diabetes, any active anticoagulation use, National Institute of Health Stroke Scale (NIHSS) > 25, and a multilobar infarction on CT scan are warnings if tPA is going to be used at > 3 hours after symptoms onset.

Some of the relative contraindications are related to increased risk of bleeding, such as:

- Major surgery
- History of hemorrhage
- Recent arterial puncture
- Post-MI pericarditis

The concern with recent surgery is for significant bleeding at the surgical site, but in one study, they found only 2 patients with hemorrhage requiring blood products and no adverse outcomes.[28] The timeline for these contraindications is somewhat arbitrary and set by the AHA.[26]

Post-MI pericarditis is a concern because there is risk for hemorrhagic conversion and destruction of a stable ventricular thrombus. If the thrombus is broken down to smaller clots, it potentially can lead to a shower of emboli. One case report hypothesizes that hemorrhage into the infarcted myocardium led to death of a 93-year-old patient.[36] Patients with relative contraindications should have a neurologic consultation and employ a shared decision-making model with the patient and family.

Q#4: What is the frequency of stroke mimics, and is there a significant risk of bleeding if thrombolytics are administered to these patients?

Before tPA administration, it is important to differentiate a stroke from a stroke-like illness. There are many medical problems that can mimic stroke and muddy the clinical picture. The percent of stroke mimics ranges from 1–16%.[37]

Stroke mimics include:

- Hypoglycemia
- Intracranial mass lesion
- Intracranial hemorrhage
- Migraine
- Seizure +/- Todd's paralysis (focal weakness following a seizure)
- Sepsis
- Syncope
- Transient global amnesia
- Panic attack/hyperventilation
- Conversion disorder
- Demyelinating diseases
- Bell's palsy
- Drug toxicity[1]

Seizures can easily be confused with stroke, especially when strokes cause the seizure or when there is Todd's paralysis following the seizure. Typically, Todd's paralysis resolves quicker than true stroke symptoms. Similarly, Bell's palsy presents with facial paralysis, but the facial droop involves the forehead, unlike stroke-induced facial droop that spares the forehead. Complex migraines, brain tumors, and demyelinating diseases can present with any number of focal neurologic symptoms. Complex migraines are typically associated with a headache, potentially with an aura, and there may be a history of similar symptoms. Brain tumors are another stroke mimic but are typically seen on imaging. In demyelinating diseases, the onset of symptoms is usually gradual, instead of abrupt, as with strokes. Drug toxicity can also present with neurologic findings. For example, phenytoin toxicity can present with cerebellar findings such as ataxia and tremors. Typically, it will present as part of a toxidrome, and levels should be checked.

Distinguishing between a stroke mimic and CVA can be difficult. A study published in Lancet Neurology used a scale to highlight potential mimics, the "Recognition of Stroke in the Emergency Room" (ROSIER) Scale (Table 1). If the score is greater than 0, the sensitivity and specificity of predicting a CVA was 92% and 86%, respectively. It has a positive predictive value of 88% and a negative predictive value of 91%. This study was prospectively validated.[38] It is a potential tool to help delineate between strokes and their mimics.[39]

Recognition of Stroke in the Emergency Room (ROSIER) Scale	
Loss of consciousness or syncope	-1
Seizure	-1
New facial droop	+1
New arm weakness	+1
New leg weakness	+1
New speech disturbance	+1
New visual field defects	+1

Adapted from Nor AM, Davis J, Sen B, et al. The recognition of stroke in the emergency room (ROSIER) scale: Development and validation of a stroke recognition instrument. Lancet Neurol. 2005;4(11):727-34 at 730.

Another study looked at distinguishing strokes and stroke mimics, collectively calling them brain attacks and defining them as "apparently focal brain dysfunction of abrupt onset." They had 30% stroke mimics (of these 20% were seizures, 13% sepsis, 11% toxicologic, 9% tumors and 9% syncope). They found certain characteristics predicting true CVA: known cognitive impairment (OR 0.33), clear time of onset (OR 2.59), definite history of focal neurologic symptoms (OR 7.21), any abnormal vascular findings (OR 2.54), higher NIHSS (1–4: OR 1.92; 5–10: OR 3.14; > 10: OR 7.23), signs lateralizing to one side of the brain (OR 2.03), and Oxford Community Stroke Classification (OCSP)* was possible (OR 5.09).[40]

**Note: The OCSP classification is the Oxford Community Stroke Classification is a stroke classification used to stratify stroke patients in clinical trials.*[41]

Although giving tPA to a stroke mimic is not ideal, the literature suggests that harm is minimal. One multicenter study enrolled 5,518 patients who received tPA for stroke, and of those, approximately 1.8% were later diagnosed with a stroke mimic. Thankfully, the rate of intracranial hemorrhage in the stroke mimic population was only 1%, compared to 7.8% in tPA recipients with acute stroke.[37]

One retrospective review of 512 patients who received tPA in the ED over a 4-year period at a single institution found a 14% incidence of stroke mimics. Only one of the stroke mimic patients had a complication related to receiving thrombolytics. That patient was ultimately diagnosed with a cervical spinal epidural mass with bleeding which required surgery, but there was no adverse outcome. Of note, there were no instances of symptomatic ICH amongst the stroke mimic patients, but a 6% rate in the patients with true CVA.[42]

A prospective study of 516 consecutive patients treated with tPA for possible stroke at a single institution over a 5-year period found 75 stroke mimic cases (14.5%). This study had only one patient with symptomatic intracranial hemorrhage, and this patient was also hypertensive and had a history of alcoholism.[43] The same authors also conducted a meta-analysis of 13 studies comprising 8,492 total patients and 392 stroke mimics (4.4%). The pooled rate of symptomatic intracranial hemorrhage among the stroke mimics was 0.5%.[43] These studies suggest that complications due to the administration of tPA in patients without ischemic strokes are relatively rare.

AHA/ASA Time Recommendations for Acute Ischemic Stroke

Intervention	Time Goal (from ED arrival)
Begin ED physician evaluation	10 min
Activation of stroke team	15 min
Begin head CT	25 min
Complete head CT interpretation	45 min
Begin rtPA administration	1 h
Admission to stroke unit	3 h

What did the actual provider do?

After a quick beside exam, ECG and point of care glucose, the patient is sent to CT. Results return quickly:

CT angiogram head with and without contrast (18:15): L MCA block at the M1/M2 junction with early L temporal-parietal infarct

Labs:
CBC: unremarkable except for Plt 116
Chem: unremarkable except for Glc 232
Trop: 0.08
PT/INR: normal

ED course:
18:22: Neuro Specialist on call (tele-neurology) started

Patient Re-checks:
18:29: Repeat neuro exam: The patient continues to have aphasia, but now is following commands. Condition is improved.
18:48 Discussed with neurology, and they recommended tPA.

Though the neurologist recommends tPA, you have some reservations based on clinical improvement, history of a prescription for anticoagulation, and history of drug use which could be contributing to the altered mental status or may have even caused a traumatic fall in the bathroom. We are at:

DECISION POINT B – YOU ARE FACED WITH 4 QUESTIONS:

1. **Should CT angiography and perfusion be done to evaluate for a large vessel occlusion (LVO)?**
2. **What are the pros and cons of neurointervention for clot retrieval?**
3. **Should we reassess the patient for improvement before giving a thrombolytic?**
4. **What laboratory tests are needed prior to giving thrombolytics?**

What does the literature say?

Q#1: Should CT angiography and perfusion be done to evaluate for a large vessel occlusion (LVO)?

Although the following studies were only able to show benefit for mechanical thrombectomy up to 6 hours after symptom onset, patients that have a target mismatch (a significant amount of ischemic but not infarcted brain tissue) on perfusion imaging may benefit from endovascular therapy after 6 hours.

The CRISP investigators conducted a multicenter cohort study at 6 U.S. hospitals between 2012 and 2015. They enrolled consecutive acute stroke patients who underwent endovascular therapy after a CT perfusion scan. Of the 190 enrolled patients with adequate CT perfusion studies, the 131 patients with target mismatch had better outcomes at 30 days (improvement of $>$ 8 points on the NIHSS or NIHSS $<$ 1). This result was seen up to 18 hours after symptom onset.[44]

The DAWN trial prospectively enrolled 206 patients with an LVO with a target mismatch on imaging (CT perfusion or diffusion weighted (DW) MRI) between 6 and 24 hours of onset, and randomized them to mechanical thrombectomy or usual care; the treatment group had greater improvement in mRS at 90 days (5.5 vs. 3.4) and no significant increase in ICH or mortality.[45] Finally, the DEFUSE-3 trial was a prospective multicenter US study that enrolled patients with LVO and favorable target mismatch on perfusion imaging 6–16 hours after symptom onset. Patients were randomized to thrombectomy vs. usual care. This study showed a higher percentage of functionally independent patients in the treatment group (45% vs. 17%) and was stopped early for efficacy.[46]

Q#2: What are the pros and cons of neurointervention for clot retrieval?

Intravenous tissue plasminogen activator (tPA) alone frequently does not result in significant reperfusion in a proximal LVO (distal internal carotid artery, first or second segment middle cerebral artery, or anterior cerebral artery). Early studies for endovascular management of stroke did not show a benefit of intra-arterial fibrinolysis or first generation mechanical embolectomy over IV tPA alone.[26,47-50] However, five studies published in the New England Journal of Medicine in 2015 and two more studies in 2017 provided good evidence that patients with this type of occlusion benefit from endovascular clot retrieval.

- The MR CLEAN study enrolled patients at 16 medical centers in the Netherlands. 500 patients with LVO were enrolled, 233 were assigned to the intervention group, with 190 of those undergoing mechanical embolectomy. Patients were enrolled if they presented within 6 hours of symptom onset. The primary outcome was modified Rankin Score (mRS) at 90 days, and more patients achieved functional independence (mRS 0–2) in the treatment group (33% vs. 19%). MR CLEAN did have a relatively low percentage of patients who achieved functional independence at 90 days compared to other trials but also had broad inclusion criteria based on time since stroke onset and included some patients with likely relatively poor outcomes at baseline.[51]
- The ESCAPE trial enrolled patients at 22 centers worldwide. Patients were enrolled up to 12 hours after symptom onset and all enrolled patients had an LVO with a small infarct core of irreversibly damaged tissue defined as an ASPECTS score 6–10 (ASPECTS values range from 0–10, with higher numbers indicating less infarct burden). 316 patients were randomized

to standard stroke care or standard care plus thrombectomy with the available device. The trial was stopped early for efficacy. The intervention group had a 2.6 adjusted common odds ratio of achieving a 1 point improvement on mRS and a higher percentage of patients in the intervention group achieving functional independence (53% vs. 29%).[52]

- The REVASCAT study was conducted at four centers in Spain. It was similar in design to the ESCAPE trial, enrolling patients with LVO without evidence of large infarct core based on CT or magnetic resonance imaging (MRI). Patients were enrolled up to 8 hours after symptom onset and were randomized to standard stroke care vs. standard care plus thrombectomy using the Solitaire device. Results were similar to the ESCAPE study, with the treatment group showing improved functional independence (44% vs. 28%).[53]
- The EXTEND-IA study enrolled patients at 14 centers in Australia and New Zealand. Patients were randomized to alteplase plus endovascular therapy with the Solitaire FR stent retriever or alteplase alone. All patients had an LVO and target mismatch on perfusion imaging (a large area of salvageable brain tissue with a small area of irreversibly damaged tissue). Endovascular therapy had to be initiated within 6 hours of symptom onset. The trial was stopped early after 70 patients were enrolled because of the increased probability of reperfusion without symptomatic ICH in the endovascular therapy group (89% vs. 37%). The treatment group also had improved functional outcomes with more patients achieving functional independence at 90 days (71% vs. 40%). The high rate of reperfusion seen in the intervention group (86% of patients with flow > 50% of previous) was attributed to patient selection with perfusion imaging and rapid time to intervention.[54]
- The SWIFT PRIME investigators performed a similar study at 39 centers in the United States and Europe. Patients with an LVO and target mismatch on perfusion imaging or small infarct core were randomized to treatment with intravenous tPA alone versus tPA plus thrombectomy with the Solitaire revascularization device. 196 patients underwent randomization (98 in each study arm). Thrombectomy plus tPA reduced disability and improved functional outcomes at 90 days.[55]
- A later study done in France, THRACE, continued to show similar benefit.[47,56] An additional study, THERAPY, assessed the penumbra device (aspiration thrombectomy). It showed potential for benefit but was stopped early for ethical considerations given the multiple other positive studies published and was thus underpowered.[57]

(Tables on next page...)

Major Studies of Mechanical Thrombectomy in CVA				
Study	**Year**	**CVA Type**	**Intervention**	**Result**
MR CLEAN[48]	2015	Anterior Circulation LVO < 6 hours	Intraarterial treatment (82% with thrombectomy) vs usual care	Improved functional independence at 90 days in the treatment group (33% vs 19%)
ESCAPE[49]	2015	LVO with small infarct core < 12 hours	Thrombectomy vs usual care	Improved functional independence at 90 days in the intervention group (53% vs 29%)
REVASCAT[50]	2015	LVO with small infarct core < 8 hours	Thrombectomy (solitaire device) vs usual care	Improved functional independence at 90 days in the intervention group (44% vs 28%)
EXTEND-IA[51]	2015	LVO with target mismatch on perfusion imaging or small infarct core < 6 hours	Thrombectomy (solitaire device) vs usual care	Improved functional independence at 90 days in the intervention group (71% vs 40%)
SWIFT PRIME[52]	2015	LVO with target mismatch on perfusion imaging or small infarct core	Thrombectomy (solitaire device) vs usual care	Improved functional independence at 90 days in the intervention group (60% vs 35%)
DAWN[56]	2018	LVO with small infarct size < 24 hours	Thrombectomy vs usual care	Improved functional independence in the intervention group (49% vs 13%)
DIFUSE 3[57]	2018	LVO with small infarct size < 16 hours	Thrombectomy vs usual care	Improved functional independence in the intervention group (45% vs 17%)

Given these data, in patients presenting within 6 hours of symptom onset and otherwise meeting criteria for intervention, angiography should be done (after a non-contrast head CT and consideration of tPA administration) to determine if there is an LVO.[26,27] For most EDs, this will be CT angiography rather than MR angiography, given the availability of imaging and time sensitive nature.

AHA/ASA* indications for endovascular therapy with a stent retriever
Patients should receive endovascular therapy with a stent retriever if they meet all the following criteria (Class I; Level of Evidence A):
a. Prestroke mRS score 0 to 1
b. Acute ischemic stroke receiving intravenous tPA within 4.5 hours of onset according to guidelines from professional medical societies
c. Causative occlusion of the internal carotid artery (ICA) or proximal middle cerebral
artery (MCA) (M1)
d. Age ≥ 18 years
e. NIHSS score of ≥ 6
f. ASPECTS of ≥ 6
g. Treatment can be initiated (groin puncture) within 6 hours of symptom onset

**ASA is the American Stroke Association*

The major trials supporting endovascular therapy for stroke cited above did not show any difference in significant adverse events, including symptomatic ICH or mortality, between treatment versus control groups.

Procedure-related complications in the various studies were similar, with variations in reporting. The MR CLEAN study noted embolization into distal territories of the treated vessel (8.6%), vessel dissection (1.7%) and vessel perforation (0.9%).[51] The ESCAPE study reported 3 patients with hematomas at the vascular access site and 1 patient with MCA perforation.[52] The EXTEND-IA trial reported 1 vessel perforation, embolization into a different vascular territory in 2 patients (but notes these were not symptomatic), and 1 groin hematoma requiring a blood transfusion.[54] The THRACE study stated the most common complications seen with intervention were vasospasm (23%) and embolization into a distal territory (6%).[56]

How about cost? The UK National Health Service did a cost-effectiveness analysis and found an estimated increased cost of mechanical thrombectomy was around $12,000 per patient; however, given greater likelihood of improvement and decreased costs of ongoing treatment later, they concluded that it was a cost-effective therapy when compared to IV tPA alone.[58]

Consulting editor comments (Weingart):

These new vessel-opening therapies have been the most profound change in the management of stroke. I have seen patients who are devastated with high NIHSS and are fully functional immediately after their intervention. This is a real therapy. Now, if we screen every potential stroke patient with CT angio and perfusion, it would take an enormous number of patients to find appropriate candidates, but we are looking for a large vessel occlusion, and there are simple screening exams that can be done. One is the Los Angeles Motor Scale (LAMS) which is being used in New York City and available on MD Calc. It is not the ridiculous stroke scale we are used to, it's simple; for example: "Do you have drift?" "Are you slurring your words?" That way you screen for who gets CT angio plus or minus perfusion. And I think you'll have a much smaller number of patients who need screening. To summarize, this is a small subset of our strokes, but finding them is absolutely critical—to the point where the screening should probably be done by EMS, and they should not be transported to centers without advanced stroke techniques available.

Q#3: Should we reassess the patient for improvement before giving a thrombolytic?

Rapidly improving stroke symptoms or low NIHSS score are frequently cited reasons to not give tPA.[59-61] Our patient appeared to have some improvement in his symptoms even before getting tPA; should he still have received it?

A retrospective review of a single institution's "Get With the Guidelines" Stroke Registry showed that 60% of patients not receiving IV tPA who were within the appropriate time frame were judged "too good to treat" (84% with low NIH score, median 2, 16% with rapidly improving stroke symptoms). Surprisingly, 32% of these patients ultimately required rehabilitation, skilled nursing facility or hospice services. When these cases were matched with similar patients who did get tPA, the tPA group did significantly better (30% vs. 37% poor outcomes).[60] This suggests that even patients with mild or rapidly improving symptoms may not follow a benign course.

In addition, the evidence for tPA suggests that it works better if administered early. In a large meta-analysis, the odds of an excellent clinical outcome was increased by 75% if tPA was given within 3 hours of symptom onset.[59,61-63]

Currently the recommendation is to observe patients for recovery only as long as it takes to mix and administer tPA, even if the patient is showing some improvement. Thrombolysis should be administered to patients with potentially disabling deficits, in the absence of other contraindications.[27]

Q#4: What laboratory tests are needed prior to giving thrombolytics?

The administration of tPA in the setting of a known coagulopathy is generally considered unsafe. However, waiting for laboratory assessment of INR and platelet count is an unnecessary delay in a patient with no history of malignancy, liver disease, renal disease, alcoholism or drug abuse and who is not taking an anticoagulant. In a review of more than 2,000 patients in an institutional "Get with the Guidelines" stroke database, only 2 of 470 (0.4%) patients eligible for tPA had a coagulopathy that was unsuspected.[64] Another retrospective review of stroke patients found only 6 of 1752 (0.3%) had an unsuspected platelet count < 100; the authors proposed that the benefit of early thrombolysis might outweigh the very low risk of treating a patient with unsuspected thrombocytopenia.[65]

Though each case should be considered individually, in a patient at low risk for coagulopathy, the only lab necessary prior to the administration of thrombolysis is point of care glucose.

What did the actual provider do?

18:50: The nursing coordinator is at the bedside asking why tPA has not yet been given.

The physician responds: "I am calling the pharmacy to verify that the patient did not fill his oral anticoagulant." Pharmacy verifies—the patient did not fill the prescription.
The patient's symptoms are starting to improve—he is saying his name. The physician decides to call back the neurologist.

Physician: "Hi Dr. Neurology, I just wanted to confirm your recommendation to give tPA as I did repeat the neuro exam and he seems minimally improved."

Neurologist: "We already decided to give the tPA so why has it not been given? The risks are greater than the benefits and we need to give it immediately. I will not be the one blamed for this delay!"

You decide to be strong… sort of… Physician: "Also, I am a bit concerned about a stroke mimic; this guy is a big-time drug user…"

Neurologist: "If I had a dollar for each time you ER folks try and get out of giving tPA. The crazy part is that studies have shown that it isn't even dangerous to give to a stroke mimic. Just give it. Now!!" they say, hanging up.

DECISION POINT C – YOU ARE FACED WITH 3 QUESTIONS:

1. **Is the legal risk higher with giving or withholding thrombolytics?**
2. **Is there a risk to the EP with neurology recommendations if the patient has a poor outcome?**
3. **What care is necessary after giving thrombolytics?**

Q#1: Is the legal risk higher with giving or withholding thrombolytics?

The small amount of data available suggests the potential medicolegal risk to the EP by omitting tPA when indicated is greater than by giving tPA to a stroke mimic. In a review of seven legal databases, 33 cases were found involving tPA ischemic stroke therapy. The majority of these cases (88%) involved failure to treat with tPA rather than complications associated with giving tPA. The defendants won 64% of the cases. Of the 12 cases that were favorable to the plaintiff, 83% were associated with failure to treat with tPA.[66]

The authors agree that based on the patient's history of A-fib, his presentation with facial droop and aphasia, and his CT findings, that he probably has a true stroke and we concur with the decision to give tPA. However, in the less likely event that he did have a stroke mimic, treatment with tPA is unlikely to have significant complications.

Q#2: Is there a risk to the EP with neurology recommendations if the patient has a poor outcome?

Even with neurology recommendation, there is still risk to the EP provider. In the above review of legal cases, six cases involved neurologists as defendants, and all six cases also involved the EP as a defendant.[66] Just having the neurologist on board doesn't get you off the hook!

Q#3: What care is necessary after giving thrombolytics?

tPA is a serine protease that cleaves plasminogen to plasmin, dissolving clots. It also disrupts the endothelial basal lamina and extracellular matrix, compromising the blood-brain barrier and potentially leading to hemorrhage.[63] The administration of tPA in acute ischemic stroke increases the risk of symptomatic intracranial hemorrhage by 6–10%, depending on multiple factors. Most hemorrhagic conversion will occur in the first 24 hours.[63] For this reason, patients should be admitted to an intensive care setting for close monitoring for at least 24 hours after receiving tPA. In this setting, patients are also monitored for the development of other complications like cerebral edema, seizures, GI hemorrhage, and angioedema.

What did the actual provider do?

The physician hangs up the phone and the stroke coordinator, standing anxiously next to the pharmacist at the bedside, looks her in the eye. The physician says, "OK, let's give the tPA."

The pharmacist pauses while mixing the medication. "Wait, it has been more than 3 hours since symptom onset now, are we still ok to give this?"

Physician: "Yes, the study ECASS-3 showed that we can extend the length of time to administer tPA to 4.5 hours."[23]

Patient Re-Checks:

18:57 tPA administered.

18:59: Spoke with neurointerventionalist. No intervention needed now.

21:00 The patient is able to speak now. He provides additional history that prior to onset of symptoms, he was in the bathroom, potty-training his baby, when he was unable to speak and became very frightened. He does not remember if he had any weakness but does remember having a headache just prior to symptoms starting.

21:12 Spoke with medical intensive care unit (ICU) for admission.

MDM: 53-year-old male with hx methamphetamine abuse and recent cardioversion out of A-fib with rapid ventricular response (RVR) presents with expressive aphasia, most likely due to CVA given laboratory, radiographic, and historical and physical exam features. Initial NIHSS score was 12.

Patient likely had an embolic event after his cardioversion from A-fib. Considered wide differential for patient's presentation, including metabolic disturbance (electrolytes, hypo/hyperglycemia), ICH, seizure, vascular issue, acute coronary syndrome, large brain mass, encephalitis/meningitis —less/not consistent with history and exam and supportive studies. Patient's troponin elevated, likely from cardioversion yesterday. Doubt acute coronary syndrome at this time as no chest pain or signs of ischemia of ECG.

Stat tele-neurology consultation completed, recommended tPA. Patient consented by tele-neurologist. Patient, although with aphasia, appeared to understand the risks/benefits. He was able to express yes and no. He never received anticoagulation yesterday (either in the department or after) and he never filled his rivaroxaban prescription. Guaiac negative. tPA given with significant improvement in symptoms. Neurointerventionalist consulted and recommends no intervention.

Final diagnosis:
1. CVA due to occlusion
2. Elevated troponin

Disposition:
Patient will be admitted to ICU for further management.

Hospital course:
The patient was admitted to the medical ICU for close monitoring after tPA. He had no hemorrhagic conversion. While in the ICU, he had an in-person neurology consult, echocardiogram with bubble study, and MRI of his brain. Echo showed a reduced ejection fraction (EF) of 45–50% but no septal defects or other significant abnormalities. MRI of his head showed an acute left parietal infarct with no evidence of hemorrhagic conversion.

On day 2, he was transferred to the telemetry floor. On the floor, a cardiology consult was placed as he had paroxysmal A-fib while in the hospital. Cardiology recommended anticoagulation with dabigatran as well as a high-dose statin, metoprolol, and lisinopril. Speech therapy evaluated him and recommended no physical therapy or rehabilitation as the patient had no deficits on day 2. He was also counseled regarding substance abuse while on the floor. He was discharged on hospital day 4 with no residual deficits.

He had appointments made for him at his primary care doctor, cardiology, and neurology for a week after discharge. Unfortunately, the patient did not show up to any of his appointments and was unable to be reached by telephone.

Case summary/debrief:
In this case, it appears that cardioversion was appropriate and unavoidable as it occurred prehospital and EMS providers felt that patient was unstable. There was some uncertainty regarding the patient's actual rhythm that could have been better addressed. Despite a technically low CHADS2 score, the patient was offered anticoagulation after discussion with cardiology. This seems appropriate, as the patient did not routinely seek medical care, was hypertensive in the ED, and engaged in drug use that could have led to undiagnosed heart failure (his BNP was mildly elevated, though he did not have heart failure symptoms). His risk of stroke was potentially greater than at first glance.

When the patient returned with stroke-like symptoms, the administration of tPA was delayed as the provider was trying to determine whether the patient was indeed a candidate. This decision was complicated by the prescription of an oral anticoagulant during the first visit. However, tPA was still given within 4.5 hours of symptom onset. The patient had rapid resolution of his symptoms and was appropriately observed in the ICU for 24 hours. He recovered uneventfully. In this case the care by the physicians during both visits was good, and the stroke complication more an unlucky turn of events. It is impossible to know if the stroke would have been prevented had the patient filled his prescription and taken the medication provided, or if the first dose of anticoagulant had been provided in the ED.

Teaching points:

- Three groups of patients with A-fib should be cardioverted: those that are unstable, those that have onset less than 48 hours, and those that are already effectively anticoagulated.
- Stroke mimics include hypoglycemia, migraine, intracranial mass lesion, conversion disorder, seizure, Bell's palsy and drug toxicity. Although giving tPA to a stroke mimic is not ideal, the literature suggests that harm is unlikely.
- Blood pressure management:
  - Blood pressure should be below 185/110mmHg prior to the administration of tPA to reduce the risk of hemorrhagic conversion.
  - If tPA is not being administered, higher blood pressures are acceptable. Antihypertensives should be started if the blood pressures is $> 220/120$mmHg, and the overall decrease in blood pressure should be limited to 15% in the first 24 hours.
- The only lab necessary prior to the administration of thrombolysis is point-of-care glucose.
- Intravenous tPA alone frequently does not result in significant reperfusion in a proximal LVO; in patients who meet criteria, consider angiography to determine eligibility for mechanical intervention.

References:

1. Cline D, Ma OJ, Meckler GD, et al. eds. Tintinalli's emergency medicine: A comprehensive study guide. 8th ed. New York, NY: McGraw Hill, 2016.
2. Pollock G. Atrial fibrillation in the ED: Cardioversion, rate control, anticoagulation, and more. Emerg Med Pract 2002;4(8):1-28.
3. Goralnick E, Bontempo LJ. Atrial fibrillation. Emerg Med Clin North Am 2015;33(3):597-612.
4. Atzema CL, Barrett TW. Managing atrial fibrillation. Ann Emerg Med 2015;65(5):532-9.
5. January CT, Wann LS, Alpert JS, et al. 2014 AHA/ACC/HRS guideline for the management of patients with atrial fibrillation: Executive summary. A report of the American College of Cardiology/American Heart Association task force on practice guidelines and the Heart Rhythm Society. Circulation 2014;130(23):2071-104.
6. von Besser K, Mills AM. Is discharge to home after emergency department cardioversion safe for the treatment of recent-onset atrial fibrillation? Ann Emerg Med 2011;58(6):517-20.
7. Michael JA, Stiell IG, Agarwal S, et al. Cardioversion of paroxysmal atrial fibrillation in the emergency department. Ann Emerg Med 1999;33(4):379-87.
8. Stiell IG, Healey JS, Cairns JA. Safety of urgent cardioversion for patients with recent-onset atrial fibrillation and flutter. Can J Cardiol 2015;31(3):239-41.
9. Stiell IG, Clement CM, Rowe BH, et al. Outcomes for emergency department patients with recent-onset atrial fibrillation and flutter treated in Canadian hospitals. Ann Emerg Med 2017;69(5):562-71.e2.
10. Nuotio I, Hartikainen JE, Gronberg T, et al. Time to cardioversion for acute atrial fibrillation and thromboembolic complications. JAMA 2014;312(6):647-9.
11. Fromm C, Suau SJ, Cohen V, et al. Diltiazem vs. metoprolol in the management of atrial fibrillation or flutter with rapid ventricular rate in the emergency department. J Emerg Med 2015;49(2):175-82.
12. Demircan C, Cikriklar HI, Engindeniz Z, et al. Comparison of the effectiveness of intravenous diltiazem and metoprolol in the management of rapid ventricular rate in atrial fibrillation. Emerg Med J 2005;22(6):411-4.
13. Stiell IG, Clement CM, Perry JJ, et al. Association of the Ottawa Aggressive Protocol with rapid discharge of emergency department patients with recent-onset atrial fibrillation or flutter. CJEM 2010;12(3):181-91.
14. Kirchhof P, Eckardt L, Loh P, et al. Anterior-posterior versus anterior-lateral electrode positions for external cardioversion of atrial fibrillation: A randomised trial. Lancet 2002;360(9342):1275-9.
15. Wolf PA, Abbott RD, Kannel WB. Atrial fibrillation as an independent risk factor for stroke: The Framingham Study. Stroke 1991;22(8):983-8.
16. Coppens M, Eikelboom JW, Hart RG, et al. The CHA2DS2-VASc score identifies those patients with atrial fibrillation and a CHADS2 score of 1 who are unlikely to benefit from oral anticoagulant therapy. Eur Heart J 2013;34(3):170-6.
17. Pisters R, Lane DA, Nieuwlaat R, et al. A novel user-friendly score (HAS-BLED) to assess 1-year risk of major bleeding in patients with atrial fibrillation: The Euro Heart Survey. Chest 2010;138(5):1093-1100.
18. Fang MC, Go AS, Chang Y, et al. A new risk scheme to predict warfarin-associated hemorrhage: The ATRIA (AnTicoagulation and Risk factors In Atrial fibrillation) study. J Am Coll Cardiol

2011;58(4):395-401.
19. Gage BF, van Walraven C, Pearce L, et al. Selecting patients with atrial fibrillation for anticoagulation: Stroke risk stratification in patients taking aspirin. Circulation 2004;110(16):2287-92.
20. Batmanian JJ, Lam M, Matthews C, et al. A protocol-driven model for the rapid initiation of stroke thrombolysis in the emergency department. Med J Aust 2007;187(10):567-70.
21. Nazir FS, Petre I, Dewey HM. Introduction of an acute stroke team: An effective approach to hasten assessment and management of stroke in the emergency department. J Clin Neurosci 2009;16(1):21-5.
22. Fugate JE, Rabinstein AA. Absolute and relative contraindications to IV rt-PA for acute ischemic stroke. Neurohospitalist 2015;5(3):110-21.
23. Hacke W, Kaste M, Bluhmki E, et al. Thrombolysis with alteplase 3 to 4.5 hours after acute ischemic stroke. N Engl J Med 2008;359(13):1317-29.
24. Stern GM, Van Hise N, Urben LM, et al. Thrombolytic therapy in wake-up stroke patients. Clin Neuropharmacol 2017;40(3):140-6.
25. Jauch EC, Saver JL, Adams HP, Jr, et al. Guidelines for the early management of patients with acute ischemic stroke: A guideline for healthcare professionals from the American Heart Association/American Stroke Association. Stroke 2013;44(3):870-947.
26. Powers WJ, Derdeyn CP, Biller J, et al. 2015 American Heart Association/American Stroke Association focused update of the 2013 guidelines for the early management of patients with acute ischemic stroke regarding endovascular treatment: A guideline for healthcare professionals from the American Heart Association/American Stroke Association. Stroke 2015;46(10):3020-35.
27. Powers WJ, Rabinstein AA, Ackerson T, et al. 2018 guidelines for the early management of patients with acute ischemic stroke: A guideline for healthcare professionals from the American Heart Association/American Stroke Association. Stroke 2018;49(3):e46-e110.
28. Meretoja A, Putaala J, Tatlisumak T, et al. Off-label thrombolysis is not associated with poor outcome in patients with stroke. Stroke 2010;41(7):1450-8.
29. Kvistad CE, Logallo N, Thomassen L, et al. Safety of off-label stroke treatment with tissue plasminogen activator. Acta Neurol Scand 2013;128(1):48-53.
30. Gorelick PB, Aiyagari V. The management of hypertension for an acute stroke: What is the blood pressure goal? Curr Cardiol Rep 2013;15(6):366.
31. Sandset EC, Murray GD, Bath PM, et al. Relation between change in blood pressure in acute stroke and risk of early adverse events and poor outcome. Stroke 2012;43(8):2108-14.
32. Aiyagari V, Gorelick PB. Management of blood pressure for acute and recurrent stroke. Stroke 2009;40(6):2251-6.
33. National Institute of Neurological Disorders and Stroke rt-PA Stroke Study Group. Tissue plasminogen activator for acute ischemic stroke. N Engl J Med 1995;333(24):1581-7.
34. Topakian R, Gruber F, Fellner FA, et al. Thrombolysis beyond the guidelines: Two treatments in one subject within 90 hours based on a modified magnetic resonance imaging brain clock concept. Stroke 2005;36(11):e162-4.
35. Frank B, Grotta JC, Alexandrov AV, et al. Thrombolysis in stroke despite contraindications or warnings? Stroke 2013;44(3):727-33.
36. Dhand A, Nakagawa K, Nagpal S, et al. Cardiac rupture after intravenous t-PA administration in acute ischemic stroke. Neurocrit Care 2010;13(2):261-2.

37. Zinkstok SM, Engelter ST, Gensicke H, et al. Safety of thrombolysis in stroke mimics: Results from a multicenter cohort study. Stroke 2013;44(4):1080-4.
38. Jackson A, Deasy C, Geary UM, et al. Validation of the use of the ROSIER stroke recognition instrument in an Irish emergency department. Ir J Med Sci 2008;177(3):189-92.
39. Nor AM, Davis J, Sen B, et al. The recognition of stroke in the emergency room (ROSIER) scale: Development and validation of a stroke recognition instrument. Lancet Neurol 2005;4(11):727-34.
40. Hand PJ, Kwan J, Lindley RI, et al. Distinguishing between stroke and mimic at the bedside: The brain attack study. Stroke 2006;37(3):769-75.
41. Pittock SJ, Meldrum D, Hardiman O, et al. The Oxfordshire Community Stroke Project classification: Correlation with imaging, associated complications, and prediction of outcome in acute ischemic stroke. J Stroke Cerebrovasc Dis 2003;12(1):1-7.
42. Chernyshev OY, Martin-Schild S, Albright KC, et al. Safety of tPA in stroke mimics and neuroimaging-negative cerebral ischemia. Neurology 2010;74(17):1340-5.
43. Tsivgoulis G, Zand R, Katsanos AH, et al. Safety of intravenous thrombolysis in stroke mimics: Prospective 5-year study and comprehensive meta-analysis. Stroke 2015;46(5):1281-7.
44. Lansberg MG, Christensen S, Kemp S, et al. Computed tomographic perfusion to predict response to recanalization in ischemic stroke. Ann Neurol 2017;81(6):849-56.
45. Nogueira RG, Jadhav AP, Haussen DC, et al. Thrombectomy 6 to 24 hours after stroke with a mismatch between deficit and infarct. N Engl J Med 2018;378(1):11-21.
46. Albers GW, Marks MP, Kemp S, et al. Thrombectomy for stroke at 6 to 16 hours with selection by perfusion imaging. N Engl J Med 2018;378(8):708-18.
47. Rodrigues FB, Neves JB, Caldeira D, et al. Endovascular treatment versus medical care alone for ischaemic stroke: Systematic review and meta-analysis. BMJ 2016;353:i1754.
48. Broderick JP, Palesch YY, Demchuk AM, et al. Endovascular therapy after intravenous t-PA versus t-PA alone for stroke. N Engl J Med 2013;368(10):893-903.
49. Kidwell CS, Jahan R, Gornbein J, et al. A trial of imaging selection and endovascular treatment for ischemic stroke. N Engl J Med 2013;368(10):914-23.
50. Ciccone A, Valvassori L, Nichelatti M, et al. Endovascular treatment for acute ischemic stroke. N Engl J Med 2013;368(10):904-13.
51. Berkhemer OA, Fransen PS, Beumer D, et al. A randomized trial of intraarterial treatment for acute ischemic stroke. N Engl J Med 2015;372(1):11-20.
52. Goyal M, Demchuk AM, Menon BK, et al. Randomized assessment of rapid endovascular treatment of ischemic stroke. N Engl J Med 2015;372(11):1019-30.
53. Jovin TG, Chamorro A, Cobo E, et al. Thrombectomy within 8 hours after symptom onset in ischemic stroke. N Engl J Med 2015;372(24):2296-306.
54. Campbell BC, Mitchell PJ, Kleinig TJ, et al. Endovascular therapy for ischemic stroke with perfusion-imaging selection. N Engl J Med 2015;372(11):1009-18.
55. Saver JL, Goyal M, Bonafe A, et al. Stent-retriever thrombectomy after intravenous t-PA vs. t-PA alone in stroke. N Engl J Med 2015;372(24):2285-95.
56. Bracard S, Ducrocq X, Mas JL, et al. Mechanical thrombectomy after intravenous alteplase versus alteplase alone after stroke (THRACE): A randomised controlled trial. Lancet Neurol 2016;15(11):1138-47.
57. Mocco J, Zaidat OO, von Kummer R, et al. Aspiration thrombectomy after intravenous alteplase versus intravenous alteplase alone. Stroke 2016;47(9):2331-8.

58. Ganesalingam J, Pizzo E, Morris S, et al. Cost-utility analysis of mechanical thrombectomy using stent retrievers in acute ischemic stroke. Stroke 2015;46(9):2591-8.
59. Tsivgoulis G, Kargiotis O, Alexandrov A. Intravenous thrombolysis for acute ischemic stroke: A bridge between two centuries. Expert Rev Neurother 2017;17(8)819-37.
60. Ali SF, Siddiqui K, Ay H, et al. Baseline predictors of poor outcome in patients too good to treat with intravenous thrombolysis. Stroke 2016;47(12):2986-92.
61. Haršány M, Tsivgoulis G, Alexandrov AV. Intravenous thrombolysis in acute ischemic stroke: Standard and potential future applications. Expert Rev Neurother 2014;14(8):879-92.
62. Emberson J, Lees KR, Lyden P, et al. Effect of treatment delay, age, and stroke severity on the effects of intravenous thrombolysis with alteplase for acute ischaemic stroke: A meta-analysis of individual patient data from randomised trials. Lancet 2014;384(9958):1929-35.
63. Maldonado NJ, Kazmi SO, Suarez JI. Update in the management of acute ischemic stroke. Crit Care Clin 2014;30(4):673-97.
64. Rost NS, Masrur S, Pervez MA, et al. Unsuspected coagulopathy rarely prevents IV thrombolysis in acute ischemic stroke. Neurology 2009;73(23):1957-62.
65. Cucchiara BL, Jackson B, Weiner M, et al. Usefulness of checking platelet count before thrombolysis in acute ischemic stroke. Stroke 2007;38(5):1639-40.
66. Liang BA, Zivin JA. Empirical characteristics of litigation involving tissue plasminogen activator and ischemic stroke. Ann Emerg Med 2008;52(2):160-4. Rost NS, Masrur S, Pervez MA, et al. Unsuspected coagulopathy rarely prevents IV thrombolysis in acute ischemic stroke. Neurology 2009;73(23):1957-62.
67. Cucchiara BL, Jackson B, Weiner M, et al. Usefulness of checking platelet count before thrombolysis in acute ischemic stroke. Stroke 2007;38(5):1639-40.
68. Liang BA, Zivin JA. Empirical characteristics of litigation involving tissue plasminogen activator and ischemic stroke. Ann Emerg Med 2008;52(2):160-4.

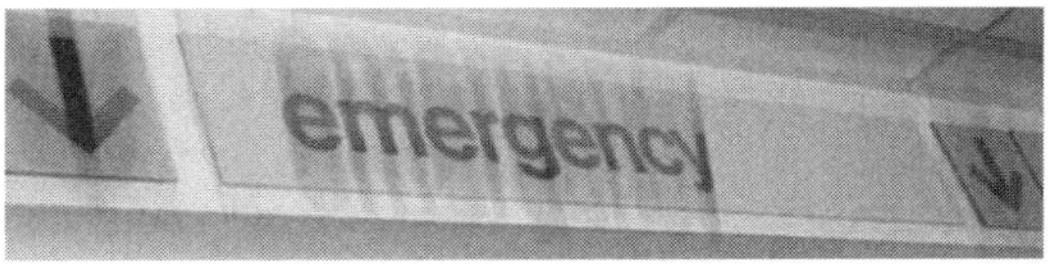

SECTION E – NEURO & SEPSIS

Chapter 23: A 70-year-old man from an ECF with abdominal pain

Steven Kornweiss, MD
Attending Emergency Physician
Spartanburg Regional Healthcare System
Spartanburg, SC

Section editor:
Tiffany M. Osborn, MD, MPH
Professor of Surgery and Emergency Medicine
Surgical/Trauma Critical Care
Department of Surgery
Washington University
St. Louis, MO

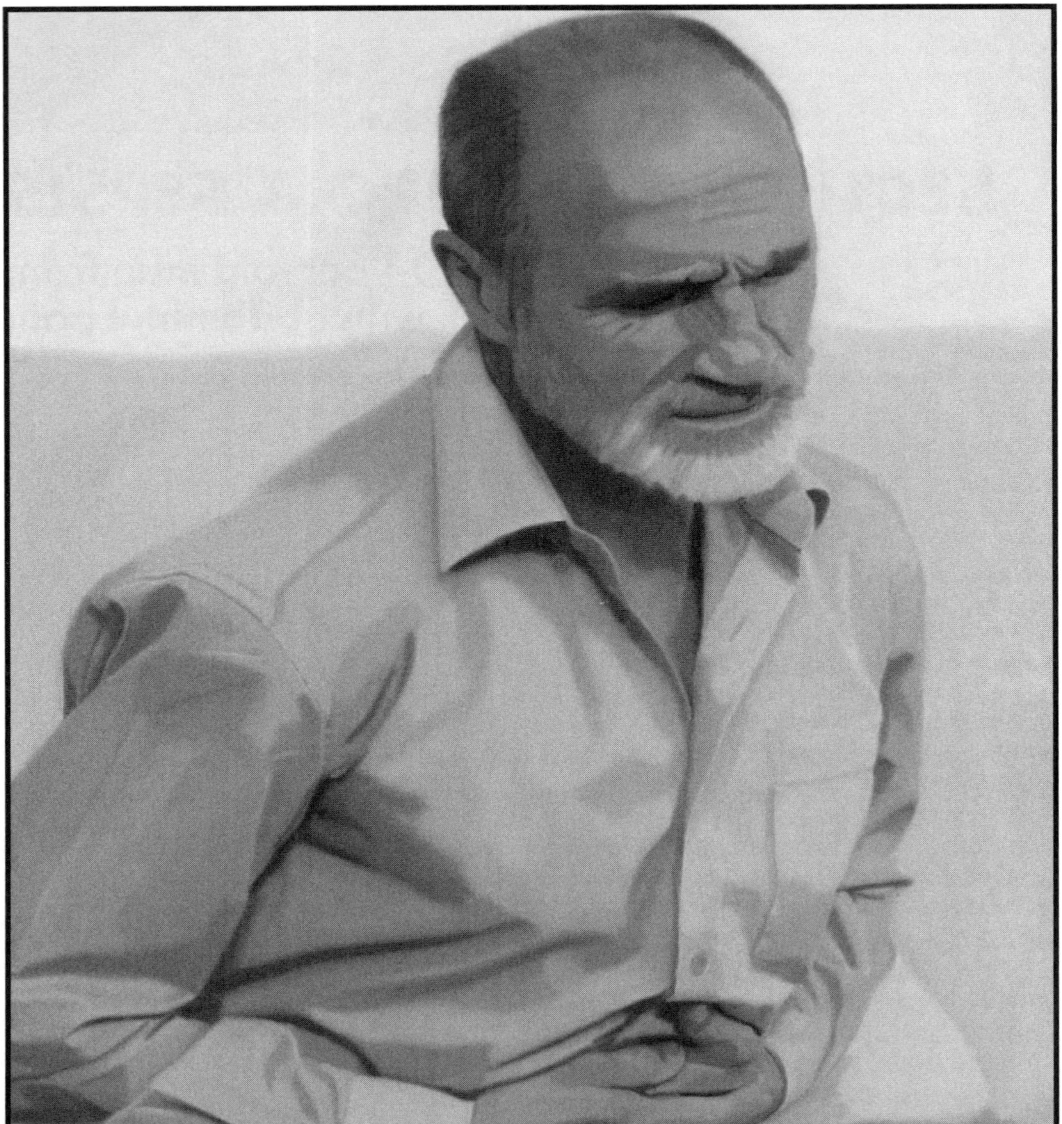

"I THINK IT'S JUST CONSTIPATION."

SECTION E / CHAPTER 23

A 70-year-old man from an ECF with abdominal pain

INITIAL ED VISIT

CC (12:15): Abdominal pain

Vitals:

Time	Temp (F)	Pulse	Resp	Syst	Diast	O2 Sat	O2%	Pain
12:15	98.5	93	16	172	84	96	RA	7/10

Triage/nursing: Arrives by EMS from nursing home. Abdominal pain and possible constipation today
PMH: diabetes, dementia
Allergies: NKDA
Medications: Metformin
PSH: None

HPI (12:40): Epigastric pain and nausea since yesterday. Denies fever, vomiting, lower abdominal pain and dysuria. History is limited by dementia.

Exam:
CONSTITUTIONAL: A&Ox2, well-nourished, NAD
HEAD: Normocephalic, atraumatic
EYES: PERRL, EOMI, no scleral icterus
ENT: Oropharynx clear and symmetric, mucous membranes moist
HEART: Regular rate and rhythm, no murmurs rubs or gallops
LUNGS: Clear to auscultation B/L, no wheezes rales or rhonchi
ABD: Epigastric tenderness, no rebound or guarding, normal bowel sounds
SKIN: Warm, dry, no rashes

DDX: Obstruction, gastritis, GERD, hepatitis, nonspecific pain, pancreatitis, PUD, pyelonephritis and UTI

Orders (12:53):
CBC, CMP, Lipase, UA with Micro, 1 VW abdominal x-ray
4 mg morphine IVP, 4 mg Zofran IVP, 1L NS Bolus

RESULTS (14:12):
CBC, CMP, Lipase are all WNL
UA:

- SG 1.020
- -Ketones
- +Protein
- Large LE
- - Nitrites
- Negative Blood
- No Bacteria
- TNTC WBF/hpf [too numerous to count]

Abd x-ray: large stool burden, non-obstructive bowel gas pattern

ED COURSE (14:57): The patient had a bowel movement and his pain is improved.

Orders (15:06): Macrobid 100mg PO

Diagnosis (15:07): constipation, UTI

DISPOSITION (15:10): Discharge to nursing home. Follow up with PCP 1-2 days. Rx Macrobid 100mg PO BID for 7 days. Miralax 1 cap full PO once daily for 7 days. Instructions for UTI and constipation.

Initial visit discussion:
On face value, the initial visit seems reasonable given a well-appearing patient, normal vital signs, a reassuring exam, normal labs, a diagnosis of UTI and constipation, and improving symptoms in the ER after a bowel movement. The pitfalls are in the differential diagnosis, the age of the patient, the location of the pain, the lack of urinary symptoms, and perhaps the failure to send a urine culture.

1. What is an appropriate differential diagnosis for abdominal pain in the elderly?

Constipation is extremely common in the elderly with a prevalence of up to 75% for nursing home patients. Constipation can cause abdominal pain, nausea, and a sense of fullness.[1] However, the emergency department differential should consist of life-threatening diagnoses first, and less dangerous diagnoses second, even if they may be more likely. This strategy will help avoid diagnostic anchoring, in which a provider chooses a readily available diagnosis and fails to consider dangerous alternatives. For upper abdominal pain in the elderly patient, consider:

Emergency Medicine Differential Diagnosis (ddx) (immediately life-threatening diagnoses):

- viscus perforation
- obstruction
- cholecystitis with or without cholangitis or obstruction
- cholangitis
- pancreatitis
- mesenteric ischemia

- ruptured or dissecting abdominal aortic aneurysm (AAA)
- myocardial infarction

Secondary ddx composed of diagnoses that are not usually life-threatening:

- non-perforated peptic ulcer disease
- biliary colic
- gastritis
- colitis
- duodenitis
- constipation
- hiatal hernia without obstruction or perforation
- diverticulitis which, although most commonly presents with low abdominal pain, can occur at any location along the colon and even occasionally in the duodenum and jejunum.[2]

The clinician in this case diagnosed constipation and UTI as the causes of the patient's pain. Ostensibly, constipation was the primary diagnosis explaining the upper abdominal pain and UTI a secondary diagnosis. Constipation is common but creates a large diagnostic pitfall in a population with a high incidence of surgical pathology (as high as 45% in patients over age 65).[3,4]

Section editor comments (Osborn):

Agree that diagnosis of abdominal pain in the elderly is challenging; for example, in order to have a physical exam finding of a rigid abdomen, there is a need for abdominal musculature, often not present in the elderly. In deconditioned patients we may not see the rigid abdomen present in a 25-year-old. Additionally, relying on presence of a fever or increased white blood cell count in the elderly is more challenging.

2. Interpreting the urinalysis:

Complicating this case is the abnormal urinalysis. What should we make of this? The abnormal urinalysis is often discounted, without acknowledgement that this test is rich with potential diagnostic information. The UA needs to be interpreted in the context of the clinical picture and pre-test probability. In this instance, the UA was ordered as a component of an "abdominal pain" order-set. Without a pre-test rationale, the clinician fell victim to availability bias and chose a diagnosis of UTI when presented with an abnormal UA. Consider now that this patient had no urinary complaints, but rather upper abdominal pain and nausea. Now consider that the UA, while demonstrating WBCs on microscopy and positive leukocyte esterase, did not show any bacteria and is nitrite negative. Certainly, this UA could indicate a urinary infection, but based on the microscopy, it is a sterile sample showing no bacteria. This finding constitutes sterile pyuria and could have generated a new branch on the differential.

Sterile pyuria is the presence of white blood cells in the urine without the presence of bacteria, and can be caused by systemic infections like pneumonia or bacteremia, intra-abdominal infections like ruptured appendicitis and other intra-abdominal catastrophes.[5] If the clinical presentation does not suggest a urinary tract infection and there are no bacteria seen on microscopy, then consider other systemic or intraabdominal infections.[6] This brings us to the next question; should a culture have been sent? Urine cultures can help ensure proper antimicrobial therapy, but if negative, they can also help redirect subsequent providers away from an erroneous diagnosis of UTI in repeat visits like this one.

3. **Should this patient have received abdominal x-rays or a CT scan?**
   Before CT was widely available, plain abdominal radiography was both the gold standard as well as the *only* standard, but it turns out that plain films of the abdomen are nearly useless in the evaluation of acute abdominal pain in the absence of a high pre-test probability for pneumoperitoneum, bowel obstruction, or an ingested metallic foreign body. Other diagnoses or subtle presentations of perforation or obstruction will not be identifiable on plain film, and even if they are, CT may be subsequently necessary to understand the full extent of the pathology.[7-11] If there is a concern about contrast-induced nephropathy or contrast allergy, recent studies suggest that non-contrast enhanced CT abdomen/pelvis is nearly as sensitive, specific, and accurate as CT with IV contrast in the vast majority of cases.[12] In time-sensitive cases or those in which the patient will have difficulty tolerating oral contrast, recent radiology literature suggests that even patients with a low BMI do not require oral contrast.[13] If IV Contrast enhanced CT is urgently or emergently indicated, consider volume expansion and performing the CT expediently even if there is risk for contrast induced nephropathy, the incidence of which is likely overestimated.[14]

RETURN ED VISIT (16:24: 4 days later)

CC: DKA

Vitals:

Pulse	BP	RR	Sat
128	135/76	32	98% RA

Moans and grasps abdomen continuously
Cannot provide history due to change in mental status
Pre-hospital blood glucose >500 per EMS

What did the actual provider do?

16:32: 1L NS, 4mg Morphine IVP, 4mg Zofran IVP
16:40: ECG – Sinus tachycardia
17:00: CXR – No acute abnormality
17:54: Labs:

- CBC – WBC 16, Hgb 12.3, Plt 156
- Lytes – Na+ 127, K+ 4.6, Cl 97, Bicarb 11
- Anion Gap – 19
- BUN/Cr – 38/2.6
- Glucose – 430
- Acetone – Negative
- VBG – pH 7.25, pCO_2 = 20, pO_2 = 135
- Troponin – Negative
- LFTs – WNL

- Lipase – Normal
- UA – SG 1.030, +LE, Small Ketones, Neg. Nitrite, Innumerable WBCs, No bacteria

Author comments (Weinstock):

We are in the footsteps of the emergency medicine provider, faced with an altered bounceback patient who is acidotic, hyperglycemic with severe abdominal pain. We are at:

DECISION POINT A – YOU ARE FACED WITH 3 QUESTIONS:

1. **What is the differential diagnosis for hyperglycemia and altered mental status (AMS)?**
2. **How should we proceed with the initial evaluation?**
3. **Does the patient have DKA as the medic suggests?**

Q#1: What is the differential diagnosis for hyperglycemia and altered mental status (AMS)?

The differential diagnosis for hyperglycemia and altered mental status (AMS) is extremely broad. Taken together, it is tempting to blame the latter on the former, as diabetic ketoacidosis (DKA) and hyperosmolar hyperglycemic state (HHS) are well known to present with varying degrees of AMS due to the myriad metabolic derangements associated with the pathophysiologic states. However, especially in cases lacking a clear inciting event, such as cessation of insulin use, we need to exercise caution in presuming causation or chronology. It is quite common for a separate process such as infection, myocardial infarction, stroke, seizure, or a toxic ingestion to cause directly and simultaneously the development of altered mental status and hyperglycemic crisis.[15] Additionally, consider that a decline in mental status is likely to accompany a decrease in medication compliance which may also lead to a secondary hyperglycemic crisis.

In patients with hyperglycemia and AMS, consider the following differential.[15,16]
Toxic ingestion: Opiates, benzodiazepines, acetaminophen, salicylates, calcium channel blocker
Endocrine: DKA, HHS, thyroid storm, pheochromocytoma, pancreatitis
Ischemia: Myocardial infarction, stroke, mesenteric ischemia
Infectious: Pneumonia, UTI, cellulitis, necrotizing fasciitis, bacteremia, cholangitis, intra-abdominal catastrophe, meningitis, encephalitis
Inflammatory: Sepsis, autoimmune
Neurologic: Intracranial hemorrhage

Section editor comments (Osborn):

This is an important point to emphasize—if the patient is in DKA—why? Also, I am often told, Type II DM can't get DKA—which of course is false but a frequently cited myth. See "Trends in Hospital Admission for DKA in adults with Type 1 and Type 2 Diabetes in England" (2018). Common causes are infection and myocardial infarction (MI). MI in diabetics may present without chest pain, especially if they have altered mental status.

Q#2: How should we proceed with the initial evaluation?

The standard work-up to evaluate for hyperglycemic crisis consists of a CBC, CMP, urinalysis, acetone/beta-hydroxybutyrate level, and a blood gas.[15] Expanding this work-up in scenarios of diagnostic uncertainty should likely prompt the addition of an ECG and a chest x-ray.

- The CBC will be necessary for cues and clues to help manage infectious, hematologic, and hemorrhagic conditions that often coexist in critically-ill patients.
- The CMP is useful for evaluation of electrolytes, anion gap, bicarbonate level, and renal and hepatic function.
- The urinalysis is used to evaluate for ketonuria and can also reveal urinary infection, dehydration, the ability of the kidneys to concentrate urine, and the presence or absence of blood and crystals to suggest alternative diagnoses.
- The blood gas (may be venous) will help to delineate the patient's acid-base physiology.
- Chest x-ray and ECG are relatively inexpensive and easy tests to perform which can assess for alternative diagnoses, such as, but not limited to, pneumonia and myocardial ischemia.

Consider adding a toxicology work-up including acetaminophen, salicylate, and alcohol levels and a urine drug screen. Sending a troponin to look for myocardial infarction, myocarditis or pericarditis in select patients may be useful as well as a lactate level to evaluate for mesenteric ischemia or sepsis, if suspected. A brain CT is indicated for any focal neurologic deficits, signs of head trauma, or history or physical findings suggestive of stroke or intracranial hemorrhage. Consider a lipase level and thyroid testing for consideration of pancreatitis, thyroid storm, or myxedema coma.[16]

Q#3: Does the patient have DKA as the medic suggests?

Based on the diagnostic criteria for DKA and HHS, the patient has neither of these conditions. The primary characteristic of DKA, elevated serum ketones, is absent. The diagnostic criteria for HHS includes a serum glucose threshold of 600mg/dL.[15] This patient does not meet these criteria. He certainly does not have DKA but is nearing the diagnostic criteria for HHS. A more accurate description would be stress-induced hyperglycemia, which can be a normal physiologic response to stress even in the non-diabetic patient. In fact, hyperglycemia is very common in critically ill patients due to the release of catecholamines, glucocorticoids and glucagon, and the concurrent decrease in insulin secretion and sensitivity.[17]

- Patients on SGLT2 Inhibitors (drug names with the suffix "gliflozin") may present with euglycemic DKA. That is, they may have clinical and laboratory criteria for DKA, yet may have a normal serum glucose. Euglycemic DKA can also occur in patients who are on insulin therapy.

What did the actual provider do?

18:00: 2nd L NS bolus, 4mg morphine IVP, 1g ceftriaxone ordered, insulin infusion of 0.01 u/kg/h ordered for DKA.
18:05: Re-examination reveals a distended and exquisitely tender abdomen with rebound and guarding. He continues to moan intermittently and hold his stomach.
18:06: Family arrives and reveals the patient has been anorexic for the past 5 days complaining of upper abdominal pain, has been vomiting constantly, and has had a gradually worsening mental status.
18:06: Repeat vitals: HR 138, BP 86/57, sat 94%.
18:10: Blood cultures, lactate level, CT abdomen/pelvis with IV contrast ordered.

Were these actions appropriate?

There is no documentation to explain the physician's thought process, but based on the orders and ED course updates, we can infer a concern for DKA, UTI, and sepsis from an intra-abdominal source. Ceftriaxone is a dubious selection—if septic shock was considered, then broad spectrum antibiotics are indicated. The patient remains tachycardic, is now hypotensive, and based on the updated abdominal exam, appears to have an acute or surgical abdomen. This author's assessment of an opportunity for improvement would be 3 considerations: surgical consultation, consideration of a central line or expanded IV access, and broad-spectrum antibiotics and blood cultures. The clinician opted to wait for results of a CT and attempt a 2nd fluid bolus. The insulin infusion is a debatable intervention at this point in the absence of DKA and HHS.

Author comments (Weinstock):

The patient has had a lot of testing and interventions, but his condition is worsening; all of the initial problems are still present including altered mental status (AMS) and severe abdominal pain, and now he is hypotensive. We are now at:

DECISION POINT B – YOU ARE FACED WITH 3 QUESTIONS:

1. **What is the next step in evaluation of our patient's abdominal pain—could it be from DKA/HHS?**
2. **What is the cause of the patient's hypotension?**
3. **What is the next step in managing the patient's conditions?**

Q#1: What is the next step in evaluation of our patient's abdominal pain—could it be from DKA/HHS?

It is common for patients with hyperglycemic crises to have severe abdominal pain; in the majority, especially those with DKA, it can be attributed to ketosis and acidosis and seems to correlate with the latter, though the relationship is not clearly causal. In one study, a serum bicarbonate of < 5mmol/L was associated with abdominal pain in 86% of patients, whereas only one-third of patients with a serum bicarbonate from 10–15mmol/L had abdominal pain.[18] Fifteen percent of the patients in the same study were thought to have a primary intra-abdominal process as the cause of their pain and hyperglycemic crisis. Given our patient's pH of 7.25, the absence of ketones, the lack of a clear UTI, and the patient's declining clinical condition, a separate, unaddressed, abdominal process is likely. Our patient's serum bicarbonate is 11, but recall, this must be due to something other than ketoacidosis, as serum ketones are negative. Therefore, the abdominal pain cannot be definitively attributed to ketoacidosis, diabetic or otherwise, and alternative explanations must be considered.

Q#2: What is the cause of the patient's hypotension?

Given the suspicion for infection, septic shock is the most readily available explanation; do not be fooled by the absence of fever. SIRS criteria to aid the diagnosis of sepsis does not require a fever, and in elderly patients or immunosuppressed patients, fever may be absent. Up to 13% of bacteremic patients > 65-years-old may present without fever.[19] Despite the cognitive availability of septic shock as an explanation for hypotension, we should avoid anchoring and consider other causes of hypotension including pericardial tamponade, ruptured AAA, GI loss, tension pneumothorax, or MI.

Classification of shock:[20]
Hypovolemic: volume depletion (diarrhea, DKA), hemorrhage (GI bleed, trauma)
Distributive: vasoplegic (septic, neurogenic), vasodilatory (anaphylactic)
Cardiogenic: myocardial infarction, cardiac depressant ingestion, cardiomyopathy
Obstructive: inflow obstruction (PE, tamponade, tension pneumothorax), outflow obstruction (aortic dissection/stenosis)
Multifactorial: adrenal insufficiency

Consider a reassessment with family members who may have now arrived, discussion with the ECF staff, repeat physical exam, and perhaps a bedside ultrasound exam of the heart, lungs, abdomen, vena cava, and lower extremity deep veins.[21,22] In this case, the suspicion of an intra-abdominal process such as infection, perforation or obstruction should make us consider most highly a distributive shock related to sepsis, but also remember that sepsis can cause myocardial dysfunction and varying degrees of cardiogenic shock.[23] Additionally, prolonged severe hyperglycemia, even in the absence of DKA or HHS, causes a hyperosmolar diuresis, especially with decreased oral intake likely resulting in hypovolemia in our patient as well.

Q#3: What is the next step in managing the patient's conditions?

Given the conclusion that the patient has hyperglycemia without DKA or HHS and possibly distributive shock from sepsis, the initial steps are to provide aggressive IV hydration in the form of a 30mL/kg NS bolus followed expeditiously by vasopressor initiation starting with norepinephrine if a MAP of 65 is not achieved with fluids alone.[24] Broad-spectrum antibiotics should be given. The source should be identified, and in this case, a CT with IV contrast is ideal. Though, as mentioned above, CT without contrast is nearly as good especially for perforation and obstruction. If biliary pathology is suspected based on physical exam and lab results, an abdominal (RUQ) ultrasound would be reasonable as well.

Section editor comments (Osborn):

I am not sure that sepsis is established just yet. Abdominal pain out of proportion to exam in the elderly = rule out mesenteric ischemia, and we are awaiting CTA and lactate results. However, I agree that hypotension + possible infection = antibiotics.

As hyperglycemia is a normal stress response, initially reverse the causes of shock and check blood glucose periodically during key points in the resuscitation, such as after each stage of fluid resuscitation, before vasopressor initiation, after goal MAP is achieved, and any time there is an acute change in hemodynamic or mental status, to evaluate the need for an insulin infusion. In a patient who is able to produce endogenous insulin, hyperglycemia may correct significantly with resuscitation. Using stop points in the resuscitation to re-evaluate the patient's glycemic status can be a useful cognitive tool and can improve physician and nursing workflow. If the patient is an insulin-dependent diabetic, the argument could be made to initiate an insulin infusion right away with a target blood glucose of 180mg/dL even in the absence of meeting diagnostic criteria of DKA or HHS. Following an algorithm developed for hyperglycemic crisis to avoid hypoglycemia and electrolyte imbalance is prudent.[15,25,26]

ED course:

20:07: CT Scan Result–Free fluid in the pelvis and inflammation around the stomach and duodenum suggestive of gastritis or duodenitis. No perforation or obstruction. There are no abnormalities seen in the liver, spleen, kidneys, small or large bowel. The gallbladder is surgically absent. There is no intra or extra-hepatic biliary ductal dilatation. The pelvic organs appear normal. The appendix is surgically absent.
Impression: likely gastritis and duodenitis with small to moderate amount of fluid in the pelvis.
20:15: BP 75/35, HR 147
20:30: ICU team consulted and CVC placed, norepinephrine initiated.
20:35: The patient has a large maroon colored bowel movement which is heme positive.

DECISION POINT C – YOU ARE FACED WITH 4 QUESTIONS:

1. **What is the new differential diagnosis given the new symptom of massive GI bleed?**
2. **How does a perforated viscus appear on CT?**
3. **How should you manage the GI bleed including resuscitation, pharmacotherapy, and transfusion?**
4. **Who should be called first, gastroenterology (GI), interventional radiology (IR), or surgery?**

Q#1: What is the new differential diagnosis given the new symptom of massive GI bleed?

Perforated gastric and duodenal ulcers usually result in peritonitis and sepsis if not treated quickly, but they are not necessarily accompanied by GI bleeding.[27] However, peptic ulcers can result in varying degrees of bleeding. Mucosal erosion can result in chronic occult blood loss or acute blood loss in the form of melena. Ulcers can also erode through neighboring arteries causing massive GI bleed defined as a GI bleed with hemodynamic instability (SBP < 90mmHg) or requiring a transfusion of greater than 4 units of PRBCs over 24 hours.[28] Despite having an anatomic origin in the upper GI tract (proximal to the Ligament of Treitz), the rapidity of the bleeding can present as melena (maroon colored stool) or hematochezia (bright red blood per rectum). Other causes of abdominal pain and massive GI bleed include ruptured esophageal varices, aortoenteric fistula, angiodysplasia, and diverticular bleeding. The most likely diagnosis in our patient is a perforated ulcer with peritonitis, sepsis, and now complicated by a GI bleed.

Q#2: How does a perforated viscus appear on CT?

Most of the time, a perforated viscus will result in pneumoperitoneum. Other findings include free fluid, inflammatory changes such as thickening or fat stranding, and extraluminal leakage of PO contrast. On a supine CT of the abdomen/pelvis, look for free air against the anterior wall of the peritoneum and around the gastric wall, duodenum, and bowel wall for extraluminal foci of air. Using the bone and lung windows may enhance the ability to notice extraluminal air by increasing the contrast between the air and its surroundings.[29] In one retrospective study, 97% of patients who had surgically verified gastroduodenal perforations demonstrated free air on CT,[30] but if a perforation is suspected clinically, the absence of free air does not completely rule out this diagnosis.[30,31]

Q#3: How should you manage the GI bleed including resuscitation, pharmacotherapy, and transfusion?

1. First, obtain resuscitative IV access with at least 2 large-bore peripheral IV catheters or an 8.5 Fr. single lumen central catheter; note that triple lumen central venous catheters have slower infusion rates than equal-bore peripheral IVs due to the positive correlation between length and resistance. Resuscitate using a combination of crystalloid and blood transfusions with special attention to reversing intrinsic or medication-induced coagulopathy.
2. Consider permissive hypotension (which has been studied in trauma) allowing for an SBP goal of 80–100mmHg to avoid clot disruption. This strategy has not been specifically studied in GI bleed but may be reasonable during the initial phase of resuscitation.
3. Blood transfusion: Target clinical signs of perfusion as the Hgb will not reflect massive blood loss or massive transfusion in real time.
4. Perform resuscitation before intubation attempting to optimize oxygenation and hemodynamics prior to performing RSI.[32] This includes obtaining a systolic blood pressure of at least 80mmHg, preferably nearer 100mmHg and performing pre-oxygenation and apneic oxygenation with a nasal cannula at 15L/m or greater prior to and during intubation.[33]
5. If the patient has an upper GI bleed and hematemesis, consider placing an NG tube prior to intubation to reduce the risk of blood obscuring the airway. Be ready with 2 suction catheters.
6. The administration of a proton pump inhibitor (PPI) bolus and infusion for acute GI bleed is controversial. One study demonstrates increased mortality in a group receiving omeprazole[34,35] while another suggests a decreased need for endoscopic intervention.[34]
7. Octreotide for variceal bleeding is also debatable, with the most recent meta-analysis showing no mortality benefit, but a decrease in failure of hemostasis and transfusion requirements.[36]
8. Use Prothrombin Complex Concentrate (PCC), FFP, Platelets, and cryoprecipitate to treat coagulopathy. PCC is preferred in patients who are anticoagulated with warfarin or a novel anticoagulant.[37] Massive transfusion protocols have been developed for traumatic bleeding but have not been widely adopted or demonstrated to improve morbidity or mortality for non-traumatic bleeding. Consider adding platelets and FFP to your transfusion regimen once you have surpassed 4 units of PRBCs within 4 hours to avoid transfusion-induced coagulopathy.[38]

Section editor comments (Osborn):

Octreotide falls into the "won't hurt but might help" category. I agree that with a dying "GI bleed" patient, giving octreotide is wise; there's not too much downside. Other times I would give octreotide is with an unexplained elevated INR that's not dying, or if their LFT's are all whacked, or their albumin is in the toilet; anything that makes you think this could be a cirrhotic patient—just empirically give octreotide.

Consulting editor comments (Weingart):

Now, is there a role for "permissive hypotension" with GI bleeds? We don't know. But we do know definitively that there is no role for *hypertension*, and yet we find many GI bleeders, the second they receive a unit of blood, they spring up to an SBP of 160mmHg, and then they drop, and then they spring. And, that is because they are so replete with endogenous catecholamines that their vessels are like violin strings, so they will bounce back and forth.

I try to stay away from the term "permissive hypotension" because it makes you feel like you're doing something wrong. When you think about it, what is the MAP we're using for patients with critical illness? It's 65mmHg. That's not *hypo*tension, that is our bare minimum *normo*tension. Do that on all your GI bleeders. Don't shoot for a MAP of 100. Shoot for the MAP of 65 or 70 and that is the lowest point of normotension, the perfect place for a resuscitation goal.

Finally, we have clear evidence that with variceal cirrhotic bleeds, patients die by translocation of bacteria, so I would absolutely give a third-generation cephalosporin, like ceftriaxone, to any GI bleeder I suspect or confirm to be a result of varices. I would include any liver failure GI bleeding patient also.

Predict and Prepare

An excellent resuscitation occurs in the mind of the resuscitationist before it occurs in reality; ***begin mobilization of resources with onset of care***, especially if these resources are hard or not timely, such as a consultant an hour away from the hospital.

Categories of preparation:

1. Gathering equipment
2. Initiating relevant protocols
3. Calling consultants
4. Mobilizing staff

Access and Protect

IV access:
At least 2 peripheral IVs 18g or larger. Central access if needed - prefer 8.5F single lumen catheters over smaller gauge triple lumen catheters.

Gastric access:
Consider NGT placement to reduce vomiting and clear gastric contents in preparation for intubation.

Airway Protection:
Reduce critical variables in the resuscitation by intubating and controlling the airway and breathing. This step may need to be delayed if hemodynamics do not allow for safe RSI.

Set and Measure Goals

Have a clear set of goals for the resuscitation and communicate them with your team.

This step occurs simultaneously with the following step

The resuscitation goals should be based on clinical measures that respond in real time.

Suggested goals:
Improvement or stability in HR
SBP 80-100mm/hg
MAP >= 60mm/hg
Maintain or improve mental status

DO NOT use Hgb as a real time measure of success as it is a delayed measure.

Transfuse and Treat

Initiate ***massive transfusion protocol***. If you do not have one, transfuse PRBc and consider introducing FFP and Platelets if you exceed 4 units.

Correct coagulopathy: Use FFP and Cryoprecipitate if volume is needed. If not, consider using PCC. Consider reversal agents for anticoagulants.

Consider PPIs for bleeding ulcers though there is controversy for benefit in the setting of active bleeding.

Consider octreotide for bleeding related to portal hypertension.

Definitive management - Endoscopy, interventional radiology (IR), surgery

Q#4: Who should be called first, gastroenterology (GI), interventional radiology (IR), or surgery?

Endoscopy should be the initial intervention for both upper and lower GI bleed; therefore, the first call should be to GI. However, patients presenting with shock, hemoglobin less than 10, or who have had greater than 6 units of blood transfused, may fail to have bleeding controlled by endoscopy.[39] In this setting, consult IR as well. Additionally, in patients with cirrhosis and variceal bleeding, IR may be needed to place a transjugular, intrahepatic, portosystemic shunt (TIPS), which if done early, may confer a mortality benefit.[40,41] Large perforated ulcers or those located on the posteriorduodenal bulb may also be predictors of endoscopic failure.

It is unusual for a peptic ulcer to present simultaneously with perforation and massive bleeding. So, there are no clear recommendations for this scenario, but in the setting of a perforation with peritonitis and sepsis, surgical intervention is universally necessary.[27] This author's opinion is that in a patient this critically ill, it would be reasonable to consult all three services.

Hospital course:

- A re-read of the CT scan shows free air around the stomach and duodenum with concern for perforation.
- Surgery is consulted and repairs a large duodenal ulcer in the operating room.
- Hospital discharge 2 weeks later with return to baseline status.

Chapter summary:

1. Elderly patients presenting with acute abdominal pain have very high rates of surgical pathology CT scan is frequently indicated and should not be delayed for hydration or oral contrast. Non-contrast CT is highly sensitive (> 92%) for acute intra-abdominal pathology.
2. Not all hyperglycemia in diabetic patients is DKA or HHS.
   a. The diagnostic criteria for DKA includes ketonemia.
   b. HHS requires a glucose level > 600 mg/dL and a serum mOsm/kg > 320 and bicarbonate > 15mEq/L.
   c. Consider precipitating factors such as MI, CVA, and sepsis.
3. Not all shock is septic shock.
4. The CT scan is 97% sensitive for perforation, but clinical findings may trump test results; in the case of a conflict, discuss with the radiologist.
5. With a massive GI bleed, obtain adequate IV access early with 2 large peripheral IVs or a large-bore central catheter (not a triple lumen). Consider early initiation of transfusion in unstable patients with ongoing blood loss, despite a normal Hb level.
6. Consider aortoenteric fistula in patients with severe abdominal pain and massive GI bleed, more likely in patients with a known AAA or who have had recent aortic surgery.

References:

1. Rao SSC, Go JT. Update on the management of constipation in the elderly: new treatment options. Clin Interv Aging 2010;5:163-71.
2. Robinson DA, Lin E. Review of: Cope's early diagnosis of the acute abdomen: 20th Ed. Ann Surg 2001;233(4):594.
3. Perkins J, Perkins K, Mattu A, et al. Pearls and pitfalls in the evaluation of nonspecific abdominal pain. Trauma 2012;26(9):61-72.
4. Kamin RA, Nowicki TA, Courtney DS, et al. Pearls and pitfalls in the emergency department evaluation of abdominal pain. Emerg Med Clin North Am 2003;21(1):61-72.
5. Dieter RS. Sterile pyuria: A differential diagnosis. Compr Ther 2000;26(3):150-52.
6. Longo DL, Wise GJ, Schlegel PN. Sterile pyuria. N Engl J Med 2015;372(11):1048-54.
7. Hickey HPM, Caldwell EW, Gore RM, et al. Helical CT in the evaluation of the acute abdomen. AJR Am J Roentgenol 2000;174(April):901-13.
8. Furukawa A, Sakoda M, Yamasaki M, et al. Gastrointestinal tract perforation: CT diagnosis of presence, site, and cause. Abdom Imaging 2005;30(5):524-34.

9. Strömberg C, Johansson G, Adolfsson A. Acute abdominal pain: Diagnostic impact of immediate CT scanning. World J Surg 2007;31(12):2347-54.
10. Gans SL, Stoker J, Boermeester MA. Plain abdominal radiography in acute abdominal pain; past, present, and future. Int J Gen Med 2012;5:525-33.
11. Smith JE, Hall EJ. The use of plain abdominal x rays in the emergency department. Emerg Med J 2009;26(3):160-63.
12. Hill BC, Johnson SC, Owens EK, et al. CT scan for suspected acute abdominal process: Impact of combinations of IV, oral, and rectal contrast. World J Surg 2010;34(4):699-03.
13. Kessner R, Barnes S, Halpern P, et al. CT for acute nontraumatic abdominal pain-is oral contrast really required? Acad Radiol. 2016;24(7):840-845.
14. Luk L, Newhouse JH. Overestimating the risk of intravenous contrast medium-induced nephropathy: A pitfall in imaging the genitourinary system. Semin Roentgenol 2016;51(1):12-16.
15. Kitabchi AE, Umpierrez GE, Miles JM, et al. Hyperglycemic crises in adult patients with diabetes. Diabetes Care 2009;32(7):1335-43.
16. Morrissey T. Altered mental status | CDEM Curriculum. CDEM. https://cdemcurriculum. com/altered-mental-status/. 2008. Accessed July 20, 2017.
17. McCowen KC, Malhotra A, Bistrian BR. Stress-Induced Hyperglycemia. Crit Care Clin. 2001;17(1):107-24.
18. Umpierrez G, Freire AX. Abdominal pain in patients with hyperglycemic crises. J Crit Care 2002;17(1):63-7.
19. Girard TD, Opal SM, Ely EW. Insights into severe sepsis in older patients: From epidemiology to evidence-based management. Clin Infect Dis 2005;40(2):719-27.
20. Proctor LD. Shock. 2019:Accessed at: https://www.merckmanuals.com/professional/critical-care-medicine/shock-and-fluid-resuscitation/shock
21. Ghane MR, Gharib MH, Ebrahimi A, et al. Accuracy of rapid ultrasound in shock (RUSH) exam for diagnosis of shock in critically ill patients. Trauma Mon 2015;20(1):1-5.
22. Farkas JD, Anawati MK. Bedside ultrasonography evaluation of shock. Hosp Med Clin 2015;4(2):135-49.
23. Kakihana Y, Ito T, Nakahara M, et al. Sepsis-induced myocardial dysfunction: pathophysiology and management. J Intensive Care 2016;4(1):22.
24. Rhodes A, Evans LE, Alhazzani W, et al. Surviving sepsis campaign. 2017; doi:10.1097/CCM.0000000000002255.
25. Clain J, Ramar K, Surani SR. Glucose control in critical care. World J Diabetes 2015;6(9):1082-91.
26. Yatabe T, Inoue S, Sakaguchi M, et al. The optimal target for acute glycemic control in critically ill patients: a network meta-analysis. Intensive Care Med 2017;43(1):16-28.
27. Lee CW, Sarosi GA, Jr. Emergency ulcer surgery. Surg Clin North Am 2011;91(5):1001-13.
28. Yoon W, Jeong YY, Shin SS, et al. Acute massive gastrointestinal bleeding: Detection and localization with arterial phase multi-detector row helical CT. Radiology 2006;239(1):160-67.
29. Broder J. ed. Diagnostic imaging for the emergency physician. Philadelphia, PA: Saunders, 2011.
30. Lee D, Park MH, Shin BS, et al. Multidetector CT diagnosis of non-traumatic gastroduodenal perforation. J Med Imaging Radiat Oncol 2016;60(2):182-186.
31. Wong CH, Chow PKH, Ong HS, Chan WH, Khin LW, Soo KC. Posterior perforation of

peptic ulcers: Presentation and outcome of an uncommon surgical emergency. Surgery 2004;135(3):321-25.
32. Levitan RM. Timing resuscitation sequence intubation for critically ill patients. Available at: http://www.acepnow.com/article/timing-resuscitation-sequence
33. Weingart SD, Levitan RM. Preoxygenation and prevention of desaturation during emergency airway management. Ann Emerg Med 2012;59(3):165–75.
34. Sreedharan A, Martin J, Leontiadis GI, et al. Proton pump inhibitor treatment initiated prior to endoscopic diagnosis in upper gastrointestinal bleeding. Cochrane Database Syst Rev 2010;(7):CD005415.
35. Hasselgren G, Lind T, Lundell L, et al. Continuous intravenous infusion of omeprazole in elderly patients with peptic ulcer bleeding. Results of a placebo-controlled multicenter study. Scand J Gastroenterol1997;32(4):328-33. http://www.ncbi.nlm.nih.gov pubmed/9140154.
36. Gøtzsche PC, Hróbjartsson A. Somatostatin analogues for acute bleeding oesophageal varices. Cochrane Database Syst Rev 2008;(3).
37. Dworzynski K, Pollit V, Kelsey et al. Guideline Development Group. Management of acute upper gastrointestinal bleeding: summary of NICE guidance. BMJ. 2012;344:e3412. http://www.ncbi.nlm.nih.gov/pubmed/22695897. Accessed July 20, 2017.
38. Sihler KC, Napolitano LM. Complications of massive transfusion. Chest 2010;137(1):209- 20.
39. Ramaswamy RS, Choi HW, Mouser HC, et al. Role of interventional radiology in the management of acute gastrointestinal bleeding. World J Radiol 2014;6(4):82-92.
40. García-Pagán JC, Caca K, Bureau C, et al. Early Use of TIPS in patients with cirrhosis and variceal bleeding. N Engl J Med 2010;362(25):2370-79.
41. Ramaswamy R. Role of interventional radiology in the emergent management of acute upper gastrointestinal bleeding. Semin Intervent Radiol 2012;29(3):169-77.

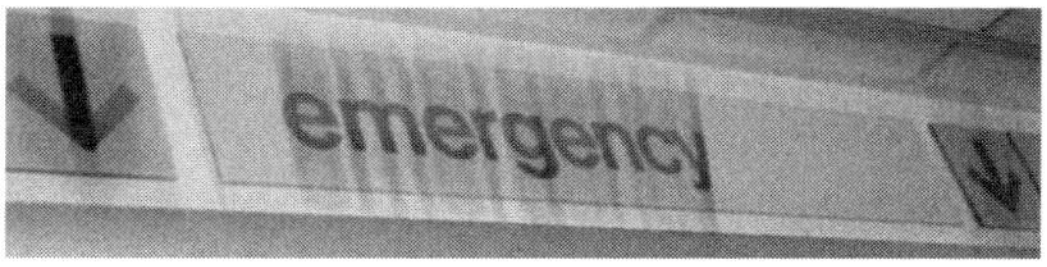

SECTION E – NEURO & SEPSIS

Chapter 24: A 29-year-old male quadriplegic trach patient with fever and respiratory distress

Stephen Villa, MD
Clinical Instructor
Medical Education Fellow
Department of Emergency Medicine
David Geffen School of Medicine at UCLA
Ronald Reagan UCLA Medical Center/Olive View UCLA Medical Center
Los Angeles, CA

Esther H. Chen, MD
Professor
Clinical Emergency Medicine
Department of Emergency Medicine
Director of Graduate Medical Education at ZSFG
University of California, San Francisco/Zuckerberg San Francisco General Hospital
San Francisco, CA

Section editor:
Tiffany M. Osborn, MD, MPH
Professor of Surgery and Emergency Medicine
Surgical/Trauma Critical Care
Department of Surgery
Washington University
St. Louis, MO

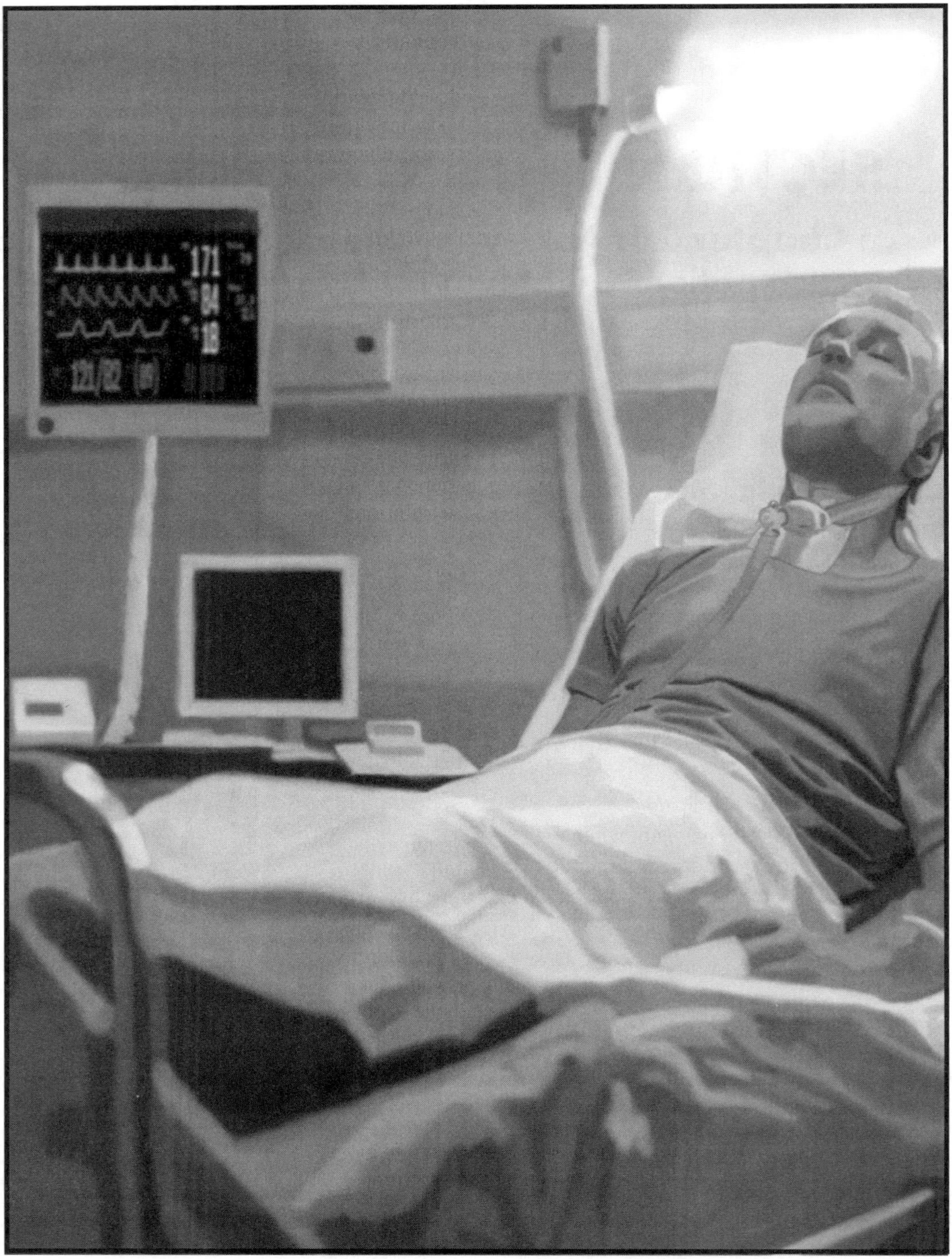
171

SECTION E / CHAPTER 24

A 29-year-old male quadriplegic trach patient with fever and respiratory distress

INITIAL ED VISIT

The patient's story:
Bob Gallant is a 29-year-old man with a history of sickle cell disease. He is a permanent resident of an extended care facility (ECF) after recently being resuscitated after an overdose which left him in a permanent vegetative state with anoxic brain damage and quadriplegia. He has a trach and requires around-the-clock care.

On September 1st, he presents to the emergency department (ED) and is admitted with a diagnosis of healthcare associated pneumonia (HCAP) and is placed on broad-spectrum antibiotics. After a 5-day hospital stay, his fever improves, and he is transferred back to the ECF.

The patient's parents are still working through their stages of grief and are unable to accept the fact that their son, previously happy and animated, will never walk or speak again. Despite multiple multidisciplinary conversations with the family, the patient remains full code.

Chapter author commentary on the initial visit:
At the initial visit, it seems like the patient was managed appropriately: broad-spectrum antibiotics and hospital admission until clinical improvement. If admitted after the year 2016, he would no longer have been diagnosed with HCAP (although knowledge translation may not occur until years later) because in 2016, the Infectious Disease Society of America and the American Thoracic Society changed their guidelines and eliminated HCAP as a separate entity distinct from Hospital-Acquired Pneumonia and Ventilator-Associated Pneumonia (VAP).[1] This patient was likely treated with agents that covered methicillin-resistant *Staphylococcus aureus* (MRSA) and *Pseudomonas aeruginosa*, such as vancomycin and piperacillin-tazobactam, respectively. These current guidelines do recommend that patients with VAP should receive a 7-day course of antibiotics, although a shorter or longer duration may also be appropriate depending on clinical improvement. Since the patient improved clinically in the hospital after 5 days, it was reasonable to send him back to the ECF.

The patient's story (continued):
Upon return to the ECF, he remains afebrile for several weeks, until just after midnight on September 21st, when the night shift nurse's aide notices an increased respiratory rate and a heart rate of 123 beats per minute. She notifies the night shift nurse but is unable to contact the ECF doctor. At the 7AM shift change, the day-shift aide finds the patient severely tachycardic and tachypneic with a temperature of 101°F. EMS is notified and the patient is transported to the ED.

ED RETURN VISIT

CC-RN (08:09): fever, respiratory distress

HPI: The patient is a 29-year-old man with a history of brain injury who is nonverbal at baseline and presents from the ECF. I did see the patient immediately upon arrival and spoke with EMS personnel who were called because the patient had a high temperature and heart rate. The patient is not able to give any history secondary to his medical condition. I did review the previous record. The patient has no known allergies. He was admitted to the hospital last month with a similar presentation and had a heart rate of 171 bpm at that time.

Social history: Extended care facility. I reviewed the nurse's notes.

ROS: Unable to obtain secondary to altered level of consciousness and nonverbal status

NKDA
PMH:
Tracheostomy present
Acute kidney failure
Embolism - per ECF report, "venous thrombosis and embolism"
Encephalopathy/brain injury
Gastrostomy in place
Iron deficiency anemia due to chronic blood loss
MDRO (multiple drug resistant organisms) resistance - sputum lung. Pseudomonas aeruginosa MDRO
Pneumonia
Respiratory failure with hypoxia
Sepsis due to methicillin resistant Staphylococcus aureus
Sickle cell disease, type S beta-plus thalassemia
TIA (transient ischemic attack)

Medications:
FentaNYL 25 mcg/hr transdermal film, Flexeril 10 mg, LevETIRAcetam 100 mg/ml oral solution, Nystatin Oral Susp, baclofen 10 mg, calcium acetate 667 mg, famotidine 20 mg, lactulose 10 gm/15 ml, oxyCODONE, traZODone 50 mg, valproic acid 250 mg/5 ml oral syrup, warfarin 5 mg

Surgical history:
Tracheostomy
Jejunostomy tube placement

PE:

Vitals:

Time	Temp	Pulse	Resp	Syst	Diast	Sat
08:45	100.5	171	30	109	79	95% vent

CONSTITUTIONAL: He is diaphoretic and a trach is in place
EYES: PERRL, no scleral icterus
RESP: Normal chest excursion with respiration; breath sounds clear and equal bilaterally; no wheezes, rhonchi, or rales
CARDIO: Tachycardic, but regular rhythm without murmurs, rub or gallop
ABD: Non-distended; with some involuntary guarding which is generalized, there is a tube from the stomach which looks like a G-tube draining green drainage
SKIN: Normal for age and race; warm and dry; no apparent lesions
EXTREMITIES: Padding in place on the extremities, pulses are 2+ and equal in all 4 extremities; no lower extremity peripheral edema or any signs of ulcerations, erythema, skin lesions
NEURO: His eyes are open, but he does not respond to verbal or tactile stimuli

Author comments (Weinstock):

The patient is nonverbal with a recent history of sepsis and now presents with tachycardia, tachypnea, diaphoresis and is hypotensive-*ish*. We are at:

DECISION POINT A – YOU ARE FACED WITH 5 QUESTIONS:

1. **The patient has a fever and tachycardia; what are the initial orders?**
2. **What is the initial antibiotic selection for a patient recently admitted and treated with piperacillin/tazobactam (Zosyn) and vancomycin?**
3. **What does the literature recommend for initial IVF rate and route?**
4. **Branch point: Would fluid administration change if our patient had a history of ESRD or heart failure?**
5. **What is unique about a tracheostomy patient with respiratory distress?**

Expert recommendations and literature review:

Q#1: The patient has a fever and tachycardia; what are the initial orders?

A medical student could have clinched the diagnosis; symptoms of fever, tachycardia, and respiratory distress scream pneumonia with sepsis. His presentation mirrors a classic oral boards-style case, at which point one would resuscitate with fluids, order antibiotics, and admit. After the initial bedside evaluation, our priorities would include obtaining large-bore peripheral intravenous (IV) access for fluid administration and providing supplemental oxygen therapy to support his tachypnea and hypoxia. The most useful initial diagnostic test would be point-of-care venous blood gas with lactate, to help with risk stratification—we know this patient is sick, but is he sick enough that he needs intensive care unit level of care? But this "obvious" diagnosis of a respiratory source of sepsis may trick us; we should still think broadly as chronically debilitated patients may have other potential etiologies such as urine (catheter associated), skin and soft tissue (decubitus ulcerations), abdominal (SBO or perforation), and central nervous system infections. Antibiotics without source control may not be helpful at all.

Other tests typically include a complete blood count (CBC), comprehensive metabolic panel, 2 sets of blood cultures, chest radiograph, urinalysis, urine culture, and electrocardiogram. Since he does have green fluid oozing from his G-tube and involuntary abdominal guarding, an abdominal and pelvis computed tomography scan (ACT) may identify an intra-abdominal infection. In patients with paraplegia, examine the skin for ulcers that may extend into the deep tissues (think sacral area…), causing abscess formation, necrotizing fasciitis, or osteomyelitis.

In 2016, Singer, et al. proposed new definitions for sepsis[2,3] and some of the recommendations were updated.[4] In case you skipped a few pages of the 74-page document, here are some highlights:

- *Sepsis:* life-threatening organ dysfunction due to a dysregulated host response to an infection.
- *Septic shock:* Sepsis + either a lactate greater than 2mmol/L in the absence of hypovolemia or requiring vasopressors to maintain a mean arterial pressure (MAP) of 65.
- *Sequential Organ Failure Assessment (SOFA)* can be used to predict in-hospital mortality, but it's cumbersome, requires diagnostic tests, and is less useful for the ED.
- *qSOFA* is a modified SOFA score [altered mental status (GCS < 15), respiratory rate ≥ 22, and systolic blood pressure ≤ 100mmHg]; the higher the score, the higher the risk of in-hospital mortality.

Section editor comments (Osborn):

This is a pandora's box; ACEP does not recognize the definitions, globally, only one emergency medicine organization signed off on them, and none from North America agreed enough to endorse. Neither third-party quality organizations, the CDC nor CMS recognize the definitions. Quality metrics are based on the Mortality Index = observed/expected mortality. So, if we classify a patient on three vasopressors with a normal lactate (or not drawn) as sepsis, but quality is judged on the previous definition (sepsis not so sick), your MI will appear much worse than someone using the CMS definitions. In other words, by choosing to use the new definitions, your care appears worse no matter how good your care is because of how the patient's illness is defined.

Q#2: What is the initial antibiotic selection for a patient recently admitted and treated with piperacillin/tazobactam (Zosyn) and vancomycin?

Our patient was treated with broad-spectrum antibiotics during his first hospitalization. Vancomycin covers gram-positive pathogens, including MRSA, and piperacillin-tazobactam covers anaerobes and some gram-positive and gram-negative bacteria, including *Pseudomonas*.[1] Given his recent hospitalization and presence of tracheostomy, those are still the primary organisms to consider, particularly multi-drug resistant *Pseudomonas* (even if our patient did not have a documented history of MDR *Pseudomonas*). Per the 2016 IDSA guidelines (in the setting of antibiotics within 90 days and septic shock), the best antibiotic coverage would double cover for *Pseudomonas*, using piperacillin-tazobactam or cefepime or carbapenem AND a fluoroquinolone or aminoglycoside, in addition to covering for MRSA with vancomycin or linezolid.[1] His bounce back to the ED suggests he was either re-infected with a new pathogen from a different source, developed a complication from his pneumonia (i.e., parapneumonic effusion), or was inadequately treated during the first hospitalization with possibilities including vancomycin-resistant *Entercoccus*, extended-spectrum β-Lactamase bacteria, and fungal infections. However, if your shop is like ours, you may have to ask for approval from an infectious disease specialist for the appropriate agents (which may not happen until the next morning), so it's OK simply to cover the most likely organisms first.

Q#3: What does the literature recommend for initial IVF rate and route?

While most of us would probably automatically give a 2-liter fluid bolus (because it's in the sepsis bundle in the electronic medical record), the current recommendation for a septic patient is a rapid infusion of 30mL/kg of crystalloid within the first 3 hours.[4] This is a strong reminder for clinicians to adjust according to the patient's weight.

Q#4: Branch point: Would fluid administration change if our patient had a history of ESRD or heart failure?

Now, what about those special clinical considerations when giving a fluid bolus may be harmful? As it turns out, the goal of giving 30mL/kg of crystalloid in the first 3 hours holds true even for those patients in whom we worry about respiratory decompensation after a rapid fluid challenge. For patients with pneumonia or other acute lung injury requiring oxygen support, or patients with renal failure or congestive heart failure, we recommend giving smaller boluses of fluid less rapidly and with more frequent reassessments of oxygenation, respiratory status, and volume status.[4,5] In addition to frequent monitoring of vital signs, we also use urine output, point-of-care cardiac and inferior vena cava (IVC) ultrasound, hemodynamic response and IVC compressibility to passive leg raise, and repeat lactate levels to help guide additional fluid administration.

Q#5: What is unique about a tracheostomy patient with respiratory distress?

Acute respiratory distress already has a broad differential diagnosis, but in a tracheostomy patient, it's critical to consider the tracheostomy-related conditions. Take a look at this trach management algorithm[6] (Figure 1 on page 553).

When faced with a possible trach problem, consider the following questions:

1. When was the trach placed? Replacement is much easier (and safer) with a mature tract (usually > 7 days post-op); otherwise a false tract may be created during tube replacement.
2. Is the tube cuffed or uncuffed? If the hypoxia is due to pathology that requires more positive pressure ventilation, consider swapping an uncuffed for a cuffed tube.
3. What size is the tube? If you cannot find the same tube, use a 6–0 endotracheal tube.
4. Why was it placed? The indications for the tracheostomy may alert you to potential complications or considerations.
5. Has the patient had a laryngectomy? These patients cannot be orally intubated or oxygenated.

Recommendations for initial critical interventions:

1. Apply high flow oxygen to the face and tracheostomy site.
2. Remove speaking valve or cap (if present) and inner tube and pass a suction catheter to clear mucus.
3. If you are unable to pass a suction catheter, deflate the cuff and listen for air exchange, as the tube may be partially obstructed or displaced. If patient improves, then scope through the trach.

4. If steps 1–3 do not improve the patient's clinical status or at any time the patient stops breathing, then the tube will need to be exchanged or oral intubation attempted.

The bottom line is that we are the airway experts. If the patient ever becomes unstable (and is not s/p laryngectomy), follow your usual oral airway algorithm and intubate from above.

Authors comments (Weinstock):

We are aware that this figure appears twice in the book, but if you have it memorized or are bored with seeing it again... all the more power to you!

(Figure on next page...)

Figure 1. Emergency Tracheostomy Management[6]

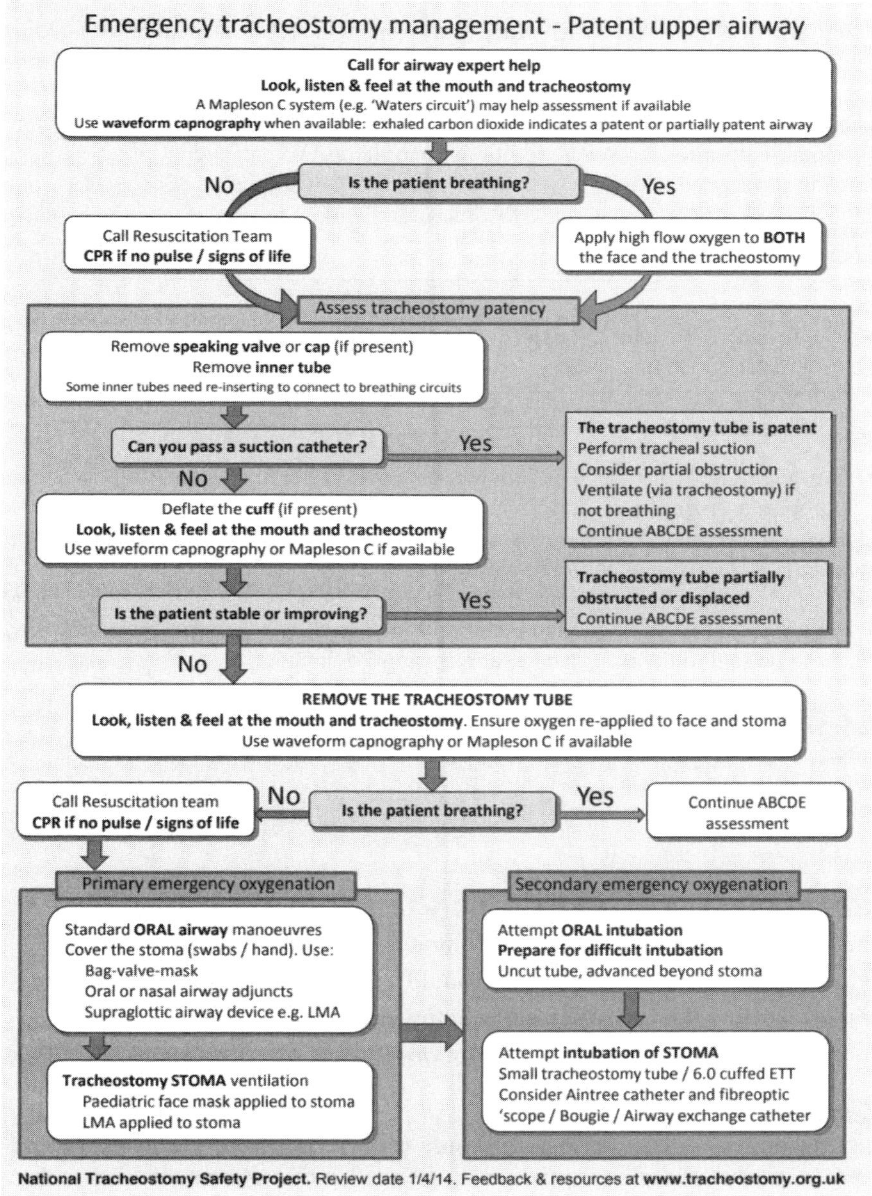

McGrath BA, Bates L, Atkinson D, Moore JA. National tracheostomy safety project. Multidisciplinary guidelines for the management of tracheostomy and laryngectomy airway emergencies. Anaesthesia. 2012;67(9):1025-41. Copyright © 2012 John Wiley & Sons. Used with permission.

What did the actual provider do?

MDM (09:06): I reviewed the ECG which shows sinus tachycardia with rate of 175bpm and nonspecific ST changes. The patient does have reported temperature of 103° F—this is sepsis. His oxygen status is good; however, he is quite tachypneic. He is nonverbal and this does appear to be chronic based on my review of the previous record. Patient did have 1, 20-gauge IV in the right upper extremity; however, additional peripheral IV lines were not able to be placed despite using ultrasound. He did have initial orders for IV fluid bolus 30cc/kg, IV Zosyn, and vancomycin. I will add on Levaquin, CXR, monitor. Pending results of testing, the patient will be admitted to the intensive care unit.

Vitals:

Time	Temp	Pulse	Resp	Syst	Diast	Sat
09:12	104.1	150	50	83	52	95%

Chapter author note: Great job! The provider recognized that this patient was "sick" and ordered all the appropriate diagnostics. Antibiotics were started quickly, including double coverage for *Pseudomonas,* which gets at source control. Although our patient's tachycardia has improved, his blood pressure is clearly headed in the wrong direction. He will need better IV access and given the multiple failed attempts at placing a US-guided line, the next best option will be central venous access. Having a central line will also be helpful in case he needs vasopressors. Seems he is not quite ready to be sent to the ICU; we are at Decision Point B:

Section editor comments (Osborn):

I would reconsider this approach; this is a hypotensive patient you are placing back on the ventilator. He is ready for the ICU. What if the ICU bed is not ready yet? We shouldn't give the ICU these kinds of outs. Depending on the volume and acuity of the ED, the patient may not be tied into a pretty bow, but he needs ICU care now!

DECISION POINT B – YOU ARE FACED WITH 4 QUESTIONS:

1. **The respiratory rate has increased; should he be sedated and placed on a vent?**
2. **BP is decreasing even with the IVF. Should we give more IVF or start pressors?**
3. **Does decreasing the fever with antipyretics change prognosis?**
4. **Does our patient need a central line for vasopressor administration?**

What does the literature say?

Q#1: The respiratory rate has increased; should he be sedated and placed on a vent?

It depends…on what's causing the worsening tachypnea. Once we've established that the trach itself is not dislodged or displaced, then we can consider and reverse the non-respiratory causes of tachypnea, such as metabolic acidosis. The indications for taking over a patient's respiratory effort are the same with or without a trach; our patient will unlikely be able to maintain a respiratory rate of 50 or may be developing acute respiratory disease syndrome (ARDS), so positive pressure ventilation may decrease his work of breathing. Use of lung protective ventilation would be optimal (i.e., 6–8mL/kg ideal body weight, as measured by height), keeping plateau pressures ≤ 30cm H_2O.[4,7] Caution should be exercised with sedation, especially with benzodiazepines. Long-term sedation disrupts sleep and can lead to delirium, which is an independent predictor of mortality in mechanically ventilated patients.[8] Instead, relieve the discomfort of mechanical ventilation with a fentanyl infusion (note that morphine metabolites and hydromorphone can accumulate in renal failure).[9] This may be enough to make the patient comfortable. However, if the patient continues to be agitated, then sedation with small IV boluses of short-acting benzodiazepines (i.e., midazolam) may be required. A propofol or dexmedetomidine infusion may be used, although both can worsen hypotension. For the aggressively agitated and/or hypotensive patient, consider a bolus of ketamine, followed by an infusion.

Section editor comments (Osborn):

Given this patient has devastating cerebral anoxia, I am not sure any sedation would be necessary, and with his hypotension, it could be harmful. Note that prolonged benzodiazepine use can cause dependence and result in withdrawal if tapered off too quickly, but this is typically an ICU issue.

If he is agitated and needs sedation:

- If propofol (or dexmitomidine) is available in the ED + if normotensive > start a drip.
- If not available in ED + the patient will be in ED for several hours—use benzodiazepines (BDZ) and order a propofol drip.
- If hypotensive, consider BDZ or ketamine.
- If expected to leave soon—within next 1–2 hours—a dose of benzodiazepines is ok.

Q#2: BP is decreasing even with the IVF. Should we give more IVF or start pressors?

After the initial fluid bolus is given, the next management step will be guided by other dynamic measurements, such as point-of-care cardiac and IVC ultrasound, hemodynamic response to passive leg raise, and lactate level clearance.[5] If the patient has a compressible IVC on ultrasound, a persistently elevated lactate level, or a positive passive leg raise test, then give more fluid. Alternatively, if the IVC is plethoric, in the context of reasonable cardiac function, then start vasopressor support. Norepinephrine is the initial vasopressor of choice, followed by vasopressin.[4] Of note, the use of lactate level clearance as a target in sepsis is not entirely clear. There is evidence that an elevated lactate level reflects the degree of activation of the stress response to the severity of illness (via endogenous epinephrine stimulating aerobic glycolysis), rather than a marker of anaerobic metabolism.[10] If the patient is started on epinephrine as the next vasopressor, it's entirely possible that the lactate level may increase. So, like everything in medicine, assess the entire patient including urine output, blood pressure, heart rate, and mental status, instead of simply relying on "lactate clearance" as the sole indicator of patient improvement.

Q#3: Does decreasing the fever with antipyretics change prognosis?

"Doc, what are you going to do about that temp?" Understandably, a high temperature makes everyone nervous, but actually, a low temperature is even worse. Hypothermia (≤ 36.5° C) is independently associated with increased mortality and organ failure in patients hospitalized for sepsis whereas higher temperatures were associated with a lower in-hospital mortality.[11,12] In hospitalized patients with fever and suspected infection, treatment with IV acetaminophen did not decrease 90-day mortality compared to placebo[13] and neither did IV ibuprofen.[14]

Even worse, one study found that treatment with either a non-steroidal anti-inflammatory drug or acetaminophen was associated with an increased 28-day mortality in septic patients.[15] So, unless the patient is distressed or uncomfortable because of the fever, treating with an anti-pyretic may not affect mortality and at least one study showed that there is potential harm.

Q#4: Does our patient need a central line for vasopressor administration?

Vasopressors can be given safely through a large peripheral vein such as an antecubital vein, in the short term.[16] So, do not delay starting vasopressors simply because the patient does not have central venous access. Once you've decided that central access is needed, which site should you pick? The common teaching is that femoral vein catheters are more likely to be become infected as compared to internal jugular or subclavian catheters; however, a meta-analysis that included more recent studies showed similar infection rates with all 3 sites.[17] A systematic review comparing internal jugular to subclavian lines showed a higher rate of arterial punctures and bloodstream infections with jugular catheters, a lower rate of malpositions with jugular catheters, and a similar rate of hemo- or pneumothorax. However, the articles used in this review were published prior to 2002, before the routine use of ultrasound guidance.[18] What about bleeding risk? Some providers arbitrarily use cutoffs for INR > 1.5 and platelet count < 50,000 even though the bleeding risk is actually very low.[19]

Bottom line: Choose the site that you're most comfortable with and when possible, use an ultrasound to guide your placement.

Section editor comments (Osborn):

If using an 18G in solid vein, for example an AC fossa, I do agree, but it can't be a 22G in the wrist, as this will infiltrate. I have seen the tissue necrosis that occurs when this happens. Regarding the femoral CVP placement and infection rates, there may be some extenuating circumstances, for example *C.diff* diarrhea, precluding placement of a catheter in this site.

What did the actual provider do?

Procedure (09:33): I placed a right femoral central line placed under ultrasound guidance. The area was prepped and draped in the usual sterile fashion. Using the Seldinger technique I did initially puncture the right femoral artery and then later successfully cannulated the right femoral vein. It was difficult to thread the wire and the needle needed to be re-advanced several times before the central line was successfully inserted. This was all done under sterile conditions. The patient received IV fluids and antibiotics through the central line.

The labs have returned:

Lab	Results	Ref range
WBC	25.2 (H)	4.6–10.2
Hb	7.3 (L)	12.0–16.0
Platelets	64 (L)	142–424

Lab	Results		Ref range
NA	159 (H)	MMOL/L	136–145
K	4.0	MMOL/L	3.6–5.1
CL	121 (H)	MMOL/L	98–107
CO_2	17 (L)	MMOL/L	22–32
BUN	58 (H)	MG/DL	8–20
CREAT	3.6 (H)	MG/DL	0.6–1.3
GLUC H	251 (H)	MG/DL	70–110
Lactic acid	8.6 (H)	MMOL/L	

Urine: WNL except protein

ABG: 7.12/28/50/16

CXR (per radiology): Denser opacity at the medial right base. Some clearing of the left base compared to the prior study.

MDM (09:52): The patient has been rechecked on multiple occasions and labs have been reviewed. His temperature is 104.1° F. I did give acetaminophen 975mg per rectum. Lactate level is 8.6. Because of the patient's tachypnea he is placed on the ventilator. I did give Ativan 1mg IV to help with sedation. He does not seem uncomfortable at the time. Patient will be admitted to intensive care unit. I will get an abdominal CT as the G-tube is draining green fluid and there is some involuntary guarding in the abdomen.

ED course (10:08): The nurse finds the physician to inform that the blood pressure is now 60/palp. Documentation of: "Awaiting orders from doctor."

Vitals:

Time	Temp	Pulse	Resp	Syst	Diast	Sat
10:09		152	16	60	palp	92% vent

MDM (10:42): The patient remains hypotensive and levophed is running at 10mcg/minute. I will add on epinephrine drip. Pt. has been placed on the vent but is trying to breath above the vent so I will give additional Ativan 0.5mg IV.

10:59: Respiratory therapist finds the doctor, "The patient is still bucking the vent. Can we have something more for sedation?"

DECISION POINT C – YOU ARE FACED WITH 4 QUESTIONS:

1. **The patient remains hypotensive after IV fluids and vasopressors; what is the next step?**
2. **The patient is now bucking the vent. What are additional choices for sedation?**
3. **If patient arrests, is ECMO indicated?**
4. **When should the patient be sent to the ICU?**

Q#1: The patient remains hypotensive after IV fluids and vasopressors; what is the next step?

- Vasopressor doses and dose ranges are very institution-dependent. Some patients may require higher doses based on the clinical response.
- After giving 30mL/kg of crystalloid, assess IVC compressibility on US, response to passive leg raise, and urine output to guide further fluid administration.[4]
- Blood transfusion is not indicated unless there are signs of acute cardiac ischemia or active bleeding. A restrictive strategy (transfuse at hemoglobin 7g/dL) has been shown to have similar 90-day mortality and rates of ischemic events compared to a liberal strategy (hemoglobin 9g/dL).[20]
- If the patient does not respond to fluid administration and 2 vasopressor agents, add on a 3rd vasopressor (i.e., vasopressin or phenylephrine) to maintain MAP at 65mmHg, then give IV hydrocortisone at 200mg/day.[4]

Section editor comments (Osborn):

We may want to consider a little more nuance here. Prior to 1999, low Hb (then considered < 10) was thought to produce great harm. With Hébert's Canadian trial (Hébert PC, et al. A Multicenter, Randomized, Controlled Clinical Trial of Transfusion Requirements in Critical Care. N Engl J Med 1999; 340:409-417), the thought was that transfusion was the enemy, producing great harm. Then caveats began to arise.

SOAP I – transfusion bad
SOAP II – transfusion good – difference leukoreduction of blood.
Sakr – transfusion = reduced mortality, especially in the elderly and CAD
Park – lower mortality with CAP sepsis
TRISS – no difference in septic shock for all comers

Here are some things to consider. Perhaps the need to transfuse is patient-dependent; for example, perhaps 9 should not have been applied to every patient and neither should 7. Another specific group, CT surgery patients with restrictive transfusion, equals higher mortality at 90 days. Why is this population different?

Regarding TRISS—median lactate 2.2. Does that equate to septic shock with a lactate of 5? If the baseline Hb is 13 and now they are 7.5 on 3 vasopressors with a H/O CAD, should we consider it? These are difficult to tease out—especially as this study was started in the ICU after significant resuscitation was done in the ED. CAD + elderly + shock—the sample size of this population in TRISS was too small to make definitive statements.

Regarding medications, if there is global myocardial dysfunction due to sepsis, try norepinephrine. If it works, then great, if not may need inotrope.

Bottom line: The data supports an approach for most patients of waiting, so we should probably wait until 7. However, that does not absolve us from thinking clinically of how individual patients are responding and taking into consideration individual response to treatment and potential requirements.

Q#2: The patient is now bucking the vent. What are additional choices for sedation?

Stop giving the Ativan boluses and instead try first giving small boluses of IV fentanyl. If he continues to buck the vent, then try to give small boluses of ketamine to avoid dropping his pressures.

Consulting editor comments (Weingart):

At this stage in the game, the sedation regimen at most emergency departments is propofol. When these folks are paralyzed and intubated, they stop moving, but the main cause for their misery is the fact that they have a large plastic object shoved in the back of their throat. And you can experience this yourself right now at home while you're reading, just stick two fingers in the back of your throat and leave them there for a few hours and see how you feel...

Propofol at general anesthetic doses will eventually stop the patient reacting from to pain because they will just be totally blunted. But on some level, they're still probably perceiving the pain and there's probably still a sympathetic upregulation. But, if on the other hand, you actually gave them an analgesic-first approach, with a dose of hydromorphone or morphine, you have now treated the pain. What you will find is then your sedative requirements are remarkably lower or nonexistent. We have had patients who are on a well-titrated regimen of oxycodone—we had already switched to oral agents—and they didn't require any sedatives. You could talk to these patients and say, "How ya doing?" And they'd be responsive and give you a thumbs up. You definitively need analgesics until that endotracheal tube is taken out or converted to a trach.

Q#3: If patient arrests, is ECMO indicated?

The practice of ED ECMO is supported by the American Heart Association for medically refractory cardiac arrest.[21] At this time, ED ECMO is primarily performed in academic institutions, but patient selection, devices, and techniques are highly variable. Even if available, our patient is excluded from most uses of ED ECMO.

Exclusion criteria for many institutions include:

- Age
- Unwitnessed arrest
- > 10 minutes of downtime without bystander CPR
- Pre-arrest co-morbidities for which ECMO is unlikely to improve the patient's quality of life.[21,22]

Q#4: When should the patient be sent to the ICU?

This question needs to be addressed early, as the argument that a patient is "too sick for transport" to the intensive care unit is irrational. Once you've obtained IV access, initiated fluid resuscitation, given antibiotics, started vasopressors, and placed the patient on mechanical ventilation, they are ready for transport. A note should be made about the provider's decision to transport the patient to CT as a decompensating patient leaving a critical care area is potentially problematic. Our [the chapter author's] opinion is that we would have advised against transport to CT, as diagnostic imaging would be unlikely to change our patient's management. Even if he had an intra-abdominal infection, no surgeon will take him to the operating room until he has been stabilized.

What did the actual provider do?

MDM (11:32): Patient does have chronic anemia as well as chronic renal failure. I did add on liver function tests, lipase, Depakote level, INR. I did speak with ID and they will review the patient's culture results. He did have a respiratory culture on September 5th which showed *Pseudomonas* and MRSA. I did review the repeat ECG showing sinus tachycardia with rate of 125bpm and some nonspecific T-wave changes. This does not show any evidence of SVT or ischemic changes. I did review the CT result showing "consideration of aspiration pneumonia." No signs of surgical or infectious intra-abdominal process. I have spoken with the hospitalist and ICU doctor for the admission.

CT abd/pelvis (radiology interpretation):
1. Dependent lower lobe consolidation on the right and atelectasis on the left. These findings are suggestive of aspiration pneumonia.
2. Otherwise normal unenhanced CT exam of the abdomen and pelvis.

Vitals:

Time	Temp	Pulse	Resp	Syst	Diast	Sat
12:12		147	16	56	palp	90% vent

Chapter author commentary (Villa and Chen): This patient is not doing well at all. He received appropriate care in the ED, and the emergency physician has communicated an appropriate handoff to the ICU doctor, hospitalist, and infectious disease specialist. Although still relatively unstable, he needs to go to the ICU for further care.

Big picture: This patient will likely not recover during his hospitalization. The most important conversation to have with the family as the "best" care may be to maximize comfort. While emphasizing that we will continue to "do everything possible" for their family member, it's just as important to convey the severity of his condition, the unlikelihood of clinical improvement, and the futility of the interventions. We would also emphasize that he may suffer even more as a result of all our interventions to keep him alive. Would this have been the life that he would have wanted for himself?

Diagnosis (12:02): Septic shock, pneumonia, tachycardia and tachypnea, altered level of consciousness.

Outcome: The intensivist has accepted the patient and asked that he "just get sent up to the unit". You inform the nurse, but there is a conflict with the ED nurse and the ICU nurse, who is concerned the patient has not been stabilized. The ED nurse goes to speak with the EP who states that they have placed a central line, given fluids and pressors, placed the patient on a vent, and at this point the patient needs ICU care. Additionally, "I have already spoken with the ICU doctor, in fact, it was about 30 minutes ago, and I thought the patient was on the way upstairs."

The patient is eventually brought to the ICU, but as they are leaving the elevator, the patient becomes asystolic and is unable to be resuscitated. He is pronounced dead at 14:33.

Chapter summary:

- Although the sepsis definitions have changed, management has not. Give 30mL/kg within the first 3 hours, broad-spectrum antibiotics for source control, and frequently reassess to determine need for more IVF vs. vasopressors to maintain MAP $\geq$ 65mmHg.
- In the trach patient with respiratory distress, consider obstruction and displacement as possible causes.
- Beware of the immature tract (< 7 days), in which the trach could go into a false tract during replacement.
- Don't forget that a patient with a laryngectomy CANNOT be intubated orally.
- For the mechanically ventilated ICU patient, sedation can lead to delirium and worse outcomes. Treat with analgesia first (fentanyl) and add small boluses of versed (if normotensive) or ketamine (if hypotensive) as needed for agitation.
- Once the patient is adequately resuscitated with IVF, treat hypotension with norepinephrine, as first line, followed by vasopressin, then epinephrine. At the time of the 3rd pressor, give a dose of steroids.
- Do not delay giving vasopressors because the patient does not have a central line. You can infuse vasopressors through a large peripheral line short-term.
- All ultrasound-guided central lines have similar complication rates. Choose the one you are most comfortable with and try to use an ultrasound whenever possible.
- Engaging the family in a multi-disciplinary conversation about goals of care can be accomplished in the ED, with the help of a palliative care consultant, if available.

References:

1. Kalil AC, Metersky ML, Klompas M, et al. Management of adults with hospital-acquired and ventilator-associated pneumonia: 2016 clinical practice guidelines by the Infectious Diseases Society of America and the American Thoracic Society. Clin Infect Dis 2016;63(5).
2. Singer M, Deutschman CS, Seymour CW, et al. The third international consensus definitions for sepsis and septic shock (Sepsis-3). JAMA 2016;315(8):801-10.
3. Seymour CW, Liu VX, Iwashyna TJ, et al. Assessment of clinical criteria for sepsis: For the third international consensus definitions for sepsis and septic shock (Sepsis-3). JAMA 2016;315(8):762-74.
4. Rhodes A, Evans LE, Alhazzani W, et al. Surviving sepsis campaign: International guidelines for management of sepsis and septic shock: 2016; Intensive Care Med 2017;43(3):304-77.
5. Dellinger RP, Schorr CA, Levy MM. A users' guide to the 2016 surviving sepsis guidelines. Crit Care Med 2017;45(3):381-5.
6. McGrath BA, Bates L, Atkinson D, et al. Multidisciplinary guidelines for the management of tracheostomy and laryngectomy airway emergencies. Anaesthesia 2012;67(9):1025-41.
7. Weingart SD. Managing initial mechanical ventilation in the smergency department. Ann Emerg Med 2016;68(5):614-17.
8. Ely EW, Shintani A, Truman B, et al. Delirium as a predictor of mortality in mechanically ventilated patients in the intensive care unit. JAMA 2004;291(14):1753-62.

9. Patel SB, Kress JP. Sedation and analgesia in the mechanically ventilated patient. Am J Respir Crit Care Med 2012;185(5):486-97.
10. Marik PE, Bellomo R. Lactate clearance as a target of therapy in sepsis: a flawed paradigm. OA Critical Care 2013;1(1):3.
11. Kushimoto S, Gando S, Saitoh D, et al. The impact of body temperature abnormalities on the disease severity and outcome in patients with severe sepsis: An analysis from a multicenter, prospective survey of severe sepsis. Crit Care 2013;17(6):R271.
12. Sunden-Cullberg J, Rylance R, Svefors J, et al. Fever in the emergency department predicts survival of patients with severe sepsis and septic shock admitted to the ICU. Crit Care Med 2017;45(4):591-9.
13. Young P, Saxena M, Bellomo R, et al. Acetaminophen for fever in critically ill patients with suspected infection. N Engl J Med 2015;373(23):2215-24.
14. Bernard GR, Wheeler AP, Russell JA, et al. The effects of ibuprofen on the physiology and survival of patients with sepsis. The Ibuprofen in Sepsis Study Group. N Engl J Med 1997;336(13):912-8.
15. Lee BH, Inui D, Suh GY, et al. Association of body temperature and antipyretic treatments with mortality of critically ill patients with and without sepsis: Multi-centered prospective observational study. Crit Care 2012;16(1):R33.
16. Loubani OM, Green RS. A systematic review of extravasation and local tissue injury from administration of vasopressors through peripheral intravenous catheters and central venous catheters. J Crit Care 2015;30(3):653 e9-17.
17. Marik PE, Flemmer M, Harrison W. The risk of catheter-related bloodstream infection with femoral venous catheters as compared to subclavian and internal jugular venous catheters: A systematic review of the literature and meta-analysis. Crit Care Med 2012;40(8):2479-85.
18. Ruesch S, Walder B, Tramer MR. Complications of central venous catheters: Internal jugular versus subclavian access—a systematic review. Crit Care Med 2002;30(2):454-60.
19. Baron RM. Point: Should coagulopathy be repaired prior to central venous line insertion? Yes: Why take chances? Chest 2012;141(5):1139-42.
20. Holst LB, Haase N, Wetterslev J, et al. Lower versus higher hemoglobin threshold for transfusion in septic shock. N Engl J Med 2014;371(15):1381-91.
21. Tonna JE, Johnson NJ, Greenwood J, et al. Practice characteristics of emergency department extracorporeal cardiopulmonary resuscitation (eCPR) programs in the United States: The current state of the art of emergency department extracorporeal membrane oxygenation (ED ECMO). Resuscitation 2016;107:38-46.
22. Extracorporeal Life Support Organization. ELSO guidelines for cardiopulmonary extracorporeal life support. 2017;Version 1.4: Accessed 11/13/2017: https://www.elso.org/Portals/0/ELSO%20 Guidelines%20General%20All%2 0ECLS%20Version%201_4.pdf

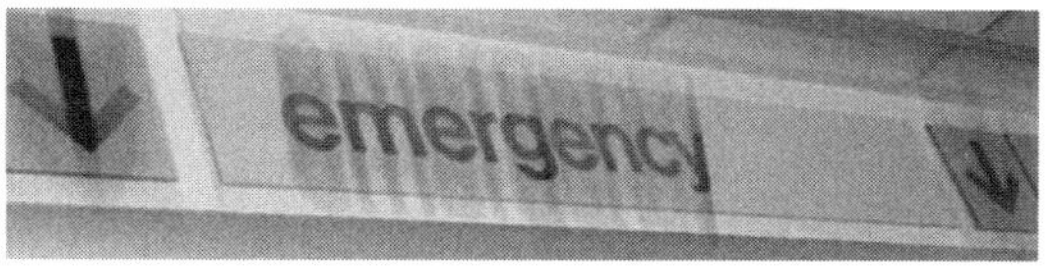

SECTION E – NEURO & SEPSIS

Chapter 25: A 51-year-old diabetic woman with vertigo

Katherine Mayer, MD, FACEP

Assistant Professor, Department of Emergency Medicine
Division of Pulmonary Medicine
University of Colorado Anschutz Medical Campus
Aurora, CO

Karina Reyner Pauly, MD

Associate Professor of Medicine
Texas A&M College of Medicine Department of Emergency Medicine
Baylor University Medical Center
Dallas, TX

Alan C. Heffner, MD

Co-Director of Critical Care, ECMO Medical Director
Pulmonary and Critical Care Consultants
Department of Internal Medicine and Department of Emergency Medicine
Carolinas Medical Center, UNC School of Medicine – Charlotte Campus
Charlotte, NC

Section editor:

Evie Marcolini, MD, FAAEM, FACEP, FCCM

Associate Professor
Emergency Medicine and Neurocritical Care
Geisel School of Medicine at Dartmouth
Board of Directors
American Academy of Emergency Medicine
Hanover, NH

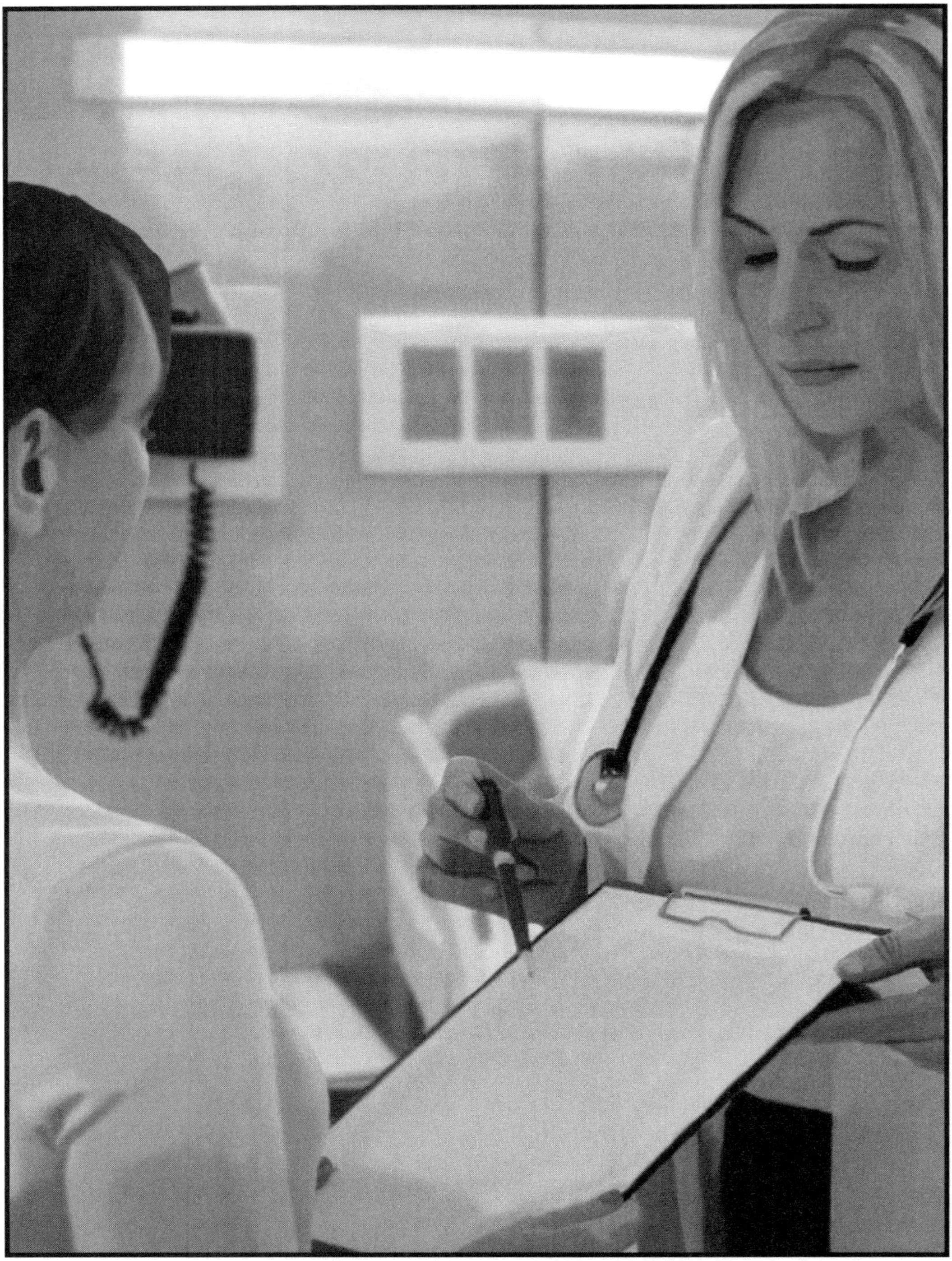

SECTION E / CHAPTER 25

A 51-year-old diabetic woman with vertigo

INITIAL ED VISIT

CC: (Monday, February 21 at 12:05 PM): Dizziness

Nursing note: 51-year-old woman complaining of temporal and periorbital headache and vertigo like room is spinning when she opens eyes or moves, on and off for a couple of weeks. She also had dry heaves today.

HPI: 51-year-old woman presented to the emergency department with "dizziness". The patient states that she's been feeling ill all week and then developed nausea and vomiting the morning of her presentation. She describes the dizziness as if the room is spinning. She states that her symptoms are worse when she moves around, but there is no specific position that makes her symptoms more severe. In addition to the nausea and vomiting which started this morning, she also notes diarrhea, which she relates to her Glucophage. Accu-Check this morning read 342. The patient also describes a gradual onset, mild, diffuse headache. She says that she thinks the headache is due to the frequent emesis today.

PMH:
Allergies: NKDA
Medications: Glucophage
Past medical history: History of MI, Diabetes, Hepatitis C
Social history: No smoking. She drinks 2 glasses of wine per night. She does not use any illegal drugs.

ROS: No abdominal pain, chest pain, SOB, confusion, lethargy, numbness, tingling, weakness.

PE:

Vitals:

Time	Temp	Pulse	Resp	Syst	Diast	O2
	96.6	112	18	169	83	97% RA

GA: Nontoxic appearing female, age appropriate
HEAD AND NECK: Her head is unremarkable; pupils equal and reactive to light, EOMI, sclera and conjunctiva are normal; oropharynx is normal, palate rise is symmetrical, tongue protrudes to midline; neck supple/no meningeal signs.

RESP: Chest is nontender, breath sounds are equal bilaterally, no respiratory distress
CARDIO: Heart is regular rate and rhythm, no JVD, heart sounds are normal
GI: Abdomen nontender, no masses, no distention, no peritoneal signs
NEURO: GCS 15, no focal motor deficit, no focal sensory deficit. Vertigo symptoms are reproduced with Dix-Hallpike maneuver (slight nystagmus is seen with the right ear toward the bed). The patient becomes diaphoretic during the maneuver.

Laboratory values:
WBC count 9.8, hemoglobin 13.3, platelet count 220
Chem-7 is normal except glucose of 268
Troponin I is normal
EKG: Normal sinus rhythm with no acute ST or T wave changes, no ischemia noted

ED course: The patient had a positive Dix-Hallpike maneuver and was given 25 mg of Antivert orally. Additional meds: Compazine 10mg IV. Cogentin 1mg PO. 0.9NS 2L IV.

Re-examination: Improved. Discharge vital signs: blood pressure 126/66, pulse 104, respiratory rate 20. She was able to walk down the hall without difficulty. Vertebrobasilar insufficiency was considered, but given that the patient's symptoms were easily reproducible on exam, and there were no other neurological symptoms such as dysarthria, diplopia, or ataxia, peripheral vertigo is much more likely. I discussed treatment options for benign paroxysmal positional vertigo. Discharged with Rx for Phenergan and Antivert.

Diagnosis: BPPV
Discharge instructions given for benign paroxysmal positional vertigo:
You should seek medical attention immediately, either here or the nearest emergency department if any of the following occur:

- You feel numbness tingling or weakness in your arms, legs, or face
- If you have difficulty with speech
- If you have difficulty with walking or with balance
- If your symptoms become worse even with taking the prescribed medication
- If you have a severe headache
- If you have vomiting that makes it hard for you to take, or keep down the prescribed medications

Discussion:
Wow, this is a tough one! There are so many reasons to suspect a peripheral etiology, specifically the fact that her symptoms are reproduced with motion of the head, even to the point that it causes diaphoresis. But what if she *did* have vertebrobasilar insufficiency (VBI), as appropriately discussed in the MDM note—wouldn't a patient with a cerebellar infarct also get worse when their head was turned?

Discussion points:

Dizziness is a common presenting complaint in the ED and remains a challenge; patients often use the term *dizziness* to describe a variety of symptoms referable to lightheadedness, generalized weakness, disbalance, and sensation of movement. The etiology of dizziness is broad and ranges from benign to life threatening, including peripheral vertigo, orthostatic hypotension, cardiac presyncope, disequilibrium, and ischemic or hemorrhagic stroke. Vertigo is a symptom, not a diagnosis.

The first differentiation is to stratify patients experiencing true vertigo. Patients with vertigo usually perceive an illusion of movement, involving themselves or the environment moving around them. This spinning sensation can occur at rest or more commonly with head movement. Vertigo is caused by central or peripheral processes with symptom exacerbation with head movement commonly attributed to benign peripheral causes of vertigo, but this is unreliable as most patients with central etiologies are equally intolerant to movement.

A provocative maneuver like the Dix-Hallpike test may provoke vertigo and nystagmus as a distinguishing feature of peripheral vertigo and may be useful in patients who are asymptomatic at rest. The test involves moving the patient from a sitting to lying position with the head tilted off the table and rotated at 45 degrees to one side. A positive test has a sensitivity of 79% and a specificity of 75% in the diagnosis of benign paroxysmal positional vertigo (BPPV), but these findings are dependent on the physician performing the exam.[1] The HINTS exam was developed to help prevent the misdiagnosis of posterior fossa infarcts. In a prospective, cross sectional study, investigators performed 3 clinical oculomotor tests, **H**ead **I**mpulse, **N**ystagmus, and **T**est of **S**kew (HINTS). Positive results included:

- A normal horizontal head impulse test
- Direction-changing nystagmus in eccentric gaze
- Skew deviation

These findings were 100% sensitive and 96% specific for posterior fossa stroke,[2] but note that the HINTS exam in this study was performed by specialty trained neuro-ophthalmologists rather than emergency physicians. The HINTS exam has performed well in subsequent studies, with a high sensitivity and NPV for excluding stroke. While early evidence is promising, emergency providers likely need specialty HINTS exam training to correctly interpret the results.[3]

Section editor comments (Marcolini):

Don't try to risk stratify your dizzy patients by asking them if the room is spinning vs. feeling lightheaded; patients are terrible at answering this question, and it is not specific. Instead, put these patients into the broad category of "vestibular syndrome" and further categorize them into "triggered, episodic or acute vestibular syndrome."

It's helpful to determine if our patient's symptoms resolve when she is *not* moving. If they do, she has "triggered vestibular syndrome," consistent with BPPV or dehydration among other diagnoses. If she has no resolution in between movement, she has "acute vestibular syndrome" which points toward posterior stroke vs. a peripheral cause such as labyrinthitis or vestibular neuritis. This will more effectively guide your workup and help to avoid missing the dangerous diagnoses such as TIA and CVA.

The neuro exam in a patient with a vestibular syndrome should evaluate for signs of posterior stroke, including finger to nose, heel to shin, Rhomberg and gait testing. We would not expect our patient to have a focal motor deficit; the most important testing is for posterior signs. Even though the HINTS exam was studied with neuro-ophthalmologists, we should be utilizing it in the emergency department, and practicing it to become better.

It's unclear to me whether there was an Epley maneuver performed, or just a diagnostic Dix-Hallpike, and then treatment with meclizine, Compazine, Cogentin and IVF. If this was truly BPPV, the preferred treatment is to mobilize the canalith out of the semicircular canal with repositioning maneuvers such as with the Epley maneuver.

Let's go back to our patient: this history of diabetes, peripheral arterial disease, coronary artery disease, hypertension, and renal insufficiency all raise concern that the vertigo could be central rather than peripheral. A few curious features about this case remain, one being the single troponin ordered. Though her dizziness in the setting of diarrhea, recent nausea and vomiting suggests possible hypovolemia and presyncope, the timeline of "feeling ill" is unclear, and the dizziness started shortly prior to presentation. Based on these features, a one-time troponin assay is likely insufficient to rule out acute coronary syndrome.

This history was also inadequate; there was not sufficient exploration of her complaint of headache, diarrhea, or hyperglycemia. Lastly, the patient was discharged with tachycardia. It is prudent to explain abnormal vital signs in patients deemed suitable for discharge. Persistent abnormal vital signs are associated with unexpected death following ED discharge.[4]

ED BOUNCEBACK

Return visit: Wednesday, February 23 10:47 a.m.

Triage (10:47): Patient seen 2 days ago for vertigo returns. Per EMS report, the patient got up to go to the bathroom at approximately 4 a.m. and found that she couldn't walk. She fell to the floor and remained there until this am, when her friend arrived. EMS found the patient with slurred speech and left-sided weakness. EMS describes left grasp weaker than right, speech slurred, left facial droop. Accu-Check 244 prior to arrival.

HPI (10:52): 51-year-old woman discharged from the ED two days ago with BPPV, presents for evaluation of weakness, slurred speech, ataxia, L facial droop, L arm weakness, L leg weakness. History obtained from patient. Patient went to bed at 12:00 a.m., awoke at around 4 a.m. with symptoms. She describes most of her symptoms were present upon awakening. She tried to go to the bathroom and fell to the floor. She was found by a friend who then called 911. Accu-Chek prior to arrival was 244. The patient denies chest pain, shortness of breath, confusion, abdominal pain, headache, or back pain.

PE: (shortened)

Vitals:

Time	Temp	Route	Pulse	Resp	Syst	Diast	O2 sat (RA)	Weight
10:52	99	Oral	102	18	171	73	94%	72kg

HEAD AND NECK: Pupils with dysconjugate gaze and persistent nystagmus
NEUROLOGIC EXAM: The patient is alert and oriented x 3; cranial nerve testing demonstrated a left 7th nerve palsy, dysarthria, and a diminished gag reflex; motor testing demonstrates weakness of the left hand and left leg. She has a pronator drift on the left, and horizontal nystagmus bilaterally. Cerebellar exam difficult to perform because of left-sided weakness.

Author comments (Weinstock):

This scenario is all too familiar; a patient arrives with stroke symptoms. But this is just a little different, as she was seen in your ED just 2 days ago and diagnosed with BPPV. We need to get *everything* right this time... not only diagnosis, but timing too. We are at:

DECISION POINT A – YOU ARE FACED WITH 4 QUESTIONS:

1. **What are the most important aspects of the history and physical exam to obtain immediately upon arrival?**
2. **What are the most common stroke mimics?**
3. **What other important alternative diagnoses may present with similar symptoms?**
4. **Does posterior circulation stroke alter the timeline or consideration of peripheral thrombolysis or endovascular clot retrieval?**

What does the literature say?

Q#1: What are the most important aspects of the history and physical exam to obtain immediately upon arrival?

As the mantra *time is brain* suggests, rapid identification of stroke patients is crucial and depends on a brief but thorough history and physical exam. The most important feature of the history is time of symptom onset. This is strategically reduced to the time that a patient was *last seen normal,* recognizing that symptom onset may not be witnessed. Salient features of the history include weakness, sensory symptoms, aphasia, or vision changes. Accompanying symptoms such as fever, seizure, headache, medication or drug usage may point to other potential stroke mimics, such as CNS infection, Todd's paralysis, complicated migraine, or drug toxicity.[5] While obtaining a history, be sure to simultaneously check the blood sugar, since hypoglycemia may present with a variety of neurological symptoms including focal weakness mimicking acute stroke.

Strokes involving the posterior circulation, defined as those involving branches supplied by the vertebrobasilar arterial system, are less common, accounting for approximately 20% of ischemic events. Historical symptoms such as vertigo, ataxia, dysphagia, and oculomotor palsies suggest involvement of the posterior circulation. A 1990 study of 85 patients with angiographically-proven complete occlusion of the basilar artery (or with bilateral vertebrobasilar occlusion and stroke) found that more than half of these patients had premonitory symptoms, the majority of which occurred in the 2 weeks prior to sudden onset or progression of the stroke. The most common symptoms in this data set were vertigo, headache, or both in combination.[6] In a 2004 registry of 87 patients with severe basilar artery occlusive disease, decreased level of consciousness, tetra-paresis, and abnormal pupils were most associated with poor prognosis. The most common symptoms in this registry, however, were bulbar and pseudo-bulbar symptoms (74%), followed by weakness (56%), and vertigo or dizziness (54%).[7] Patients presenting with vertigo along with any other neurologic symptom should be assumed to have a vascular etiology for vertigo until proven otherwise.[8]

The first step in the physical exam of suspected stroke patients is assessing the patient's airway, breathing, and circulation. Following confirmation of cardiopulmonary stability, rapid completion of a physical exam, including a complete neurologic assessment, should be performed. The National Institute of Health Stroke Scale (NIHSS) is a useful tool, but it is heavily weighted toward anterior circulation neurologic function; posterior circulation strokes can be missed if the NIHSS is used in lieu of a focused neurologic examination.[9]

- Cranial nerves, including extraocular movements are particularly important; vertical and bidirectional nystagmus typically represent central nervous system disease process, with oculomotor palsies localizing brainstem involvement.
- The HINTS exam can be used in vertiginous patients to rule in a posterior circulation stroke.
- Evaluate for signs of trauma, seizure activity, carotid bruits, cardiac murmurs or arrhythmias.[10]

A small retrospective review of misdiagnosed cerebellar infarction showed that two-thirds of medical records did not document gait or ocular movements.[11] We advise that all patients presenting with dizziness have a detailed neurologic exam, paying close attention to extraocular movements, nystagmus, gait, and truncal and limb ataxia. Recall that on this patient's first visit there was no documentation of gait, cranial nerves or limb ataxia in the physical exam. Although a positive Dix-Hallpike test was reported, this finding is not specific enough to exclude central vertigo.

Q#2: What are the most common stroke mimics?

Certain non-vascular clinical conditions that present with acute focal neurologic symptoms mimic stroke including hypoglycemia, seizure, metabolic imbalances, complicated migraine, hypertensive encephalopathy, syncope, infection, drug toxicity, and psychogenic. The proportion of stroke mimics varies between different clinical registries. In a large prospective study of patients seen by the NIH stroke program over a 10-year period, a third were ultimately diagnosed with a stroke mimic. Factors associated with the diagnosis of a stroke mimic included younger age, arrival to the ED by private vehicle, and absence of cardiovascular risk factors.[12] Stroke mimics complicate the management of potential stroke patients, and it is not uncommon for these patients to receive thrombolytics. In a registry of 512 patients treated with IV tPA for presumed stroke, 14% were ultimately diagnosed with a stroke mimic, with the most common etiologies being seizure (38%), migraine (37%), and conversion disorder (21%). Thankfully, ICH rates are very low in this group and most patients are functionally independent at discharge.[13] In fact, current data suggests that patients treated with IV tPA who had an alternative discharge diagnosis other than stroke did not sustain higher complication rates.[14]

How can we avoid being fooled by a stroke mimic?

- First and foremost, obtain a blood sugar on all potential stroke patients, since hypo- and hyperglycemia may present with focal neurologic deficits.
- Seizure, the most common stroke mimic, is associated with focal weakness, also known as Todd's paralysis and should be considered in patients with a history of epilepsy or witnessed seizure-like activity.
- Complicated migraines can be associated with neurologic deficits, including hemiplegia. These patients usually have a headache accompanied by aura.
- Metabolic derangements such as hyperammonemia, hyponatremia and hypernatremia can also cause neurologic deficits.
- Consider hyperammonemia in patients with cirrhosis, who may have telangiectasias, an ascitic fluid wave, flapping tremor, jaundice or caput medusae.
- There are several infections that can mimic stroke, including CNS infections such as meningitis, encephalitis, and intracranial abscess. These patients usually manifest signs and symptoms of infection that can be identified by history, vital signs or physical exam.
- Psychiatric disease is the most challenging stroke mimic to recognize.[15] In cases of incongruences of the neurologic exam, we should document objectively, but withhold language such as "conversion disorder" initially as it is a diagnosis of exclusion and requires a multi-disciplinary approach. Consider psychiatric causes in patients who are younger, have a history of psychiatric disease, and lack risk factors for stroke.

Q#3: What other important alternative diagnoses may present with similar symptoms?

Other important illnesses can present similarly to our patient. Carotid and vertebral artery dissection should be considered in young patients presenting with signs or symptoms suggestive of stroke. In a systematic review of approximately 2000 patients with acute vertebral artery dissection, the most common symptoms were vertigo (58%), headache (51%) and neck pain (46%).[16] Dissection is most commonly linked to hyperextension of the neck, chiropractic manipulation, or trauma, but can also occur spontaneously and less commonly from a prothrombotic state. Symptoms depend on the arterial branch involved.[17] Our patient did not have any risk factors for cerebrovascular dissection. Aortic dissection is another challenging diagnosis, with many presenting with focal neurologic deficits. Acute neurologic deficit accompanied by history of chest or back pain should trigger consideration of aortic dissection as a unifying diagnosis. An important corollary is that 20% of aortic dissections do not have chest pain, making it even more challenging to diagnose.[18] Pulse deficit, new aortic regurgitation murmur, and focal neurologic deficits are suggestive of aortic dissection.

Q#4: Does posterior circulation stroke alter the timeline or consideration of peripheral thrombolysis or endovascular clot retrieval?

Ischemia involving the posterior circulation is difficult to diagnose, as common symptoms and signs of posterior circulation stroke, such as nystagmus, truncal ataxia, and cranial neuropathies, are not accounted for in the NIHSS.[19] Cerebellar infarction, a subset of posterior circulation strokes, has a high morbidity and mortality. Although the FDA has not yet approved expanding the time interval to administer IV tPA from 3 hours to 4.5 hours post-symptom onset, the American Heart Association has published a Class I recommendation for the administration of tPA to eligible stroke patients 3 to 4.5 hours post-symptom onset.[20] The efficacy of tPA is time dependent, and data shows that patients with a posterior circulation stroke have a prolonged door-to-needle time.[21] Delays in diagnosis and treatment are attributed to the nonspecific presentation, including vertigo, nausea and vomiting, which can be seen in a number of disease processes.[22] The indication and time window for tPA in posterior circulation stroke is the same as that for the anterior circulation.

Occlusion of the basilar artery, with a high morbidity and mortality, is a special subset of posterior circulation thrombosis that requires special management. In a prospective study of 184 patients with angiography-proven basilar artery occlusion, most patients were treated with IV alteplase up to 48 hours after onset of symptoms, but a delay in the onset to treatment time was not associated with an increased rate of symptomatic intracranial hemorrhage.[23] Endovascular therapies have been shown to be effective, with a therapeutic window that far exceeds that of systemic tPA. In the largest registry of patients with posterior circulation strokes from acute basilar artery occlusion, poor neurologic outcomes were associated with interventions > 9 hours post-symptom onset.[24]

Section editor comments (Marcolini):

Cerebellar hemorrhage is more concerning than the same size bleed in the cortex. The posterior fossa doesn't have as much room for swelling, and small increases in hematoma size can be disastrous. In these cases, always be prepared for the worst and consult neurosurgery to evaluate the patient and be on standby for exam changes indicative of hematoma expansion or swelling causing herniation. This is the time when I will be most vigilant to the neurologic exam, and I will use succinylcholine instead of a non-depolarizing agent because the exam is just that important.

DECISION POINT A – ***What did the actual provider do?***

Author comments (Weinstock):

We resume the ED course with the MDM note/ED course [which was recorded later]:

MDM (11:17): Head CT scan was negative. Shortly after returning from the study, the patient became significantly less responsive and developed sonorous respirations. Pupils are less reactive, and she appears to have an L-sided gaze. The paralysis seemed to be now affecting both sides of her body. The decision is made to intubate the patient.

ED course: Now things begin to move quickly; the crash cart is brought to the room, respiratory is paged overhead, pharmacy is called to the bedside. The nurse looks up and asks simply, "Which meds are you going to use?"

Author comments (Weinstock):

Are there unique issues with administering induction and paralytic and intubating an acute stroke patient? And how about post-intubation management? We are at:

DECISION POINT B – YOU ARE FACED WITH 4 QUESTIONS:

1. **What are the considerations when intubating a stroke patient?**
2. **What are appropriate induction and paralytic agents?**
3. **Are there any techniques to prevent a spike (or drop) in BP during intubation?**
4. **What are appropriate vent settings and sedative medications post-intubation?**

What does the literature say?

Q#1: What are the considerations when intubating a stroke patient?

Strokes are not momentary brain injuries but rather evolve and usually worsen over time, including sudden decompensation which may require airway management. The sedating and paralyzing agents used for rapid sequence intubation (RSI), can confound the neurologic exam. There is not a specific GCS score which requires intubation; we don't want to act too early, and we don't want to wait too long. Published guidelines from the Neurocritical Care Society recommend intubation in patients with large hemispheric infarcts and the following:

- impaired level of consciousness
- decreased respiratory drive
- loss of protective reflexes
- development of dysphagia

Other clinical features that support consideration of airway intervention include GCS < 10, signs of increased ICP, midline shift on imaging, or the co-existence of pulmonary edema.[25]

Airway manipulation can result in two responses that increase ICP:

1. The reflex sympathetic response (RSR) increases heart rate and BP, which in turn increases ICP.
2. The direct laryngeal reflex may increase ICP independent of the RSR.

Just as important as an increased ICP, systemic hypotension and a drop in cerebral perfusion pressure can be equally harmful. The sudden drop in sympathetic drive following most induction agents may lead to a dramatic fall in vasomotor tone. Be ready to temporarily support the vasculature with an agent like phenylephrine.[26]

Important "rules of thumb" include:

- A concern for increasing ICP with laryngoscopy should not prevent airway protection.
- The presence of coma is not an indication to forego sedatives or paralytics for RSI. Patients may appear unresponsive but can still develop increased ICP without appropriate induction agents.
- Minimize airway manipulation, and thus ICP elevation, by using the most experienced operator.
- Be prepared for sudden swings in blood pressure (both high and low) during intubation procedures.

Consulting editor comments (Weingart):

We certainly need to be really careful on stroke patients to avoid spiking the blood pressure as well as to avoid dropping it. For the crash rapid sequence intubation (RSI); for example, the patient with a traumatic brain injury (TBI) or the stroke patient who is vomiting from their big middle cerebral artery (MCA) stroke due to increased intracranial pressure (ICP), you can't do a 6 minute titration of blood pressure stabilizing agents because the major thing that's going to kill them is hypoxemia. So, intubate in your normal style.

But, if you have a patient whose ICP is getting worse and there is time to actually plan out the intubation, it'd be really nice to blunt their sympathetic response, as well as prevent their blood pressure from dropping.

For these patients, we get everything ready including both nicardipine and push-dose vasopressors. We will give a big dose of fentanyl—something like 250, 300 micrograms to blunt the sympathetic response. As soon as the fentanyl is administered, intubation materials need to be ready as some of the patients will have apnea. If they spike their blood pressure, start the nicardipine; if the blood pressure drops, consider small doses of push-dose pressors.

In terms of agents, I don't care with succinylcholine vs. rocuronium. Etomidate is a very good choice because it is pretty neutral in these patients; it will leave their BP where it started.

Q#2: What are appropriate induction and paralytic agents?

1. Etomidate: The short-acting induction agent Etomidate has an excellent hemodynamic profile which is important in patients with known or suspected ICP elevation as cerebral perfusion pressure is dependent on MAP. (CPP = MAP – ICP).
2. Ketamine: The dissociative agent Ketamine was once believed to raise ICP; however, this concern has been refuted. Most research evaluating Ketamine as an induction agent and its effect on ICP has been done in patients with traumatic brain injury. A 2014 systematic review on the use of Ketamine in TBI reveals no increase in ICP with bolus dosing, and a trend toward a reduction in ICP.[27, 28]
3. Paralytics: In terms of paralytic agents, we get to choose between the depolarizing agent succinylcholine, and the non-depolarizing agent rocuronium. The benefit of succinylcholine includes a rapid onset and short duration of action, generally making it the preferred agent for RSI paralysis in acute brain injury. Succinylcholine is associated with transient increases in ICP, but this effect is not clinically significant. Succinylcholine-induced hyperkalemia is a risk for patients with serious neurologic and neuromuscular diseases, but this becomes clinically important greater than 72 hours following injury. Succinylcholine is a reasonable choice in this clinical situation.[29]

Section editor comments (Marcolini):

When thinking about ICP, the holy grail is really CPP, which is optimized by optimizing MAP. So when you increase HR and BP (such as in using ketamine or with the reflex sympathetic response) you are increasing MAP, which will help to overcome ICP to maintain CPP. CPP=MAP-ICP. Having said that, there are discreet blood pressure goals for intracerebral hemorrhage, and ketamine can increase blood pressure beyond those targets.

What if?...

Note that with a spontaneous intracerebral hemorrhage (ICH), the blood pressure goals are different from the acute ischemic stroke (AIS). With ICH, we want the blood pressure to definitely be <180, and it would be safe to push it to <140, but if they are chronically hypertensive you might consider targeting <160 because their core is used to a higher pressure head for perfusion (think renal perfusion). In the patient without evidence of chronic hypertension, a goal of <140 might be more efficacious in preventing the hematoma from expanding. With AIS, we want the systolic blood pressure to be <185 to get tPA, and then <180 for 24 hours after that, but we want it to stay on the higher side to increase the benefits of collateral circulation to the penumbra.

I would be very hesitant to use ketamine in the ICH patient—it's great for a traumatic brain injury (TBI), to maintain CPP, but the ICH patient wants lower blood pressure, and in the acute period is not likely to be battling ICP issues. You are more concerned about preventing hematoma expansion, and less likely to have increased ICP, as the perihematomal edema hasn't developed yet.

Q#3: Are there any techniques to prevent a spike (or drop) in BP during intubation?

Just as airway manipulation causes an increase in ICP through the direct laryngeal reflex, it also causes an increase in the heart rate and BP through the reflex sympathetic response (RSR). Using lidocaine to attenuate the direct laryngeal reflex has fallen out of favor, and we do not have quality trials to support its use as a pre-RSI medication. Fentanyl, at a dose of 2–3mcg/kg eases the RSR that occurs with intubation and can be given about a minute before laryngoscopy. This approach should only be used in patients that have sufficient BP reserve, or those that are hypertensive.

Particularly in patients that do not have significant BP reserve, and even those that do, the emergency provider should be prepared for hypotension to occur during intubation. Small fluid boluses or the temporary initiation of phenylephrine to support vasomotor tone are reasonable approaches to have available during intubation attempts.[26]

Section editor comments (Marcolini):

I totally agree that lidocaine is out, fentanyl is in!

Q#4: What are appropriate vent settings and sedative medications post-intubation?

The goals with our patient are twofold: normalization of cerebral blood flow and oxygenation. The ventilator should be set to a volume-cycled mode, using lung-protective volumes set at 6–8cc/kg ideal body weight. Even in the case of suspected ICP elevation, if no rapid surgical resolution is planned, aim for a pCO_2 of 30–40mmHg. To prevent neuronal damage from hyperoxia, dial down the FiO_2 as low as possible to achieve a SaO_2 of 94%.

Hyperventilation can be an acutely temporizing intervention, but is only rarely helpful in the short run. Hyperventilation causes cerebral vasoconstriction (with maximal vasoconstriction occurring at a pCO_2 of 30 mmHg), which decreases cerebral blood flow and thus ICP. This intervention, however, risks surrounding tissue ischemia. The only scenario when hyperventilation beyond a pCO_2 of 30 mmHg will be helpful is in the acutely deteriorating patient with new signs of elevated ICP, and you need to temporize the situation. For example, a patient with an acute rise in BP, bradycardia, and blown pupil already rolling to the OR for surgical decompression. In this situation, one should employ an end-tidal CO_2 monitor. But even in the case of known elevated ICP, aim for a pCO_2 of 30–40mmHg.[30]

Pain, agitation, and fear will only work to increase ICP, so maximize use of analgesic and sedative medications. Fentanyl is short-acting, hemodynamically protective, and a good first choice for analgesia. Propofol is also short-acting and has been shown to decrease ICP but can cause hypotension and myocardial depression. In general, the goal MAP should be > 80mmHg, in order to maintain cerebral perfusion pressure (CPP) > 60mmHg. Propofol is a good agent for sedation, as long as administration does not adversely affect MAP. Depending on the hemodynamic profile of the patient, using ketamine for continuous sedation is also an option. Maintain the head-of-bed at 30 degrees to lower ICP and prevent aspiration.[26]

Section editor comments (Marcolini):

I think of using hyperventilation in the patient who is showing signs of herniation (blown pupil, acute significant deterioration) *and* is imminently going to have a decompressive procedure such as ventriculostomy or craniectomy. Prolonged hyperventilation very effectively vasoconstricts cerebral arteries by blowing off CO_2 but once the brain reads the alkalosis, it adjusts to normalize the pH and then vasodilation ensues, thus increasing intracranial hypertension. Also, the prolonged vasoconstriction increases the risk of ischemic stroke. So if someone is going to have room to swell, such as with a craniectomy or ability to decrease ICP by draining CSF, then temporizing hyperventilation can be appropriate.

DECISION POINT B – ***What did the actual provider do?***

MDM: Additional information from boyfriend [was obtained] after patient intubated. He states that the patient had been feeling well after discharge 2 days prior. Patient did complain of some intermittent dizziness but had no definite ataxia.

The patient was successfully intubated without complication using succinylcholine and etomidate. The endotracheal tube position was confirmed by capnography.

Author comments (Weinstock):

So good job, the patient is intubated, and she is getting bundled up for transport to the ICU. There are many pathways which can occur prior to the patient leaving the ED; following are a few "what if" scenarios. We are at:

DECISION POINT C – YOU ARE FACED WITH 5 QUESTIONS:

1. **What are the other possibilities for bilateral paralysis?**
2. **What is the best approach to a posterior stroke in evolution?**
3. **What is the best management of a cerebellar hemorrhage?**
4. **What are the priorities of acute blood pressure management in spontaneous intracerebral hemorrhage?**
5. **How does elevated ICP affect our management and timeliness of care? What is the Monroe-Kellie doctrine?**

What does the literature say?

Q#1: What are the other possibilities for bilateral paralysis?

Our patient rapidly decompensated, developing paralysis of both extremities and airway compromise. She was quickly intubated for airway protection, leaving no time for a repeat neurologic examination.

The differential for acute bilateral paralysis is broad:

- Weakness can be localized anatomically based on history and physical exam. Lesions can involve the cerebral cortex, spinal cord, anterior horn cell, peripheral nerve, neuromuscular junction, or muscle.
- Cortical causes include intraparenchymal hemorrhage, stroke, and seizure.
- A special subset of stroke caused by ischemia or hemorrhage of the brainstem known as locked-in syndrome, presents with rapid onset tetraplegia and aphasia with no cognitive involvement. Patients with sudden onset tetraplegia or paraplegia may have spinal cord compression, which can occur spontaneously or as a result of trauma.
- Non-traumatic causes of myelopathy include compression of the cord, which can be seen in epidural abscess, spontaneous epidural hematoma, or mass.
- Ischemia and demyelination can also produce bilateral myelopathy. Paralysis occurs below the level of the spinal cord lesion involved. While most demyelinating processes occur gradually over time, ischemia and hemorrhage involving the cord progress more rapidly. Severe disease processes cause proximal greater than distal weakness.
- Myopathies and neuromuscular diseases such as Myasthenia Gravis and Lambert Eaton Syndrome typically have a more gradual clinical course.
- Diseases involving the anterior horn cell, such as ALS and polio, present with motor weakness and can be differentiated by the presence of infectious symptoms.
- Peripheral neuropathies and myopathies also generally have a more subacute clinical course compared to cortical and spinal cord etiologies.[31]

Q#2: What is the best approach to a posterior stroke in evolution?

Institutions will vary in terms of "code stroke" protocols for imaging, but most will include CT angiography. Importantly, patients with posterior vascular abnormalities (stenosis or occlusion) that may be outside the systemic tPA window of 4.5 hours, may still be candidates to undergo endovascular intervention, so recognizing subtle signs of posterior stroke evolution is vital. As time to recanalization increases, the risk of poor neurologic function also increases, particularly 9 hours post-symptom onset.[32] In a recently published multicenter, observational retrospective trial, 202 consecutive patients with basilar artery occlusion were studied, all of whom underwent thrombectomy within 12 hours of stroke symptom onset. This study reported that reperfusion was successful in 91.5% of patients, and 44.8% of patients had favorable neurologic recovery (modified Rankin scale 0-2).[33] The important "take home" is that posterior strokes, particularly those in evolution, may still have therapeutic options outside the usual 3–4.5 hour "window." Consulting a neurointerventional specialist is appropriate.

Q#3: What is the best management of a cerebellar hemorrhage?

Following the recognition of an intracerebral hemorrhage, three immediate questions must be considered.

1. What is the BP?
2. Is the patient coagulopathic?
3. Is the hemorrhage supra or infra-tentorial?

There is some equipoise on surgical decompression and hematoma evacuation in supra-tentorial ICH, but the Society of Neurocritical Care and the American Heart Association guidelines endorse surgical decompression for cerebellar ICH > 3cm, those associated with brainstem compression, or hydrocephalus.[34–36] In this case, evolving obstructive hydrocephalus precipitated acute decompensation. This is easily reversible with surgical intervention. In short, the first phone call following diagnosis of a cerebellar ICH should go to the neurosurgeon.

A 2009 *Stroke* study evaluated long-term outcomes of 57 consecutive patients with malignant cerebellar infarctions treated with decompressive suboccipital craniectomy. At a mean follow-up period of 4.7 years, 40% of patients were functionally independent.[37]

Q#4: What are the priorities of acute blood pressure management in spontaneous intracerebral hemorrhage?

Acute BP control in intracerebral hemorrhage has been the focus of several important randomized controlled trials. The INTERACT and ATTACH trials demonstrated the safety of lowering BP < 140mmHg in patients with ICH. Based on the results from the INTERACT2 and ATACH-2 trials, outcomes are not better with SBP goal of < 140mmHg over the goal of < 180mmHg. It is generally accepted that the goal of < 180mmHg is desired in ICH to mitigate the risk of hematoma expansion and neurologic deterioration. Rapidly titratable medications such as nicardipine or labetalol are first line agents.[38,39] If your patient with ICH has normal blood pressure at baseline, it is safe and feasible to lower the SBP to < 140.

Q#5: How does elevated ICP affect our management and timeliness of care? What is the Monroe-Kellie doctrine?

Intracranial hypertension is defined as a sustained rise (> 5 min) of ICP to > 20–22cm H_2O. As such, we have little time to act before brain damage occurs. The Monroe-Kellie doctrine explains that the sum of the intracranial contents (brain, blood, and CSF) represent a fixed volume, held in constraint by the inflexible cranial vault. The proportional volume of these contents can change in response to a new space-occupying lesion, but at a certain point, the low compliance of the cranial vault causes a precipitous rise in ICP.[40]

In the ED, it's unlikely a patient will have an intracranial device to measure ICP; therefore, we must rely on clinical signs to recognize elevated ICP.

- In the awake patient, these signs include severe headache, nausea/vomiting, or altered mentation.
- In the comatose patient, these signs include hypertension, bradycardia, and irregular respirations. Clinical signs of brain herniation include acute coma, pupillary dilatation, and hemiparesis or posturing.

In these situations, emergency use of osmotherapy agents can temporarily reduce ICP to identify potential for surgical intervention.

Section editor comments (Marcolini):

If your patient has an abnormal exam, and it is not explained by findings on the CT, consider the possibility of intracranial hypertension, and consider giving an osmotic agent such as mannitol or hypertonic saline to quickly and temporarily reduce intracranial pressure. You should also consider the possibility of subclinical seizure and give a loading dose of an anti-epileptic agent such as fosphenytoin, phenytoin or levetiracetam. The CT has to match the exam, and if not, consider the possibility that something else is going on like seizures or edema.

DECISION POINT C – *What happened?*

- The patient was evaluated by neurology. Due to the uncertain time of onset of symptoms and the duration of symptoms, she was deemed to be not a candidate for thrombolytics. The patient was transferred for an emergent MRI and then taken to the MICU.
- The MRI ultimately demonstrated brainstem infarction. Support was withdrawn and the patient expired later that day.

Case summary:

- While there is intense interest in early identification of acute ischemic stroke, it is important to maintain a broad differential diagnosis. As an example, cephalgia, vomiting, and dizziness can represent acute carbon monoxide poisoning.
- Inform patients of diagnostic uncertainty so they can return if symptoms change or worsen.
- In patients with posterior circulation stroke, sudden deterioration may indicate stroke in evolution or secondary injury from brainstem compression due to local mass effect or obstructive hydrocephalus.
- Brainstem and cerebellar infarcts are uncommon and historically associated with poor outcomes. Nonetheless, rapid identification and surgical intervention can still achieve survival with good neurologic recovery.

References:

1. Halker RB, Barrs, DM, Wellick KE, et al. Establishing a diagnosis of benign paroxysmal positional vertigo through the Dix-Hallpike and Side-Lying Maneuvers: A critically appraised topic. Neurologist 2008;14(3):201-04.
2. Kattah JC, Talkad AV, Wang DZ, et al. HINTS to diagnose stroke in the acute vestibular syndrome: three-step bedside oculomotor examination more sensitive than early MRI diffusion-weighted imaging. Stroke 2009;40(11):3504-10.
3. Cohn B. Can bedside oculomotor (HINTS) testing differentiate central from peripheral causes of vertigo? Ann Emerg Med 64(3):265-68.
4. Sklar DP, Crandall CS, Loeliger E, et al. Unanticipated death after discharge home from the emergency department. Ann Emerg Med 2007:49(6);735-45.
5. Jauch EC, Saver JL, Adams Jr. HP, et al. Guidelines for the early management of patients with acute ischemic stroke. A guideline for healthcare professionals from the American Heart Association/American Stroke Association Stroke 2013;44(3):870-47.
6. Ferbert A, Bruckmann H, Drummen R. Clinical features of proven basilar artery occlusion.

Stroke 1990;21(8):1135-42.
7. Voetsch B, DeWitt LD, Pessin MS, et al. Basilar artery occlusive disease in the New England Medical Center Posterior Circulation Registry. Arch Neurol 2004;61(4):496-04.
8. Demel SL, Broderick JP. Basilar occlusion syndromes: An update. Neurohospitalist 2015;5(3):142-50. doi:10.1177/1941874415583847.6
9. Martin-Schild S, Albright KC, Tanksley J, et al. Zero on the NIHSS does not equal the absence of stroke. Ann Emerg Med 2011;57(1)42 - 5.
10. Schneider JI, Olshaker JS. Vertigo, vertebrobasilar disease, and posterior circulation ischemic stroke. Emerg Med Clin North Am 2012;30(3):681–93.
11. Savitz SI, Caplan LR, Edlow, JA. Pitfalls in the diagnosis of cerebellar infarction. Acad Emerg Med 2007;14(1):63-8. doi:10.1197/j.aem.2006.06.060.
12. Merino JG, Luby M, Benson RT, et al. Predictors of acute stroke mimics in 8187 patients referred to a stroke service. J Stroke Cerebrovasc Dis 2013;22(8):e397-03.
13. Chernyshev OY, Martin-Schild S, Albright KC, et al. Safety of tPA in stroke mimics and neuroimaging-negative cerebral ischemia. Neurology 2010;74:1340-45.
14. Zinkstok SM, Engelter ST, Gensicke H, et al. Safety of thrombolysis in stroke mimics: Results from a multicenter cohort study. Stroke 2013;44(4):1080-84.
15. Magauran BG, Nitka M. Stroke mimics. Emerg Med Clin North Am 2012;30(3):795-04.
16. Gottesman RF, Sharma P, Robinson KA, et al. Clinical characteristics of symptomatic vertebral artery dissection. A systematic review. Neurologist 2012;18(5):245-54.
17. Debette S, Grond-Ginsbach C, Bodenant M, et al. Differential features of carotid and vertebral artery dissections: the CADISP study. Neurology 2011;77(12):117481.
18. Pape LA, Awais M, Woznicki EM, et al. Presentation, diagnosis, and outcomes of acute aortic dissection: 17-year trends from the International Registry of Acute Aortic Dissection. J Am Coll Cardiol 2015;66(4):350-8.
19. Inoa V, Aron AW, Staff I, et al. Lower NIH stroke scale scores are required to accurately predict a good prognosis in posterior circulation stroke. Cerebrovasc Dis 2014;37(4):251-5.
20. Powers WJ, Rabinstein AA, Ackerson T, et al. 2018 Guidelines for the early management of patients with acute ischemic stroke: A guideline for healthcare professionals from the American Heart Association/American Stroke Association. Stroke 2018;49(3):e46-e110.
21. Sarraj A, Medrek S, Albright K, et al. Posterior circulation stroke is associated with prolonged door-to-needle time. Int J Stroke. 2015;10(5):672-8.
22. Merwick Á, Werring D. Posterior circulation ischaemic stroke. Br Med J 2014;19;348:g3175.
23. Strbian D, Sairanen T, Silvennoinen H, et al. Thrombolysis of basilar artery occlusion: impact of baseline ischemia and time. Ann Neurol 2013;73(6):688-94.
24. Vergouwen MD, Algra A, Pfefferkorn T, et al. Time is brain(stem) in basilar artery occlusion. Stroke 2012;43(11):3003-6.
25. Torbey MT, Bosel J, Rhoney DH, et al. Evidence-based guidelines for the management of large hemispheric infarction, a statement for health care professionals from the Neurocritical Care Society and the German Society for Neuro-Intensive Care and Emergency Medicine. Neurocrit Care 2015;22(1):146-64.
26. Rajajee V, Riggs B, Seder DB. Emergency neurologic life support: airway, ventilation and sedation. Neurocrit Care 2017; https://doi.org/10.1007/s12028-017-0451-2.
27. Zeiler FA, Teitelbaum J, West M, et al. The ketamine effect on ICP in traumatic brain injury. Neurocrit Care 2014;21:163-73. https://doi.org/10.1007/s12028-013-9950-y.

28. Himmelseher S, Durieux ME. Revising dogma: ketamine for patients with neurological injury? Anesth Analg 2005;101(2):524-34.
29. Patanwala AE, Erstad BL, Roe DJ, et al. Succinylcholine is associated with increased mortality when used for rapid sequence intubation of severely brain injured patients in the emergency department. Pharmacotherapy 2016;36(1):57-63. doi:10.1002/phar.1683.
30. Coles JP, Fryer TD, Coleman MR, et al. Hyperventilation following head injury: effect on ischaemic burden and cerebral oxidative metabolism. Crit Care Med 2007;35(2):568-78.
31. Caulfield AF, Flower O, Pineda JA, et al. Neurocrit Care 2017;27(Suppl 1):29. https://doi.org.ezproxy.library.tamu.edu/10.1007/s12028-017-0450-3.
32. Vergouwen MD, Algra A, Pfefferkorn T, et al. on behalf of the Basilar Artery International Cooperation Study (BASICS) study group. Time is brain(stem) in basilar artery occlusion. Stroke 2012;43(11):3003-6.
33. Kang DH, Jung C, Yoon W, et al. Endovascular thrombectomy for acute basilar artery occlusion: A multicenter retrospective observational study. J Am Heart Assoc 2018;7(14):e009419. Published 2018 Jul 7. doi:10.1161/JAHA.118.009419.
34. Hemphill JC, Lam A. Emergency neurologic life support: intracerebral hemorrhage. Neurocrit Care 2017; https://doi.org/10.1007/s12028-017-0453-0.
35. Hemphill JC, Greenberg SM, Anderson CS, et al. Guidelines for the management of spontaneous intracerebral hemorrhage: a guideline for healthcare professionals from the American Heart Association/American Stroke Association. Stroke;2015:46:2032-60.
36. Kirollos RW, Tyagi AK, Ross SA, et al. Management of spontaneous cerebellar hematomas: A prospective treatment protocol. Neurosurgery 2001;49(6):1378-86.
37. Pfefferkorn T, Eppinger U, Linn J, et al. Long-term outcome after suboccipital decompressive craniectomy for malignant cerebellar infarction. Stroke 2009;40(9):3045-50.
38. Anderson CS, Heeley E, Huang Y, et al. Rapid blood-pressure lowering in patients with acute intracerebral hemorrhage. New Engl J Med 2013;368:2355–65.
39. Qureshi AI, Palesch YY, Barsan WG, et al. Intensive blood- pressure lowering in patients with acute cerebral hemorrhage. New Engl J Med 2016;375:1033-43.
40. Cadena R, Shoykhet M, Ratcliff JJ. Emergency neurologic life support: Intracranial hypertension and herniation. Neurocrit Care 2017; https://doi.org/10.1007/s12028-017-0454-z.

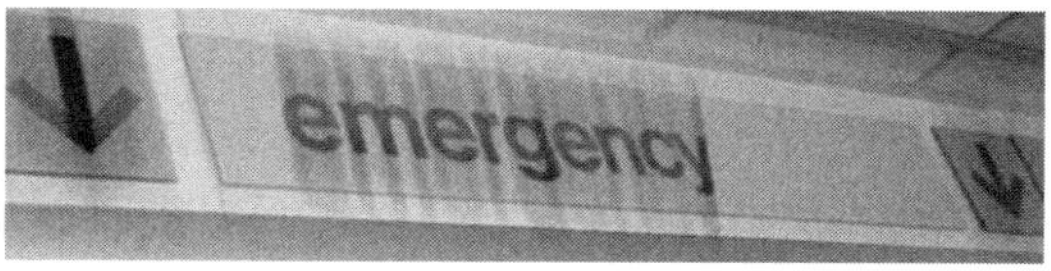

SECTION F – TRAUMA, DM, HEME, GI, HTN

Chapter 26: A 22-year-old diabetic woman with sinus pain

Brit Long, MD
Assistant Professor
Emergency Medicine
San Antonio Uniformed Services Health Education Consortium
Ft. Sam Houston, TX

Alex Koyfman, MD
Assistant Program Director
Clinical Assistant Professor
Emergency Medicine
University of Texas Southwestern Medical Center
Dallas, TX

Section editor:
Joseph Shiber, MD, FACEP, FACP, FCCM
Professor
Emergency Medicine, Neurology and Surgery
Director ECMO/Acute Lung Service
Co-director NSICU and UF North ICU
UF College of Medicine–Jacksonville
Jacksonville, FL

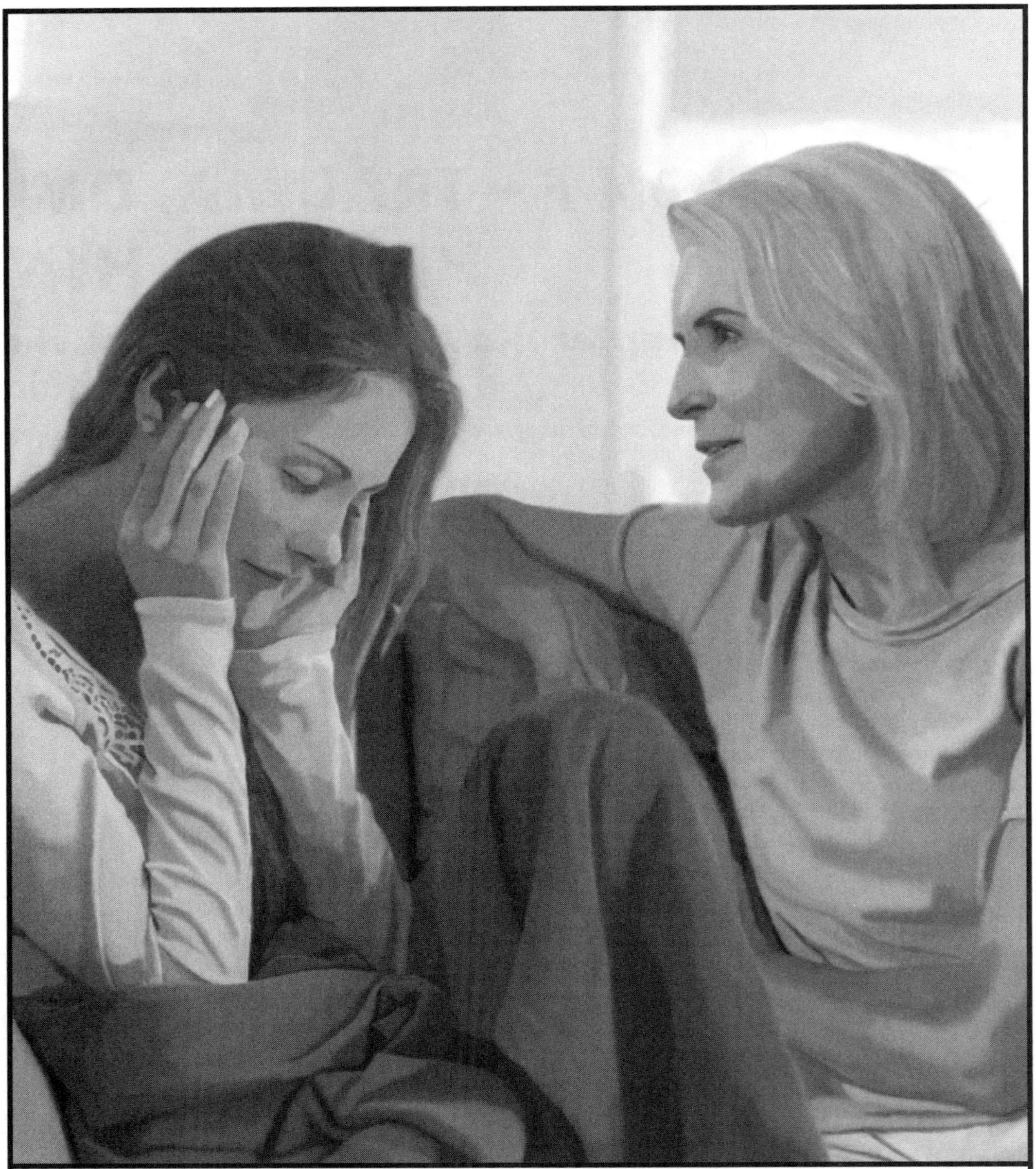

"MY SINUSES HURT!"

SECTION F / CHAPTER 26

A 22-year-old diabetic woman with sinus pain

"Can I have some antibiotics for my sinusitis?"

Sinusitis is a common condition managed in the ED, and though most commonly due to a viral infection, patients often ask for antibiotics. Though sinusitis in the healthy can be straightforward, the management in patients with comorbidities can be complicated. For example, what happens when sinusitis and hyperglycemic crisis occur simultaneously? This chapter will explore evaluation and management of sinusitis, hyperglycemic crisis, altered mental status, and seizures.

INITIAL ED VISIT

CC (06:14): Sinus pain and nasal congestion

Vitals:

Time	Temp	Rt.	Pulse	Resp	Syst	Diast	Pos.	O2 Sat
06:14	97.9	0	130	18	154	88	S	95

O2%	Pain Scale
ra	10/10

Triage/nursing: Arrives from private auto. Has sinus congestion and pain for the past 3 days. No fevers. Reports yellow sinus drainage. Took acetaminophen.

PMH: Diabetes, type 1
Allergies: NKDA
Medications: Diabetic pills, BCP
PSH: Negative

HPI (06:50): Patient states maxillary and right frontal sinus pain for the past three days. Patient states she has been severely congested. Denies visual problems or pain with movement of eyes. Denies vomiting or chest pain. Resting comfortably on exam. She is type 1 diabetic. Denies shortness of breath. No fever, unexplained weight change or malaise. No cough, n/v/d, abdominal pain, urinary symptoms, HA, rash.

EXAM (06:52):
CONSTITUTIONAL: Alert and oriented X3, well-nourished, well appearing, in no apparent distress.
HEAD: Normocephalic; atraumatic.
EYES: PERRL, no scleral icterus.
NOSE: The nose is normal in appearance without rhinorrhea. Tender to palpation over right maxillary sinus.
RESP: Normal chest excursion with respiration; breath sounds clear and equal bilaterally; no wheezes, rhonchi, or rales.
CARDIO: Regular rhythm, without murmurs, rub, or gallop.
ABD: Non-distended; non-tender, soft; no rigidity, rebound, or guarding.
SKIN: Normal for age and race; warm and dry; no apparent lesions.

DIAGNOSIS (06:55): Maxillary sinusitis, acute

ORDERS (07:14): Check pulse

DISPOSITION: Discharge home ambulatory. Follow up with family practice in 2–3 days. Rx amoxicillin 500mg PO TID #30, ultram 50mg #20. After care instructions for sinusitis. Record released from tracking board at 07:17.

Initial visit discussion:

1. How is sinusitis diagnosed, and does she need antibiotics?

Acute sinusitis is defined as inflammation of the nasal cavity and sinuses which lasts less than 4 weeks. This is most commonly due to a viral infection, with a bacterial infection occurring in less than 2% of cases, and complications are rare.[1,2] A variety of medication cocktails can be used, with treatment including analgesics and antipyretics, saline irrigation, decongestants, intranasal steroids/decongestants, and mucolytics, with symptoms typically improving within 10 days.[1,2] Antibiotics are not recommended in acute, uncomplicated sinusitis, with a number needed to harm of 1 in 8 due to medication side-effects.[3-5] The American Academy of Otolaryngology-Head and Neck Surgery (AAO-HNS) in 20152 and Infectious Diseases Society of America (IDSA) 2012 guidelines differ slightly in terms of treatment.[1]

- The AAO-HNS recommends patients with uncomplicated acute sinusitis be treated symptomatically and observed, with no antibiotics.[2]
- The IDSA states antibiotics should be given to patients with persistent symptoms > 10 days, those with severe symptoms (fever greater than 39o C and purulent nasal drainage/facial pain for greater than 3 days), or patients who were better and then worsened (Double sickening).[1]

Note that over 80% of patients improve within 2 weeks without antibiotics.[2,3]

Patients with a bacterial source tend to have symptoms lasting over 10 days with greater severity. Purulent nasal discharge and severe pain or pressure demonstrate greater sensitivity and specificity for a bacterial source.[1-3]

What group defines complicated sinusitis? This includes patients with fever greater than 102° F, cranial nerve palsy, periorbital edema or erythema, severe headache, confusion, or vision changes. These symptoms or findings require head CT with IV contrast and ENT consultation.[1,2]

Our patient does not have a normal immune status due to her diabetes. Should she receive antibiotics? Societies recommend consideration on a case-by-case basis as well as consideration of the affected sinus. Frontal, ethmoid, and/or sphenoid sinusitis is more concerning, particularly in diabetics, compared to maxillary sinus involvement and is associated with a higher incidence of complications. Whereas most cases do not require antibiotics, with our patient, we agree that antibiotics are warranted.

2. Does our patient truly have sinusitis? What else should we consider?

Our patient is a diabetic, which means that we need to keep our antennae raised for dangerous infections.

- Rhinocerebral mucormycosis is an infection of the nasal and paranasal sinuses by mold species (*Mucor, Rhizopus,* and several others), which ultimately invade the vasculature, erode bone, and result in tissue necrosis.[6] These fungi thrive in hyperglycemic environments, particular ketoacidosis. Patients commonly present with headache, nasal discharge, and sinus pain. Sound familiar? Compared to patients with simple sinusitis, these patients will appear toxic, and close evaluation of their sinuses often reveals palatal eschars, turbinate destruction, perinasal swelling, and erythema or cyanosis of the face. Orbital involvement will result in periorbital edema, proptosis, and blindness. This infection spreads rapidly. CT is needed for diagnosis, with rapid ENT consultation, and amphotericin B or liposomal amphotericin B.[6]
- Malignant otitis externa is another life-threatening consideration which typically affects diabetics older than 35 years. It is usually caused by *Pseudomonas*. Patients present with ear pain and otorrhea, with infection that begins in the external auditory canal, followed by spread to cartilage, bone, and soft tissue.[7] Similar to mucormycosis, this requires IV antibiotics for toxic patients, CT, and ENT consultation.

What are the take home points? Be wary of diagnosing sinusitis in the diabetic. Close evaluation of the nose, oropharynx, palate, and cranial nerves is required. Any concern for a complicated course, including fever, toxic appearance, altered mental status, or cranial nerve abnormality, warrants imaging.

3. Wait…why wasn't a blood glucose checked? Do we need to know what medications she takes for her diabetes?

Type 1 diabetes is defined by absolute insulin deficiency. Thus, these patients are on some form of insulin. Today's medical technology allows for insulin pumps or regimens that involve subcutaneous insulin.[8-10] In this case, the physician did not evaluate a blood glucose level or document the patient's medications. There is no standard that states checking blood glucose is absolutely necessary, or that a full medication list is required.[10-12] However, a quick point-of-care glucose may assist the physician in evaluating for diabetic complications such as hyperglycemic crisis (including diabetic ketoacidosis (DKA) and hyperosmolar hyperglycemic state (HHS)). Hyperglycemia does not mean the patient is in DKA.[10-12] However, a quick glucose can provide a glimpse into the patient's glucose control. If this is not done, questioning the patient on polyuria, polyphagia, and polydipsia can assist, as the presence of these may indicate hyperglycemia. Weight loss, profuse vomiting, and abdominal pain are other symptoms suggestive of hyperglycemic crisis.[11]

One of the primary causes of hyperglycemic crisis is noncompliance. A patient who is not regularly taking her medications is at risk for DKA or HHS.[12, 13] Evaluating for a potentially life-threatening complication is important, and assessment of the patient's medication regimen and serum glucose is quick and easy.

Section editor comments (Shiber):

Are we certain this is Type 1 Insulin-dependent as she is on an oral agent, and metformin is only used for Type 2? She may be a Type 2 that is now insulin-requiring. She was diagnosed at an early age which previously was uncommon for Type 2, but since obesity has become rampant in children and adolescents, it is not at all uncommon. Anytime a Type 1 diabetic has a glucose > 250, it is likely they are in DKA (even early, mild) as if they are lacking in insulin (not resistant as Type 2) then when they are truly hyperglycemic it is associated with DKA.

4. What about her tachycardia?

Vital signs are vital! Various factors are associated with death after discharge. One major factor is the presence of abnormal vital signs upon discharge. The presence of abnormal vital signs is consistently associated with death after discharge, along with chronic disease exacerbation, atypical presentations, and substance abuse.[14,15] A classic study in *Annals of Emergency Medicine* reviewed death after ED discharge.[15] Tachycardia was associated with unexpected deaths. The charts in the study often revealed little to no explanation for this tachycardia. Abnormal vital signs are a sensitive, but nonspecific, marker for risk and should trigger the search for a cause. Abnormal vital signs could be an indicator of decompensated chronic disease or severe, acute disease. Thus, physicians should work to determine the underlying cause of tachycardia.

Putting it all together:

This patient has a history of diabetes and a clinical diagnosis of acute sinusitis. The history did not include further delineation of the patient's diabetic medications. However, the patient denied headache, rash, and other systemic symptoms. She had no fever. The provider diagnosed her with sinusitis, prescribed antibiotics and Tramadol, and discharged her. No prescriptions were provided for other sinusitis symptoms, and no blood glucose was obtained, as she appeared well otherwise with no description of diabetic symptoms, though it is unclear whether these were specifically asked. This seems straightforward, except for the tachycardia of 130. There was an order for a repeat pulse check shortly prior to discharge, but it seems that this "fell through the cracks."

ED RETURN VISIT (2 days later)

CC: Alt LOC

HPI text (20:19): Pt has a history of diabetes mellitus diagnosed at age 16-17 according to her mother who is at the bedside. Her diabetes has been treated with metformin. She does not use insulin. Three years ago reportedly she was in diabetic ketoacidosis. She reportedly has had "a cold" for the last 2-3 weeks including a nonproductive cough, nasal congestion and some rhinorrhea. Five days ago she developed a right-sided headache and was evaluated here and was given a prescription for amoxicillin and tramadol. According to her mother, she's been anorexic, vomiting and has not been taking food and fluids for approximately four days. Pt is unable to provide details of why she is here. Her mother is at the bedside and provides historical details. She arrived by ambulance. Paramedics were unable to establish a peripheral IV. They report that glucometer read "high."

PE:

Vitals:

Pulse	BP	Sat
154	158/96	100%

CONSTITUTIONAL: Alert but poorly conversant. She tries to follow commands, but does so poorly.
EYES: No scleral icterus. Pupils are 4 mm and reactive. She will not follow commands to evaluate extraocular muscle movement.
NECK: Soft and supple without meningeal signs.
MOUTH: Mucous membranes are very dry.
RESP: Normal chest excursion with respiration; breath sounds clear and equal bilaterally; no wheezes, no rhonchi, or rales.
CARDIO: Regular rhythm, without rub or gallop.
ABD: Non-distended; diffusely tender, soft; no rigidity, rebound, or guarding. There is no CVAT.
SKIN: Normal for age and race; warm and dry; no apparent acute lesions.
NEURO: Cranial nerves III-XII grossly intact. Motor exam of the upper and lower extremities is intact. Romberg's are downward bilaterally.
VASCULAR: Radial and posterior tibial pulses are intact and symmetric bilaterally. Femoral and carotid pulses are symmetric bilaterally.

ED course: (20:40) 2L Normal saline

Labs (21:36)

- CBC – WNL
- Electrolytes – K+ = 4.6, serum bicarbonate = 9
- BUN/creatinine = 32/1.6
- Glucose = 662

- Acetone = Moderate
- UA – WNL

ABG

- pH = 7.12
- pCO_2 = 15
- pO_2 = 151

Author comments (Weinstock):

Our patient certainly seems to be in DKA, is an ABG required or is a VBG adequate? And how about the fluids—is cerebral edema a consideration? We are at:

DECISION POINT A – YOU ARE FACED WITH 3 QUESTIONS:

1. **Is she in DKA or HHS?**
2. **What is the best management strategy for DKA and HHS?**
   a. **What are the initial resuscitation steps before administration of insulin?**
   b. **How should fluids be administered?**
   c. **Is bolus insulin required before starting the insulin infusion?**
   d. **What about bicarbonate?**
3. **Can we obtain VBG instead of ABG?**

What does the literature say?

Q#1: Is she in DKA or HHS?

What's one of the first rules in evaluation of altered mental status? Check a glucose! Hyperglycemia and hypoglycemia may result in severe alterations in neurologic status. DKA and HHS are severe complications that occur in diabetics.[8,11]

- DKA occurs due to insulin deficiency with hyperglycemia and counter-regulatory hormone production. It is diagnosed by serum glucose > 250mg/dL, ketonuria or ketonemia, serum pH < 7.3, and serum bicarbonate < 15mEq/L.
- On the other hand, HHS is diagnosed with altered sensorium, serum glucose > 600mg/dL, minimal or no ketonuria or ketonemia, serum osmolality > 320mOsm/kg, pH > 7.3 (usually), and bicarbonate > 15 mEq/L.[8,11]

This differentiation is not always straightforward, as HHS may display acidemia from shock (most commonly hypovolemic). However, ketones should be absent or mild. Patients with HHS have some pancreatic beta cell function, and thus, there is still some insulin production. HHS patients will present with severe mental status changes, though coma may not be present. DKA will demonstrate greater acidemia with at least moderate ketonemia/ketonuria.[8,11] We should keep in mind, however, that not all DKA will present with glucose > 250mg/dL, as up to 10% of patients will present with levels less than 250mg/dL (known as euglycemic DKA).[16]

Section editor comments (Shiber):

Euglycemic DKA can occur with the use of Na-Glucose Cotransporter Inhibitors (SGLT2) which induce glycosuria and are associated with DKA even at glucose levels of 150–250mg/dL. An additional note is that we now know that this patient, who in the history of the return visit states that she does not use insulin, is a Type 2 diabetic. The fact that she does not use insulin rules out Type 1. This was previously called MODY—maturity onset diabetes in the young—when it was uncommon, but now we know obese adolescents do get Type 2 DM.

Q#2: What is the best management strategy for DKA and HHS?

The difference between DKA and HHS can affect management, mainly during the initial resuscitation. The typical water deficit is 6L in DKA and 9L in HHS. Both display large total body losses of electrolytes, though measurements with intravascular contraction may offer falsely normal results. DKA typically occurs in Type 1 diabetics, with HHS occurring in older patients with Type 2 diabetes,[11] but the delineation is not always clear, as Type 2 diabetics can still experience DKA.

A large number of triggers result in DKA, with one of the primary goals to find the underlying etiology. Infection and insulin noncompliance are the most common causes of exacerbation, but other etiologies may occur including intraabdominal pathology, medication changes, toxins/drugs, pregnancy, trauma, surgery, and other shock states. DKA is itself an inflammatory state and a cause of endothelial injury, which may result in intracerebral hemorrhage, pulmonary edema, stroke, PE, and MI.[12,13,17]

Bedside evaluation of glucose is the first step. ECG is needed to evaluate for ischemia. Other testing includes CBC, urinalysis, ketones, electrolytes, liver and kidney function, lipase, serum osmolality (if concerned for HHS), and a pregnancy test in females. Additional testing should be based on the patient and situation. Troponin, DIC panel, thyroid function, aspirin and acetaminophen levels, and cultures may be needed. Imaging should also be based on the presentation. For example, a chest x-ray is fast and easy to obtain, with little patient risk.

So, we have covered the initial evaluation, but what about treatment? The two top priorities in hyperglycemia management include fluid and electrolyte repletion. Notice, we didn't say anything about insulin. While the work-up is ongoing, fluid resuscitation should begin. A bolus of 0.9% normal saline can be provided over 1 hour at 20mL/kg, which can be repeated based on patient hemodynamics.[8,11,13]

Q#2a: What are the initial resuscitation steps before administration of insulin?

Fluid resuscitation and electrolyte evaluation are more important than insulin. In hyperglycemic crisis, total body potassium is decreased due to vomiting as well as dehydration with redistribution; repletion may be required to avoid a fatal cardiac dysrhythmia.[18,19] If laboratory results are delayed, one trick is to obtain an ECG to assess for changes from hypokalemia and hyperkalemia. Over 80% of patients will have normal or elevated potassium levels on labs.[12,18] Those with normal or low potassium require repletion, as treatment with insulin will result in hypokalemia up to 60% of the time. At initiation of therapy, over 5% of patients will be hypokalemic.[20] Those hypokalemic on initial check (<3.3mEq/L) require IV potassium in addition to IV fluids at 20–30mEq/hr. If potassium levels are between 3.3 and 5.2mEq/L, then 20–30mEq/L of potassium should be added to each liter of fluid. If levels are greater than 5.2mEq/L, potassium supplementation is not needed, though serum checks should occur at 2 hr intervals.[8,11,13] For patients who are PO tolerant, oral repletion is possible.

Key point: Potassium levels should be checked prior to administration of insulin.

Section editor comments (Shiber):

Prior to the discovery of insulin, the mortality of DKA was 100%. Fluid resuscitation and electrolyte balance are important, but insulin administration is critical and should begin immediately when true DKA is diagnosed (not simply with hyperglycemia). The sicker the DKA patient, the more critical that the IVF and insulin start, as the pH will be lower. Most literature supports that > 90% of actual DKA patients have serum hyperkalemia on presentation and that the average serum value in a large database was 5.6mEq/L. In my 22 years (17 working plus 5 residency) I have never seen a DKA patient with a K+ < 3.5 on presentation and have challenged any of my colleagues and residents to find one case. Both the lack of insulin and acidosis cause hyperkalemia. While osmotic diuresis from hyperglycemia-causing glucosuria can cause K+ losses, this process should be of short duration in a Type 1 diabetic since they are critically ill almost immediately. Type 2 diabetics in DKA or HHS may have a longer course of illness prior to presentation, with more K+ losses and less (or no) acidosis, so they may be more likely to be hypokalemic; they are also less in need of immediate insulin therapy which can be delayed while aggressive IVF and electrolyte replacement is accomplished.

Q#2b: How should fluids be administered?

Resuscitation at 20mL/kg/hr should be started, with hydration status re-evaluated every hour. Repeat boluses may be required based on hemodynamic status, urine output, and examination findings. Once hemodynamic signs normalize, remaining fluid deficits can be replaced over 24 to 48 hours. Normal saline (NS) is quick, cheap, and easy and is the usual "go-to" fluid for resuscitation.[18,19] However, in DKA and HHS, we have better options. A common phenomenon found with NS in DKA resuscitation is worsening of acidemia with decreasing bicarbonate, even though the anion gap may improve.[13,18,21] This occurs with hyperchloremic metabolic acidosis with NS boluses. A randomized trial compared NS and lactated ringers (LR) for DKA resuscitation and found a trend towards faster pH improvement with LR, and patients receiving NS demonstrated a decrease in serum bicarbonate by 0.6mEq/L.[21] Patients with LR experienced an increase in bicarbonate by 1mEq/L. Plasma-lyte, which is a balanced crystalloid with similar pH to LR, demonstrates faster improvement in bicarbonate, as well as less hyperchloremia compared to NS.[22]

Summary: Normal saline's tendency towards hyperchloremic metabolic acidosis and decrease in bicarbonate during initial phase of DKA resuscitation makes it second choice to LR or Plasma-lyte.[18,19]

Consulting editor comments (Weingart):

The cerebral edema "concern" was a thing that happened in the pediatric world; I've never worried about it in adults. We have an ultra-aggressive DKA clearance protocol and there's countless examples in the emergency medicine world of very rapid clearance protocols and no one's seeing cerebral edema. I don't know if this really happens in adults. In fact, I don't know if it really happens in peds... but, I don't speak to peds, I will just say it's not really a big concern of mine in adult patients.

Q#2c: Is bolus insulin required before starting the insulin infusion?

In the past, patients received a bolus of insulin with the goal to overcome the insulin deficiency in DKA to suppress lipolysis, hepatic gluconeogenesis, and acidosis. However, this bolus can lead to hypoglycemia, hypokalemia, and cerebral edema.[18,19] Goyal, et al. conducted a study evaluating insulin bolus versus no bolus and found no difference in rate of change of serum glucose, anion gap, and ED or hospital length of stay,[23] but found that the risk of hypoglycemia was increased in the group receiving a bolus. Kitabchi, et al. found no difference in time to normalization of glucose, pH, or bicarbonate.[24] Both recommend against a bolus. Kitabchi, et al. recommended an initial rate of 0.14units/kg/hr IV.[23,24] Blood glucose checks every hour should occur, and if the glucose has not decreased by 10%, then a bolus can be provided, ranging from 0.1units/kg to 0.14units/kg.[11] Serum glucose is expected to decrease by 50–100mg/dL/hr. If serum glucose levels do not decrease as expected, the insulin infusion can be increased by 1unit/hr.

Most centers will hold the patient's chronic long-acting insulin until the patient and labs have improved, then administer subcutaneous insulin with IV insulin infusion overlapping for several hours. However, recent UK guidelines recommend continuing the long-acting insulin throughout hyperglycemic crisis management.[18,25,26] For example, if the patient is on 10units glargine (i.e. Lantus) and has not had any glargine for several days, this full dose can be given when the patient receives the insulin infusion. The long-acting insulin protects against us stopping the insulin infusion during an episode of hypoglycemia (which should be corrected by giving more glucose). Second, the long-acting insulin improves the transition from infusion to subcutaneous insulin.[18] It also reduces hyperglycemia when the admitting team discontinues the insulin infusion.

Section editor comments (Shiber):

The more severe the DKA the more benefit from an insulin bolus (yes, to stop lipolysis and acidosis). There is good literature supporting it and showing no increase in hypoglycemia, and it is still recommended by the ADA. If a bolus is not given, then the infusion should be started at 0.14u/kg/hr.

Consulting editor comments (Weingart):

Don't wait until clearance to start long-acting insulin. That requires another 90–120 minutes to allow an overlap of the drip with the insulin. We can give long-acting insulin at any point during the regimen, and when you're at the point of clearance you can just turn the drip off and be done. That cuts hours if you're going to clear them in the ED. But we should give the long-acting insulin at reasonable times because these agents are going to be given every 12 or 24 hours, and if you give it at 3 AM, it makes it really hard for the team upstairs. So, 9 PM or 10 PM rolls around and the DKA treatment is occurring, we'll just give the long-acting insulin then, even though it might be another 4 or 5 hours before they are done fully clearing their keto acids.

Q#2d: What about bicarbonate?

The primary foundation of hyperglycemic crisis management involves fluid and electrolyte therapy. Patients in DKA may develop severe acidemia, but does bicarbonate improve patient outcomes, while increasing the pH? The 2009 ADA guidelines recommend bicarbonate (100mmol in 400mL of sterile water) for patients with arterial pH < 6.9.[10,11] However, several studies have shown bicarbonate therapy is ineffective and may even be detrimental.[22,27,28]

- Morris, et al. evaluated patients with pH < 7.14 with DKA and found no improvement in glucose, ketone levels, or time to improvement in pH or glucose.[28]
- A large retrospective study of DKA patients with pH < 7.0 found no difference in time to resolution of acidemia, time to discharge, or time on IV insulin with bicarbonate.[27]
- Chua, et al. conducted a systematic review of 44 articles, finding no improvement in glycemic control, but there was an increased risk for cerebral edema and prolonged hospitalization in children who received bicarbonate.[29]

Not only does bicarbonate fail to improve these numbers, but it may harm patients.[18,19] Okuda, et al. found a 6-hour delay in ketosis improvement in patients receiving bicarbonate, as well as worsened hypokalemia and increased intracellular and central nervous system acidosis.[30] We should be wary of relying on bicarbonate to improve pH or patient outcomes and instead focus on rehydration, electrolyte replacement, and insulin.[11,18,26] If the patient is hyperkalemic with ECG changes, bicarbonate may have a limited role, but our administered insulin and fluids will go a long way to correcting hyperkalemia. However, bicarbonate may assist in treating hyperchloremic non-anion gap acidosis.[18]

Q#3: Can we obtain VBG instead of ABG?

How many times have you heard "What did the ABG show?" The ABG is thought to be more accurate than VBG, especially when assessing pH and bicarbonate levels.[18,26,31,32] However, VBGs are less painful, can be obtained at the time of IV insertion, and have less complications such as radial artery injury, nerve injury, and pain.[18,19,31,32] In terms of pH, Brandenburg, et al. compared ABG and VBG and found pH differences of less than 0.03.[33] Gokel, et al. found a mean difference in pH of 0.05 and bicarbonate of -1.88,[34] while Kelly in 2000 found a mean difference of pH of 0.02 and difference of bicarbonate of -1.4.32 Similar to pH, bicarbonate levels between ABG and VBG do not clinically differ, with a difference of 1–2mmol/L.[31,32,34,35]

Summary: Patients with DKA (or a critical illness) do not require ABG, as pH and bicarbonate readings obtained from VBG are accurate.

Consulting editor comments (Weingart):

Beta hydroxybutyrate is our main monitoring technique for our DKA protocols; it's a very clean representation, as opposed to all the other things that could be causing their anion gap to remain elevated. It is much better than pH because often times as the DKA gets better—if you were using hyperchloremic fluids like normal saline—they will continue to clear their DKA and never affect their pH because they will convert their anion gap acidosis to a hyperchloremic acidosis and their pH will stay high. If we use anion gap exclusively, many patients don't clear because they have other reasons for anion gap acidosis, like end-stage renal disease. So, I don't like anion gap. Beta hydroxybutyrate is beautiful. It's a clean representation of their keto acids. We use beta hydroxybutyrate of less than 1 as a marker that the patient has finished clearing their DKA.

Back to the case:
What did the actual provider do?

- 20:47: Regular insulin 8 units IVP and regular Humulin insulin drip at 5mg/hr
- 20:50: Potassium 20meq IVPB
- CXR: WNL
- ECG: NSR without abnormality
- Vital sign recheck (21:58): Pulse 166, BP 106/80, sat 98%
- ED course: Altered consciousness worsens—she responds to painful stimuli only

Were the provider's actions appropriate? The patient appears to be in DKA based on the blood gas and laboratory results, and she is tachycardic and altered. The physician gave 2L NS, insulin, and potassium. However, the patient's heart rate is above 160, and she remains altered after 3 hours in the ED. In fact, her mental status is worse. There is no mention in the documentation for consideration of why the patient is in DKA and why she is altered. The patient's status is declining, and now we are at a crossroads for management.

DECISION POINT B – YOU ARE FACED WITH 2 QUESTIONS:

1. **The patient is altered. Is a head CT indicated, even with no history of trauma?**
2. **What other items are on the differential for altered mental status in a patient with DKA?**

Q#1: The patient is altered. Is a head CT indicated, even with no history of trauma?
Patients in DKA or HHS can certainly present with altered mental status. In fact, altered mental status is one of the requirements for HHS. The provider's suspicion will be a determining factor. If the patient demonstrates focal neurologic findings such as unilateral weakness or cranial nerve deficit, emergent head CT should be obtained. If the patient does not respond to resuscitation, strong consideration should be given to obtaining head CT. Most sources say obtain imaging when appropriate.[10,11,26] We recommend obtaining head CT with focal findings, those with severe alterations in mental status, and in those who do not improve with resuscitation.

Q#2: What other items are on the differential for altered mental status in a patient with DKA?
A large differential exists for altered mental status. To help us with that differential, there are several mnemonics.[36] One of the more popular mnemonics is AEIOU TIPS.
A: Alcohol
E: Epilepsy, Electrolytes, Endocrine, Encephalopathy
I: Insulin
O: Opioids, Oxygen, Overdose
U: Uremia (liver and kidney)
T: Trauma, Temperature, Toxin
I: Infection, Ischemia (MI), Intracranial process
P: Psychiatric, Poisoning
S: Stroke, Seizure

This is a significant number of potential etiologies, but this can be narrowed with common and easily obtainable tests including glucose, pulse oximetry, and ECG. A focused history and focused exam may reveal additional clues, but history may be only obtainable from family, co-inhabitants, or EMS in altered patients. Neurologic exam should evaluate pupils, cranial nerves, tone, motor activity, sweat production, clonus, and if able, sensation, cerebellar, and gait testing. Work-up includes CBC, chemistry, urine, ECG, chest x-ray, head CT, LFT's, pregnancy test in females, thyroid function, and ASA/acetaminophen levels. Concern for meningitis or encephalitis warrants lumbar puncture.

Back to the patient…

MDM: While arranging for the patient to be transferred to the ICU, she began to seize. I gave Ativan 2mg IVP with rapid resolution of the seizure. She remains altered, responding to painful stimuli only, even with resuscitation measures.

ED diagnosis:
- DKA (Diabetic ketoacidosis)
- Seizures
- Persistent vomiting
- Dehydration (hypovolemia)

DECISION POINT C – YOU ARE FACED WITH 3 QUESTIONS:

1. **How should the seizures in diabetics be managed?**
2. **When should she be intubated?**
3. **How do we maximize success for intubation in the patient with severe metabolic acidosis, and what ventilator settings should be used?**

What does the literature say?

Q#1: How should the seizures in diabetics be managed?

Seizures are more common in diabetics, with up to 25% experiencing seizure at some point during their lifetime, with even greater risk in those with DKA.[37] Immune dysfunction, cerebral microvascular changes, and other metabolic factors play a role. Most seizures resolve in under 1 minute. Beyond this point, benzodiazepines are the first line therapy. If an IV is not present, midazolam 10mg IM should be used for those over 40kg. Lorazepam (Ativan) at 0.1mg/kg can be used if IV is available. Benzodiazepines can be given repeatedly; however, when a second dose is necessary, consideration should be given to additional medications. The longer the seizure persists, cerebral perfusion and oxygenation worsen, resulting in metabolic decompensation and neurologic injury.[38,39]

If benzodiazepines fail to control the seizure, airway protection may be needed,[40] with induction by propofol 2–5mg/kg IV, ketamine 1–2mg/kg IV, or midazolam 0.2mg/kg IV, which all demonstrate antiepileptic properties. If the physician feels intubation can be avoided, other second line medications include fosphenytoin 20–30mg/kg IV at 150 mg/min. This can also be given intramuscularly, unlike phenytoin. Levetiracetam 45–60mg/kg (maximum 4500mg), valproate 20–40mg/kg at 5mg/kg/min, and phenobarbital 20mg/kg are other second line medications.[39-41]

Q#2: When should she be intubated?

Airway is our initial step in the ABC's; however, intubation in DKA can worsen the patient's status, potentially ending in those infamous words "Code Blue." Intubation is dangerous on several levels for patients with severe DKA, first being the actual act of intubation.[40-45] Critical DKA patients have low bicarbonate levels and metabolic acidosis, and they compensate with their respiratory drive. A difficult intubation may result in rapid $PaCO_2$ rise, resulting in a decrease in pH. Even with an "easy" airway, the patient's physiologic status makes intubation extremely dangerous.[40-45] Another aspect is ventilator management following successful intubation. Patients who are critically ill before intubation are actively inhaling and exhaling to compensate, while a ventilator switches this physiology to active inhalation and passive exhalation. This allows $PaCO_2$ to further increase.[40-45]

As long as the patient can protect the airway, intubation should be avoided. Mental status changes solely due to DKA should resolve with resuscitation. Close evaluation and reassessment are required. If intubation is required, be ready for decompensation. The most skilled provider should intubate. This is not the time for the first-year resident to take a crack. Post-intubation management is critical to avoid dramatic changes in ventilation and associated metabolic and hemodynamic complications.

Section editor comments (Shiber):

You need to match their minute ventilation L/min and not just the respiratory rate. The tidal volumes are typically large with Kussmaul breathing, which is the patient's respiratory alkalosis compensating for the metabolic acidosis. When DKA is improving or resolves, then either reduce the minute ventilation (MV) if on an MV mode such as volume or pressure control or else you will overshoot and cause an alkalosis. It may be simpler and safer to keep the MV on a spontaneous mode (such as pressure support or APRV) so that although receiving ventilatory support, the patient will control his/her own breathing and MV based on his/her needs and pH, as long as oversedation is avoided.

Q#3: How do we maximize success for intubation in the patient with severe metabolic acidosis, and what ventilator settings should be used?

Resuscitation before intubation is key. These patients should receive IV fluids to replace intravascular depletion. NIPPV should be attempted first, and if the patient improves, intubation may be avoided,[40-45] but if the patient continues to decompensate, intubation will be needed. Preoxygenation and NO DESAT principles are essential.[41, 43-45] An $EtCO_2$ monitor should be utilized. Once ready to intubate, the question centers on induction with paralysis versus induction only. Most emergency providers are comfortable with induction and paralysis to optimize the airway approach. Paralysis can result in rapid worsening of acidemia due to CO_2 buildup. Some advocate a ketamine-only approach, as ketamine protects the respiratory drive, allowing respiratory compensation to continue.

What are other means of ensuring the patient does not code during intubation? Sodium bicarbonate will not help if the patient is breathing at his/her maximum, as they are already compensating. Bicarbonate generates further CO_2, which will not be blown off.[40, 41, 43-45] To avoid cardiac arrest from acidemia, we need to match their respiratory effort. First, watch the patient and count accurately the RR before intubation. After the patient is on the ventilator, match the patient's pre-sedation respiratory drive with a high RR. Before and during the intubation, several strategies can reduce the risk of worsening acidosis, including the use of a non-invasive ventilation mask and SIMV respiratory settings, or awake intubation with topical anesthesia and ketamine. These strategies allow clinicians to match the patient's respiratory effort.

What happened to the patient?

Hospital course:

- Encephalopathy worsens
- MRI brain normal
- Encephalopathy improves
- Hospital discharge after 4 days

Final diagnosis:

1. Diabetic ketoacidosis (DKA)
2. Altered level of consciousness
3. Acute sinusitis

Chapter summary:

- Antibiotics should be given to sinusitis patients with persistent symptoms > 10 days, those with severe symptoms, or to patients who were better and then worsened.
- The diagnosis of sinusitis in immunocompromised patients should involve consideration of mucormycosis and malignant otitis externa.
- Hyperglycemic crisis consists of DKA and HHS. DKA is diagnosed by serum glucose > 250mg/dL, ketonuria or ketonemia, serum pH < 7.3, and serum bicarbonate < 15mEq/L. HHS is diagnosed with altered sensorium, serum glucose > 600mg/dL, minimal or no ketonuria or ketonemia, serum osmolality > 320mOsm/kg, pH > 7.3 (usually), and bicarbonate > 15mEq/L.
- Insulin should not be started until the potassium level is established. If hypokalemic on initial check (< 3.3mEq/L), provide IV potassium in addition to IV fluids. If the patient is PO tolerant, provide potassium by mouth.
- Insulin should be provided at 0.14units/kg/hr infusion, rather than bolus.
- Even in severe acidosis, sodium bicarbonate may worsen patient outcomes. It does not improve pH or glucose levels.
- VBG should be used, rather than ABG, as it demonstrates similar pH and bicarb levels.
- Intubation is dangerous in DKA; if the patient is protecting their airway, avoid intubation.

References:

1. Chow AW, Benninger MS, Brook I, et al. IDSA clinical practice guideline for acute bacterial rhinosinusitis in children and adults. IDSA Guidelines. Clin Infect Dis 2012;54(8)e72-e112.
2. Rosenfield RM, Piccirillo JF, Chandrasekhar SS, et al. Clinical practice guideline (update): Adult sinusitis. Otolaryngol Head Neck Surg 2015;152(2S):S1-S39.
3. Lemiengre MB, van Driel ML, Merenstein D, et al. Antibiotics for clinically diagnosed acute rhinosinusitis in adults. Cochrane Database Syst Rev 2012;17:10:CD006089.
4. Berg O, Carenfelt C, Rystedt G, et al. Occurrence of asymptomatic sinusitis in common cold and other acute ENT-infections. Rhinology 1986;24(3):223-5.
5. Gwaltney JM Jr. State of the art: Acute community-acquired sinusitis. Clin Infect Dis 1996;23(6):1209-23.
6. Long B, Koyfman A. Mucormycosis: What emergency physicians need to know? Am J Emerg Med 2015;33(12):1823-5.
7. Pfaff JA, Moore GP: Otolaryngology in Marx JA, Hockberger RS, Walls RM, et al. eds:

Rosen's emergency medicine: Concepts and clinical practice, 8th ed. St. Louis, MO: Mosby, Inc., 2014; Ch 72.
8. Kitabchi AE, Umpierrez GE, Miles JM, Fisher JN. Hyperglycemic crises in adult patients with diabetes. Diabetes Care 2009;32(7):1335-43.
9. Centers for Disease Control and Prevention. National Diabetes Fact Sheet 2011. United States Department of Health and Human Services. Available at: http://www.cdc.gov/diabetes/pubs/factsheet11.htm. Accessed January 2017.
10. American Diabetes Association. Standards of medical care in diabetes—2011. Diabetes Care 2011;34(suppl 1):S11–61.
11. Van Ness-Otunnu RV, Hack JB. Hyperglycemic Crisis. J Emerg Med 2013;45(5):797-05.
12. Nyenwe EA, Kitabchi AE. Evidence-based management of hyperglycemic emergencies in diabetes mellitus. Diabetes Res Clin Pract 2011;94(3):340-51.
13. Trachtenbarg DE. Diabetic ketoacidosis. Am Fam Physician 2005;71(9):1705-14.
14. Gabayan GZ, Sun BC, Asch SM. Qualitative factors in patients who die shortly after emergency department discharge. Acad Emerg Med 2013 Aug;20(8):778-85.
15. Sklar DP, Crandall CS, Loeliger E. Unanticipated death after discharge home from the emergency department. Ann Emerg Med 2007;49(6):735-45
16. Munro JF, Campbell IW, McCuish AC, et al. Euglycaemic diabetic ketoacidosis. Br Med J 1973;2(5866):578-80.
17. Barski L, Nevzorov R, Rabaev E, et al. Diabetic ketoacidosis: Clinical characteristics, precipitating factors and outcomes of care. Isr Med Assoc J 2012;14(5):299-03.
18. Farkas J. PulmCrit – Four DKA Pearls. May 2014. https://emcrit.org/pulmcrit/four-dka-pearls/. Accessed March 2017.
19. Rezaie S. Diabetic ketoacidosis (DKA) myths. REBEL EM 2015. http://rebelem.com/diabetic-ketoacidosis-dka-myths/. Accessed March 2017
20. Arora S, Cheng D, Wyler B, et al. Prevalence of hypokalemia in ED patients with diabetic ketoacidosis. Am J Emerg Med 2012 Mar;30(3):481-4.
21. Van Zyl DG, Rheeder P, Delport E. Fluid management in diabetic-acidosis—Ringer's lactate versus normal saline: a randomized controlled trial. Q J Med 2012;105(4):337-43.
22. Mahler SA, Conrad SA, Wang H, et al. Resuscitation with balanced electrolyte solution prevents hyperchloremic metabolic acidosis in patients with diabetic ketoacidosis. Am J Emerg Med 2011;29(6):670-4.
23. Goyal N, Miller JB, Sankey SS, et al. Utility of initial bolus insulin in the treatment of diabetic ketoacidosis. J Emerg Med 2010;38:422-7.
24. Kitabchi AE, Murphy MB, Spencer J, et al. Is a priming dose of insulin necessary in a low-dose insulin protocol for the treatment of diabetic ketoacidosis? Diabetes Care 2008;31(11):2081–5.
25. Joint British Diabetes Societies Inpatient Care Group. The management of diabetic ketoacidosis in adults. https://www.diabetes.org.uk/Documents/About%20Us/What%20we%20say/Management-of-DKA-241013.pdf. Accessed February 2017.
26. Savage MW, Dhatariya KK, Kilvert A, et al. Joint British Diabetes Societies. Joint British Diabetes Societies guideline for the management of diabetic ketoacidosis. Diabet Med 2011;28(5):508-15.
27. Duhon B, Attridge RL, Franco-Martinez AC, et al. Intravenous sodium bicarbonate therapy in severely acidotic diabetic ketoacidosis. Ann Pharmacother 2013;47(7-8):970-5.

28. Morris LR, Murphy MB, Kitabchi AE. Bicarbonate therapy in severe diabetic ketoacidosis. Ann Intern Med 1986;105(6):836-40.
29. Chua HR, Schneider A, Bellomo R. Bicarbonate in diabetic ketoacidosis – A systematic review. Ann Intensive Care 2011;1(1):23.
30. Okuda Y, Adrogue HJ, Field JB, et al. Counterproductive effects of sodium bicarbonate in diabetic ketoacidosis. J Clin Endocrinol Metab 1996;81(1):314-20.
31. Kelly AM. Review Article: Can venous blood gas analysis replace arterial in emergency medical care. Emerg Med Australas 2010;22(6):493-8.
32. Ma OJ, Rush MD, Godfrey MM, et al. Arterial blood gas results rarely influence emergency physician management of patients with suspected diabetic ketoacidosis. Acad Emerg Med Aug 2003;10(8):836-41.
33. Brandenburg MA, Dire DJ. Comparison of arterial and venous blood gas values in the initial emergency department evaluation of patients with diabetic ketoacidosis. Ann Emerg Med 1998;31(4):459-65.
34. Gokel Y, Paydas S, Koseoglu Z, et al. Comparison of blood gas and acid-base measurements in arterial and venous blood samples in patients with uremic acidosis and diabetic ketoacidosis in the emergency room. Am J Nephrol 2000 Jul-Aug;20(4):319-23.
35. Zeserson E, Goodgame B, Hess JD, et al. Correlation of venous blood gas and pulse oximetry with arterial blood gas in the undifferentiated critically ill patient. J Intensive Care Med 2016. pii: 0885066616652597.
36. Huff JS. Ch. 168: Altered mental status and coma. In Tintinalli J, ed. Emergency medicine: A comprehensive study guide. 8th ed. New York, NY: McGraw-Hill, 2016.
37. Yun C, Xuefeng W. Association between seizures and diabetes mellitus: A comprehensive review of literature. Curr Diabetes Rev 2013;9(4):350-4.
38. Chapman MG, Smith M, Hirsch NP. Status epilepticus. Anaesthesia 2001;56(7):648-59.
39. Glauser T, Shinnar S, Treimen DM. Evidence-based guideline: Treatment of convulsive status epilepticus in children and adults: Report of the guideline committee of the American Epilepsy Society. Epilepsy Curr 2016;16(1):48-61.
40. Farkas J. Rapid sequence termination (RST) of status epilepticus. EMCrit June 2014. https://emcrit.org/pulmcrit/rapid-sequence-termination-rst-of-status-epilepticus/. Accessed March 2017.
41. Weingart S. Podcast 155 – Status epilepticus with Tom Bleck. EMCrit Aug 2015. https://emcrit.org/podcasts/status-epilepticus/. Accessed March 2017.
42. Santos C. Airway subtleties in critically ill patients. emDocs. June 2014. http://www.emdocs.net/airway-subtleties-critically-ill-patients/. Accessed March 2017.
43. Weingart S. Podcast 3 – Laryngoscope as a murder weapon (LAMW) series – Ventilatory kills – Intubating the patient with severe metabolic acidosis. EMCrit May 2009. https://emcrit.org/podcasts/tube-severe-acidosis/. Accessed March 2017.
44. Weingart S, Levitan RM. Preoxygenation and prevention of desaturation during emergency airway management. Ann Emerg Med Mar 2012;59(3):165-75.
45. Weingart S. Rapid sequence awake – An awake intubation update. EMCrit Jul 2016. https://emcrit.org/wee/awake-intubation-update/. Accessed March 2017.

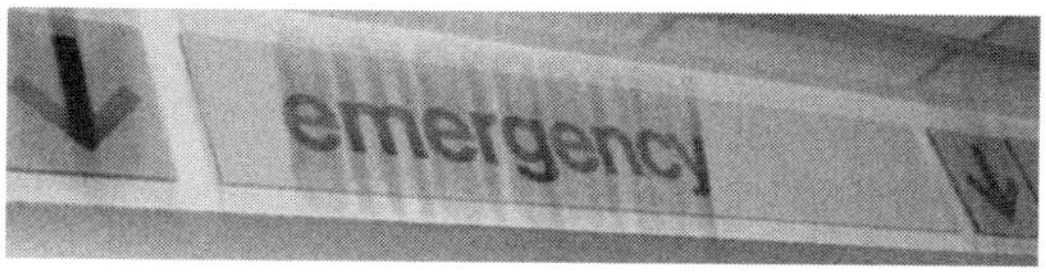

SECTION F – TRAUMA, DM, HEME, GI, HTN

Chapter 27: A 55-year-old healthy man with elevated blood pressure

Richard M. Pescatore, DO, FAAEM
Assistant Professor
Emergency Medicine
Drexel University College of Medicine
Chief Physician
Delaware Division of Public Health
Dover, DE

Haney Mallemat, MD
Associate Professor
Internal Medicine and Emergency Medicine
Cooper Medical School of Rowan University
Camden, NJ

Section editor:
Joseph Shiber, MD, FACEP, FACP, FCCM
Professor
Emergency Medicine, Neurology and Surgery
Director ECMO/Acute Lung Service
Co-director NSICU and UF North ICU
UF College of Medicine–Jacksonville
Jacksonville, FL

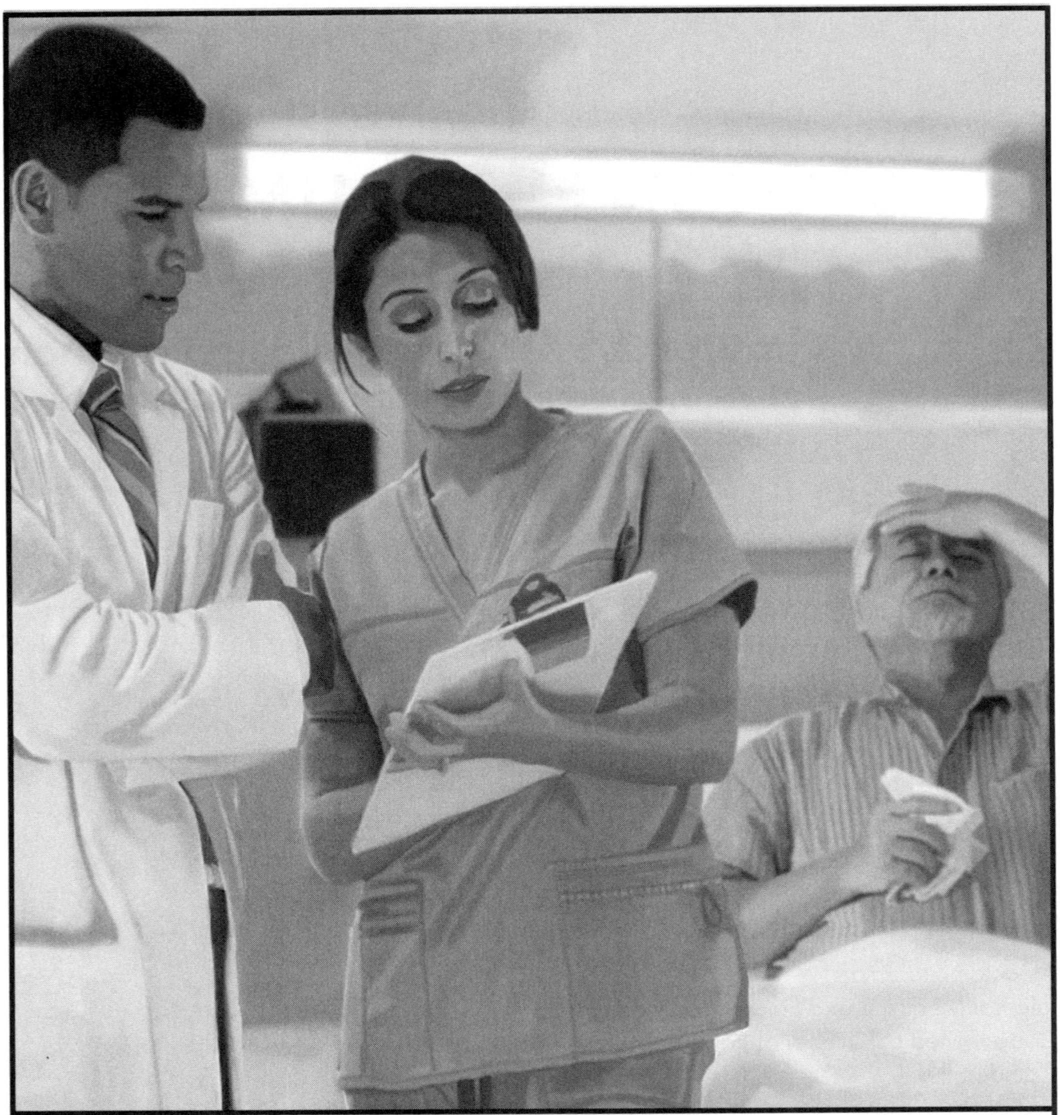

"WE NEED TO GET THE BP DOWN ASAP!"

SECTION F / CHAPTER 27

A 55-year-old healthy man with elevated blood pressure

Hypertension (HTN) is a staggeringly common condition throughout the world, thought to affect a third of Americans and an even greater fraction of patients presenting to the emergency department.[1, 2, 3] An ED patient with an elevated blood pressure (BP) presents a diagnostic and therapeutic challenge, as the spectrum of disease can span from the asymptomatic, chronic patient who needs little more than primary care referral, to the critically ill who require prompt and expert intervention. Furthermore, inconsistent terminology has compounded uncertainty and practice variation. Hypertensive emergency is diagnosed when end-organ injury (i.e., cardiovascular, renal, or neurologic) occurs in the setting of markedly elevated BP.[4]

In the absence of treatment, hypertensive emergency has a very poor prognosis, with 1-year mortality rates reported as high as 79%.[5] Even with prompt treatment the residual risk for end-stage renal disease and cardiovascular complications remains high.[6] In 1939, Keith, et al. found that the mean survival of patients with hypertensive emergency was 10.5 months, with no survivors at 5 years.[7] Appropriate treatment has dramatically reduced immediate deaths and 1-year mortality, with rates ranging between 4% in one European registry and 7–10% in U.S. cohorts.[8, 9, 10]

This case is real, including the documentation and medical decision-making. We start with this patient's initial presentation and—yes—the bounceback just one day later.

INITIAL ED VISIT

HPI (21:22): The patient is a very pleasant 53-year-old gentleman with no documented past medical history (nonsubscriber to routine medical care) who presents with complaint of high BP. He reports checking his BP today via a local pharmacy's automated cuff and became alarmed when it read "over 200," and thus he opted to present for emergency evaluation. Otherwise, the patient is without complaint. Specifically, he denies chest pain, shortness of breath, visual changes, or headache. He is well-appearing.

Allergies: NKDA
Social history: Patient denies tobacco abuse, EtOH abuse, or IVDA
Family history: Reviewed and not pertinent
ROS: All other systems reviewed and are negative except as noted. Nursing triage notes were reviewed
PMH: None
PSH: None

PE:

Vitals:

Temp	Pulse	Resp	BP	SpO2
97.8	86	16	202/135	99% (RA)

GA: A&OX3, WA/WN
HEENT: NC/AT, PERRL, TMI, nares patent, trachea midline
CV: RRR s m/r/g/t
RESP: CTAB s wheezes, rales, or rhonchi
ABD: Soft, NT/ND. No palpable midline abdominal mass
BACK: No CVA tenderness
SKIN: No rashes or lesions
NEURO: CN II-XII grossly intact

EKG (21:28): Reviewed and interpreted by me. NSR at 80bpm. LAD, LVH. Normal intervals. No acute ischemic changes, no STEMI.

MDM (21:45): Patient presents with asymptomatic hypertension. There is no evidence of Hypertensive Emergency—no chest pain, SOB, neurologic deficit. Per ACEP guidelines, no indication for further testing. Will refer patient to f/u with PCP.

IMPRESSION (21:52): Hypertension, unspecified

PLAN: F/u with PCP in 48-72h. RTER with worsening symptoms.

At face value, this appears to be a relatively simple and well-documented encounter. It is a complaint we face on a regular basis, so common, in fact, that the American College of Emergency Physicians (ACEP) has developed a clinical policy,[11] which the treating physician even cites in their medical decision-making! Nonetheless, there are multiple areas where the management and documentation can be improved.[7]

Documentation and patient safety issues:

1. **Speed of disposition:** We are often pressured to rapidly evaluate and manage the disposition of patients, but occasionally, the waiting room thins and the department hums along at top efficiency, allowing for rapid management and disposition of patients with lower-acuity complaints. This patient was discharged 30 minutes after arrival. We are held to task for moving too slowly, but moving too quickly may retrospectively be interpreted as being careless.
2. **There's only one set of vital signs recorded:** With the exception of minor complaints, patient vitals should be trended, and nearly always repeated prior to discharge. This is especially true in a patient presenting with a complaint so pertinent to vital signs—an elevated BP! Subsequent BP readings taken in the ED—more often than not—will demonstrate a reduction from triage vitals, which helps to establish a reassuring trend and justifies lack of intervention. If the next BP is 160/90, great… if it is 260/160, maybe our management would be different.
3. **Physical exam:** "CN II-XII grossly intact" is an inadequate neurologic evaluation for this

patient in whom the diagnosis is predicated upon an exclusion of focal neurologic deficits. There is no documentation regarding cerebellar motion testing, the presence or absence of papilledema or spontaneous venous pulsations, or the patient's gait.

4. **MDM:** At first glance, citing the ACEP clinical policy regarding asymptomatic elevated BP seems like a good strategy; however any benefit to such charting is nullified (and, indeed, likely destructive) when this statement is incorrect. What? We'll discuss in more detail below.
5. **Patient discharge instructions:**
   - It is unclear whether the importance of follow-up for the commencement of antihypertensive therapy was discussed with the patient.
   - There is uncertainty of his ability to obtain timely follow-up. The physician had discussed the patient's non-participation in medical care earlier in the documentation—one would assume that means he doesn't have a primary care provider.
   - Most importantly, the patient is instructed to "RTER with worsening symptoms." What symptoms, exactly? Isn't his whole plan of care predicated upon the fact that this is *asymptomatic* HTN?

Were the decisions regarding the patient's evaluation and management appropriate? For such a common presentation, there is significant practice variation as well as confusion regarding clinical recommendations.

1. What is the role of the emergency clinician in managing patients with asymptomatic HTN?

The majority of patients who present to the ED with elevated BP receive no intervention or instructions regarding their HTN. Recognizing the frequency of ED visits and the paucity of evidence regarding management, the American College of Emergency Physicians (ACEP) released a clinical policy addressing critical issues in the evaluation and management of asymptomatic HTN in 2006 and later amended the document in 2013.[11]

The ACEP clinical policy offers a Level "C" recommendation (i.e., there is an absence of any adequate published literature and is based on panel consensus) that patients with asymptomatic elevated BP do not require routine screening for acute target organ injury, nor do they require routine intervention with antihypertensive medications. It is recommended that patients should be referred for timely outpatient follow-up.[11]

2. What, if anything, changes when the patient is uninsured, has no primary care provider, or is known to be noncompliant with medical care?

The ACEP policy makes specific exceptions for patients in whom poor follow-up or medical noncompliance is anticipated with a consensus recommendation that screening for end-organ injury and/or initiation of antihypertensive therapy may reduce the rate of adverse outcomes related to HTN. Several studies have demonstrated higher rates of kidney disease in populations at higher risk for medical noncompliance, suggesting that ED screening and intervention may offer benefit.[12]

3. Should antihypertensive medications be initiated from the ED?

Generally speaking, initiation of antihypertensive therapy from the ED is unnecessary. There are compelling data, however, to suggest that prescription of antihypertensive medications from the ED is associated with improved BP management at follow-up without any increased risk of adverse events or hypotension, and most experts recommend this approach, particularly in at-risk populations.[13,14]

Putting it all together:

The patient who presents to the emergency department with a chief complaint of "high BP"—that is, the patient with asymptomatic HTN—presents a "fork in the road" for work-up and management. The dearth of high-quality literature examining this population is somewhat reconciled by the ACEP Clinical Policy Statement. HTN represents a chronic issue best managed through primary care resources; however, the unique position of the ED as both the first line for acute care and a safety net for all care, means that the idiosyncrasies of each presentation must be weighed when considering the need for screening or management from the ED. Most patients do not require lab testing, electrocardiograms, or imaging and can be discharged with a plan for appropriate and expedient follow-up. Where social, situational, or other factors might delay or derail that approach, consideration should be given to escalation of intervention in the ED.

Section editor comments (Shiber):

Note that the patient's MAP is ~160. At this rate they are above cerebral vascular autoregulation; the cerebral blood flow (CBF) will be high leading to edema and an elevated intracranial pressure (ICP). A hypertensive emergency WILL happen, it is only a matter of time. Consider that the non-invasive cuff only truly measures a MAP and then uses an algorithm to calculate the SBP and DBP, so that the MAP is actually more accurate. The exam documented the heart exam as RRR s m/r/g/t. Often an S4 is present at this BP indicating a stiff LV as a result of a very high aortic arterload. Finally, I agree with the authors on the minimal neurologic exam; it is very easy to test their gait, as well as other aspects of cerebellar function such as smooth tracking movements and rapid alternating movements.

ED BOUNCEBACK

The patient did not initiate follow-up with primary care. The morning after ED discharge the complained to his wife of headache and had several episodes of vomiting. The following evening his wife found him seizing in a downstairs bathroom, and EMS arrived to find the patient with persistent seizures.

ED VISIT #2 (one day after initial ED visit)

HPI (23:02): The patient is a 53-year-old male who presents BIBA with seizures, no known seizure disorder. He was seen here yesterday evening with asymptomatic HTN and referred to f/u with his primary care doctor. Per the patient's wife, he has been complaining of headache and nausea with vomiting since shortly after discharge. He was found seizing shortly PTA. EMS responded and administered 2mg IV Lorazepam without improvement.

Allergies: NKDA
Social history: Patient denies tobacco abuse, EtOH abuse, or IVDA
Family history: Reviewed and not pertinent
ROS: ROS unobtainable due to severity of condition. Nursing triage notes were reviewed

PMH: None
PSH: None

PE:

Vitals:				
Temp	Pulse	Resp	BP	SpO_2
99.8	126	8	224/140	94% (RA)

GA: Acutely ill. Afebrile
HEENT: NC/AT, pupils 6mm, sluggish.
CV: Tachycardic, no murmur
RESP: CTAB s wheezes, rales, or rhonchi
ABD: Soft, NT/ND. No palpable midline abdominal mass
BACK: No CVA tenderness
SKIN: No rashes or lesions
NEURO: Active tonic-clonic seizure activity.

MDM (23:15): Patient presents with seizures, hypertension, recent complaint of headache. Presumed SAH. Will control seizure activity and proceed immediately to CT.

Author comments (Weinstock):

We are faced with a patient who needs emergent neuroimaging, but the seizures need to be controlled first. While the team establishes IV access and you gather additional history from EMS, we arrive at:

DECISION POINT A – YOU ARE FACED WITH 3 QUESTIONS:

1. **What is the differential diagnosis for the patient presenting with seizures and HTN?**
2. **What is the recommended strategy for anti-epileptic therapy?**
3. **In the patient with recalcitrant status epilepticus requiring endotracheal intubation, what is the best approach to medication selection?**

What does the literature say?

Q#1: What is the differential diagnosis for the patient presenting with seizures and HTN?

Establishing a focused but thorough differential diagnosis is critical to help direct initial therapy. While we are most suspicious for subarachnoid hemorrhage, alternate possible diagnoses include:

- hypertensive emergencies such as intraparenchymal hemorrhage or posterior reversible encephalopathy syndrome
- an intracranial mass
- head trauma
- an underlying seizure disorder
- alcohol withdrawal seizures and delirium tremens
- severe electrolyte abnormalities (especially hyponatremia or hypoglyecmia)
- drug overdose
- meningoencephalitis

Q#2: What is the recommended strategy for anti-epileptic therapy?

ACEP's clinical policy on seizures[15] is concordant with guidelines by the American Academy of Neurology and Neurocritical Care Society with a recommendation to use a parenteral benzodiazepine as first line therapy, with Level A data supporting the use of lorazepam (0.1mg/kg/dose, max: 4mg/dose) or midazolam (5–10mg).[16] IV lorazepam has classically been employed to reasonable effect; however, lessons from the RAMPART Trial (a sentinel trial regarding EMS management of status epilepticus published in the *New England Journal of Medicine* in 2012), have suggested that intramuscular midazolam may lead to more rapid seizure control in situations where IV access is not already established.[17]

The use of anti-epileptic medications in patients who have failed multiple doses of benzodiazepines is less clear. Emergency physicians may consider intravenous administration of the following medications, which offer similar efficacy and carry Level B recommendations:

- phenytoin
- fosphenytoin
- phenobarbital
- valproate

The use of levetiracetam for patients who have failed initial abortive therapy has grown, and several small studies have suggested that it is likely as effective as more traditional therapies such as phenytoin, with a lower incidence of adverse effects.[18,19]

Q#3: In the patient with recalcitrant status epilepticus requiring endotracheal intubation, what is the best approach to medication selection?

Patients who have received large doses of benzodiazepines, or who continue to seize despite a secondary anti-epileptic agent, often require endotracheal intubation in anticipation of respiratory failure or for airway protection. If further sedation is needed, etomidate (0.3mg/kg) is a hemodynamically neutral hypnotic agent with rapid onset.[20]

Long-acting paralytics are contraindicated in patients with status epilepticus unless continuous EEG can be expeditiously implemented due to the risk of unrecognized continued seizure activity. There are no data to suggest that the use of depolarizing neuromuscular blockade may precipitate critical hyperkalemia as it is unlikely that the muscle activity induced by neuromuscular blockade will be of any significance in a patient with prolonged seizure activity.

Section editor comments (Shiber):

Rapid sequence intubation (RSI) for any seizure should preferably use succinylcholine so that a clinical seizure can be detected. Additionally, many SZ patients are intubated primarily for airway protection from the sedation due to the benzodiazepines and their postictal state; these patients do not need ongoing sedation but to simply "wake up" in order to be evaluated for extubation.

DECISION POINT A – ***What did the actual provider do?***

(23:05): Upon patient arrival, the provider administered a second dose of 2mg IV lorazepam (first dose administered by EMS). Labs including CBC, BMP, UA, Troponin, CK, PT/PTT, and bedside glucose—this was reported by the RN as 86mg/dL. When seizures did not abate, a third dose of lorazepam was given and 1000mg of levetiracetam ordered; however, the patient became hypoxic and the decision was made to intubate for airway protection and further anti-epileptic management.

(23:15): The patient was given etomidate 20mg and succinylcholine 100mg and then intubated via direct laryngoscopy with an 8.0 endotracheal tube. The intubation was uneventful.

The story continues: The patient is now intubated, but the encounter is not over. Sedation and analgesia are required before transfer to the CT scanner. What are the best options? Should this be done with concomitant BP management? We are at:

DECISION POINT B – YOU ARE FACED WITH 2 QUESTIONS:

1. **What is the best approach for post-intubation analgesia and sedation?**
2. **Should the blood pressure be treated prior to imaging?**

What does the literature say?

Q#1: What is the best approach for post-intubation analgesia and sedation?

Many common sedative and amnestic agents possess no analgesic properties, and analgesia should be prioritized in post-intubation care. Fentanyl, a synthetic opioid with rapid titratability and short half-life is a good choice, either as an infusion (0.7–10mcg/kg/h) or in boluses.

A comprehensive review of sedation in the critically ill patient concluded that despite nearly 100 trials examining different sedation regimens, no drug was clearly superior to its comparators.[21] Propofol infusion (5–50mcg/kg/min), is the most commonly used anesthetic for sedation in critically ill patients as well as for general anesthesia in the United States.[22] Its rapid rate of clearance, short duration of action and ease of titration offer distinct advantages in the emergency setting. The use of propofol in patients with status epilepticus is generally regarded as an ideal agent for sedation and further treatment.[23] Propofol is a global CNS depressant and GABA agonist, which has been well-demonstrated to suppress epileptiform activity within seconds after administration.24 It may cause hypotension due to both vasodilatation and a negative inotropic effect, which may limit application in hypovolemic and hypotensive patients.

Section editor comments (Shiber):

Only if the patient has a concomitant painful condition, as having an ETT and being restrained may not be comfortable but it is not painful; the minute volume (MV) should be adjusted to support the patient comfortably so that you are not simply making them tolerate the ventilator. All opiates suppress spontaneous respirations which is not the goal for our patient nor the majority of patients intubated in the ED. Fentanyl and all opiates will induce sedation, but this is actually a side-effect; a general tenet of medicine is to use a medication for its primary intended effect and not for its side-effects.

Q#2: Should the blood pressure be treated prior to imaging?

Empiric antihypertensive treatment likely offers little benefit in the undifferentiated hypertensive emergency because the goal BP and medications of choice vary depending on diagnosis; the concept that "minutes count" lacks validity in light of the potential harm of overcorrection. With intracerebral hemorrhage, the best available data suggest that aggressive anti-hypertensive therapy leads to no difference in outcomes of death or disability,[25] and most cohorts consistently demonstrate around a 10% incidence of iatrogenic hypotension following initiation of antihypertensives,[26] suggesting that risk outweighs benefit until a condition amenable to therapy can be identified.

DECISION POINT B – *What did the actual provider do?*

Lorazepam 4mg IV was administered for post-intubation sedation. No antihypertensives were administered prior to imaging.

The story continues:
(23:53): The patient is taken to CT by nursing and respiratory therapy. The treating physician reviews the images in real time and documents "wet read by emergency physician: no large intracranial hemorrhage identified." Initial lab results have returned:

WBC 12.1 (H)
Hgb 11.8gm/dL (L)
Plt 248thou/mcl

Na 147mEq/L (H)
Cl 107mEq/L
K 6.3mEq/L (H)
HCO3 12mEq/L (L)
Creat 4.8mg/dL (H)

Trop 0.05 (H)
CK 4300 (H)

ED course: When patient returns from CT he is noted to have irregular shaking movements. There is debate among the treating physician and resident as to whether this represents seizure activity or agitation and inadequate sedation. Repeat vitals are taken and an ECG ordered which is not able to be interpreted due to patient movement.

T 99.8 **P** 126 **R** 32 **BP** 228/142 SpO2 99%

MDM (00:44): The levetiracetam has arrived we have started the infusion. I ordered propofol infusion to be started at 20mcg/kg/min. CT brain negative for acute intracranial pathology. Patient was noted to have acute renal failure and mild rhabdomyolysis, likely due to prolonged seizure activity.

Author comments (Weinstock):

How should the blood pressure be managed? We are at:

DECISION POINT C – YOU ARE FACED WITH 3 QUESTIONS:

1. **What is the management of hyperkalemia in the setting of acute renal failure?**
2. **What is the patient's presumed diagnosis?**
3. **What is the best approach to emergent antihypertensive therapy?**

What does the literature say?

Q#1: What is the management of hyperkalemia in the setting of acute renal failure?

The emergency treatment of severe hyperkalemia is generally independent of its etiology, and because the therapy is safe, maintain a low threshold for starting treatment.[27] Any ECG manifestations of severe hyperkalemia demand immediate therapy. Electrocardiographic changes are generally progressive and proportional to the rate of rise of potassium; however, ventricular fibrillation may be the first ECG disturbance of hyperkalemia.[28] Treatment should be initiated at 6.5mEq/L, the point at which most patients will begin to manifest ECG changes beginning with peaked T waves, progressing to widening of the QRS complex at potassium levels above 7mEq/L. The risk of sudden cardiac arrest rises significantly at levels above 8mEq/L.

Treatment begins with:

1. IV calcium, usually as 1 amp (1000mg) of calcium gluconate. Calcium directly antagonizes the myocardial effects of hyperkalemia without lowering serum potassium and is beneficial even in patients with normal calcium levels.[29] Calcium should always be given when ECG manifestations of severe hyperkalemia are noted (a widening QRS); however, routine use of calcium based on the absolute potassium values or with isolated peaked T waves is discouraged, as intravenous calcium can lead to cardiac dysrhythmias, tachycardia, and elevated BP.
2. Insulin and dextrose – Efforts to force potassium to redistribute intracellularly should be undertaken, typically with regular insulin (10U IV) (with dextrose administered prior to insulin when blood glucose is < 350mg/dL to support blood glucose levels).
3. Beta-agonists (albuterol) given as nebulization solution (20mg over 10 minutes), and occasionally.
4. Sodium bicarbonate when the pH of the blood is acidotic.

Note that all of the above interventions are temporizing solutions intended to shift potassium intracellularly as kaliuria corrects the systemic potassium overload. Enhanced renal elimination in the non-anuric patient is potentially definitive, and it may be accomplished with loop diuretics. The oliguric or anuric patient may occasionally require emergent hemodialysis. Exchange resins such as sodium polystyrene sulfonate (Kayexalate) have never demonstrated efficacy in decreasing serum potassium levels acutely. Additionally, a serious but infrequent side-effect—the development of colonic necrosis in about 2% of patients receiving SPS—make it a poor choice for hyperkalemia.[29]

Q#2: What is the patient's presumed diagnosis?

In the presence of normal imaging and the patient's history of headache, seizure, and altered mental status, the lack of compelling evidence for infection, and his severely elevated BP, the patient most likely has Posterior Reversible Encephalopathy Syndrome, or PRES. Once termed hypertensive encephalopathy, that nomenclature has been eschewed since a landmark paper in 1996 married the clinical diagnosis of hypertensive encephalopathy with the radiologic syndrome of posterior leukoencephalopathy to arrive at PRES.[30] PRES is a disorder of reversible subcortical vasogenic edema in patients with acute neurologic symptoms and characteristic radiographic features. Clinical manifestations include:

- non-localized headache unresponsive to analgesics
- visual disturbances
- altered mental status
- seizures in the setting of acute HTN or cytotoxic therapies[31]

Aside from ICU admission and critical care consultation, our patient would benefit from specialist evaluation by neurology for the presumed diagnosis of PRES as well as nephrology for his acute renal failure.

Q#3: What is the best approach to emergent antihypertensive therapy?

The short-term goal for treatment of PRES is to reduce the systolic BP by 10–15% within the first hour and by 25% within the following several hours.[32] Some sources recommend a target of less than 160/100mmHg; however, no randomized clinical trials have been undertaken assessing therapeutic interventions or BP goals.[33] As such, the choice of antihypertensive agent is left to the discretion of the treating physician. Nicardipine (at a starting dose of 2.5–5mg/h, max dose: 15mg/h) is commonly used, though Clevidipine, another dihydropyridine calcium channel blocker, has gained traction due to its rapid action and ease of titration.[34]

Pronounced fluctuations of BP should be avoided, as they may exacerbate cerebral edema and ischemia. Note that hypertensive states are thought to induce an abnormal pressure natriuresis mechanism, which in the setting of acute BP elevation and hypertensive emergencies may contribute to a fluid-contracted state.[35] Initiation of medications to decrease systemic vascular resistance may lead to overshoot in BP targets as a "clamped down" but hypovolemic circulatory system is forced to suddenly relax. Administration of a small volume (500–1000mL) of isotonic fluid prior to the antihypertensives may mitigate this drop.[36]

DECISION POINT C – *What did the actual provider do?*

MDM (01:14): The patient was administered 1g of calcium gluconate, as well as 50mEq sodium bicarbonate, 10U regular insulin, and 25mg of dextrose. Nephrology was consulted and advised commencement of isotonic bicarbonate infusion, 150mEq of sodium bicarbonate in 1000mL of 0.9% NS infused at 125mL/hr.

MDM (01:49): Patient with presumed hypertensive encephalopathy. I have started antihypertensive therapy with nicardipine and paged neurology as well as the ICU team for admission. The patient was started on a nicardipine infusion at 5mg/hr. The dose was steadily increased by the bedside nurse to 15mg/hr. Repeat BPs were documented in the treatment record:

2302—224/140
2312—212/138
2324—238/148
2350—225/139
0028—228/142

0044—230/138
0110—244/140
0145—236/130
0155—232/126
0205—228/126
0224—136/74
0226—119/68

Consulting editor comments (Weingart):

Though there was an adverse outcome, I maintain that nicardipine is the agent of choice for arterial vasodilation. For other patients such aortic catastrophes where an agent is needed to block the heart rate and inotropy; use esmolol. But the vasodilator of choice for everything else is nicardipine, meaning that we only need to learn about one drug. But we need to use it right, which means we can't leave the patient at the same dose that decreased their BP initially. Nicardipine should be given as a push which is repeated, if necessary. And then when the blood pressure's at goal, we decrease the dose to 3mg/hour, and work from there.

If we leave the nicardipine at the initial dose, we are bound to fail. For example, everyone's called away for a cardiac arrest and then return 1 hour later and the patient's blood pressure is 60/40. This can't happen.

Regarding the goal BP, we need to separate out those diseases which need rapid BP lowering, such as the hypertensive patient with aortic dissection or abdominal aortic aneurysm; we'll bring those patients immediately down to 120, 110, systolic without a second thought. Versus, the neuro hypertensive emergencies where we shoot for 25 or 30% decrease in BP. With these patients—hypertensive emergency, stroke, intercranial hemorrhage, or a PRES patient—we need a balance; not too high, but not too low. For these patients a 25–30% reduction, or less than the 180mmHg is a very reasonable goal.

Author comments (Weinstock):

In the "olden days" we used to pinprick a nifedipine capsule and squirt it under the tongue to decrease the BP... until we found out that this was causing more harm than good. This case strikes to the heart of "first do no harm." We "won the BP battle," but lost the war. There are not many patients who require bedside attendance or every 5 minute checks, but management of the hypertensive emergency/posterior reversible encephalopathy syndrome (PRES) patient does. We have taken him from 224/140 to 119/68. We are at:

DECISION POINT D – YOU ARE FACED WITH 2 QUESTIONS:

1. **What immediate corrective actions can be undertaken when patients suffer iatrogenic *hypo*tension?**
2. **What is the role of push-dose pressors in immediate BP control?**

What does the literature say?

Q#1: What immediate corrective actions can be undertaken when patients suffer iatrogenic *hypo*tension?

Antihypertensive agents should be discontinued immediately upon recognition of hypotension, as supratherapeutic dosing is a common complication of infusion of vasoactives with longer half-lives. Sedative infusions should also be lowered significantly or halted, as most sedating agents cause a decrease in systemic vascular resistance and are associated with vasoplegia. IV fluids should be administered to support the BP.

Section editor comments (Shiber):

Yes! Stopping sedatives is something that many forget to do in the ED and simply start or increase vasopressor infusions while the propofol drip continues!

Q#2: What is the role of push-dose pressors in immediate BP control?

Bolus administration of intravenous vasopressors and inotropics, or push-dose pressors, is a technique that has been used for decades in anesthesia environments and has gained recent traction in the emergency medicine community.[37] Phenylephrine, for example, is a pure alpha-1 agonist with a broad safety profile which can rapidly correct hypotension due to iatrogenic vasoplegia. While literature surrounding this technique continues to emerge, it appears to be a safe and effective intervention which can be lifesaving in temporizing critically low BP's.[38]

DECISION POINT D – ***What did the actual provider do?***

ED course: The patient suffered a profound drop in BP as a consequence of the propofol and nicardipine infusions. The patient's nurse noted the decline and stopped all medications immediately before informing the physician, who ordered 2L of IV fluid to be administered. BP slowly recovered.

0231—128/74
0240—145/90
0252—166/92
0300—169/90

(03:04): The patient was transferred to the ICU.

What was the patient's outcome?

BP was controlled with nicardipine and the patient was eventually transitioned to enteral antihypertensive therapy. MRI later demonstrated hyperintensity and restricted diffusion of the bilateral frontoparietal region consistent with watershed infarction, as well as subcortical vasogenic edema in the bilateral parieto-occipital region consistent with PRES.

The patient was unable to be weaned from mechanical ventilation due to depressed mental status and ataxic respirations and ultimately underwent tracheostomy and PEG placement prior to transfer to a long-term acute care facility for prolonged ventilator management.

Chapter author debrief: This was a difficult case—an unexpected and rapid deterioration of a seemingly benign complaint that was further complicated and compounded by the consequences of intervention. Certainly, the treating physician did a commendable job in rapid control of the patient's presenting status epilepticus, expert control of the airway, and expedient diagnosis. The proper interventions were ordered and implemented within minutes of the patient's arrival to the ED, and a complex case full of critical care decision points was skillfully dispositioned. Nonetheless, the ED environment is defined by the high risk of serious disease and advanced intervention. While reduction of the patient's BP was the correct and necessary intervention, aggressive up-titration of antihypertensives and rapid BP lowering adds complexity and danger without increased benefit. Caution should be the rule when medications are used to manipulate patients' BP, and slow and deliberate reduction of MAP by no more than 15% can ensure efficacy without compromising safety.

Chapter summary:

- Management of asymptomatic high BP is nuanced, requiring a patient-specific approach.
- Utilization of clinical practice guidelines demands a thorough understanding and proper application (especially before citing them in the MDM).
- Posterior Reversible Encephalopathy Syndrome (PRES) is the new term for hypertensive encephalopathy where there is a neurologic consequence of end-organ damage in hypertensive emergency.
- Hypertensive emergencies are often fluid-depleted states, and initiation of parenteral antihypertensives can cause rapid and dangerous reductions in BP. Consider administration of IV fluid prior to vasoactive therapy in the patient with evidence of volume contraction and target MAP reduction between 10–20%.

References:

1. Nwankwo T, Yoon SS, Burt V, et al. Hypertension among adults in the United States: National health and nutrition examination survey, 2011-2012. NCHS Data Brief 2013;133:1-8.
2. Anchala R, Kannuri NK, Pant H, et al. Hypertension in India: A systematic review and meta-analysis of prevalence, awareness, and control of hypertension. J Hypertens 2014;32(6):1170-7.
3. Wang J, Zhang L, Wang F, et al. Prevalence, awareness, treatment, and control of hypertension in China: Results from a national survey. Am J Hypertens 2014;27(11):1355-61.
4. Chobanian AV, Bakris GL, Black HR, et al. Seventh report of the Joint National Committee on Prevention, Detection, Evaluation and Treatment of High Blood Pressure: The JNC 7 report. JAMA 2003;289(19):2560-72.
5. Rodriguez MA, Kumar SK, De Caro M. Hypertensive crisis. Cardiol Rev 2010;18(2):102-7.
6. Cremer A, Amraoui F, Lip GYH, et al. From malignant hypertension to hypertension-MOD: A modern definition for an old but still dangerous emergency. J Hum Hypertens 2016;30(8):463-6.
7. Keith NM, Wagener HP, Barker NW. Some different types of essential hypertension: Their course and prognosis. Am J Med Sci 1974;268(6):336-45.
8. Monnet X, Marik PE. What's new with hypertensive crises? Intensive Care Med 2015;41(1):127-30.
9. Leiba A, Cohen-Arazi O, Mendel L, et al. Incidence, aetiology and mortality secondary to hypertensive emergencies in a large-scale referral centre in Israel (1991-2010). J Hum Hypertens 2016;30(8):498-02.

10. González-Pacheco H, Morales-Victorino N, Núñez-Urquiza JP, et al. Patients with hypertensive crises who are admitted to a coronary care unit: Clinical characteristics and outcomes. J Clin Hypertens (Greenwich) 2013;15(3):210-4.
11. Wolf SJ, Lo B, Shih RD, et al. (2013). Clinical policy: critical issues in the evaluation and management of adult patients in the emergency department with asymptomatic elevated blood pressure. Ann Emerg Med 2013;62(1):59-68.
12. Nishijima DK, Paladino L, Sinert R. Routine testing in patients with asymptomatic elevated BP in the ED. Am J Emerg Med 2010;28(2):235-42.
13. Brody A, Rahman T, Reed B, et al. Safety and efficacy of antihypertensive prescription at emergency department discharge. Acad Emerg Med 2015;22(5):632-5.
14. Karras DJ, Kruus LK, Cienki JJ, et al. Evaluation and treatment of patients with severely elevated blood pressure in academic emergency departments: a multicenter study. Ann Emerg Med 2006; 47(3):230-36.
15. Huff SJ, Melnick E, Tomaszewski CA, et al. Clinical policy: Critical issues in the evaluation and management of adult patients presenting to the emergency department with seizures. Ann Emerg Med 2014;63(4):437-47.
16. Brophy, Gretchen M., et al. Guidelines for the evaluation and management of status epilepticus. Neurocrit Care 2012;17(1):3-23.
17. Silbergleit R, Durkalski V, Lowenstein D, et al. Intramuscular versus intravenous therapy for prehospital status epilepticus. N Engl J Med 2012;366(7):591-600.
18. Mundlamuri RC, Sinha S, Subbakrishna DK, et al. Management of generalised convulsive status epilepticus (SE): A prospective randomised controlled study of combined treatment with intravenous lorazepam with either phenytoin, sodium valproate or levetiracetam–pilot study. Epilepsy Res 2015;114:52-8.
19. O'Connor J, Levy P, Wilson SS. Levetiracetam is as effective as phenytoin for status epilepticus with less adverse events in the ED. Crit Care Med 2015;43.12(Suppl.):6.
20. Oglesby AJ. Should etomidate be the induction agent of choice for rapid sequence intubation in the emergency department? Emerg Med J 2004;21(6):655-9.
21. Reade MC, Finfer S. Sedation and delirium in the intensive care unit. N Engl J Med 2014;370(5):444-54.
22. Makii JM, Mirski MA, Lewin JJ 3rd. Sedation and analgesia in critically ill neurologic patients. J Pharm Pract 2010;23(5):455-69.
23. Carley S, Crawford I. Towards evidence based emergency medicine: Best BETs from the Manchester Royal Infirmary. Propofol for resistant status epilepticus. Emerg Med J 2002;19(2):143-4.
24. Brown LA, Levin GM. Role of propofol in refractory status epilepticus. Ann Pharmacother 1998;32(10):1053-9.
25. Qureshi AI, Palesch YY, Barsan WG, et al. Intensive blood-pressure lowering in patients with acute cerebral hemorrhage. N Engl J Med 2016;375(11):1033-43.
26. Peacock WF, Varon J, Baumann BM, et al. CLUE: A randomized comparative effectiveness trial of IV nicardipine versus labetalol use in the emergency department. Crit Care 2011;15(3):R157.
27. Weisberg LS. Management of severe hyperkalemia. Crit Care Med 2008;36(12):3246-51.
28. Dodge HT, Grant RP, Seavey PW. The effect of induced hyperkalemia on the normal and abnormal electrocardiogram. Am Heart J 1953;45(5):725-40.
29. Chamberlain MJ. Emergency treatment of hyperkalaemia. Lancet 1964;1(7331):464-7.

30. Hinchey J, Chaves C, Appignani B, et al. A reversible posterior leukoencephalopathy syndrome. N Engl J Med 1996;334(8):494-500.
31. Min Z, Gnann JW Jr. Reversible posterior leukoencephalopathy syndrome. Intern Emerg Med 2014;9(3):341-2.
32. Fugate JE, Claassen DO, Cloft HJ, et al. Posterior reversible encephalopathy syndrome: Associated clinical and radiologic findings. Mayo Clin Proc 2010;85(5):427-32.
33. Liao PY, Lee CC, Chen CY. Hypertensive brain stem encephalopathy. Am J Emerg Med 2015;33(1):131.e5-7.
34. Finger JR, Kurczewski LM, Brophy GM. Clevidipine versus nicardipine for acute blood pressure reduction in a neuroscience intensive care population. Neurocrit Care 2016;26(2):167-73.
35. Hall JE, Mizelle HL, Hildebrandt DA, et al. Abnormal pressure natriuresis. A cause or a consequence of hypertension? Hypertension 1990;15(6 Pt 1):547-59.
36. Haas AR, Marik PE. Critical care issues for the nephrologist: Current diagnosis and management of hypertensive emergency. Semin Dial 2006;19(6):502-12.
37. Holden D, Ramich J, Timm E, et al. Safety considerations and guideline-based safe use recommendations for "bolus-dose" vasopressors in the emergency department. Ann Emerg Med 2018;71(1):83-92.
38. Weingart S. Push-dose pressors for immediate blood pressure control. Clin Exp Emerg Med 2015; 2(2):131-W2.

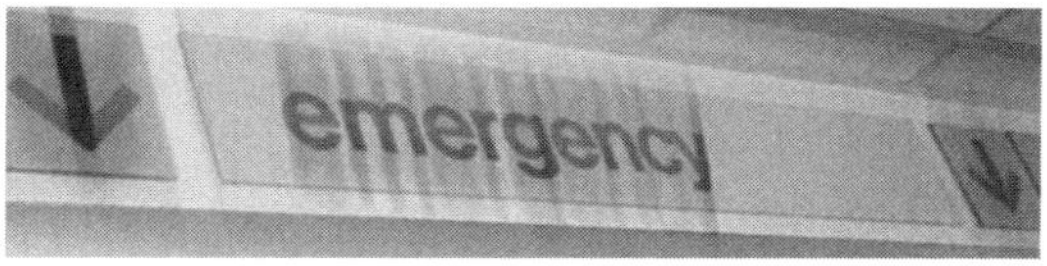

SECTION F – TRAUMA, DM, HEME, GI, HTN

Chapter 28: A 75-year-old woman with head and neck pain and vomiting

Annahieta Kalantari, DO, FACEP, FACOEP, FAAEM

Assistant Professor Emergency Medicine
Associate Program Director
Emergency Medicine Residency
Penn State Health Milton S. Hershey Medical Center
Hershey, PA

Elizabeth Barrall Werley, MD, FACEP

Assistant Professor
Program Director, Emergency Medicine Residency
Penn State Health Milton S. Hershey Medical Center
Hershey, PA

Section editor:

Joseph Shiber, MD, FACEP, FACP, FCCM

Professor
Emergency Medicine, Neurology and Surgery
Director ECMO/Acute Lung Service
Co-director NSICU and UF North ICU
UF College of Medicine–Jacksonville
Jacksonville, FL

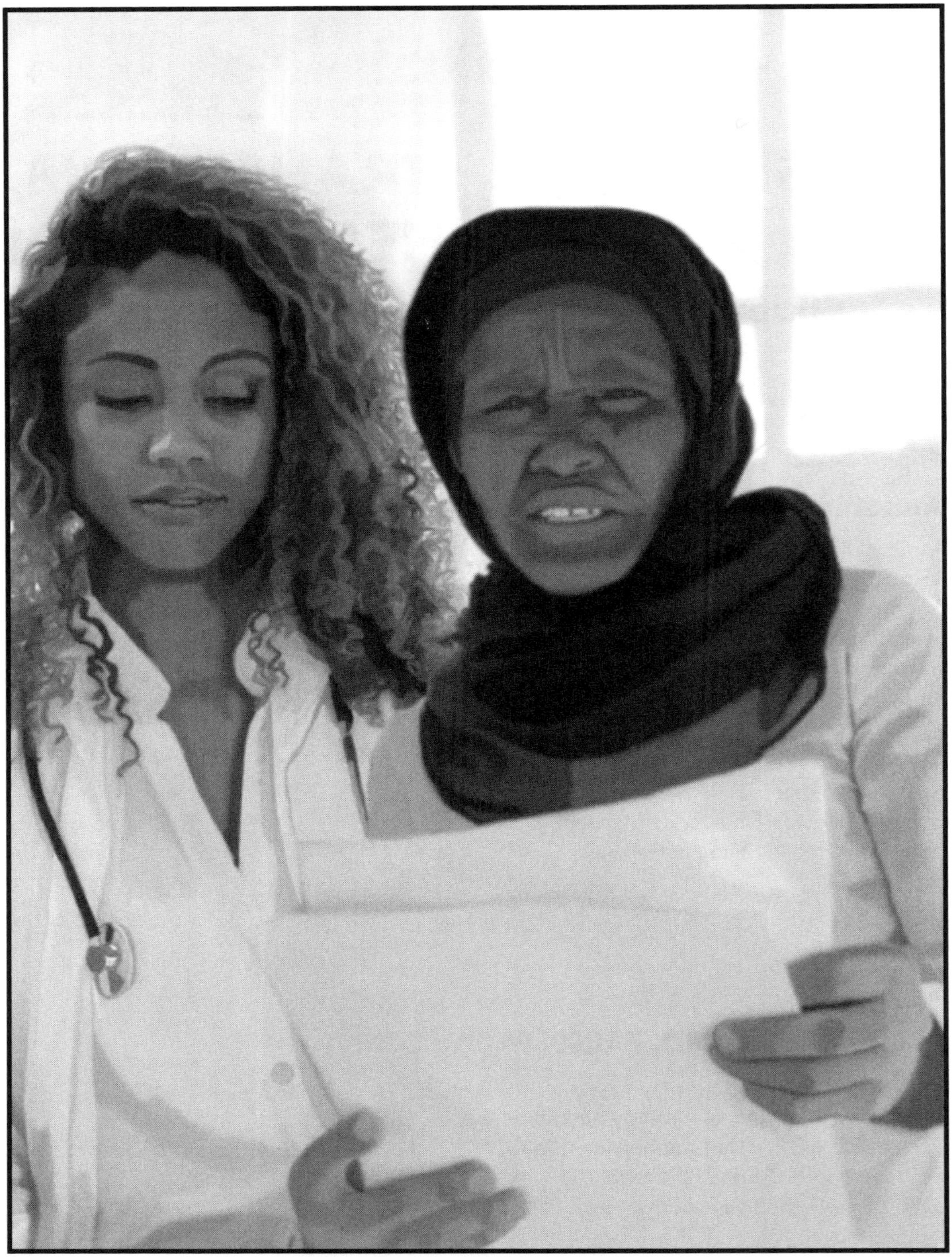

SECTION F / CHAPTER 28

A 75-year-old woman with head and neck pain and vomiting

INITIAL ED VISIT

CC: Head pain, neck pain-no trauma, vomiting, ear pain

Vitals:

Time	Temp	Rt	Pulse	Resp	Syst	Diast	Pos.	O2%	Pain
97.8	100.4	O	106	16	107	53	S	ra	10/10
23:19	103.3	O							
02:08	102.8	O							

TRIAGE (22:11): Symptoms for several days with worsening today. "What is your biggest concern during your ER visit today?" See what is wrong with her. Non-English speaking – language line waiver signed

PAST HISTORY:
NKDA
PMH: HTN
PSH: Neg
Medications: None

HPI (00:52): 75-year-old female with history of hypertension, otherwise in good general health, she does not smoke cigarettes. Several days ago, onset myalgias, chills but no documented fever, mild sore throat, nonproductive moderate cough with waxing and waning headache. Headache is generalized, gradual onset, has gone away completely and then returned. Nausea with occasional vomiting, denies diarrhea. Denies urinary symptoms, chest pain, shortness of breath, back pain or abdominal pain, blood in urine/stool, bruising, rash.

EXAM (00:54):
GA: Well-appearing; well nourished; awake, alert and cooperative, in mild pain distress
THROAT: Mildly red pharynx with no tonsillar hypertrophy.
NECK: Supple; able to touch chin to chest without difficulty or complaint. Anterior and posterior cervical chain lymphadenopathy bilaterally which is moderately tender
CARDIO: Regular rate and rhythm, no murmurs, rubs or gallops
RESP: Breath sounds clear and equal bilaterally; no wheezes, rhonchi, or rales.
Respirations are easy, no retractions or accessory muscle use.

ABD: Non-distended; non-tender, without rigidity, rebound or guarding.
SKIN: Normal for age and race; warm and dry
NEURO: Cranial nerves III-XII are intact. Sensory and motor functions are intact. Strength is 5/5 for flex/ext. in 4 extremities. Patellar DTR's are equal and intact. F > N testing is equal and nl.

Orders: IVF NS 500ml bolus then 125ml.hr, Benadryl 25mg, Morphine 4mg IVP, Reglan 10mg IVP, Ibuprofen 600mg po, Ceftriaxone 1 Gram IVPB, Zithromax 500mg IVPB

RESULTS (reviewed 02:57):
RSS – Negative, Flu A/B – negative. UA – negative, urine legionella and pneumococcus - negative

Test	Flag	Value	Units	Ref. Range
WBC		9.7	K/uL	4.6-10.2
HGB		12.9	G/DL	12.0-16.0
PLT	L	81	K/uL	142-424

Lytes: Sodium 124 and others nl. BUN/creat – WNL. Blood Cx ordered and pending

TWO VIEWS OF THE CHEST, 04/10/2010: Patchy bibasilar density, may represent atelectasis

Progress Note (02:58): The patient appears nontoxic and diagnostic studies did not suggest sepsis or a toxic state. She can be d/c home. With a history of cough and fever will continue to treat with zithromax.

DIAGNOSIS (02:59): Bronchitis

Follow-up: Follow-up with your family physician of choice or [the doctor on call] if not improved in 2-3 days. Rx Azithromycin. ACI bronchitis in English and Somali.

Discussion:

A. Questions about the history:

This patient reports a headache (HA). There is no mention of a migraine diagnosis in her past; this requires further investigation. Does she have a prior history of HA? If yes, is this one different? Does she have a headache because she is febrile or a complaint of "fever and headache," concerning for an intracranial infection? The history is cursory: "Headache is generalized, gradual onset, has gone away completely and then returned." She was given a migraine "cocktail" and that is the last we hear about the headache. In fact, though this is first item in the chief complaint, it is not even reflected in the diagnosis.

B. Is the data "lost in translation?"
She is not English speaking. In the setting of fever, this should trigger a cascade of travel history questions directed to infectious sources, as well as travel diagnoses which can present with fever, such as deep vein thrombosis (DVT) or pulmonary embolism (PE). Has she recently visited a malaria hot zone? Did she recently return from the Sub Saharan Africa meningitis belt? Are her immunizations up-to-date? Is she at risk for tuberculosis? What about questions regarding other causes of fever, such as recent instrumentation? There is no social history documented. Though admittedly uncommon in a 75-year-old, does she inject drugs or heavily consume alcohol?

The note says: "language line waiver signed," which is likely EMR-specific, but to an outsider, does this mean she signed a waiver to use a medical translator service or to decline one? And if translator services were declined, how did we determine that she understood enough to decline? Perhaps a family member was used? It is curious that the answer to the question: "What is your biggest concern during your ER visit today?" was "See what is wrong with her"—an answer given by a family member and *not* by the patient. Patients need an interpreter, yet they are frequently not utilized by healthcare providers. "Language concordance" and interpreter use likely influences a patient's comprehension of their disease process.[1]

C. Questions about documentation:
The patient has one documented heart rate of 106 but her physical exam states: "CARD: Regular rate and rhythm." Did her vitals improve at the time of the exam or was this just a "templated" exam? We do not know because there is only one full set of vitals documented. We assume the patient is being treated for a migraine given the medications that were given but we are not certain because there is not a medical decision-making note reflecting approach to diagnosis or response to therapy. There are no comments or interpretations of the lab abnormalities. All of these documentation errors are a golden egg wrapped in diamond encrusted paper to a plaintiff's attorney; a test is done, it is abnormal, the results are not acknowledged or explained.

D. Questions about medical decisions:
Our patient has an extensive ED problem list including:
- Neck pain
- Fever
- Cough
- Thrombocytopenia
- Hyponatremia

E. The diagnosis is succinct: DIAGNOSIS (02:59): Bronchitis. But how do we even know she *has* bronchitis? The Tmax was 103.3; unless there is now a secondary bacterial infection, bronchitis rarely presents with such a high fever.[2] The chest x-ray is not completely normal; it demonstrates bibasilar opacities. Possible pneumonia with tachycardia and fever meets the Sepsis 2.0 definition of severe sepsis[3] and should trigger a cascade of events including obtaining a lactate level per the Center for Medicare and Medicaid guidelines.[4] Additionally, if pneumonia is a viable diagnosis, utilizing the CURB-65 score[5] would have demonstrated that the patient falls into the moderate risk group (age and low diastolic blood pressure) and observation should have been considered.[6]

F. Lab abnormalities:

Let's say the patient does not have pneumonia (spoiler alert: she does not). What about her hyponatremia and thrombocytopenia?

1. **Hyponatremia:** The sodium level of 124 is a significant hyponatremia.[7] Is this acute or chronic? Are prior lab values available? If yes, there is no comparison noted. Her chief complaint includes headache and vomiting, perhaps these are due to the low sodium. Further discussion of the ddx of hyponatremia is detailed below, but at this point, it does not appear the provider has discovered an etiology, or even appreciated this significant lab abnormality enough to mention it in an MDM or diagnosis.
2. **Thrombocytopenia:** Her platelet count is 81,000 which classifies her as moderate thrombocytopenia.[8] Are there prior labs for comparison? Is a viral illness causing her thrombocytopenia? Perhaps medications? Might she have cirrhosis; there are no liver functions tests or coagulation studies to confirm or refute this possibility. Is this evidence of end-organ dysfunction secondary to sepsis? Could her travel history contribute to the thrombocytopenia; perhaps she was in a region where Dengue fever is prominent? Could she have a thrombotic microangiopathy such as thrombotic thrombocytopenic purpura (TTP) or hemolytic uremic syndrome (HUS)—it does not seem as if these diagnoses were considered as a peripheral smear for schistocytes was not ordered.

G. Fever: Fever is due to an alteration of the hypothalamic temperature set point which may be internal or external.[9] Infectious etiologies, such as viral, bacterial, and fungal infections, can induce production of pyrogenic cytokines which alter the hypothalamic temperature set point. There are myriad non-infectious causes of fever as well, which are often a result of the disruption in normal immune, inflammatory, and hematopoietic processes including inflammatory processes such as allergic reactions, atelectasis, and transfusion reactions; metabolic derangement from alcohol or drug withdrawal or toxidromes. Neurologic issues such as stroke, hemorrhage or trauma, or dysautonomias are known to cause fever,[9] as are vascular insults such as myocardial infarction or vascular thromboembolism (pulmonary embolism, deep vein thrombosis, microangiopathy),[10] Additionally, any type of injury to the hypothalamus, such as tumor burden, hemorrhage/trauma, or inherent hypothalamic malfunction, can cause a fever.[11] Though there is a diagnosis of "bronchitis," with the extensive and unexplored differential, we do not feel this diagnosis has been definitively established.

Section editor comments (Shiber):

Hyponatremia and thrombocytopenia are both worrisome especially in a highly febrile 75 y/o and should have warranted admission. Legionnaires' disease can have a negative urine antigen test if not serogroup 1 infection.

Author comments (Weinstock):

A seemingly innocuous presentation and diagnosis... which should have been expanded by the "slew" of additional questions that our chapter authors had for this patient! It's curious how this additional history, so obvious at an M&M conference, can be omitted at the bedside. Additionally, the logical flow of an evaluation and documentation are missing here—this patient is clearly high risk, and though the diagnosis is not obvious at this point, the need to gather further data should be...

ED BOUNCEBACK (4 days later)

CC (13:22): Nausea and vomiting X 3 days, arrives per family member via wheelchair

HPI text (14:21): She has a history of hypertension and otherwise is in good health and is a nonsmoker and nondrinker. She now complains of onset about 10 days ago of myalgias, abdominal pain, cough, sore throat, headache, fever and then developed nausea, vomiting and diarrhea the past 3 days. She was seen here in the ER 4 days ago with similar symptoms and had a fever up to 103 and unremarkable workup and was discharged on Zithromax. She was kept minimal not down since then and continues to feel ill. Her rapid strep of the throat and influenza antigen were negative 4 days ago. She later did admit that she has been taking her medicine for her hypertension but does not know the name of it. Denies stiff neck, dysuria, urinary frequency, LOC, rash, bruising, malignancy, calf pain.

PAST HISTORY:
NKDA
PMH: HTN
PSH: Neg
Medications: None

PE:

Vitals:

Time	Temp Rt	Pulse	Resp	Syst	Diast	O2 sat (RA)	Weight
13:23	100.3	129	20	99	58	95	57 kg

CONSTITUTIONAL: Alert and oriented X3, well-nourished, appears sl SOB with a normal voice, 1+ ant cervical adenopathy. No neck stiffness.
HEAD: Normocephalic; atraumatic.
EYES: PERRL, no scleral icterus.
NOSE: The nose is normal in appearance without rhinorrhea
RESP: Normal chest excursion with respiration; breath sounds clear and equal bilaterally; no wheezes, rhonchi, or rales
CARDIO: Regular rhythm, without murmurs, rub or gallop
ABD: Non-distended; sl tender upper abdomen, otherwise soft, without rigidity, rebound or guarding
SKIN: Normal for age and race; warm and dry; no apparent lesions
EXT: No ankle edema or calf tenderness

Author comments (Weinstock):

So, what's the big deal? How did this case make it into a critical care book; a non-English speaking patient presents with multiple complaints... then bounces back with multiple complaints... But a look below the surface reveals some troubling signs of impending problems: she is extremely tachycardic, her blood pressure is low, and the antibiotic prescribed does not seem to be working. Is it possible that her fever is not related to infection? We are standing in the footsteps of the emergency provider without a diagnosis. We are at:

DECISION POINT A – YOU ARE FACED WITH 3 QUESTIONS:

1. **What is the differential diagnosis?**
2. **Which IV fluid is best?**
3. **What testing should be ordered?**

What does the literature say?

Q#1: What is the differential diagnosis?

Focusing just on the bounceback visit, we are faced with an elderly female complaining of myalgias, abdominal pain, cough, sore throat, headache, fever who then developed nausea, vomiting and diarrhea and who is now febrile, tachycardic and hypotensive. Her differential diagnosis is extensive. Infectious etiologies take precedence including but not exclusive to meningitis, encephalitis, bacteremia, pneumonia, urinary tract infection, ascending cholangitis or other intra-abdominal processes. However, noninfectious causes of fever should be considered including drugs and other toxins, malignancies and thrombosis. Chronic salicylate toxicity can mimic sepsis.[12] The patient speaks Somali, could she have primary HIV versus an infection secondary to immunocompromise?[13]

When we add information from the previous visit, we note a platelet count of 81,000 and sodium level of 124. Taking this into consideration, thrombotic thrombocytopenia, adrenal insufficiency, pituitary apoplexy, brain mass, cirrhosis, hemolytic uremic syndrome and antiphospholipid antibody syndrome should be added to our differential.

Q#2: Which IV fluid is best?

This patient is in shock. Given the history of vomiting and diarrhea, it is likely hypovolemic in nature. She requires intravenous fluids—but which fluid is best?

Traditionally, crystalloids have been the first line resuscitation fluids administered with normal saline being the most common.[14-16] It is abundant and inexpensive. However, multiple studies have demonstrated that normal saline is associated with hyperchloremic metabolic acidosis,[15] damage to the endothelial glycocalyx,[17] acute kidney injury, decreased glomerular blood flow[18,19] and interstitial edema with third spacing. When comparing the chemical composition of normal saline to that of human serum, it is the most physiologically *abnormal* fluid choice.[16] There has been great debate surrounding the question of whether balanced crystalloid fluids should be utilized in large volume resuscitations. Both the SALT-ED[20] and SMART[21] trials investigated this question. Both studies were single-centered, unblinded, randomized cross-over trials.

The SALT-ED trial investigated primarily hospital-free days and secondarily major adverse kidney effects in noncritically ill patients receiving either normal saline or balanced crystalloid (lactated

Ringer's solution or Plasma-Lyte A). The final sample size of the SALT-ED trial was 13,347 with 6,708 assigned to balanced crystalloid and 6,639 assigned to saline. Results demonstrated patients in the balanced-crystalloid group had low chloride and higher bicarbonate levels with less hyperchloremia and acidemia when compared to saline. There was no difference in the number of hospital-free days between the two groups but patients in the balanced-crystalloid group had a lower incidence of major adverse kidney events within 30 days and a lower composite outcome of kidney related death, renal-replacement therapy and persistent renal dysfunction.

The SMART trial investigated the proportion of patients who met one or more criteria for a major adverse kidney event within 30 days: in-hospital death before ICU discharge or at 30 days or at 60 days, ICU-free days, ventilator-free days, vasopressor-free days, days alive and days free of renal-replacement therapy during 28 days after enrollment in critically ill patients receiving either balanced-crystalloid or saline. A total of 15,802 patients were enrolled with 7,942 in the balanced crystalloid group and 7,860 in the saline. In-hospital deaths were similar between the two groups 6.6% vs 7.3% (OR 0.89; 95% CI , 0.78–1.02). There was no difference between ICU-free, vasopressor-free, ventilator-free and renal-replacement free days. However, 14.3% of the balanced-crystalloid group vs. 15.4% of the saline group had major adverse kidney event (OR 0.90; 95% CI, 0.82–0.99; P=0.04). Among patients with sepsis, the 30-day in-hospital mortality was 25.2% with balanced crystalloids and 29.4% with saline (OR 0.80; 95% CI, 0.67–0.97; P=0.02).

Consulting editor comments (Weingart):

Every ED has one fluid that's "everywhere," and then they have another fluid that's "somewhere." In most places the "everywhere" fluid is normal saline. I would like to see that switched. I would like to see LR on all the carts and then normal saline available as a few bags "somewhere." Even if you don't believe the studies yet, there's no downside to making LR the primary fluid in the ED.

Now where would you want normal saline first? One is in brain injury patients, because we don't want to decrease their sodium down to the 130, which LR will eventually do. Another is in patients who are alkalotic, for example a patient with a lot of vomiting, though nothing bad will happen from giving LR. There was a past concern about giving LR with a blood product, but that's been disproven, so if you accidentally gave LR with a blood product, it's okay. But, just to make everyone happy, consider using normal saline.

Q#3: What testing should be ordered?

For the evaluation of sepsis, our work-up will include CBC, BMP, hepatic function panel, coagulation studies, blood cultures, lactate level, a urine analysis and a chest x-ray. Procalcitonin can be considered since she was treated for a presumptive bacterial lower respiratory tract infection.[22] Depending on the results, we can consider the addition of a lumbar puncture and CT scan of the chest, abdomen and pelvis to evaluate for the source of infection which will also offer insight on end-organ dysfunction and severity of illness. To evaluate the hyponatremia, we can add serum osmolality, urine sodium and urine creatinine. Because of a consideration for brain mass and pituitary apoplexy, a head CT should be ordered, especially if considering a lumbar puncture. A salicylate level should be ordered in addition to other co-ingestants such as acetaminophen. Additionally, with the thrombocytopenia on her last visit, we should consider lactate dehydrogenase, peripheral smear for schistocytes, fibrin and fibrinogen levels.

What did the actual provider do?

Labs:

- WBC = 35 (H)
- Hb 12 (L)
- MCV 77 (L)
- Plt 8 (L)
- Na+ 121 (L)
- Ion. Ca++ 1.00 (nl. 1.15-1.37),
- ABG 7.52/25/47 (RA)

Vitals:

Time	Temp	Pulse	Resp	Syst	Diast	O2 sat (RA)
16:03		142	28	82	52	95

Author comments (Weinstock):

The BP has dropped to 82/58 and she is significantly more tachycardic at 142bpm. Her daughter has just arrived and shared that she is a lab tech, and "knows sick when I see it." You are in the room with the extended family who are trying to interpret, the patient is struggling to keep her eyes open. It is clear she is altered; her condition is worsening before your eyes.

The daughter addresses you, a bit hysterical, "Doctor, my mother is a fighter and I can't even get her to answer my questions. She is getting worse, not better—*do something!*" We are at:

DECISION POINT B – YOU ARE FACED WITH 5 QUESTIONS:

1. **She has severe leukocytosis, hyponatremia, and thrombocytopenia. Which should be addressed first?**
2. **Is she septic?**
3. **What is causing the hyponatremia?**
4. **Are additional tests indicated?**
5. **Should she receive a platelet transfusion?**

What does the literature say?

Q#1: She has severe leukocytosis, hyponatremia and thrombocytopenia. Which should be addressed first?

Her hyponatremia is the most acutely life-threatening abnormality. Hyponatremia can lead to cerebral edema, seizure and subsequent death. Chronic hyponatremia is defined as hyponatremia present for greater than 48 hours. This patient is presenting at 10+ days of symptoms. She should be given isotonic fluids with the goal of slowly correcting her sodium due to risk of osmotic demyelination.[23] This is a delicate balance because the patient is also hypotensive and requires resuscitation. Early vasopressor therapy should be considered.

It is difficult to determine whether her symptoms are secondary to her hyponatremia or a different underlying, but as yet undiagnosed problem.[24,25] Correction of hyponatremia with hypertonic saline is reserved for the severely encephalopathic patients and seizures/status epilepticus thought to be due to hyponatremia in the setting of concentrated urine and at a very calculated rate of administration.[23]

This patient's leukocytosis can be reassessed after additional testing returns. Lastly, the patient is thrombocytopenic but is not bleeding; if she starts to bleed, this will require prompt attention.

Section editor comments (Shiber):

Though the hyponatremia is certainly concerning, the circulatory shock (HR 142 and BP 82/52) is the most life-threatening problem, and 2nd would be hypoxemia (PO_2 of 47 on ABG). Spontaneous serious bleeding (intracranial hemorrhage or a GI bleed) occurs when platelets are < 10K. I agree with continuing to evaluate the underlying etiology and holding off on transfusion at this time as she does not appear to be actively bleeding.

Q#2: Is she septic?

Leukocytosis alone will not define sepsis regardless of whether we are using Sepsis 2.0,[3] Sepsis 3.0[26] or the CMS definitions4 of sepsis. Other factors come into play, for example, we must actually suspect infection! Let us assume she has an infection. If using Sepsis 2.0, she has severe sepsis at minimum with 2/4 SIRS criteria (leukocytosis, tachycardia, tachypnea but is just shy of fever) making her septic. Her thrombocytopenia and altered mental status are evidence of end-organ dysfunction elevating her to severe sepsis. If these vitals persist after receiving IV fluids, then she meets criteria for septic shock. If using Sepsis 3.0, the patient meets all 3 qSOFA criteria: altered mental status, systolic blood pressure < 90mmHg and a respiratory rate > 22 (although the authors of Sepsis 3.0 state this should not be used as a definition and should not trigger management pathways).[26] If using the CMS definitions, she will meet the definition of severe sepsis in the setting of infection. An initial lactate of 4 or hypotension after fluids would meet septic shock criteria, but again, we have not yet diagnosed an infection.

Q#3: What is causing the hyponatremia?

Hyponatremia is defined as a plasma sodium concentration <135mEq/L. It is found in 20–30% of hospitalized patients and 7.7% of outpatients.24,25 To better differentiate the etiology, it is commonly broken down to 3 categories based on the patient's volume status:

- Hypovolemic hyponatremia
- Euvolemic hyponatremia
- Hypervolemic hyponatremia[24]

Our patient does not appear to be volume-overloaded as her lung exam is clear, she does not have a gallop rhythm, there is no peripheral edema and she has no history of heart failure or cirrhosis with ascites. That leaves us with hypovolemic and euvolemic hyponatremia. Although the patient has a history of vomiting and has a fairly low blood pressure, there are no documented physical exam findings consistent with dehydration. Hypovolemic hyponatremia is further differentiated based on the urine sodium concentration. This was not tested for on either visit, so we cannot comment.

But there are some common causes of hypovolemic hyponatremia that may apply. First, she is noted to have a history of hypertension, though her record states that she is not taking any medications, but perhaps this documentation got "lost in translation." If she is dehydrated, she could also have ketonuria. Ketones in urine are associated with fat metabolism (lipolysis) when all glycogen stores have been utilized. It is due to starvation and not dehydration; pregnant women with hyperemesis may be both dehydrated and have ketosis/ketonuria so they need both fluids (IV or PO) and something to eat, which may contribute to their hyponatremia. Another possibility could be "cerebral salt wasting" due to intracranial disease.

Given the constellation of symptoms, the patient seems less likely to have a subarachnoid hemorrhage or traumatic brain injury, but given her fever and headache with nausea and vomiting, both encephalitis and meningitis are possible. She could also have nonrenal causes, such as volume loss from her vomiting and diarrhea. Euvolemic hyponatremia may be due to both stress and drugs. Another possibility is syndrome of inappropriate antidiuretic hormone (SIADH) secretion. SIADH can be caused by pulmonary infections, encephalitis or meningitis (still possible given her constellation of symptoms), malignancy, as well as nonspecific causes such as nausea, pain, stress, or an idiopathic etiology. Acute hyponatremia is likely to present with more severe symptoms, whereas chronic hyponatremia is typically less severe; the timing of onset will dictate further management.[23,24]

Thiazide diuretics are known to cause hyponatremia, especially after therapy initiation.[23-25] Angiotensin-converting enzyme inhibitors (ACEIs) and angiotensin receptor blockers (ARBs) are also known to cause hyponatremia.[7,27] Each of the above is commonly prescribed in the treatment of hypertension so it's possible we have an easy answer to the hyponatremia.

Q#4: Are additional tests indicated?

These are the results we have so far: WBC 35, Hb 12, MCV 77, Plt 8, Na+ 121, blood Cx – neg., Ion. Ca++ 1.00 (nl. 1.15–1.37), ABG 7.52/25/47 (RA). Though this is a good start, we also recommend a hepatic function panel, coagulation studies, lactate levels, urine analysis, serum osmolality, urine sodium, urine creatinine, aspirin or acetaminophen levels, lactate dehydrogenase, peripheral smear for schistocytes, fibrin or fibrinogen levels. CT brain is not completed. We cannot do a lumbar puncture at this time as we do not know if there is elevated intracranial pressure,[28,29] and in fact would not do an LP with platelet count < 50–75. A chest x-ray has also not been obtained. Yes! A whole lot of additional tests are indicated.

Q#5: Should she receive a platelet transfusion?

The American Association of Blood Banks (AABB) recommends platelet transfusions in:

- Hospitalized adult patients with therapy-induced hypoproliferative thrombocytopenia with a platelet count of 10×10^9 cells/L or less to reduce bleeding.
- Patients having elective central venous catheter placement with a platelet count of 20×10^9 cells/L or less.
- Patients having elective diagnosis lumbar puncture with platelet counts less than 50×10^9 cells/L or less.
- Patients having major neuroaxial surgery with a platelet count of 50 x 109 cells/L or less.[30]

These recommendations were based on a systematic review meta-analysis conducted by Kumar, et al.[31] So, based on the AABB, at this point the answer is… maybe. She is not actively bleeding, but she is hypotensive and has fever and altered mental status.

With that being said, does she really need a platelet transfusion at this time? The only criteria above would be for placement of a central line; if she remains hypotensive after fluid resuscitation, she will require vasopressors, but these can be administered peripherally. Loubani, et al. published a systematic review meta-analysis in the *Journal of Critical Care* in 2015 that evaluated all case reports of tissue injury and vasopressor extravasation via peripheral IV vs. a central venous catheter. The study found that 85.3% of tissue injury events occurred when vasopressor administration was located in a site distal to the antecubital or popliteal fossae. Additionally, the average duration of vasopressor infusion before tissue injury occurred was 55.9 hours with a median of 24 hours.[32] If vasopressors are needed, these should be able to be given peripherally.

What did the actual provider do?

- CT chest: CMG with some CHF, no infiltrate
- CT abd/pelvis: Negative
- Meds: Zosyn IV, gentamicin IV, vancomycin IV, Decadron 10mg ivp
- Order: Platelet transfusion 4 units

What happened to the patient?

The mental status continues to deteriorate. The etiology of her symptoms has not yet been determined. We are at:

DECISION POINT C – YOU ARE FACED WITH 4 QUESTIONS:

1. **The patient is rapidly decompensating with unstable vitals and altered consciousness. Is intubation indicated, or should NiPPV be considered?**
2. **Which meds should be used for induction and paralysis?**
3. **Could she have thrombotic thrombocytopenic purpura (TTP)?**
4. **Are there risks with the platelet transfusion in TTP?**

What does the literature say?

Q#1: The patient is rapidly decompensating with unstable vitals and altered consciousness. Is intubation indicated, or should NiPPV be considered?

A low GCS is associated with a higher risk of aspiration[33-35] and ensuing pneumonitis. Our patient has progressively worsened while in the ED; she is a candidate for intubation to prevent aspiration. But let's take a step back. First of all, does she want to be intubated? Because the patient is altered, we are unable to ask her directly but can ask her daughter who is at the bedside. If the answer is yes, let us next take note of the fact that the patient is hypotensive and tachycardic, giving her an elevated shock index with an associated higher risk of post-intubation cardiac arrest.[36-38] She is a patient where push-dose vasopressors should be considered.[39]

Maybe we should use NiPPV to help? Prior studies have demonstrated the use of NiPPV to avoid or delay intubation in critically ill patients with pulmonary edema and acute or chronic COPD exacerbation.[40] This prompted research in evaluating the use of NiPPV in critically ill patients presenting with a variety of conditions.[41-43] However, many of these studies excluded patients with a low GCS. The British Thoracic Society guidelines outright state: "NiPPV is not indicated in impaired consciousness."[44] If our patient was altered secondary to respiratory acidosis or hypoxia,

NiPPV would be a reasonable option. Her pH is 7.52. She is not hypercarbic with a PCO_2 of 25. Her PAO_2 is low at 47 leading one to question if this is a VBG instead of an ABG given that her pulse ox is 95% on room air. We do not have a cause yet for her declining mentation. Because of this, she will likely continue to decompensate, and these authors recommend against using NiPPV.

Section editor comments (Shiber):

The blood gas is unlikely a VBG since that would indicate a profound alkalosis as her arterial pH would then be ~7.60.

Q#2: Which meds should be used for induction and paralysis?

Our patient is hypotensive. It is most likely due to decreased systemic vascular resistance vs. hypovolemia. In either case, induction with any medication that would decrease sympathetic tone will likely lead to a peri-intubation cardiac arrest. Ketamine will not decrease this patient's sympathetic tone and is a good choice for an induction agent.

Q#3: Could she have thrombotic thrombocytopenic purpura (TTP)?

The classic pentad of TTP (below) is helpful to make a diagnosis, but note that up to 35% of patients do not have neurologic signs at presentation. Additionally, renal abnormalities and fever do not occur commonly.[45] Headache is included as part of the pentad under CNS Abnormalities —it is very common:

- thrombocytopenia
- microangiopathic hemolytic anemia
- neurologic abnormalities
- renal impairment
- fever

Waiting for this classic pentad results in delay of diagnosis.[46] Updated diagnostic criteria state that thrombocytopenia and microangiopathic hemolytic anemia will by themselves make the diagnosis.[45,46] If jaundice and or pallor is present, this may suggest the presence of hemolytic anemia. However, in the absence of physical exam findings, laboratory tests are required to confirm microangiopathic hemolytic anemia. Schistocytes and reticulocytes on peripheral blood smear, increased serum lactate dehydrogenase levels, elevated indirect bilirubin and a negative Coombs test are suggestive of a microangiopathic hemolytic anemia.[46] Our patient has thrombocytopenia but does not appear pale or jaundiced, and we do not have other confirmatory lab tests of TTP at this time.

Section editor comments (Shiber):

MAHA (microangiopathic hemolytic anemia) is a category of small vessel (capillary)-induced anemias that include: TTP, HUS, HELLP, DIC, and malignant hypertension; all of specific etiologies lead to endothelial injury and indiscriminate platelet activation causing in-situ thrombosis and tissue bed malperfusion and hypoxia. LDH will be elevated early and haptoglobin will decrease early, but indirect bili may not be elevated initially.

Pathophysiologically, platelets adhere creating small microthrombi that indiscriminately occlude capillary beds leading to very vague presenting signs and symptoms. The most common signs and symptoms are nonspecific and include:

- abdominal pain
- nausea, vomiting
- weakness
- headache[46]

Other signs and symptoms include bruising, bleeding, confusion, visual problems, fatigue, arthralgia, proteinuria, microhematuria, chest pain and shortness of breath.[45] Thrombocytopenia in the setting of any combination of these or other nonspecific complaints should prompt the addition of a peripheral blood smear and lactate dehydrogenase level to confirm the diagnosis of TTP and initiate treatment.

TTP is treated with plasma exchange therapy, which reduces the mortality rate from 90% to 10–20%.[8,30,31,47-49] However, the therapy cannot be initiated if the disease process is not suspected. The reason for the updated diagnostic criteria is to increase sensitivity in capturing the patients who can be treated. A peripheral blood smear is essential in order to make the diagnosis.

Q#4: Are there risks with platelet transfusion in TTP?

Yes. For the non-TTP patient, platelet transfusions are not benign due to associated allergic reactions, febrile nonhemolytic reactions and sepsis from bacterial contaminants (they are stored at room temperature putting them at risk for bacterial growth).[30]

In 1981, there were 4 reported cases of bad outcomes in patients with TTP after they were transfused with platelets. Three patients became comatose after the transfusion,[50] and 1 woman died secondary to "vascular lesions in the brain that were comprised chiefly of masses of platelets" leading authors to conclude these were secondary to platelets received in her transfusion 30 minutes prior to her CVA and subsequent death.[51] After these reports, platelet transfusions were avoided in patients with TTP.

In 2009, Swisher and colleagues reported the results of a retrospective review of the Oklahoma TTP-HUS Registry that evaluated adverse events in patients with TTP-HUS who received platelet transfusions vs. those that did not. This registry accounted for all patients who received plasma exchange at every hospital in the state of Oklahoma from January 1, 1989 to December 31, 2007. The registry included 382 consecutive patients, but after exclusion criteria were applied, 54 patients were included in the final analysis. Thirty-three patients received platelet transfusions and 21 did not. There were no significant differences between the two groups regarding demographics and clinical features. There were no p-value-based significant differences in adverse outcomes, but absolute values did demonstrate a difference. Severe neurologic abnormalities including coma, stroke, seizure, and TIA were higher in the platelet transfusion group (52% vs. 33% $p=0.190$). Mortalities were 24% for both groups.[49]

Another single-centered retrospective review evaluated adverse outcomes of platelet transfusions in patients with TTP and found no difference in complications but found a higher mortality in the group that received platelet transfusions [13% (3/23) patients vs. 3.1% (1/32) patients, $p=0.298$]. A more detailed analysis of the 4 deaths revealed none of the patients died from a thrombotic event. One patient died of acute respiratory distress secondary to graft-versus-host disease after allogeneic stem cell transplantation for acute lymphoblastic leukemia. Another had HIV infection with recurrent Burkitt's lymphoma and seizure and died of a pontine hemorrhagic infarction. Another had complicated past medical history with recent CVA and new sinonasal carcinoma with brain involvement and died of disease progression and tongue asphyxiation. The one patient without transfusion had cardiac arrest secondary to anemia and respiratory failure.[48]

Section editor comments (Shiber):

"Thrombotic" here probably means LARGE-Vessel occlusion but that is *not* the pathology in TTP—it is capillary bed occlusion and it will worsen with the more platelets that are consumed. "Fanning the flames of the Fire" is the analogy that best describes what occurs when patients with TTP are transfused.

The currently accepted treatment for TTP is plasma exchange therapy which requires placement of a large-bore CVC catheter. With regard to bleeding complications, there was no consistent relationship between platelet count and bleeding. Major bleeding risks occurred in patients who had blind catheter insertion and or had the catheter inserted in a noncompressible site.[47] Rizvi, et al. report that out of a total of 92 central venous catheter placements, major catheter-related complication occurred in one patient with a platelet count of 83,000/uL who died of hemorrhage after elective insertion of a subclavian catheter to replace an initial femoral catheter.[52]

The take away from these studies is that there is no very high quality study that definitively states platelet transfusion in TTP is safe or unsafe. Both reviews had small numbers and were from a single-patient database. A large-bore central venous catheter can be relatively safely placed under ultrasound guidance in a compressible vein in the absence of a platelet transfusion.

Section editor comments (Shiber):

Plasma exchange can also be accomplished without a temporary HD catheter by using 2 reliable, large-bore, antecubital peripheral IV's. Another option while waiting for plasmapheresis is to give FFP; while it won't remove the antibody inhibitor of ADAMTS 13, it will give some normal protein enzyme activity to help control the vWF activation. This is considered a temporizing measure while calling in personnel to do the plasma exchange.

Hospital course:
(22:27) Critical care consult: Declining mental status and respiratory failure > the patient has been intubated and pressors will be continued.

(09:35) The next morning: Hematology:

- I have personally reviewed peripheral blood film which shows significant granulocytosis with a predominance of bands with some promyelocytes and metamyelocytes, there were nucleated red cells and there was a paucity of platelets. The primary abnormality; however, was significant schistocytosis.
- The patient has a microangiopathic hemolytic anemia in the context of significant thrombocytopenia. The patient also has new neurologic changes. All of this together is convincing evidence that the patient has thrombotic thrombocytopenic purpura. I have already contacted the Red Cross, and we are going to start plasmapheresis immediately. She has already had a dialysis catheter placed by Dr. _____ who was seeing the patient concurrently with me.
- The patient clearly is critically ill, and time is of the essence so I have been in contact multiple times with the Red Cross to tell them they need to get her pheresed immediately. I am going to

pherese her with 3 liters of cryo-poor. She has already been typed and crossed. I have discussed with the staff that she should get no more platelet transfusions and we will obviously follow her along closely. We will start out with daily pheresis.

Discharge summary: 75-year-old female patient who was seen in the ED with flu-like symptoms and then returned with TTP-HUS and sepsis. Hospital course complicated by respiratory failure, ARF, and bacteremia.

Chapter summary:

1. The initial documentation could have been better, additionally there is no medical decision-making (MDM) note. Recognizing that this patient was high risk may have prompted additional history.
2. Address abnormal labs; her hyponatremia and thrombocytopenia were not explored.
3. Consider noninfectious causes of fever, especially if there are other abnormalities such as thrombocytponia.
4. The classic pentad of TTP is:
    - thrombocytopenia
    - microangiopathic hemolytic anemia
    - neurologic abnormalities
    - renal impairment
    - fever

References:

1. Baker D, Parker R, Williams M, et al. Use and effectiveness of interpreters in an emergency department. JAMA 1996;275(10):783-8.
2. Kinkade S, Long NA. Acute bronchitis. Am Fam Physician 2016;94(7):560-5.
3. Dellinger RP, Levy MM, Carlet JM, et al. Surviving sepsis campaign: International guidelines for management of severe sepsis and septic shock: 2008. Crit Care Med 2008;36(1):296-327.
4. Centers for Medicaid and Medicare Services. Sepsis Bundle Project (SEP). Specifications manual for national hospital inpatient quality measures discharges 10-01-15 (4Q15) through 06-30-16 (2Q16). https://www.qualitynet.org/inpatient/specifications-manuals#tab8 Accessed 11/11/16.
5. Lim WS, van der Eerden MM, Laing R, et al. Defining community acquired pneumonia severity on presentation to hospital: An international derivation and validation study. Thorax 2003;58(5):377-82.
6. Sharp AL, Jones JP, Wu I, et al. CURB-65 Performance among admitted and discharged emergency department patients with community-acquired pneumonia. Acad Emerg Med 2016;23(4):400-5.
7. Sra J, Repp AB. Hyponatremia. Hosp Med Clin 2012;1(2):e199-e208.
8. Williamson DR, Albert M, Heels-Ansdell D, et al. Thrombocytopenia in critically ill patients receiving thromboprophylaxis: Frequency, risk factors, and outcomes. Chest 2013;144(4):1207-15.
9. Dinarello C, Porat R. Fever. In: Harrison's principles of internal medicine. 19th ed. New York, NY: McGraw-Hill;2014.

10. Kline JA. Pulmonary embolism and deep vein thrombosis. In: Walls R, Hockenberger R, Gausche-Hill M, eds. Rosen's emergency medicine: Concepts and clinical practice. 9th ed. Philadelphia, PA: Elsevier;2018:1051-66.
11. Kayser J, Lanken P. Day-to-day management of the critical care patient. In: Lanken P, Manaker S, Kohl B, Hanson C, eds. The intensive care unit manual. 2nd ed. Philadelphia, PA: Elsevier Saunders;2014:129-33e.
12. Leatherman JW, Schmitz PG. Fever, Hyperdynamic shock and multiple-System organ failure. Chest 1991;100(5):1391-6.
13. Gokengin D, Doroudi F, Tohme J, et al. HIV/AIDS: Trends in the Middle East and North Africa region. Int J Infect Dis 2016;44:66-73.
14. Brunkhorst FM, Engel C, Bloos F, et al. Intensive insulin therapy and pentastarch resuscitation in severe sepsis. N Engl J Med 2008;358(2):125-39.
15. Madhusudan P, Tirupakuzhi Vijayaraghavan BK, Cove ME. Fluid resuscitation in sepsis: Reexamining the paradigm. Biomed Res Int 2014;2014:984082.
16. Myburgh JA, Mythen MG. Resuscitation fluids. N Engl J Med 2013;369(13):1243-51.
17. Glassford NJ, Eastwood GM, Bellomo R., et al. Physiological changes after fluid bolus therapy in sepsis: A systematic review of contemporary data. Crit Care 2014;18(6):696.
18. Chowdhury AH, Cox EF, Francis ST, et al. A randomized, controlled, double-blind crossover study on the effects of 2-L infusions of 0.9% saline and plasma-lyte(R) 148 on renal blood flow velocity and renal cortical tissue perfusion in healthy volunteers. Ann Surg 2012;256(1):18-24.
19. Yunos NM, Bellomo R, Story D, Kellum J. Bench-to-bedside review: Chloride in critical illness. Crit Care 2010;14(4):226.
20. Self WH, Semler MW, Wanderer JP, et al. Balanced crystalloids versus saline in noncritically ill adults. N Engl J Med 2018;378(9):819-28.
21. Semler MW, Self WH, Wanderer JP, et al. Balanced crystalloids versus saline in critically ill adults. N Engl J Med 2018;378(9):829-39.
22. Huang DT, Yealy DM, Filbin MR, et al. Procalcitonin-guided use of antibiotics for lower respiratory tract infection. N Engl J Med 2018;379(20):1972-3.
23. Adrogué HJ, Madias NE. The challenge of hyponatremia. J Am Soc Nephrol 2012;23(7):1140-8.
24. Mount, D. Fluid and electrolyte disturbances. In: Kasper D, Fauci A, Hauser S, et al, eds. Harrison's Principles of Internal Medicine. 19th ed. New York, NY:McGraw-Hill;2014.
25. Rondon-Berrios H, Agaba EI, Tzamaloukas AH. Hyponatremia: Pathophysiology, classification, manifestations and management. Int Urol Nephrol 2014;46(11):2153-65.
26. Singer M, Deutschman CS, Seymour CW, et al. The Third International Consensus definitions for sepsis and septic shock (Sepsis-3). JAMA 2016;315(8):801-10.
27. Mohan S, Gu S, Parikh A, et al. Prevalence of hyponatremia and association with mortality: Results from NHANES. Am J Med 2013;126(12):1127-37. e1121.
28. Gopal AK, Whitehouse JD, Simel DL, et al. Cranial computed tomography before lumbar puncture: A prospective clinical evaluation. Arch Intern Med 1999;159(22):2681-5.
29. Hasbun R, Abrahams J, Jekel J, et al. Computed tomography of the head before lumbar puncture in adults with suspected meningitis. N Engl J Med 2001;345(24):1727-33.
30. Kaufman RM, Djulbegovic B, Gernsheimer T, et al. Platelet transfusion: A clinical practice guideline from the AABB. Ann Intern Med 2015;162(3):205-13.
31. Kumar A, Mhaskar R, Grossman BJ, et al. Platelet transfusion: A systematic review of the clinical evidence. Transfusion 2015;55(5):1116-27; quiz 1115.

32. Loubani OM, Green RS. A systematic review of extravasation and local tissue injury from administration of vasopressors through peripheral intravenous catheters and central venous catheters. J Crit Care 2015;30(3):653 659-617.
33. Christ A, Arranto CA, Schindler C, et al. Incidence, risk factors, and outcome of aspiration pneumonitis in ICU overdose patients. Intensive Care Med 2006;32(9):1423-7.
34. Eizadi-Mood N, Saghaei M, Alfred S, et al. Comparative evaluation of Glasgow Coma Score and gag reflex in predicting aspiration pneumonitis in acute poisoning. J Crit Care 2009;24(3):470 479-415.
35. Miller CD, Rebuck JA, Ahern JW, et al. Daily evaluation of macroaspiration in the critically ill post-trauma patient. Curr Surg 2005;62(5):504-8.
36. Heffner AC, Swords DS, Neale MN, et al. Incidence and factors associated with cardiac arrest complicating emergency airway management. Resuscitation 2013;84(11):1500-4.
37. Kim WY, Kwak MK, Ko BS, et al. Factors associated with the occurrence of cardiac arrest after emergency tracheal intubation in the emergency department. PLoS One 2014;9(11):e112779.
38. Wardi G, Villar J, Nguyen T, et al. Factors and outcomes associated with inpatient cardiac arrest following emergent endotracheal intubation. Resuscitation 2017;121:76-80.
39. Weingart S. Push-dose pressors for immediate blood pressure control. Clin Exp Emerg Med 2015;2(2):131-2.
40. Brochard L, Mancebo J, Elliott M. Noninvasive ventilation for acute respiratory failure. Eur Respir J 2002;19(4):712-21.
41. Correa TD, Sanches PR, de Morais LC, et al. Performance of noninvasive ventilation in acute respiratory failure in critically ill patients: A prospective, observational, cohort study. BMC Pulm Med 2015;15:144.
42. Meeder AM, Tjan DH, van Zanten AR. Noninvasive and invasive positive pressure ventilation for acute respiratory failure in critically ill patients: A comparative cohort study. J Thorac Dis 2016;8(5):813-25.
43. Schnell D, Timsit J-F, Darmon M, et al. Noninvasive mechanical ventilation in acute respiratory failure: Trends in use and outcomes. Intensive Care Med 2014;40(4):582-91.
44. Baudouin S, Blumenthal S, Cooper B, et al. BTS Guideline: Non-invasive ventilation in acute respiratory failure. Thorax 2002;57(3):192-211.
45. Scully M, Hunt BJ, Benjamin S, et al. Guidelines on the diagnosis and management of thrombotic thrombocytopenic purpura and other thrombotic microangiopathies. Br J Haematol 2012;158(3):323-35.
46. George JN. Thrombotic thrombocytopenic purpura. N Engl J Med 2006;354(18):1927-35.
47. Duffy SM, Coyle TE. Platelet transfusions and bleeding complications associated with plasma exchange catheter placement in patients with presumed thrombotic thrombocytopenic purpura. J Clin Apher 2013;28(5):356-8.
48. Otrock ZK, Liu C, Grossman BJ. Platelet transfusion in thrombotic thrombocytopenic purpura. Vox Sang 2015;109(2):168-72.
49. Swisher KK, Terrell DR, Vesely SK, et al. Clinical outcomes after platelet transfusions in patients with thrombotic thrombocytopenic purpura. Transfusion 2009;49(5):873-87.
50. Gottschall JL, Pisciotta AV, Darin J, et al. Thrombotic thrombocytopenic purpura: Experience with whole blood exchange transfusion. Semin Thromb Hemost 1981;7(1):25-32.
51. Harkness DR, Byrnes JJ, Lian EC, et al. Hazard of platelet transfusion in thrombotic

thrombocytopenic purpura. JAMA 1981;246(17):1931-3.
52. Rizvi M, Vesely S, George J, et al. Complications of plasma exchange in 71 consecutive patients treated for clinically suspected thrombotic thrombocytopenic purpura-hemolytic-uremic syndrome. Transfusion 2000;40(8):896-901.

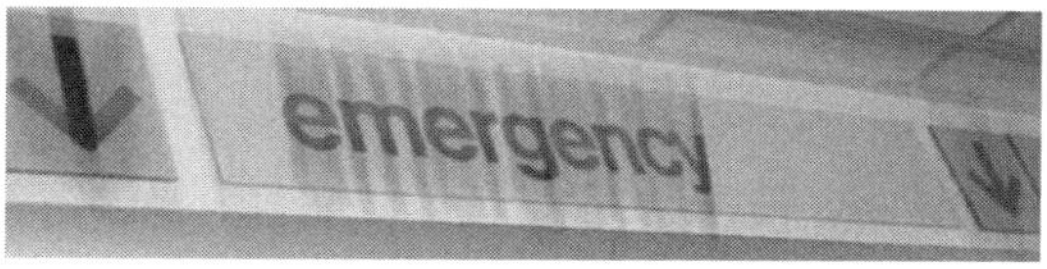

SECTION F – TRAUMA, DM, HEME, GI, HTN

Chapter 29: A 78-year-old woman with dementia and new confusion

Roya Z. Caloia, DO, MPH, FACEP, FAAEM

Emergency Physician, USACS Southeast
Core Faculty USACS, Grand Blanc, MI
Clinical Assistant Professor
Michigan State University College of Osteopathic Medicine
East Lansing, MI

Christopher A. Moore, DO, FACEP

Emergency Physician, USACS Southeast
Core Faculty and Director Undergraduate Medical Education, Ascension Genesys Hospital
Clinical Professor
Michigan State University College of Osteopathic Medicine
Clinical Faculty
AT Still University Kirksville College of Osteopathic Medicine
Kirksville, MO

Section editor:

Joseph Shiber MD, FACEP, FACP, FCCM

Professor
Emergency Medicine, Neurology and Surgery
Director ECMO/Acute Lung Service
Co-director NSICU and UF North ICU
UF College of Medicine–Jacksonville
Jacksonville, FL

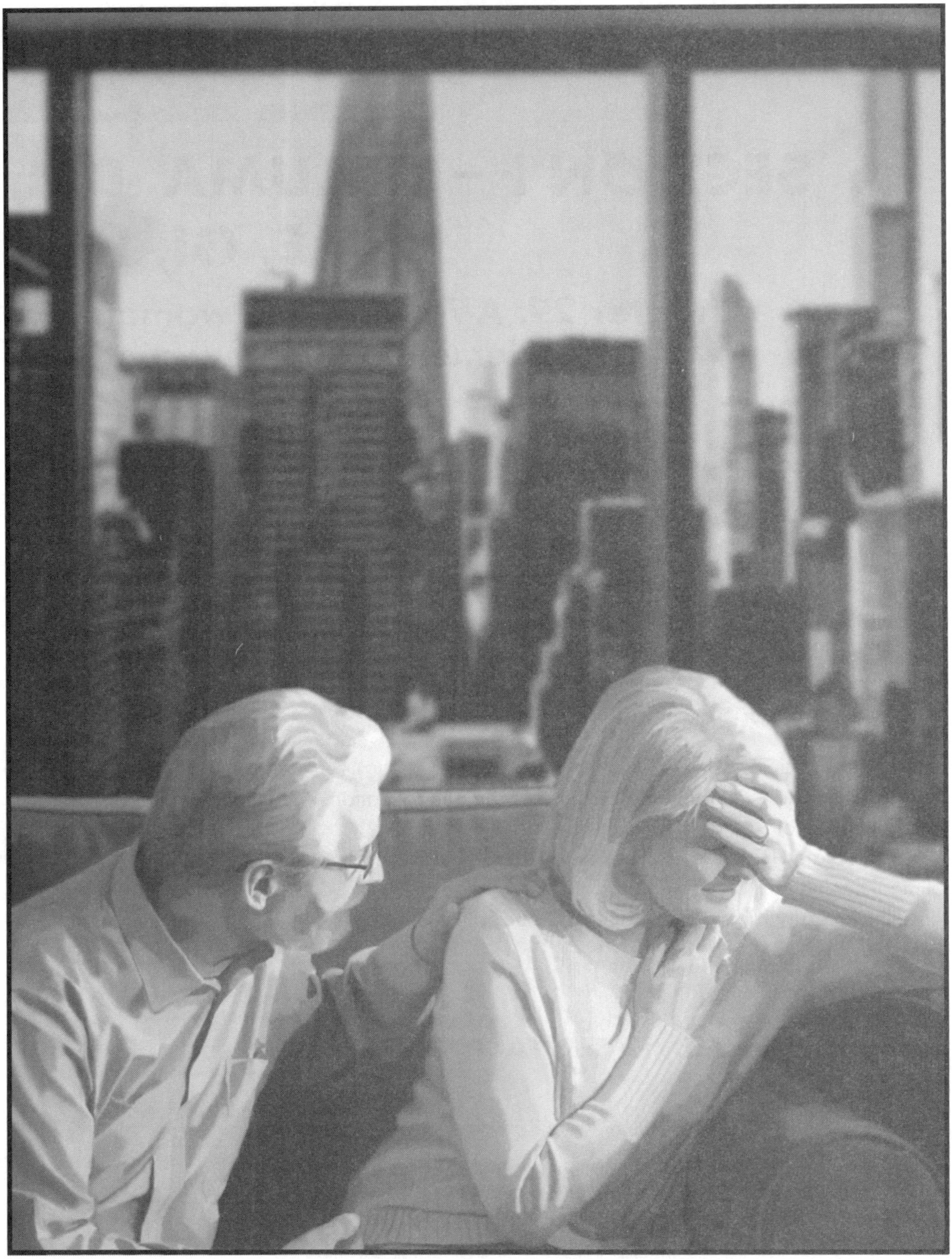

SECTION F /CHAPTER 29

A 78-year-old woman with dementia and new confusion

The patient's story:
Esther Schwartz was born in New York City, went to high school in New York City, married in New York City, and then started a family. From young adulthood to middle age, her apartment was filled with the laughter of children, relatives, and friends, but when her last son moved out for good, her life slowed… as did her cognition.

For the last 8 years, she has had a progressive decline with a gradual reversal of the traditional marital roles; her husband has stopped working and is now caring for his frail wife.

On a steamy late July morning, with his wife more confused and starting to hallucinate over the last couple of days, David decides it is time to seek medical attention. He helps his wife into the elevator, then hails a cab to a neighboring Urgent Care.

He tells the PA that he is concerned about a urinary tract infection, so a dip is performed, but when normal, they are directed to the emergency department.

INITIAL ED VISIT

CC: Altered mental status

HPI (13:17): 78-year-old female presents with acute delirium, hallucinatory events and talking and arguing with people that aren't in the room for the past 2 days. Yesterday, she states there were animals and a circus in her backyard. She's had a cough for the past 2 years but no changes, no fevers or chills. She's had no urinary complaints but husband states this has happened previously when she has had a UTI. She went to the urgent care today and was told that her urine was clean. No new medications have been started or stopped, no history of alcohol use or abuse. She has had no falls, she is on rivaroxaban. Husband states that she's had no blood in her stools, but a couple of days ago there was black stool but equated this to eating Oreo cookies. She has had 2 weeks of left shoulder pain worse with movement, no injury. He has been giving her Aleve because of her shoulder pain. No fever, rhinorrhea, blood in the urine, bruising, rash, numbness of the extremities.

Allergies: NKDA

Medications: Melatonin, ergocalciferol, HCTZ, magnesium oxide, montelukast, rivaroxaban, acetaminophen, atenolol, atorvastatin, levothyroxine, omeprazole
Past Medical History: Dementia, Afib, High cholesterol, Hypertension
Surgical history: Parathyroidectomy
Family history: No family history items have been selected or recorded.
Social history: No alcohol or tobacco

PE:

Vitals:

Temp	Pulse	Resp	Syst	Diast	Sat (RA)
97.6	71	22	107	63	95%

CONSTITUTIONAL: Alert and oriented X 1 (she knows her name and knows the month but unsure of the date or place), well-nourished, well appearing, in no apparent distress
EYES: PERRL, no scleral icterus.
RESP: Normal chest excursion with respiration; breath sounds clear and equal bilaterally; no wheezes, rhonchi, or rales
CARDIO: Regular rhythm, without murmurs, rubs or gallops
ABD: Non-distended; non-tender, soft, without rigidity, rebound or guarding
SKIN: Normal for age and race; warm and dry; no apparent lesions
NEURO: No lateralizing weakness or numbness, no facial droop, no dysarthria
MUSCULOSKELETAL: Shoulder with decreased range of motion but no overlying warmth or erythema
RECTAL: The stool is dark but not black and is heme positive

Labs (15:31): 7/11/2016 15:02 EDT

WBC Count	8.9 thou/mcL
Hemoglobin	**9.0 gm/dL LOW**
Platelet Count	243 thou/mcL
Sodium Level	140mmol/L
Potassium Level	4.4mmol/L
Chloride Level	106mmol/L
Carbon Dioxide Level	22mmol/L
Anion Gap	12.0mmol/L
Glucose Level	**112mg/dL HI**
BUN	**63mg/dL HI**
Creatinine	**2.77mg/dL HI**
Alcohol (Ethanol) Level	<0.01gm/dL
Salicylate Level	<4.0mg/dL
Lactic Acid Level	1.4mmol/L
Ammonia Level	1 mmol/L

MDM (16:04) ECG: Sinus rhythm. The patient has evidence of upper GI bleeding probably related to recent Aleve on top of rivaroxaban and this would account for her anemia and elevated BUN but not necessarily her mentation. I started a pantoprazole drip and will admit the patient to a telemetry bed.

Impression and plan:
1. UGI Bleeding
2. AMS
3. Blood loss anemia
4. Hx of dementia

Plan: Admit: to Inpatient Telemetry Unit.

Discussion points at the initial visit:

We *love* this ED patient; labs, IV proton pump inhibitor (PPI), admission and… next case. Before we explore the critical care decision points of her return visit (yes, she *did* bounceback), we will address several questions from the initial visit:

1. Which patients with GI bleeding benefit from admission?

As ED docs, we know GI bleeds and we know sick vs. not sick. Whether we use the calculators or scores, few of us would have sent this patient home. She has an upper GI bleed until proven otherwise. The approach is to start proton pump inhibitors (continuous drip versus twice daily dosing —more on the data below), hold anticoagulants, repeat hemoglobin and hematocrit and consult GI. Consideration with our patient should have been to add on a PT/PTT/INR and type and screen.

The Glasgow-Blatchford Score (GBS), AIMS65, Modified GBS, and pre-endoscopy Rockall score are some of the more commonly known tools to help with risk stratification in upper GI bleeds. If we use the GBS, our patient would have a score of 11 (with a score greater than 0 being high risk for needing medical intervention) for an elevated BUN, low Hb, and tachycardia. Other criteria that are used in the scale include presence of melena, presentation with syncope, liver disease history, or heart failure history.[1-5]

Regarding admission, we see patients with GI bleeds all the time, and many can continue their ED evaluation as an outpatient, but our patient had some factors which factor *strongly* into the decision to admit: she is on rivaroxaban and has been taking naproxen, her BUN is elevated, she has heme positive stool, is anemic (knowing her baseline hemoglobin would be useful) has borderline low blood pressure and isn't mentating well. The consideration of a worsened and rapid GI bleed, especially unrecognized in a demented patient, would make ED discharge problematic. We recommend monitoring, serial hemoglobins, and a GI consult.

2. Does a Protonix/PPI drip improve mortality/morbidity?

It is currently believed that PPIs used in patients with bleeding peptic ulcers will increase gastric pH and cause stabilization of clots. However, there is no significant improvement in mortality. In 2005, a *Cochrane Review* of 21 randomized controlled trials comprising 2,915 patients showed PPIs had no significant effect on mortality but did reduce rebleeding and surgery.[6]

In 2009, the NNT found there to be no benefit and no harm in treating patients with PPIs.[7] The decrease in rebleeding when compared to placebo or H2 Blockers was significant enough to warrant still using PPIs on presumptive upper GI bleeds. Interestingly, in 2013, Chan, et al. found that there was no significant difference in morbidity or mortality when comparing continuous IV PPI vs. twice daily IV dosing. As a result, many hospitals are moving away from the 8mg/hr continuous Protonix drip in favor of BID dosing of IV Protonix.[8]

3. Do UTIs cause confusion in elderly patients?

It seems common medical knowledge that a UTI can cause delirium in elderly patients; however, there have been no studies to confirm our perception.[9] It does seem obvious, but we have not been able to prove causality. As a result, it is imperative to look for other sources for mental status changes with a history and physical, consideration of new medications or interactions, falls, or a metabolic abnormality and to consider ordering a CT head, electrolytes, and a CXR.

What we do know is that patients with underlying brain disease, like dementia, are seemingly more susceptible to delirium.[10] Conditions that can precipitate delirium include fluid and electrolyte disturbances, infections, metabolic disorders, low perfusion states, post-operative states, drug or alcohol toxicity, and withdrawal from alcohol, barbiturates, benzodiazepines, SSRIs.[11]

So, in our patient, the alteration in mental status could be due to hypoperfusion given her underlying dementia. A curious note on the documentation: the doctor does not address the confusion in the MDM, and the results of a urinalysis, chest x-ray and CT head are not documented either, causing us to wonder if the evaluation was suspended after a decision was made to admit for GI bleed.

Final thoughts on the initial visit: GI bleeds are pretty cut and dried, right? Complicating factors include anticoagulation and the consideration of coagulopathy from chronic liver disease or esophageal varices. But we can only treat what we know, which is why it is important to ask about concomitant use of NSAIDS in patients on anticoagulation. In patients we are considering discharging, learning about NSAID or anticoagulant use could be the "game-changer" that tilts the scale toward admission. Many patients don't think it is important to mention over-the-counter medications or supplements. Consider explicitly asking about medications by name: "Do you take aspirin, ibuprofen, naproxen, Motrin, Aleve, or Advil?"

Author comments (Weinstock):

Who hasn't had a patient deny using ibuprofen... but then admit to using "Motrin?" "Doctor, is it broken or fractured?" OK. Enough said. We need to obtain appropriate data on which to base our evaluation, management and disposition decisions and asking a question in several different ways or inquiring about over-the-counter medicines can make all the difference!

Hospital course: The patient was admitted and had an EGD showing erosive gastritis and duodenitis. Her hemoglobin was stable, rivaroxaban was held; NSAIDs were discontinued. The visual hallucinations were diagnosed as encephalopathy superimposed on dementia, and they resolved while in the hospital. HCTZ and losartan were held due to their nephrotoxicity. The patient's husband was instructed to restart the rivaroxaban 1–2 days after discharge, to only give acetaminophen for the degenerative joint disease in her shoulder, and oral PPIs were added to her medication regimen.

Author comments (Weinstock):

Upon discharge from the hospital, the patient and her husband fall back into their previous routine; she wakes late and he fixes her breakfast, they have a mid-afternoon lunch and often a visit from their children, then an early evening supper. Four days after the hospital discharge, she is not up, and when her husband goes to check on her, finds she has fallen. He is unable to get her to stand despite several attempts, so he calls 911.

When the paramedics arrive, they find the patient is purplish in color, sweaty, and barely responsive. Her respirations slow and she becomes bradycardic, rapidly decompensating into full arrest. With her husband watching from the doorway, chest compressions are started, an IV is established, and she is intubated with some difficulty. She is transported with lights and sirens to the ED.

ED BOUNCEBACK (6 days after initial ED visit)

CC: Cardiac arrest

HPI (10:31): I did see the patient immediately upon arrival and also spoke with the paramedics. The patient is not able to give any history secondary to the fact that she is intubated. The patient was here recently and I did review the previous record. The patient was at home and they were called for a 'lift assist' and when they arrived the patient was upstairs and was cyanotic, tachypneic and when they got the patient down to the first floor she went into cardiac arrest. They did chest compressions for 20 minutes. They gave 2mg total of epinephrine, 2 amps of sodium bicarbonate and got a pulse back. The husband has not yet arrived. According to the paramedics, the husband told them that she was a no code, however, there was no paperwork available. I will discuss further with husband when he gets here.

PE:

Vitals:

Time	Temp (axillary)	Pulse	Resp	Syst	Diast	Sat
10:34	98.6	108	16	94	69	100% (vent)

CONSTITUTIONAL: Patient is unresponsive. Will not open her eyes to verbal commands, she is receiving no sedative medication, color is good, she is not diaphoretic
RESP: Equal breath sounds bilaterally with auscultation with bagging and no air auscultated over the stomach
CARDIO: Regular rhythm, without murmurs, rub or gallop
ABD: Non-distended; non-tender, soft, without rigidity, rebound or guarding
right femoral pulses 2+
SKIN: Normal for age and race; warm and dry; no apparent lesions
EXTREMITIES: No lower extremity peripheral edema

MDM (10:53): I did review the pre-arrival ECG as well as ECG here showing atrial fibrillation with rapid ventricular response with a rate of 108 and evidence of right bundle branch block and inferior T wave inversion. I did review the previous record. I did speak with [the cardiologist] about the ECG having the appearance of right bundle branch block and not of STEMI. I will discuss the code status with the husband when he arrives.

Author comments (Weinstock):

We are standing in the footsteps of the emergency physician caring for a profoundly unstable post-arrest patient, hypotensive, tachycardic, altered... and don't even know the code status! Did she arrest from a GI bleed? Why did the paramedics intubate if she was "no code?" We are at:

DECISION POINT A – YOU ARE FACED WITH 4 QUESTIONS:

1. **The patient is post-arrest—what is the likely etiology and how should evaluation and management be initiated?**
2. **Is emergent cardiac catheterization indicated?**
3. **She has atrial fibrillation with RVR—should her rate be managed chemically, electrically or with IV fluids?**
4. **There is word that she is a no code—does this change the management at this point?**

What does the literature say?

Q#1: The patient is post-arrest—what is the likely etiology and how should evaluation and management be initiated?

The patient was recently in the hospital for an upper GI bleed. She is supposedly back on anticoagulation. She was cyanotic on EMS arrival and lost pulses. On arrival to the ED, she is afebrile, but tachycardic and hypotensive. A logical place to start would be consideration of the Hs and Ts. Is she:

- **Hypovolemic?** Maybe she hasn't been eating or drinking well since having left the hospital. Maybe she is having another GI bleed?
- **Hypoxic?** She may have been hypoxic given her initial cyanosis.
- **Acidotic?** Labs will tell us if she is acidotic; she did respond to epinephrine as well as 2 ampules of sodium bicarbonate, so this is a possibility.
- **Hyper/hypokalemic?** Her HCTZ and losartan were stopped on discharge, but she has dementia and she may have continued taking these medications possibly leading to worsening renal failure and hyperkalemia.
- **Hypothermic?** She isn't hypothermic currently.
- **Hypoglycemic?** There is no documented blood glucose. That should be one of the first things obtained, or at least received in report from EMS.
- **Toxin?** Could there have been an unintentional overdose of medication? Certainly, a consideration, especially with older patients with dementia. Could she have taken her husband's medications? We don't know his medical history.
- **Tension pneumothorax?** Breath sounds are normal, and we will obtain a chest x-ray, so likely no tension pneumothorax.
- **Thrombotic event such as an MI or PE?** She does have t-wave inversions—could it be an MI? It seems like this was a consideration initially and involved cardiology early on. A pulmonary embolism is a strong consideration. She has a history of atrial fibrillation, was potentially off of her anticoagulation for a period of time, was recently hospitalized, and is tachycardic and hypotensive.

Q#2: Is emergent cardiac catheterization indicated?

The majority of patients with ROSC after arrest do not have ST-elevation on the post-arrest ECG,[12] though 25% have an acute occlusion and 60% have significant obstructive lesions. In July 2015, the ACC/AHA proposed and published an algorithm with guidelines for managing comatose post-arrest patients without ST-segment elevation. Patients with multiple unfavorable resuscitation features are found to be less likely to benefit from coronary intervention.[13]

Unfavorable features:

- Unwitnessed arrest
- Initial rhythm which is not ventricular fibrillation
- No bystander CPR
- > 30min to ROSC
- Ongoing CPR
- Ph < 7.2
- Lactate > 7
- Age > 85
- End stage renal disease
- Non-cardiac causes

Care should be individualized despite "numbers" which argue against intervention; sometimes family shows up and says, “she does Sudoku every day and volunteers at the local school 3 times a week and doesn’t take any medications.” These authors recommend emergently consulting interventional cardiology to discuss emergent catheterization.

Author comments (Weinstock):

In the first Chapter we detailed a 2019 *NEJM* study by Lemkes, et al. of over 551 post-arrest patients without STEMI who were randomized to emergent catheterization vs. delay until neurologic recovery —without a difference in outcomes—please refer to Chapter 1 for further detail of this study. Agree with an emergent discussion with interventional cardiology. The same Chapter also details other post-arrest management including Targeted Temperature Management (TTM).[14]

Q#3: She has atrial fibrillation with RVR—should her rate be managed chemically, electrically or with IV fluids?

Atrial fibrillation with RVR post-arrest has a significantly higher 180-day mortality rate (66% vs. 43%).[15] Our patient is technically unstable; would cardioversion (CV) be a bad thought? She has potentially been anticoagulated and there is an uncertain time of onset of atrial fibrillation. If we choose to cool, that may result in bradycardia, which could become pronounced with rate control medications. Most rhythm control medications could have adverse effects in the setting of cardiac arrest. These authors feel that with her heart rate only minimally elevated, she should not undergo interventions for her tachycardia but be reassessed after fluids and the cooling procedures.

Section editor comments (Shiber):

If she is chronically in AF then electrical CV would very unlikely be successful. It may not be harmful except for the time wasted setting up and executing the CV instead of treating her underlying medical conditions and working on rate control. To attempt to rate control her with calcium channel blockers should be avoided as they would likely cause worsened hypotension since they are negative inotrope and vasodilators; beta-blockers would also compromise her blood pressure. Although not rapidly acting, digoxin loading is the only rate controlling agent that does not cause hypotension and may improve BP by its positive inotropic effect.

Q#4: There is word that she is a no code—does this change the management at this point?

At one point or another, we all face the intubated DNR patient. A little review of the basics first: do not resuscitate orders are written instructions for healthcare providers to not perform cardiopulmonary resuscitation.

- A "DNR CC" is a Do Not Resuscitate Comfort Care: A dying patient receives any care that eases pain and suffering in the final days but no resuscitative measures to save or sustain life.
- A "DNR CC-Arrest" means a dying person receives treatment, including resuscitative efforts, if necessary, until the time he or she experiences a cardiac or respiratory arrest. Once an arrest is confirmed, all resuscitative efforts are withdrawn, and comfort care alone is initiated.
- A "full code" means all resuscitative efforts are attempted.

Every scenario, of course, is different. Sometimes, the patient has a durable power of attorney that makes the decision. Sometimes, there is paperwork signed by the patient that confirms their wishes. Sometimes, there are caveats, such as the patient who wants medicines but no compressions or no intubations. Sometimes, people change their minds when faced with impending death; if they are of sound mind and body and able to make that decision, then that decision should be honored.

For our patient, her DNR order may have been in the computer from her very recent visit. During resuscitation, staff should be employed to search the electronic medical record to find the paperwork. If it is determined that the husband is not coming, we would recommend finding paperwork to determine the next of kin or power of attorney to determine the patient's wishes. Until a definitive code status has been obtained, these authors feel that the patient should continue to undergo cardiopulmonary resuscitation.

What did the actual provider do?

MDM (11:07): I did go back and check on the patient again. At this point she is hypotensive with a pressure of 64. Rapid cooling had been started but will be stopped at this time. She will receive an IV fluid bolus. Point-of-care (POC) troponin is minimally elevated 0.09, other labs are pending. This could be from a pulmonary embolism. The patient's husband is on his way here and so I will discuss with him ongoing care when he arrives. The patient is completely unresponsive to verbal or tactile stimuli. She has not received any sedative medication.

Author's note: A recheck of her vital signs reveals:

Vitals:

Time	Temp (rectal)	Pulse	Resp	Syst	Diast	Sat
11:06	101.1	98	20	64	34	100% (vent)

DECISION POINT B – YOU ARE FACED WITH 5 QUESTIONS:

1. **The patient is now profoundly hypotensive, should she be given blood empirically?**
2. **She now has a temperature—should the sepsis protocol be initiated?**
3. **Should the rapid cooling have been stopped?**
4. **Should vasopressors be started, or do you wait for IVF? Which pressors should be first line?**
5. **Should she go to CT for a scan to evaluate for PE—how about a bedside US? How could this change management?**

What does the literature say?

Q#1: The patient is now profoundly hypotensive, should she be given blood empirically?

Thinking physiologically will keep our differential diagnoses in line; there are 4 classes of shock:

a. Obstructive (cardiac tamponade, massive PE, tension pneumothorax)
b. Distributive (neurogenic, sepsis)
c. Cardiogenic (STEMI, heart failure with poor ejection fraction)
d. Hypovolemic (hemorrhage, overt dehydration)

Utilization of point-of-care ultrasound (POCUS) and performing a rapid ultrasound for shock and hypotension (RUSH exam) can differentiate the class of shock within a matter of minutes when correlated to patient presentation.[16]

Out patient's ECG does not demonstrate an overt ischemic event, which makes cardiogenic less likely, but it is concerning for new onset right heart strain; could this be a PE?

Empiric blood transfusion could be delayed without a point-of-care hemoglobin and no active signs of exsanguination from the gastric tube suction or rectal exam—additionally the physical exam mentions skin has "good color." If the choice is made to transfuse the patient at this point, O negative or non-cross-matched blood should be selected. Our patient had a recent UGI bleed and now has a BP of 64/34, but with good color. Do we have time to wait? Hard to say... these authors recommend a rapid re-evaluation and close monitoring of the vitals as well as type and cross-match for 2 units, but to hold on transfusing at this time.[17,18]

Consulting editor comments (Weingart):

The only fluids a bad GI bleeder should be receiving are either red or yellow [plasma or FFP]; there's no "clears" [saline]. That's the first thing. Do they need a bicarb drip? No, they need adequate resuscitation with blood products that will fix their profound metabolic acidosis. Now, once they're out of the exsanguinating phase, should we give bicarb drip solely for metabolic acidosis? And the answer is... maybe. And here's what it comes down to: if you're going to give IV fluids, and they are profoundly acidotic and maybe their kidneys are already taking a hit, then there's no reason you can't make your IV fluid isotonic bicarb because you're going to be giving them fluids anyway. When you give LR or NS as fluids, the NS is going to make things worse in terms of their acidosis and the LR is not going to make things better. So, why not give bicarb isotonic as drip?

It's never a good idea to give pushes of amps of bicarb. And, if you weren't going to give crystalloid, then it's probably not a good idea to give crystalloid in the form of bicarb drip either, due to the risk of volume overload. A bicarb drip should be given with a non-anion gap acidosis and in patients who are oliguric or anuric because those patients need the bicarb. A patient with a hyperchloremic acidosis, whether from a renal tubule acidosis or iatrogenic because they got a lot of normal saline, they're profoundly acidotic and their kidneys are not going to be able to fix it on their own. In this situation, giving exogenous bicarb makes a lot of sense.

Q#2: She now has a temperature—should the sepsis protocol be initiated?

Although fever can be reactive from a number of causes, in this scenario it is reasonable to presume sepsis and initiate therapy including a 30cc/kg IV fluid bolus, lactate, blood cultures, and broad-spectrum antibiotics.[19]

Q#3: Should rapid cooling have been stopped?

Targeted Temperature Management (TTM) goal temperatures are to be met within 3–4 hours.[20] In our case, we need to get additional information from the husband regarding goals of care. A palliative care consultation is reasonable but should not stop medical management. While the work-up and management is continued, including CT brain and possibly CTA for PE, as the patient is profoundly hypotensive, the cooling process should be stopped. Also, consider the fact that this patient has not yet received optimal resuscitation. Note that an additional contraindication to cooling is sepsis.

Q#4: Should vasopressors be started, or do you wait for IVF? Which pressors should be first line?

Thinking physiologically, I'd like to know what the preload (IVC ultrasound) and cardiac exam are like with consideration of a poor EF, RV dilation and or pericardial effusion.[16] If the IVC is collapsing and flat, then more IV fluid is necessary for preload. If the IVC is dilated and not collapsing, then initiate vasopressor therapy and maintenance fluids. Norepinephrine would be the first-line vasopressor of choice presuming adequate IV fluids have been provided including 30cc/kg for current sepsis guidelines.[19] For our patient, having norepinephrine prepared and ready to infuse after the IV fluid bolus is complete would be ideal. In the meantime, attempting push-dose pressor support with epinephrine (10–20 micrograms) during initial IV fluid resuscitation may provide ideal bridging support.[21]

Q#5: Should she go to CT for a scan to evaluate for PE—how about a bedside US? How could this change management?

Dogmatic emergency medicine and oral board training would recommend against this for the simple reason that you do not send unstable patients to radiology. That is where they go to have their cardiac arrest, right? A RUSH exam with an extended bedside DVT scanning is probably the best plan of care for this patient.[16] If there is right ventricular dilation with cardiac septal bowing and positive bilateral femoral DVTs then one would have a presumptive diagnosis/concern for PE with consideration of initiating anticoagulation/thrombolysis and then to manage bleeding, if it occurs.

Section editor comments (Shiber):

This is a tough case if the patient does have a PE, we would have significant concern about initiating anticoagulation or thrombolysis in a patient with a significant recent GI bleed. It would be nice to have a diagnosis, though.

What did the actual provider do?

MDM (11:36): The rapid cooling protocol will be suspended until the patient's blood pressure has improved. The patient has completed 3 liters of IV fluid and her blood pressure systolic is now 44. She will receive epinephrine 0.5mg IV which is in the room so we can get this rapidly. Additionally, she'll be started on Levophed 5mcg/m IV, and I did speak with pharmacy and they're sending that down right now and should be down within the next several minutes. I did have a long discussion with the husband who has recently arrived who states the patient should be a no code and does not want chest compressions. He would like to keep her on the ventilator at this time. I did review her labs including blood gas showing profound metabolic acidosis.

Vitals:

Time	Temp	Pulse	Resp	Syst	Diast	Sat
11:31				44	palp	

ABG: 7.00/27/204/6.8 – **lactic acid 13.4**

WBC Count	**22.6thou/mcL HI**
Hemoglobin	**8.4gm/dL LOW**
Platelet Count	197thou/mcL

Sodium Level	14 mMol/L
Potassium Level	5.0mMol/L
Chloride Level	**110mMol/L HI**
Carbon Dioxide Level	**10mMol/L LOW**
Anion Gap	**22.0mMol/L HI**
Glucose Level	**169mg/dL HI**
BUN	**47mg/dL HI**
Creatinine	**3.80mg/dL HI**

MDM (12:07): The patient is now on Levophed at 20 mics per minute and I also started dobutamine 5 mcg/kg/m. Patient does not have significant anemia that will require transfusion. I did review her previous record again. The patient now is febrile with temperature 101.4 degrees and is likely septic and does have an additional 1L of IV fluid ordered as well as IV vancomycin and Zosyn and Levaquin, and she will also have blood cultures drawn.

Chapter author note: I'd also still like to know if a CT brain is in the works, because if there is a large intracranial hemorrhage, the best treatment may be palliative care. Xarelto was recently discontinued and then restarted; along with her recent hospitalization with immobilization, this makes PE likely as the reason for being cyanotic and unresponsive (wells score 6, PE likely). A-a gradient 475mmHg is severely elevated assuming FiO_2 100% on the vent. If there is no pneumonia seen on the CXR, then PE is much more likely. Also, the provider has not mentioned any likely source of the septic shock. The severe metabolic acidosis is likely hypoxic lactic acidosis induced and there is no account for the cause of drastic hypoxia. In this setting, if a CT brain demonstrates no bleed, we could consider tPA for PE; however, we need to take into account her relative contraindications including that she is over 75-years-old, she just underwent CPR lasting longer than 10 minutes, is currently on oral anticoagulation, and she recently had internal bleeding.[22] A POCUS RUSH exam would be helpful here to guide therapy and verify the right heart strain that was demonstrated on the ECG.

The last blood pressure was 44/palp, and there is no mention in the MDM of central line placement or arterial line placement. When a train wreck patient like this is on their second pressor, with that blood pressure, we recommend central line placement.

Overall, we believe the patient care was appropriate with a shift to sepsis, with the consideration still remaining about possible PE.

Author comments (Weinstock):

We are back at the bedside, the patient is deteriorating, and the differential still has multiple considerations. The physician is fluctuating between "no code" and "full bore" treatment. We are at:

DECISION POINT C – YOU ARE FACED WITH 4 QUESTIONS:

1. **How is persistent hypotension after pressors managed?**
2. **How should the vent setting be adjusted with the ABG results?**
3. **Could the hemoglobin be falsely reassuring due to dehydration?**
4. **Is the sepsis management appropriate?**

What does the literature say?

Q#1: How is persistent hypotension after pressors managed?

This patient is now on norepinephrine and dobutamine and not improving; she has vasopressor resistant shock, where do we go from here?

We would consider using epinephrine as a second line or additional pressor as it also has inotropic support.[23] Additionally, we need a central line and arterial lines placed with consideration given to adjunctive therapies, possibly including vasopressin and stress dose steroids.[23]

Could the vent settings be contributing to the hypotension? In patients with shock, baseline inspiration results in negative intrathoracic pressure which facilitates preload and venous return, whereas patients on a mechanical ventilator experience positive pressure intrathoracically, inhibiting venous return and hindering preload. This positive pressure will cause a relative coronary artery collapse during diastole causing worsening cardiac ischemia. Managing a ventilator in a patient with refractory shock on 2 pressors is difficult, but it is improved by placement of central and arterial lines. In theory, decreasing PEEP and tidal volume could decrease the intrathoracic pressure helping to offload the effects of the ventilator.

Section editor comments (Shiber):

Note that dobutamine is an inotrope not a vasopressor as it has vasodilatory properties as a pure beta-agonist without any alpha-agonist effects; it could be included in the larger category of vasoactive medications that includes pressors and inotropes. The authors mention that the patient meets criteria for vasopressor-resistant shock—this is certainly a consideration to take into account, though realize that she is not actually on the maximal dose of Levophed as it is only at 20 mcg/min.

Author comments (Weinstock):

See Chapter 7, "A 56-year-old healthy man with bronchitis and shortness of breath" for a discussion of the DOPES mnemonic for causes of post-intubation hypotension.

At any point during a clinical resuscitation, if the therapeutic interventions are not working, stop and rethink the case. For an excellent review, visit R.E.B.E.L. EM "Occult Causes of Non-Response to Vasopressors."[24]

- Is she acidotic? Yes.
- Does she have hypothyroidism? No; she is on levothyroxin (she has no history or other reason to suspect hypothyroidism.)
- Could this have been anaphylaxis? The story does not point to that; however, it is a possibility.
- Could this be adrenal insufficiency or failure? Sure, she was recently in the hospital, but she doesn't have hyponatremia and hyperkalemia; she is not on long-term steroids (there was no cortisol level ordered).
- Could she have ongoing bleeding? Sure.
- Other considerations include hypocalcemia or an overdose of beta-blockers, calcium channel blockers or TCAs.

Whether the clinician was able to obtain more history from the husband or EMS is unknown, but a targeted history might shine some light on other possible reasons for shock.

Q#2: How should the vent setting be adjusted with the ABG results?

Assuming that this ABG was with a FiO_2 of 100%, the only adjustment would be to wean the FiO_2 to maintain normal PaO_2. $PaCO_2$ of 27mmHg suggests the pH disturbance is metabolic, so adjusting the respiratory rate would not improve the patient's condition or pH. Consideration for a sodium bicarbonate drip may be of help.

Q#3: Could the hemoglobin be falsely reassuring due to dehydration?

A study done on 293 patients (288 Jehovah's Witness) who were prospectively observed for mortality from various post-operative states found the mortality to be 0.9% for patients with a hemoglobin of 7.1–8.0g/dL (n=232) who did not receive a transfusion.[25] However, these patients were not in severe shock. When patients are in cardiogenic shock, or unstable angina, the threshold for transfusion is < 8.0g/dL.[26] This patient's hemoglobin of 8.4g/dL is likely to drop secondary to the large IV fluid resuscitation, so it would be prudent to type and cross the patient and have blood ready for a transfusion. A repeat CBC after the resuscitation would aid in this decision-making. The American Association of Blood Banks, however, would not recommend transfusion.[26]

Q#4: Is the sepsis management appropriate?

The sepsis management of this case was appropriate and initiated within the 3-hour bundle recommendation by the Surviving Sepsis Campaign (4 liters of fluid given, Zosyn/vancomycin/levofloxacin, and then initiation of pressors). An improvement in the documentation would be to explain and delineate the potential source of the fever, as there was no mention of pneumonia, HCAP or UTI in the MDM. Additionally performing and documenting a "focused-repeat-exam" after the large IV fluid bolus was complete would have been helpful.[19]

What did the actual provider do?

Vitals:

Time	Temp	Pulse	Resp	Syst	Diast	Sat
11:08				62	48	

MDM: I feel the most likely reason for the patient's arrest at this point is sepsis. The husband did give me a history of 2 days of shortness of breath and this was not an acute, sudden onset of shortness of breath and this makes pulmonary embolism less likely. I cannot do an emergent contrast CT but a VQ scan could always be done as an inpatient if necessary. The patient will be sent to the ICU. I spoke with the [intensivist], who accepts the patient in consultation. The hospitalist service will be contacted for the admission.

Were the provider's actions appropriate?

Chapter author comments: She is febrile, her blood pressure is 62/48 on 2 pressors, receiving IV fluids per sepsis protocol as well as antibiotics but is without a clear diagnosis. We disagree with "hanging our hat"on a diagnosis of sepsis, when our patient had 2 days of shortness of breath—the diagnosis of PE is still very much in play; how about the ultrasound or a bedside echo? TPA may not be the best option given her many relative contraindications, but heparin could be started in consultation with GI. Are we certain this has nothing to do with her recent GI bleed?

We would have recommended starting a bicarbonate drip in the ED with her profound metabolic acidosis. But with all that being said, the patient is a no code. How aggressive should we get? The vasopressors alone are extraordinary measures. Central and arterial lines are invasive procedures. Our approach would have been to explain everything to the husband and go through an actual DNR sheet with him to ensure that our interventions were in keeping with her wishes.

ED diagnosis: Cardiac arrest, severe sepsis, shortness of breath and cyanosis, unresponsive, anemia, acute on chronic renal failure, profound metabolic acidosis.

Hospital course: The patient was admitted to the ICU on a sodium bicarbonate drip, pressor support, continued IV fluids and anticoagulation was held. A CT of the head, a formal echo and a CTA chest were deferred until the patient was stable. Unfortunately, the patient arrested and was pronounced dead before the studies could be performed.

Final hospital impression:

1. Cardiac arrest with acute respiratory failure and hypoxia
2. Cardiogenic shock
3. Paroxysmal atrial fibrillation with RVR

Chapter summary:

- Obtain as much history as possible from EMS and family.
- If things aren't adding up, go back to the drawing board.
- Use your ultrasound machine. There were many opportunities for use in this case. Sure, the patient may not have been stable to leave the department, but there is no reason an ultrasound could not have been performed at the bedside.
- Ensure the MDM is clear about consideration of life-saving diagnoses and interventions.
- All fever is not sepsis.

References:

1. Blatchford O, Murray WR, Blatchford M. A risk score to predict need for treatment for upper gastrointestinal haemorrhage. Lancet 2000;356(9238):1318-21.
2. Rockall TA, Logan RF, Devlin HB, et al. Risk assessment after acute upper gastrointestinal haemorrhage. Gut 1996;38(3):316-21.
3. Stanley AJ, Laine L, Dalton HR, et al. Comparison of risk scoring systems for patients presenting with upper gastrointestinal bleeding: international multicentre prospective study. BMJ 2017;356:i6432.
4. Saltzman JR, Tabak YP, Hyett BH, et al. A simple risk score accurately predicts in-hospital mortality, length of stay, and cost in acute upper GI bleeding. Gastrointest Endosc 2011;74(6):1215-24.
5. Vreeburg EM, Terwee CB, Snel P, et al. Validation of the Rockall risk scoring system in upper gastrointestinal bleeding. Gut 1999; 44:331-35.
6. Leontiadis GI, Sharma VK, Howden CW. Systematic review and meta-analysis of proton pump inhibitor therapy in peptic ulcer bleeding. BMJ 2005;330(7491):568.
7. Sreedharan A, Martin J, Leontiadis GI, et al. Proton pump inhibitor treatment initiated prior to endoscopic diagnosis in upper gastrointestinal bleeding. Cochrane Database Syst Rev 2010;(7):CD005415.
8. Chan WH, Khin LW, Chung YF, et.al. Randomized controlled trial of standard versus high-dose intravenous omeprazole after endoscopic therapy in high-risk patients with acute peptic ulcer bleeding. Br J Surg 2011;98(5):640-4.

9. Balogun SA, Philbrick JT. Delirium, a symptom of UTI in the elderly: Fact or fable? A systematic review. Can Geriatr J 2014;(1): 22-6.
10. Francis J, Martin D, Kapoor WN. A prospective study of delirium in hospitalized elderly. JAMA 1990;263(8):1097-101.
11. Francis J, Young GB. Diagnosis of delirium and confusional states. UpToDate 2014. Retrieved September 2, 2017, from https://www.uptodate.com/contents/diagnosis-of-delirium-and-confusional-states.
12. Hollenbeck RD, McPherson JA, Mooney MR, et al. Early cardiac catheterization is associated with improved survival in comatose survivors of cardiac arrest without STEMI. Resuscitation 2014;85(1):88-95.
13. Rab T, Kern KB, Tamis-Holland JE, et al. Cardiac arrest: A treatment algorithm for emergent invasive cardiac procedures in the resuscitated comatose patient. J Am Coll Cardiol 2015;66(1):62-73.
14. Lemkes JS, Janssens GN, van der Hoeven NW, et al. Coronary angiography after cardiac arrest without ST-segment elevation. N Engl J Med 2019;380(15):1397-407.
15. Thomsen JH, Hassager C, Erlinge D, et al. Atrial fibrillation following out-of-hospital cardiac arrest and targeted temperature management-are we giving it the attention it deserves? Crit Care Med 2016;44(12):2215-22.
16. Seif D, Perera P, Maihot T, et al. Bedside ultrasound in resuscitation and the rapid ultrasound in shock protocol. Crit Care Res Prac 2012; Article ID 503254.
17. National Institute for Health and Care Excellence. Acute upper gastrointestinal bleeding, 2014. Available from https:// arms.evidence.nhs.uk/resources/hub/1037665/attachment (accessed 4 May 2015)
18. Jairath V, Kahan BC, Gray A et al. Restrictive versus liberal transfusion for acute upper gastrointestinal bleeding (TRIGGER): a pragmatic, cluster randomised feasibility trial. Lancet 2015; 386: 137-44.
19. Levy MM, Rhodes A, Phillips GS, et al. Surviving Sepsis Campaign: Association between performance metrics and outcomes in a 7.5 –year study. Intensive Care Med 2014;40(11):1623-33.
20. Callaway CW, Donnino MW, Fink EL, et al. Part 8: Post-cardiac arrest care: 2015 American Heart Association guidelines update for cardiopulmonary resuscitation and emergency cardiovascular care. Circulation 2015;132(18 suppl 2):S465-82.
21. Weingart S. EMCrit podcast 205 – Push-dose pressors update. EMCrit Blog 2017;(8):https://emcrit.org/emcrit/push-dose-pressor-update
22. Kearon C, Akl EA, Ornelas J, et al. Antithrombotic therapy for VTE disease: CHEST guideline and expert panel report. Chest 2016; 149(2):315-52.
23. Farkas, J. Accelerated goal directed therapy for septic shock. EMCrit 2015;(7): https://emcrit.org/pulmcrit/accelerated-goal-directed-therapy-for-septic-shock/
24. Swaminathan A. Occult causes of non-response to vasopressors. REBEL EM 2017;(7): http://rebelem.com/occult-causes-of-non-response-to-vasopressors.
25. Shander A, Javidroozi M, Naqvi S, et al. An update on mortality and morbidity in patients with very low postoperative hemoglobin levels who decline blood transfusion (CME). Transfusion 2014;54(10 Pt 2):2688-95.
26. Carson JL, Grossman BJ, Kleinman S, et al. Red blood cell transfusion: A Clinical Practice Guideline From the AABB. Ann Intern Med 2012;157(1):49-58.

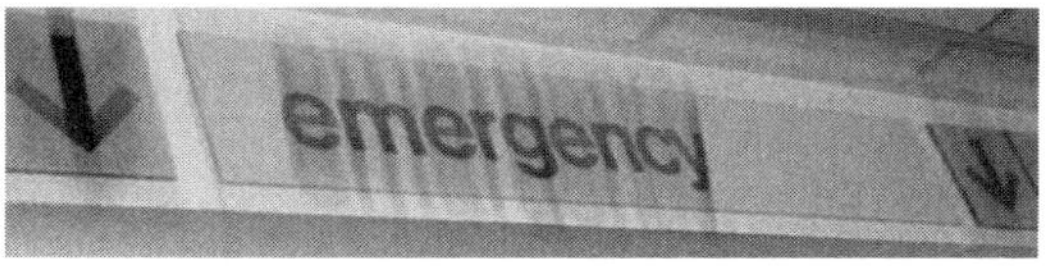

SECTION F – TRAUMA, DM, HEME, GI, HTN

Chapter 30: A12-year-old healthy girl with syncope

Ann Dietrich, MD, FAAP, FACEP

Associate Professor
Ohio University Heritage College of Medicine, Athens, OH
Editor-in-chief
Pediatric Emergency Medicine Reports
Editor-in-chief
Trauma Reports
ACEP Pediatric Emergency Medicine Committee

Jill Fitch, MD

Professor of Pediatrics
Pediatric Intensive Care Unit
Cardiothoracic Intensive Care Unit
Director of the Pediatric Analgesia and Sedation Service (PASS)
Nationwide Children's Hospital, Columbus, OH

Section editor:
Joseph Shiber, MD, FACEP, FACP, FCCM

Professor
Emergency Medicine, Neurology and Surgery
Director ECMO/Acute Lung Service
Co-director NSICU and UF North ICU
UF College of Medicine–Jacksonville, Jacksonville, FL

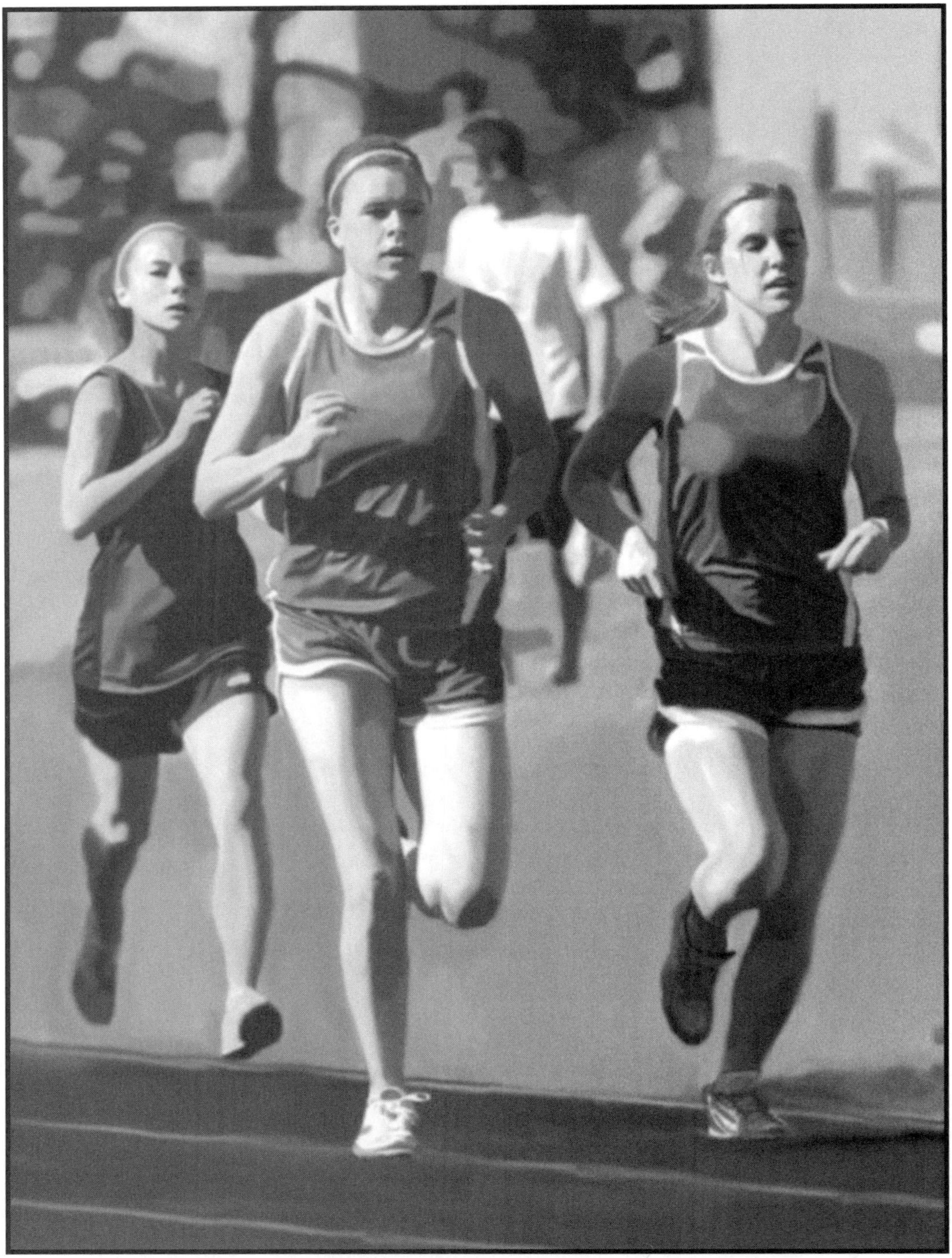

SECTION F / CHAPTER 30

A 12-year-old healthy girl with syncope

The patient's story:
Brittany is a healthy and active 12-year-old girl; she enjoys hanging out with her older sisters and playing with friends. She is competitive, playing soccer in the fall and spring and competing in "club" track, emulating her 16-year-old sister who has twice reached districts in the 400-meter dash.

On July 12th, her team was competing in a multi-city invitational. They arrive at the track early, prepared for a hot day with plenty of water and snacks. By 10 AM, it is already 83 degrees outside. Her event starts at 12:30 PM, and she has decided to wait until after the race to eat, so she will not get cramps.

When the gun goes off for her hurdling event, she hits the ground running, but she does not feel her normal amount of energy. At the 300-meter mark, she is in 3rd place and tries to turn on the speed, but finds her form is off and is passed by two runners, unusual for Brittany. At the last stretch, she tries to fend off another runner with her signature "kick," but her legs are not steady, and she falls 20 meters before the finish line, partially breaking her fall with the hurdle, before coming to a rest. She slowly gets up, and as the ultimate competitor, walks across the finish line.

INITIAL ED VISIT (visit to a dedicated Children's Hospital)

CC(13:20): Dizziness after running a race in the heat

Hx: She presented with dizziness, not feeling well at end of race. She has no headache, no vomiting, but did feel nauseated.

PMH: No medical issues. No previous hospitalizations or surgeries.

PE:

Vitals:

Time	Temp	Pulse	Resp	Syst	Diast	Sat (RA)
13:21	98.4	153	20	108	70	99%

GA: Alert and oriented, tired appearing
NECK: No c-spine pain with palpation
LUNGS: CTAB
CV: RRR without m/r/g
EXT: No tenderness with palpation

MDM/ED course (14:47): We will give oral fluids. She appears dehydrated. She should stay cool and avoid exposure to the sun for the remainder of the day. Given instructions for hydration and sent home.

Diagnosis: Dehydration

Disposition: Home with discharge instructions for heat exposure and dehydration

Author comments (Weinstock):

It was a curious chief complaint... not just dizziness but "dizziness after running a race in the heat." Certainly accurate, but did it color the provider's evaluation and management? There were presumably many kids running the same race. But there is only one in the ED.

Upon discharge from the emergency department, she returns to the meet, but according to her mother, "Her color is bad." She is tired and at one point, answered a question "slower than I would have expected." When the meet ends, Brittany stands up to leave and passes out. Her mother is close by and catches her and gently lowers her to the ground. She is only unconscious for a few seconds, and she is allowed to lay flat for a few minutes, then two teammates put her arms above their shoulders and help her to the car. On the way, she passes out again, so they lay her back down in the parking lot and dial 911.

RETURN ED VISIT (4 hours later — same ED)

HPI (17:23): The patient is a 12-year-old female with syncope. She was in the hot weather all day, sweating, but says she drank one [sports drink] and 2 water bottles. She has not eaten because she thought it would hurt her race. She fell once but has no history of head trauma or neck trauma, denies vomiting or fever. There is no history of headache or seizure activity.

Allergies: NKDA
Social history: No smoking or alcohol
Family history: No history of sudden deaths or drowning deaths in under 50-year olds
ROS: She denies sexual activity, LMP was 2 weeks ago
PMH: None
PSH: None

PE:

Vitals:

Time	Temp	Pulse	Resp	Syst	Diast	Sat (RA)	Pain	Weight
16:58	98.1	165	24	68	palp	99%	1/10	38 kg

GA: A&OX3, color is grey, answering questions but delayed response
EYES: PERRL
CV: RRR without m/r/g. Normal heart sounds. Prolonged capillary refill. No peripheral edema
PULM: CTAB, no wheezes, rales, rhonchi. Good chest excursion

BACK: Nontender, no bruises or marks
SKIN: Normal without bruises or rash
NEURO: GCS = 15, no focal deficits

Author comments (Weinstock):

We have a 12-year-old girl who now returns after a syncopal episode, with significant tachycardia and hypotension. We are at the bedside in the ED. We are at:

DECISION POINT A – YOU ARE FACED WITH 3 QUESTIONS:

1. **What is the differential diagnosis of pediatric syncope?**
2. **Which aspects of the history, exam, and testing are helpful with pediatric syncope?**
3. **The patient is hypotensive—what are the first steps in the evaluation and management?**

What does the literature say?

Q#1: What is the differential diagnosis of pediatric syncope?

Syncope is defined as the temporary loss of consciousness resulting from a reversible disturbance of cerebral function. It is characterized by a loss of consciousness due to rapid or gradual onset of the lack of cerebral blood flow, collapse, and transient symptoms with resolution. Adhering to the definition is important, as in many cases, a complaint of "syncope" is not actually syncope.

Initially, differentiate syncope from seizure which is more likely with:

- History of seizure disorder (check meds and speak with bystanders)
- Tongue biting
- Confusion for over 5–10 minutes upon regaining consciousness (postictal phase)
- Incontinence
- Preceding aura
- Observed posturing or jerking lasting over several seconds (patients with syncope may have a few "myoclonic jerks" but do not have presence of persistent generalized tonic-clonic activity.

Section editor comments (Shiber):

These myoclonic jerks stop immediately when cerebral perfusion is restored by fainting or lying down.

Syncope can be divided into 3 categories: Neurally-mediated syncope, cardiovascular syncope and non-cardiovascular syncope.

A. Neurally-mediated syncope (NMS) is the most common etiology and may be precipitated by emotional stress, a sudden change in posture, hunger, physical exhaustion or a crowded environment. It is usually preceded by a prodrome (lightheadedness, dizziness, nausea, shortness of breath, pallor, diaphoresis or visual changes) that lasts several seconds to minutes, progressing to a brief period of unconsciousness. Vasodepressor syncope associated with exercise most commonly occurs immediately after the termination of an activity, and the patient returns to normal after the event. [1,2]

B. Cardiovascular syncope falls into 2 categories: Primary cardiac and cardiac dysrhythmias. Historical features of cardiac syncope include little or no prodrome, a prolonged loss of consciousness (longer than 5 min), exercise-induced symptoms, chest pain, palpitations, or a history of familial cardiac disease including long QT syndrome, cardiomyopathy, or sudden death in a family member less than 35-years-old.

1. **A primary cardiac cause does not match our patient at all.** In addition to the lack of historical risk factors, our patient has a much more continuous course. There are no signs of left ventricular (LV) outflow tract obstruction limiting cardiac output (i.e. no systolic ejection murmur or evidence of heart failure on physical examination). She does not have a history of congenital heart disease.
2. **Cardiac dysrhythmias** are more of a concern in a child with historical risk factors, especially corrected or partially corrected congenital heart lesions. Dysrhythmias that can lead to syncope include:

- Long QT syndrome (LQTS)
- Brugada syndrome [familial ventricular fibrillation]
- Post-operative atrial flutter or ventricular tachycardia VT
- Wolff-Parkinson-White syndrome [WPW] associated with atrial tachycardia [atrial fibrillation], and rarely
- Idiopathic VT or VT associated with arrhythmogenic right ventricular dysplasia
- Medication toxicity/abuse including caffeine and cocaine

C. Non-cardiovascular syncope:

- **Could this be a heat-related illness?** Our patient has been in the sun all day, but her body temperature is normal, which would be unusual for such significant hypotension and tachycardia.
- **Could she be hypovolemic?** She is tachycardic; is she dehydrated from the heat? How about a confounding factor such as underlying eating disorder? She really doesn't have a history consistent with an eating disorder, and her weight is just less than the 50% for age, making this unlikely. She did not eat before her first race, but she did get oral fluids at her first ED visit.
- **Could she have an ectopic pregnancy?** No one likes to acknowledge that their young children might have sex, but a missed ectopic could be fatal. So, this should be included in the differential.[3,4]
- **How about anemia?** Frequently underestimated is the combination of poor iron intake; vegan diets and heavy periods may result in significant anemia. Frequently, adolescents do not wish to discuss their periods, but in this scenario, a menstrual history should be obtained, and an H/H considered.[5]
- **Could she have Epstein Barr virus (EBV)** with an associated large spleen that ruptured spontaneously or from her fall? There is no history offered of a recent viral infection, but this was not specifically addressed by the provider. The abdominal exam may offer clues.[6,7]
- **Could she be abused, physically or sexually?** Speaking to a teen by themselves and also doing a physical exam looking for bruising and suspicious marks is important. Though important as part of a pediatric-specific history, this is less likely with our patient.
- **Could she have had a seizure?** Findings suggestive of seizure include transient altered mental status, rigidity or shaking, incontinence, tongue biting, and a postictal period after the episode. The findings, as documented, were absent, but it is hard to say if all were considered.

Q#2: Which aspects of the history, exam, and testing are helpful with pediatric syncope?

A. History: History should initially differentiate between syncope and seizure, establish the onset of the syncope (sudden without premonition or gradual), duration of loss of consciousness, history of similar episodes, previous evaluation as well as associated symptoms of chest pain, back pain, headache, abdominal pain, leg swelling or menometrorrhagia, or blood in the urine or stool. Congenital deafness has been associated with PLQTS. Family history should identify risk factors such as sudden death in relatives < 35-year-old, particularly unexplained drowning events and cardiac dysrhythmias.[8] Social history should include consideration of sexual activity, illicit drug use, home situation, as well as findings of anorexia nervosa or bulimia.[8]

B. Physical exam should include:

- Overall appearance including signs of trauma as well as body habitus with consideration of a "Marfanoid appearance"
- Vital signs
- Oropharyngeal for vesicles (Coxsackie has been associated with myocarditis), tonsillar hypertrophy (mononucleosis)
- Neck for cervical lymph nodes or jugular venous distention
- Chest for scars, chest movement
- Cardiovascular for abnormal cardiac sounds (S3 or S4), any murmurs, or muffled heart tones due to pericardial effusion
- Lungs for asymmetric breath sounds, abnormal lung sounds
- Abdomen for signs of pregnancy, splenic enlargement, surgical scars, distention, or bruising
- Extremity exam for pulses, edema, clubbing
- Neuro exam including assessment of cerebellar function

C. Testing:

- A urine pregnancy should be checked with signs of puberty.
- A CBC should be considered if there is a possibility of anemia, as with a female with a history of heavy periods or potential splenic or hepatic rupture or any child without a plausible explanation for their symptoms who is hemodynamically unstable.
- An electrocardiogram (ECG) should be included in all initial evaluations of syncope in children. Emphasis should be placed on the QT interval and T wave morphology for:
    1. Long QT syndrome
    2. Voltage criteria that are consistent with left or right ventricular hypertrophy for the evaluation of obstructive cardiac lesions or cardiomyopathies
    3. Manifestations of pre-excitation such as WPW (evaluate for a delta wave, short PR, widened QRS)
    4. Brugada syndrome (RBBB with ST elevation in V1/V2)
    5. Arrhythmia including pauses, conduction disturbances or ectopy[1,2]

In a child with an isolated syncopal event, with no risk factors, a history compatible with neurally-mediated syncope and a complete return to normal, a urine pregnancy (where appropriate) and an ECG are all that are indicated.

Q#3: The patient is hypotensive—what are the first steps in the evaluation and management?

Shock is inadequate oxygen delivery to the tissues to meet metabolic demand. If the blood pressure is normal for age it's compensated shock and if not, then it's uncompensated shock.

Shock can be one of four categories:

1. Volume depletion
2. Cardiogenic
3. Distributive
4. Obstructive

It is easy when the history and physical point toward a common diagnosis such as vomiting and diarrhea with volume depletion or allergen exposure with anaphylaxis, but sometimes it's more difficult. Our patient should be a simple dehydration, but she's not.

Irrespective of the etiology, first stabilize the ABC's. Vascular access is the first challenge. If you cannot achieve intravenous access after 2 attempts, an intraosseous line should be performed. Next, determine the etiology of shock.

Progressing from the least to most likely: There is no history of heart disease, no murmur, no gallop, no enlarged liver, no edema; cardiogenic shock is not likely! Distributive shock? There are no allergic-type symptoms, and this would be an awfully expedited course for sepsis. In addition, she should have more symptoms of infection such as fever, altered mental status, etc. so it really doesn't fit.

Obstructive shock includes tension pneumothorax, pulmonary embolism (PE), SVC syndrome, or pericardial tamponade. She does not have unilateral breath sounds or tracheal deviation (tension PTX), specific risk for PE, facial edema or history of malignancy or indwelling line (SVC syndrome) or distal heart sounds and JVD (tamponade).

So, that leaves hypovolemic shock, but from what? The story does not match simple shock from ongoing losses, particularly following improvement with initial replenishment of the deficit. This doesn't match the history or response to previous treatment. Our diagnosis is still unclear.

What should be done? Start fluid resuscitation with a 20mL/kg bolus of IV crystalloid (normal saline given rapidly with a push/pull system). A fluid bolus on IV PUMP will run too slow; she needs rapid restoration of blood pressure and heart rate. This may be repeated three times up to a total fluid administration of 60mL/kg. If she remains hypotensive, the next decision is to administer vasopressors or blood products.

What did the actual provider do?

The provider orders labs including CBC, BMP and LFTs plus an ECG and a urine dip and pregnancy test plus IVF 20mL/kg (760mL) NS. The patient is not placed on a cardiac monitor.

The patient's story continues (18:01): While waiting for the lab results, Brittany's mother takes her to the bathroom, and she falls again. This time, bumping into a wall then hitting the floor. She is initially unable to be aroused and the mother yells, "My baby is not breathing!" prompting a nearby tech to call an overhead code. The emergency physician arrives just in time to see the pediatric rapid response team running down the hall from the PICU. She is placed on a stretcher, extremely pale, slow to respond, and clammy.

As she is being transferred from the stretcher to her bed, she moans "Ouch!"

"I didn't think you had any pain?" her nurse asks.

"It's my belly," the patient mumbles.

Lifting her gown, the nurse is surprised to find a large bruise in the LUQ. A repeat check of the vitals reveals her heart rate has increased to 168, a blood pressure which is not able to be auscultated, and a pale and lethargic child. We are at:

DECISION POINT B – YOU ARE FACED WITH 4 QUESTIONS:

1. **What is our differential diagnosis now?**
2. **What are imaging choices for pediatric blunt trauma?**
3. **What is the sensitivity for diagnosing a spleen injury with US vs. CT?**
4. **The patient is hypotensive with a BP unable to be auscultated; should we give blood now or wait for imaging results?**

What does the literature say?

Q#1: What is our differential diagnosis now?

OK. We now have a LUQ bruise with tenderness and associated hypotension; it's time to narrow the differential to trauma, most likely splenic trauma. We now know the reason for her hypovolemic shock. Abdominal trauma is the most common cause of unrecognized fatal injury in children, with the spleen being the most common organ injured. Unfortunately, sometimes the physical exam findings can be subtle. The most common mechanisms of injury include motor vehicle and pedestrian injuries as well as sports-related injuries, bicycle injuries, and child abuse. The normal systolic blood pressure in children is 90mmHg plus twice the child's age in years (the lower limit is below 70mmHg plus twice the child's age in years, or below 50mmHg in some studies). Severe blood loss is defined as blood loss greater than 45% of the circulating volume and results in hemodynamic instability.

Q#2: What are imaging choices for pediatric blunt trauma?[9]

FAST (Focused Assessment with Sonography for Trauma): The role of FAST for the evaluation of spleen injury in pediatrics is unclear. The sensitivity ranges from 50 to 92%, with a comprehensive meta-analysis suggesting the sensitivity to be around 66%. The specificity of this exam is low, so in a hemodynamically stable patient, a positive FAST examination should be followed by an urgent CT. Bedside FAST may have utility in hemodynamically unstable patients to rapidly identify or rule out intraperitoneal hemorrhage when patients cannot undergo CT. However, surgical consultation for the hemodynamically unstable patient should not be delayed for imaging.[10,11]

Contrast-enhanced computer tomography (CT) is the gold standard for the evaluation of blunt abdominal trauma; but patients should be hemodynamically stable. Based on the radiation risk in children, low-dose protocols are preferred (3–6mSv instead of 11–24mSv). The American Pediatric Surgical Association (APSA) guidelines recommend CT scanning in children at risk for injuries that might be missed by FAST, need for surgery, recurrent bleeding, and when other abdominal injuries (such as pancreatic or hollow viscous injury) are suspected.[12]

Q#3: What is the sensitivity for diagnosing a spleen injury with US vs. CT?[9]

The diagnostic performance of a contrast-enhanced ultrasound (CEUS) is better than that of US, as sensitivity, specificity, PPV, NPV, and accuracy were 100, 100, 100, 100, and 100 % for CEUS and 38.8, 100, 100, 12.8, and 44 % for US in one series.[13] This study concluded that CEUS is more sensitive and accurate than baseline US and almost as sensitive as CT in the identification and characterization of solid organs lesions in blunt abdominal trauma. CT was still more sensitive and accurate than CEUS in identifying prognostic indicators, such as active bleeding and urinoma.

One recent study concluded that among hemodynamically stable children treated in an ED following blunt torso trauma, the use of FAST compared with standard care did not improve clinical care, including use of resources; ED length of stay; missed intra-abdominal injuries; or hospital charges. These findings do not support the routine use of FAST in this setting.[14]

Q#4: The patient is hypotensive with a BP unable to be auscultated; should we give blood now or wait for imaging results?

This patient is clearly hemodynamically unstable and requires rapid resource activation!! Highest level of trauma activation should be initiated which will pull all resources immediately to the patient's bedside, including surgical resources, lab and blood bank.

Aggressive intravenous access, followed by fluid resuscitation, 3 boluses of 20mL/kg of crystalloid replacement should be administered before blood replacement.[15] Massive transfusion protocol in children should be applied with a ratio of 1:1:1.[16] Transfusion triggers have been debated, and although, there are no class I data to support a specific numerical threshold, it is generally agreed that transfusion should be considered when hemoglobin is less than 7g/dL.[16]

The patient's resuscitation should be monitored for improvement which is classically indicated by reduction of the heart rate, improved mental status, return of peripheral pulses and normal skin color, increase in blood pressure, and urinary output, as well as increase in extremity warmth.

Even though the benefit of thromboelastography (TEG) has not been confirmed in children, recent ATOMAC guidelines suggested that it may be useful in these patients as well (based on adult data).[17]

Section editor comments (Shiber):

An Hb level of 7g/dL is a generally accepted transfusion threshold for anemia only—but not in an actively bleeding hemodynamically unstable patient. If a patient is presumed to have ongoing hemorrhage (by ATLS nomenclature to be a non-responder or transient responder to initial crystalloid administration) then give blood products.

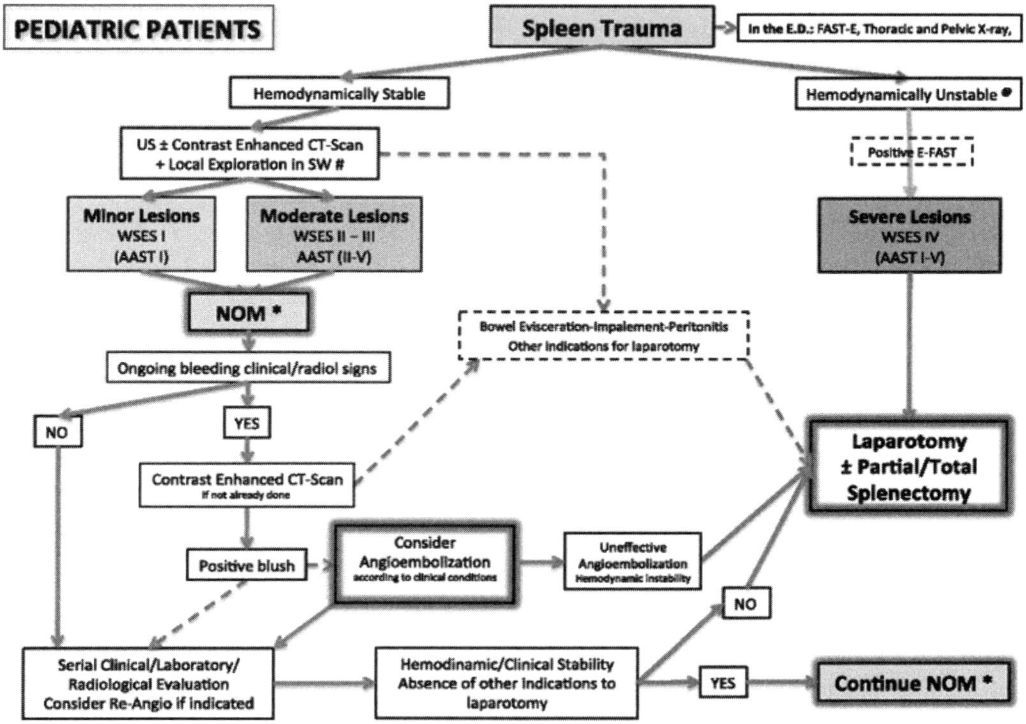

Coccolini F, Montori G, Catena, F, et al. Splenic trauma: WSES classification and guidelines for adult and pediatric patients. World J Emerg Surg 12, 40 (2017). https://doi.org/10.1186/s13017-017-0151-4; Creative Commons license, http://creativecommons.org/licenses/by/4.0/

What did the actual provider do?

The provider activated a Level I trauma because of the hemodynamic instability and the LUQ bruise. The team then held a debate over the pediatric use of ultrasound in an unstable trauma patient. The decision was made to perform a FAST exam. The patient had received 40mL/kg of 0.9NS; 10mL/kg of PRBC's were ordered. The FAST exam was positive showing free fluid.

The story continues:
Surgery is called, and the intern arrives, eventually finding you in another patient's room with a knock on the door, "I think you should come and see the patient in room 7, she is not answering questions."

As you enter the room, the mother quickly gets out of her chair and asks, "We have been here for over 2 hours and she is getting worse. Why aren't you doing anything?!"

You look down and see the patient unresponsive in the bed. Quickly checking her pulse, it is not able to be palpated, and you yell, "Code Blue" to a candy striper walking down the hall. The surgery intern finds an Ambu bag on the wall and struggles to connect it to oxygen as you begin chest compressions. You catch a glimpse of the mother to your left, tears streaming down her face. We are at:

DECISION POINT C – YOU ARE FACED WITH 4 QUESTIONS:

1. **What are the initial steps in a pediatric resuscitation?**
2. **Should she be intubated?**
3. **If unable to be resuscitated, is ECMO indicated?**
4. **Is hypothermia protocol indicated?**

Q#1: What are the initial steps in a pediatric resuscitation?

The first and most important step is CPR; recommendations, although supported by limited amount and quality of data, recommend a sequence of Circulation – Airway – Breathing (C-A-B) over the previously taught A-B-C sequence (Class IIb, LOE C-EO). The 2015 CPR guidelines recommend a chest compression rate of 100/min to 120/min for infants and children (Class IIa, LOE C-EO). Epinephrine is still the first-line pharmacologic therapy in pediatric cardiac arrest (Class IIa, LOE C-LD).[18]

However, in this situation the arrest is secondary to hemorrhage and the volume status must be immediately addressed. Intravenous access, if not already in place, should be obtained with IO being a reasonable option. Fluids should be initiated with three, 20mL/kg isotonic saline fluid boluses followed by blood products based on response. Tranexamic acid (TXA) has been shown in bleeding trauma patients over 16 years of age to decrease mortality without increasing prothrombotic complications if administered within 3 hours of injury.[19]

Though not extensively studies in the pediatric EM population, TXA has successfully reduced blood loss and transfusion requirements in pediatric cardiac surgery, scoliosis surgery, and craniosynostosis repair.[20,21]

Adverse effects include gastrointestinal effects, hypotension with rapid intravenous injection, dizziness, headache, muscle pain and spasms, and post-operative convulsions in children receiving high doses during cardiac surgery. The potential risk of thrombosis has not been identified with large doses in pediatric cardiac and spinal surgery. Although the incidence of death from hemorrhage with traumatic injuries is not as common in children, hemorrhage remains the most common cause of death in pediatric solid organ injuries and is the second leading cause of traumatic death in children.

Section editor comments (Shiber):

The CAB or Chest Compressions 1st recommendation is very specifically for out-of-hospital cardiac arrest (OHCA) caused by a primary cardiac dysrhythmia (acute coronary syndrome most often or a cardiomyopathy leading to arrhythmogenic potential) so that the "hand-only" CPR is optimal to continue circulating the well-oxygenated blood until EMS arrives and can defibrillate. All other types of cardiac arrest still require an airway and oxygenation and ventilation, preferably simultaneously as chest compressions are started.

Q#2: Should she be intubated?

The airway and oxygenation need to be supported, initially with BVM and then intubation, but in our case, the priority should be volume resuscitation.[22] In an arrest situation, rapid sequence intubation (RSI) is not required, but following return of spontaneous circulation (ROSC), it may be necessary to complete an RSI to secure the airway.

- Ketamine is a good induction agent.
- The 2015 AHA guidelines recommend targeting normoxemia after ROSC (Class IIb, LOE B-NR), and to avoid hypoxemia.
- The goal is to achieve normoxemia while ensuring that hypoxemia is strictly avoided.[18]
- Atropine is no longer routinely recommended.[18]

Q#3: If unable to be resuscitated, is ECMO indicated?

Extracorporeal membrane oxygenation (ECMO) has been utilized following major trauma for respiratory support with a national database review of extracorporeal life support (ECLS) in pediatric trauma patients, finding improved survival rates to discharge, comparable to patients not undergoing ECLS with similar injuries. ECMO would not be used with active bleeding from the spleen or other organs since anticoagulation is required to maintain patency of the circuit.[23]

Evidence from in-hospital cardiac arrest patients has shown no overall benefit to the use of CPR with ECMO (ECPR) compared to CPR without ECMO. However, it has been shown to be of benefit in children with surgical cardiac diagnoses. For children with underlying cardiac disease, ECPR has resulted in long-term survival even after more than 50 minutes of conventional CPR.[24,25]

Section editor comments (Shiber):

ECMO would not be indicated since it does not help bleeding or hypovolemic shock. Anticoagulation is not a strict requirement for V-V ECMO (we run our patients with brain injuries or open chests/abdomens without any AC for up to a week), but it is for V-A ECMO since any clot in the post-membrane circuit could cause a devastating emboli.

Q#4: Is hypothermia protocol indicated?

THAPCA-IH showed that for comatose children who survived in-hospital cardiac arrest, therapeutic hypothermia (target temperature, 33° C), as compared with therapeutic normothermia (target temperature, 36.8° C), did not confer a significant benefit with respect to survival with a good functional outcome at 1 year. For our patient, hypothermia is probably not going to be of benefit.[26,27]

AHA 2015 guidelines recommend for infants and children who are comatose after out-of-hospital cardiac arrest to either maintain 5 days of continuous normothermia (36° C to 37.5° C) or to maintain 2 days of initial continuous hypothermia (32° C to 34° C) followed by 3 days of continuous normothermia (Class IIa, LOE B-R).

Section editor comments (Shiber):

TTM would be for normothermia and to avoid hyperthermia for a post-arrest patient due to traumatic hemorrhage. Hypothermia is contraindicated for any clinically significant bleeding or ongoing hemodynamic instability.

What happened?

After 2 rounds of chest compressions and intravenous epinephrine, the patient now has a pulse. She has not yet been intubated. Blood arrives just as the pulse returns and is started through a 18g IV in the left antecubital vein with a pressure bag. The surgery intern has notified the attending. Brittany is taken to the OR and then to the ICU where she spends an uneventful night and is released the next day to the floor. Two days later she is discharged home.

Final diagnosis: Syncope secondary to traumatic splenic injury (WSES IV).

Outcome: Brittany arrives home and pulling into the driveway, sees her entire team waiting for her with flowers and cheers. Six weeks later, she begins to run again.

References:

1. Bayram AK, Pamukcu O, Per H. Current approaches to the clinical assessment of syncope in pediatric population. Childs Nerv Syst 2016;32(3):427-36.
2. Anderson JB, Willis M, Lancaster H, et al. The evaluation and management of pediatric syncope. Pediatr Neurol 2016;55:6-13.
3. Dussoix P, Hagelberg T, Vermeulen B. An unusual case of syncope. Eur J Emerg Med 2004;11(1):59.
4. Wong E, Suat SO. Ectopic pregnancy—a diagnostic challenge in the emergency department. Eur J Emerg Med 2000;7(3):189-94.
5. Cooke AG, McCavit TL, Buchanan GR, et al. Iron deficiency anemia in adolescents who present with heavy menstrual bleeding. J Pediatr Adolesc Gynecol 2017;30(2):247-50.
6. Barnwell J, Deol PS. Atraumatic splenic rupture secondary to Epstein-Barr virus infection. BMJ Case Rep 2017;2017 pii: bcr2016218405. doi: 10.1136/bcr-2016-218405. PMID:28119438.
7. Sergent SR, Johnson SM, Ashurst J, et al. Epstein-Barr virus-associated atraumatic spleen laceration presenting with neck and shoulder pain. Am J Case Rep 2015;16:774-7.
8. American Academy of Pediatrics, Policy statement: Pediatric sudden cardiac arrest. Pediatrics 2012;129(4):e1094-e1102.
9. Lynn KN, Werder GM, Callaghan RM, et al. Pediatric blunt splenic trauma: A comprehensive review. Pediatr Radiol 2009;39(9):904-16.
10. Menaker J, Blumberg S, Wisner DH, et al. Use of the focused assessment with sonography for trauma (FAST) examination and its impact on abdominal computed tomography use in hemodynamically stable children with blunt torso trauma. J Trauma Acute Care Surg 2014;77(3):427-32.
11. Scaife ER, Rollins MD, Barnhart DC, et al. The role of focused abdominal sonography for trauma (FAST) in pediatric trauma evaluation. J Pediatr Surg 2013;48(6):1377-83.
12. Stylianos S. Evidence-based guidelines for resource utilization in children with isolated spleen or liver injury. The APSA Trauma Committee. J Pediatr Surg 2000;35(2):164-9.
13. Menichini G, Sessa B, Trinci M, et al. Accuracy of Contrast-Enhanced Ultrasound (CEUS) in the identification and characterization of traumatic solid organ lesions in children: A retrospective comparison with baseline US and CE-MDCT. Radiol Med 2015;120(11):989-1001.
14. Holmes JF, Kelley KM, Wootton-Gorges SL, et al. Effect of abdominal ultrasound on clinical

care, outcomes, and resource use among children with blunt torso trauma: A randomized clinical trial. JAMA 2017;317(22):2290-96.
15. American College of Surgeons. Committee on Trauma. Advanced Trauma Life Support® (ATLS®): Student course manual. 9th ed. Chicago, IL: American College of Surgeons, 2012.
16. Notrica DM, Eubanks JW, Tuggle DW, et al. Nonoperative management of blunt liver and spleen injury in children: Evaluation of the ATOMAC guideline using GRADE. J Trauma Acute Care Surg 2015;79(4):683-93.
17. Gendreau JL, Knoll C, Adams RH, et al. The role of thromboelastography in pediatric patients with Sinusoidal Obstructive Syndrome receiving defibrotide. Biol Blood Marrow Transplant 2017;23(4):707-12.
18. de Caen AR, Berg MD, Chameides L. Guidelines Update for Cardiopulmonary Resuscitation and Emergency Cardiovascular Care. Part 12: 2015 American Heart Association Pediatric Advanced Life Support. Circulation. http://circ.ahajournals.org/content/132/18_suppl_2/S526.
19. Harvey V, Perrone J, Kim P. Does the use of tranexamic acid improve trauma mortality?Ann Emerg Med 2014;63(4):460-2.
20. McLeod LM, French B, Flynn JM, et al. Antifibrinolytic use and blood transfusions in pediatric scoliosis surgeries performed at US children's hospitals. J Spinal Disord Tech 2015;28(8):E460-6.
21. Grassin-Delyle S, Couturier R, Abe E, et al. A practical tranexamic acid dosing scheme based on population pharmacokinetics in children undergoing cardiac surgery. Anesthesiology 2013;118(4):853-62.
22. Misir A. Fluid and medication considerations in the traumatized patient. Curr Pediatr Rev 2018;14(1):9-27.
23. Watson JA, Englum BR, Kim J, et al. Extracorporeal life support use in pediatric trauma: A review of the National Trauma Data Bank. J Pediatr Surg 2017;52(1):136-9.
24. de Mos N, van Litsenburg RR, McCrindle B, et al. Pediatric in-intensive-care-unit cardiac arrest: Incidence, survival, and predictive factors. Crit Care Med 2006;34(4):1209-15.
25. Lowry AW, Morales DL, Graves DE, et al. Characterization of extracorporeal membrane oxygenation for pediatric cardiac arrest in the United States: Analysis of the kids' inpatient database. Pediatr Cardiol 2013;34(6):1422-30.
26. Bhattacharjee, S., Baidya DK, Maitra S. Therapeutic hypothermia after cardiac arrest is not associated with favorable neurological outcome: A meta-analysis. J Clin Anesth 2016;33:225-32.
27. Moler FW, Silverstein FS, Holubkov R, et al. Therapeutic hypothermia after in-hospital cardiac arrest in children. N Engl J Med 2017;376(4):318-29.